REDEMPTION—GOD'S GRAND DESIGN

BIBLE TRUTHS 6 for Christian Schools®

Third Edition
BJU PRESS
Greenville, SC 29614

Consultants
from the administration, faculty, and staff of Bob Jones University
Philip D. Smith, Ed.D., *Provost*
James R. Davis, M.A., *Director of Product Development, Bob Jones University Press*
Dan Olinger, Ph.D. *(Theology), Professor of Theology, School of Religion*
Bryan Smith, M.A., *Secondary Author, Bob Jones University Press*
Vicky Burr, *Elementary Authors Project Director, Bob Jones University Press*
Ebby E. Autry, *Grade 6 Consultant, Bob Jones Elementary School*
Abigail C. Nicholson, *Grade 6 Consultant, Bob Jones Elementary School*

Note:
The fact that materials produced by other publishers may be referred to in this volume does not constitute an endorsement of the content or theological position of materials produced by such publishers. Any references and ancillary materials are listed as an aid to the student or the teacher and in an attempt to maintain the accepted academic standards of the publishing industry.

BIBLE TRUTHS 6 for Christian Schools®
Redemption—God's Grand Design
Third Edition

Coordinating Writer
Tammie D. Jacobs

Designer
Wendy Searles

Writers
Peggy S. Alier
Marnie Batterman
Kathryn L. Bell
Eileen M. Berry
Nellie Ashe Cooper
Robin Sisney Wood

Computer Formatting
Peggy Hargis

Project Editor
Nathan Huffstutler

Photo Acquisition
Tara Swaney

Produced in cooperation with the Bob Jones University School of Education and Bob Jones Elementary School.
for Christian Schools is a registered trademark of Bob Jones University Press.

Five excerpts from *The Scofield Bible,* edited by C. I. Scofield, copyright 1937, 1945 by Oxford University Press, Inc. Used by permission of Oxford University Press, Inc. Used on pages 24, 110, 174, 177, 219.
Bible dictionary pages. Taken from the *New Unger's Bible Dictionary* by Merrill F. Unger, Moody Press, copyright 1988. Used by permission.
Entry of Ruth IV from *Williams' Complete Bible Commentary* by George Williams. Complimentary use.
Entry of Acts 2 from *Witness to Christ: A Commentary on Acts* by Stewart Custer, Bob Jones University Press, copyright 2000.

ISBN 1-57924-552-8

15 14 13 12 11 10 9 8 7 6 5 4 3

Table of Contents

UNIT 1 Before the Foundation

UNIT 2 Through the Covenant

UNIT 3 Under the Blood

Table of Contents

Table of Contents

Table of Contents

UNIT 9 To the Ends of the Earth

UNIT 10 At the Appointed Time

Table of Contents

Get the Bible Reading H.A.B.I.T.

Name ______________________________

BIBLE STUDY Skills

A habit is something that is done over and over until it becomes a part of someone's behavior. In each unit of this book, you will find a page with suggested Scriptures to help you develop the habit of reading the Bible daily. These H.A.B.I.T. guidelines will help you as you seek God in His Word and spend quiet time with Him.

Have a special time set aside each day to read your Bible. If possible, make it the same time every day.

Ask God to teach you from His Word. Remember to thank Him for helping you to understand and apply it.

Be still and give your attention to what you are reading.

Investigate the Scripture by asking yourself questions about it.

Take time to look up words and ideas you do not understand.

As you read the Scripture for each day, write the date in the box. Example: 9/2

Christ our Redeemer created all things and holds them together. **Colossians 1:12-17**	The price for sin is death, but God offers eternal life as a free gift. **Romans 6:23**	All men sinned through Adam, so everyone must die. **Romans 5:12-14**	All men can receive the free gift of righteousness through Christ. **Romans 5:15-17**	Christ's obedience made it possible for all men to have eternal life. **Romans 5:18-21**
By faith we understand the things we cannot see. **Hebrews 11:1-3**	Abel's faith allowed him to offer a better sacrifice than Cain. **Hebrews 11:4**	Without faith it is impossible to please God. **Hebrews 11:5-6**	Christ redeemed man by His own blood, not by the blood of animals. **Hebrews 9:11-12**	Christ's blood purifies believers for service. **Hebrews 9:13-14**
The Lord knows how to deliver godly people. **II Peter 2:4-9**	Scoffers are ignorant of God's past judgment of sin. **II Peter 3:1-6**	God wants none to perish but all to repent. **II Peter 3:7-9**	God's judgment will come suddenly, so believers ought to be living holy, godly lives. **II Peter 3:10-12**	While God patiently waits, we must be diligent to keep our lives clean. **II Peter 3:13-15**
God will exalt the humble person in His time. **I Peter 5:5-6**	God resists the proud but gives grace to the humble. **James 4:6-7**	Man must repent of sin and humble himself before God. **James 4:8-10**	Christians should think more of others than themselves. **Philippians 2:3-4**	Christ is the example of a humble servant's spirit. **Philippians 2:5-11**

Prayer Power

Name ______________________

The habits of daily reading and meditating on God's Word are vital to Christians. Equally important is the practice of powerful prayer.

Prayer is not—

sending up an S.O.S. when you are in trouble.

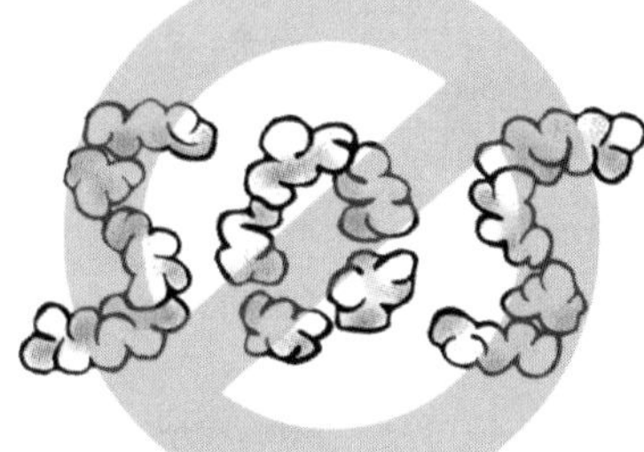
SOS

repeating the same words over and over.

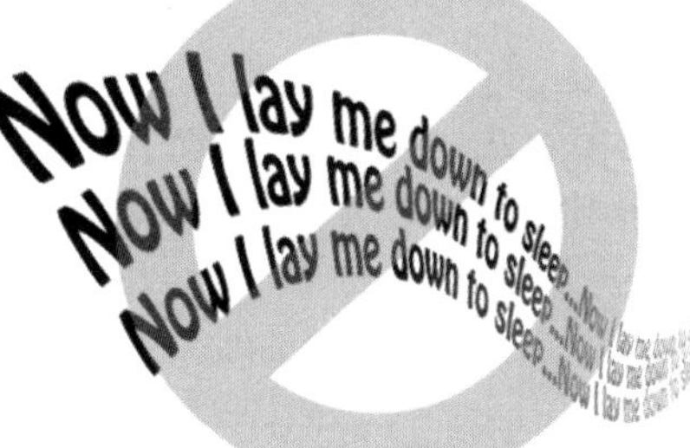
Now I lay me down to sleep...
Now I lay me down to sleep...
Now I lay me down to sleep...

giving God a list of what you want.

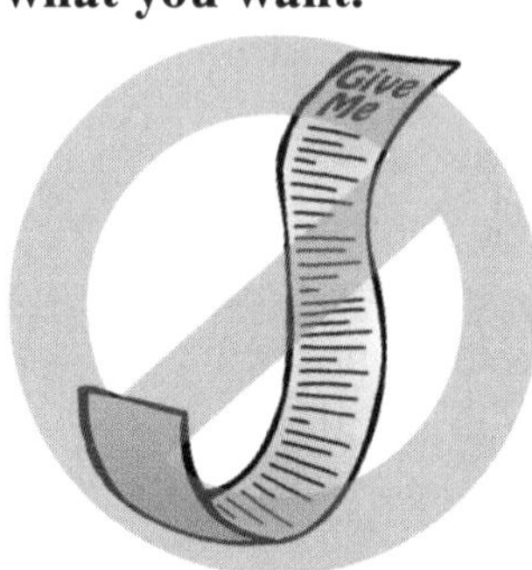
Give Me

WHERE should you pray?	**Anywhere!** Ps. 139:1-4
WHEN should you pray?	**Anytime!** I Thess. 5:17
WHAT should you pray for?	For the purposes of God's kingdom to be fulfilled. For what you need. For a right relationship with God (forgiveness). For a right relationship with others (forgiving them). For deliverance and protection. Matt. 6:9-13
WILL your prayers be answered?	**You may pray with confidence!** I John 5:14-15
WHAT IF you don't know exactly what to say?	**You have a wonderful prayer Helper!** Rom. 8:26-27
WHAT should you always include in your prayers?	**Thanksgiving!** Phil. 4:6

From the Beginning

Genesis 1-2

Name ______________________

Genesis does not argue for the existence of God or make any explanation of His activities before the beginning of time. It simply states, "In the beginning God …" and continues with the account of the Creation and God's plan to save sinful man. For a person to believe that God's Word is true and accept what it says to him, he must believe that God exists and that He has good purposes for man (Heb. 11:6).

Answer the question.

Who created all things?

Genesis 1:1	**_______________ the Father**
Hebrews 1:2	**Jesus Christ the _______________**
Genesis 1:2	**the Holy _______________**

Nothing happened by chance in God's creation of all things. Everything was perfectly designed and was known to Him from the beginning.

Beside each part of God's wonderful creation, write the letter of the purpose for which it was designed.

______ 1. Separation of light and darkness (Gen. 1:4)

______ 2. Separation of waters above and waters below (Gen. 1:6)

______ 3. Separation of dry land from waters (Gen. 1:9)

______ 4. Production of all kinds of plants and trees (Gen. 1:11)

______ 5. Placement of the sun, moon, and stars (Gen. 1:14-18)

______ 6. Man and woman (Gen. 1:27)

A. To make the atmosphere—heavens and sky
B. To provide food, soil enrichment, oxygen exchange, shade, and beauty
C. To mark seasons, days, and years, and to give light to the earth
D. To make the parts of a day—day and night
E. To make a habitable environment for land animals and man
F. To reflect the image of God; to worship and serve Him

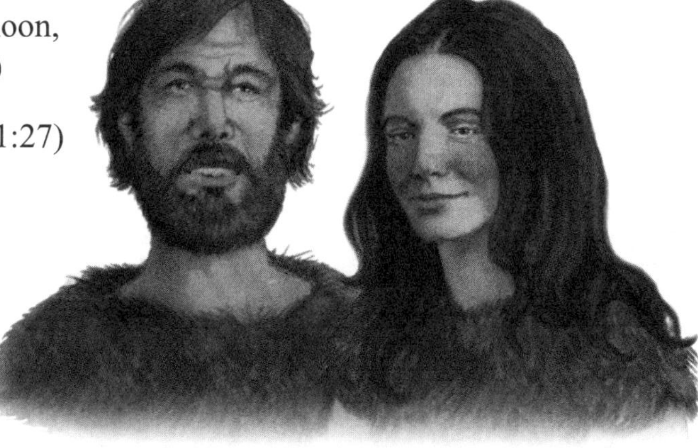

Name ______________________

What were the results of the Fall of man (the sin of Eve and Adam)?

Complete the sentences. You may use your Bible for help.

decay	guilt	pain	age
work	fellowship	disease	inherited

1. Adam and Eve experienced __________ when they saw their true unworthiness before God. Then they tried to cover their nakedness (Gen. 3:7).
2. They lost ________________ with God and hid themselves since they were no longer comfortable in God's presence (Gen. 3:8).
3. Their _________ became difficult. In order to make the earth produce crops, they had to struggle against thorns and thistles (Gen. 3:17-18).
4. The joy of having children would be accompanied by _________ (Gen. 3:16).
5. Their bodies would _________ and be subject to _________ and ____________, and finally die (Gen. 3:19).
6. Their sin would be _____________ by all who came after them (Rom. 5:12).

THINK ABOUT IT

Once sin is committed it can never be undone. God does not erase history. Adam and Eve had to leave the perfect place God had prepared for them. Cherubim, special angels associated with God's holiness and power, were set to guard the entrance so that Adam and Eve and those who came after them could not return. Sin affects not only the sinner, but others as well. The sinfulness of Adam and Eve was passed to all human beings. Man would be hopeless without God's grace, which is greater than the sin of mankind.

Is salvation in Jesus Christ "Plan B" that God made because "Plan A" failed when Adam and Eve sinned? Why or why not?

____

____

____

Why Must I Develop Christian Living Skills?

Name ____________________

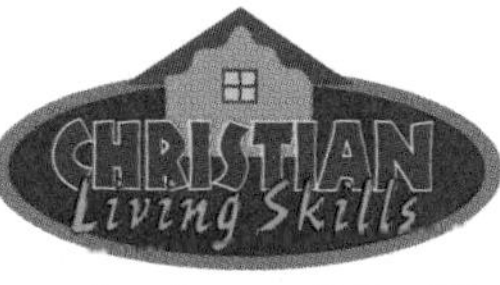
CHRISTIAN
Living Skills

Jesus commands you to be like Him. How can you do that? What does it mean to be like Him? To become like Jesus, you must be willing to change your attitudes to His. Your choices must be His choices. How will other people know that you are becoming more like Christ? They will know by watching your **testimony.**

Your **testimony** is really just how you show others what you believe about God. It is your reputation or the kind of person you are known as. What is your reputation? Do others know you live for Jesus by the choices you make? Is your reputation or testimony pleasing to God?

List several ways that others will be able to observe your testimony.

1. ____________________
2. ____________________

Why must we develop Christian Living Skills?

Read each verse and match it to the correct reason that you should be developing Christian Living Skills.

______ To please God by obeying Him

______ To be an example of Jesus Christ to others

______ To learn how to solve problems by using God's Word

______ To avoid becoming a *stumbling block* to others

A. I Timothy 4:12
B. Romans 14:13
C. II Timothy 3:16-17
D. Psalm 147:11

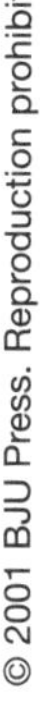

God has given Christians the responsibility of making choices that would not be stumbling blocks to others (Rom. 14:13). They must use caution so that their lives are pure, shining clearly as examples of Christlikeness.

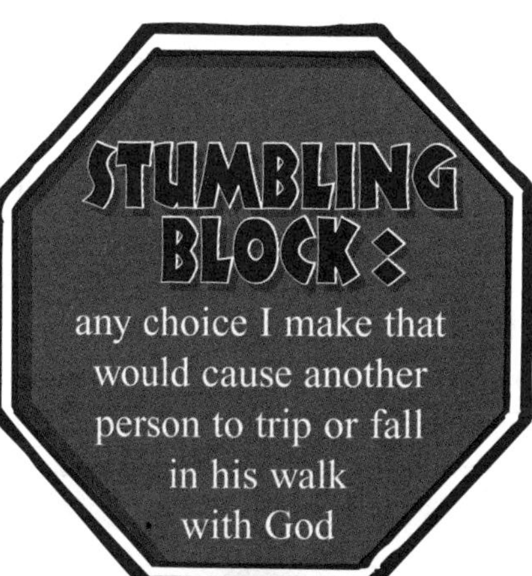
STUMBLING BLOCK:
any choice I make that would cause another person to trip or fall in his walk with God

List some choices that you should avoid so that you will not be a stumbling block to someone else.

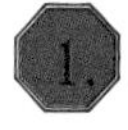
1. ____________________

2. ____________________

Something to Think About

Christlikeness

Name ______________________

CHRISTIAN Living Skills

Having a testimony that is pleasing to God means that you obey His Word by making **RIGHT CHOICES** and avoiding **WRONG CHOICES.** The choices you make will have a great influence on you and on others.

Study the chart below. Think about how each action will affect you and others. Complete the chart.

Action	Effect of Action on You	Effect of Action on Others
Cheating on a math test: Wrong Choice	• a guilty conscience • points lost on your grade	• God displeased • trust of teacher lost • parents displeased • friends' doubt of your love for Jesus Christ
Obeying parents by cleaning room: Right Choice	• a clear conscience • no punishment	• pleasing to God • pleasing to parents • clean room
Gossiping about the new student in class: ____________ Choice		
Turning in your assignments on time: ____________ Choice		

Learning how to please God by making right choices is important. However, you must also please God by making biblical changes in your actions, attitudes, words, and thoughts.

What About Me?

Take time at home to think about your actions and the effects they have on yourself and on others. Evaluate your actions from this morning. Choose one action and complete the chart.

My Action	Effect of My Action on Me	Effect of My Action on Others
____________ Choice		

Blessed and Blessing

Ephesians 1:3-4

Name ______________________

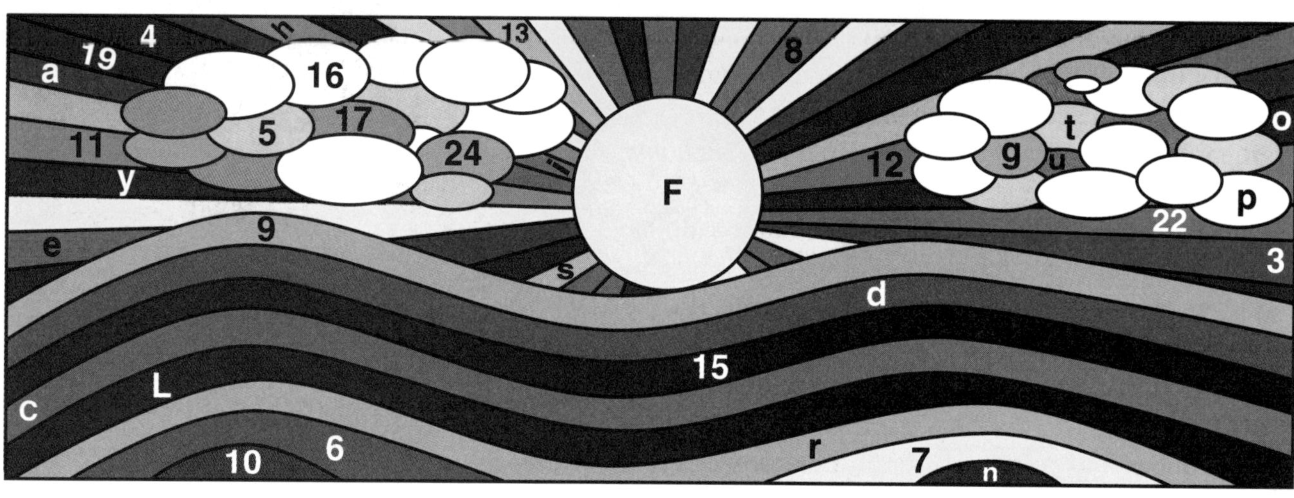

4
a
19
16
13
8
17
5
11
24
y
F
12
g
t
u
o
p
22
e
9
s
3
d
15
L
c
10
6
r
7
n

Find the matching colored letter for each number and write it in the corresponding space.

1. Who is to be praised or blessed for giving spiritual blessings? ___ ___ ___ (24 4 6)

   the ___ ___ ___ ___ ___ ___ (7 3 5 11 8 9)

2. *Heavenly places* means in the ___ ___ ___ ___ ___ ___ ___ ___ ___ (13 16 12 9 12 5 17 3 15) and ___ ___ ___ ___ ___ ___ ___ (8 5 8 9 10 3 15) realm.

3. God knew before the ___ ___ ___ ___ ___ ___ ___ ___ (22 9 8 3 5 12 4 10) of the world who would believe on the Lord Jesus Christ.

4. God's purpose is that Christians be ___ ___ ___ ___ (11 4 15 19).

Write the letter of the definition that matches the meaning of the italicized word.

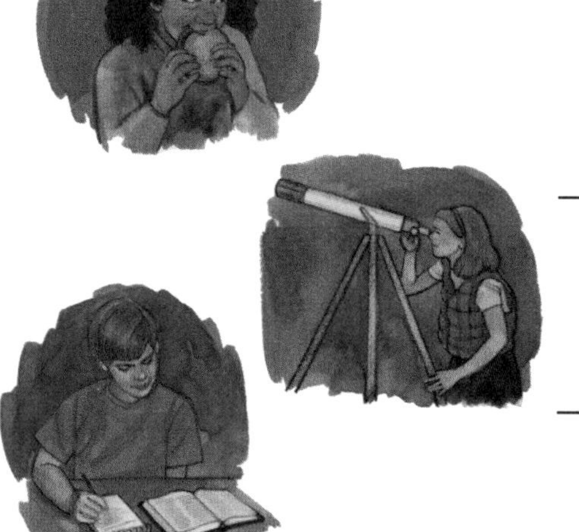

_____ 1. Natalie took a big bite of double hamburger with all the trimmings. "M-m-m," she sighed. *"Heavenly!"*

_____ 2. Lucy really enjoys using her new telescope to look for *heavenly* bodies in the night sky.

_____ 3. Kirk began keeping a list of *heavenly* blessings and the verses where he read about them.

A. having to do with the Lord

B. unusually enjoyable

C. having to do with outer space

God's Purposes

Name ______________________

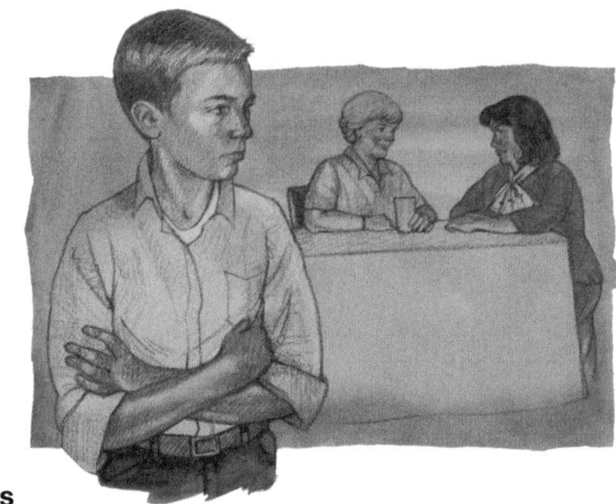

It was a sad day for Robert's family. After his cousin Nathan's funeral, the family returned to his grandparents' house. During the conversation after dinner, Robert overheard his Aunt Barb talking to Granny. "Such a waste! I've never known a person so young to be such a soul winner. Just think how many people Nathan would have led to the Lord if he had lived to grow old." Robert was confused. Was God's purpose for Nathan's life cut short by an accident? Were there people who would not hear the gospel because Nathan had died?

Choose one or more of these Scripture references and use it as a basis for answering Robert's questions in a letter to him.

Isaiah 46:9-10 Ephesians 1:7-12 II Timothy 1:9 Psalm 33:11 Proverbs 19:21

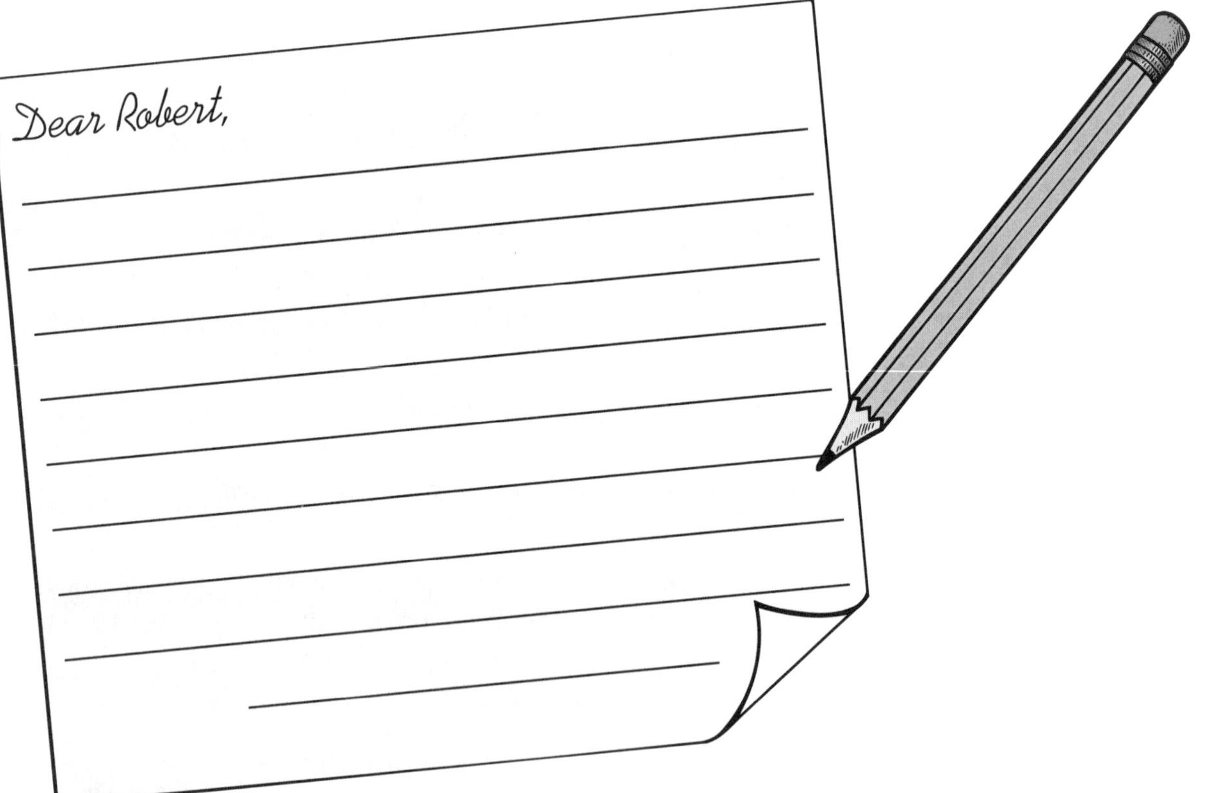
Dear Robert,

Although God works out His purposes differently in the lives of individual Christians, He has one purpose for all Christians. According to Ephesians 1:4, what is that purpose?

____

____

Adopted!
Ephesians 1:5-6

Name ______________________________

In writing Ephesians 1:5-6, Paul used a metaphor to describe the relationship that a believer has with God. When parents legally take into their family a young child who was not physically born to them, they adopt him. When God takes into His family a sinner who repents, He adopts him.

Put an *X* beside each statement that is true.

An adopted child—

______ belongs to his adoptive parents just as much as if he were born to them.

______ does not have to obey his adoptive parents.

______ is under the care and protection of his adoptive parents.

______ lives with his adoptive family.

______ must pay for the right to be adopted.

A believer in Jesus Christ—

______ belongs to the family of God.

______ is under the care and protection of God.

______ has no choice about whether or not he is adopted.

______ is an heir to the kingdom of God.

______ lives to obey his heavenly Father and bring honor to Him.

Who makes adoption into the family of God possible?

____

Suppose there is an adopted child who moves into the home of his adoptive parents and just stays in his room. He does not come out and enjoy the company of his parents. He does not ask his parents for what he needs. When they furnish good things for him, he does not thank them. He is not interested in finding out what his parents expect of him. He does not have any desire to tell them what his interests are. Is this child behaving like a member of the family? Of course not.

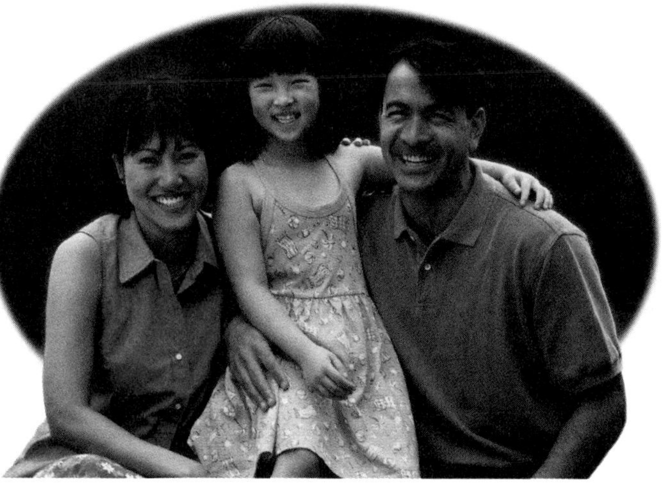

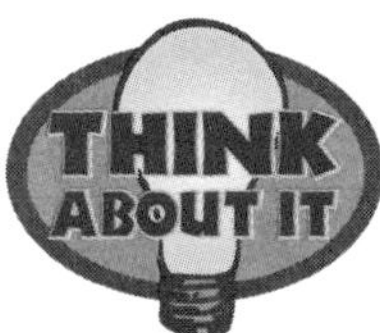
THINK
ABOUT IT

If you are an adopted member of God's family through faith in Jesus Christ, do you—

- ✔ seek to please your heavenly Father at all times?
- ✔ ask your heavenly Father for your needs?
- ✔ thank your heavenly Father for His gifts?
- ✔ read the Bible to find out what your heavenly Father expects?
- ✔ tell your heavenly Father about your interests and activities?

Singing with Understanding

"O God, Our Help in Ages Past" (vv. 1-2)

Name ______________________

The comforting idea that God is a refuge during difficult times is found throughout Scripture, especially in the Psalms. His protection and help are represented by a number of different images.

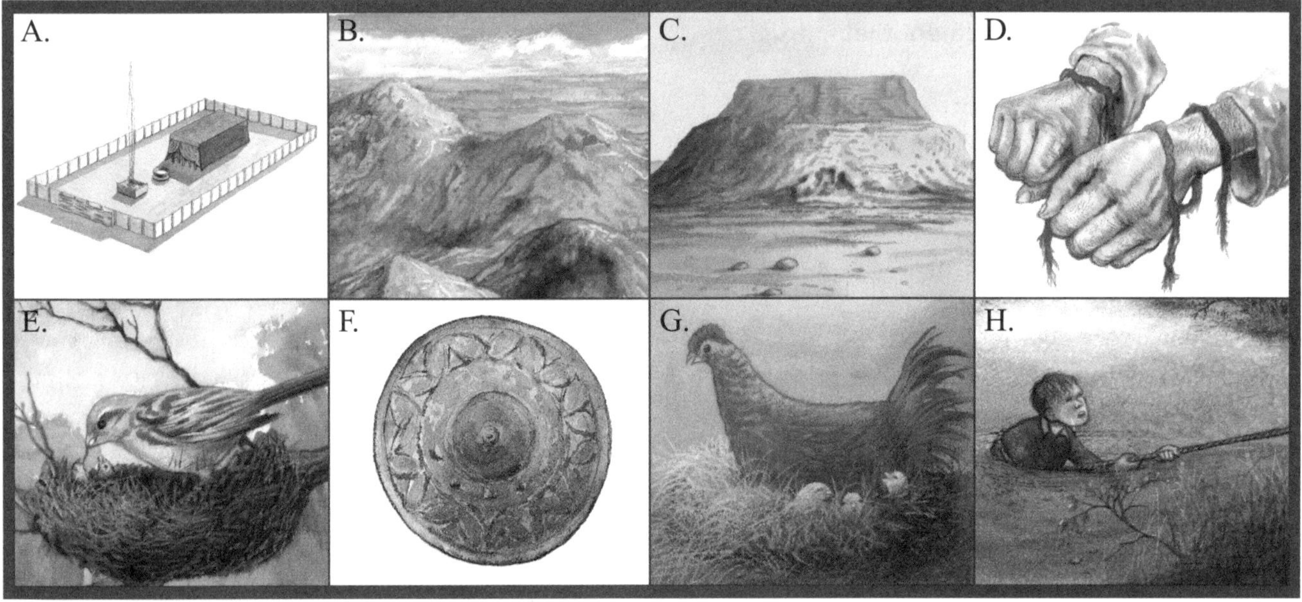
A.
B.
C.
D.
E.
F.
G.
H.

Write the letter of the matching image for each Scripture reference.

______	Psalm 3:3*a*	______	Psalm 61:4*a*	______	Psalm 121:1
______	Psalm 18:2	______	Psalm 69:14	______	Psalm 129:4
______	Psalm 36:7	______	Psalm 84:3-4		

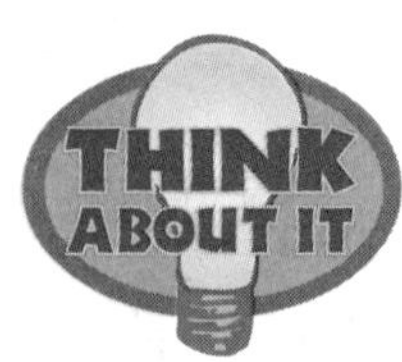
THINK
ABOUT IT

Write the answers.

1. Tell about a time when God helped you when you were in trouble.

____

____

____

2. How can thinking about what God did for you and others help you when you face a new problem?

____

____

____

Pleasing God

Genesis 4:1-16

Name ______________________

Write a *C* for Cain or an *A* for Abel in each speech bubble.

God placed a curse upon me because I murdered my brother. ◯

I offered the firstborn of my flock to the Lord. ◯

My attitude toward correction was wrong. ◯

God warned me not to let sin control me. ◯

My offering was acceptable to God. ◯

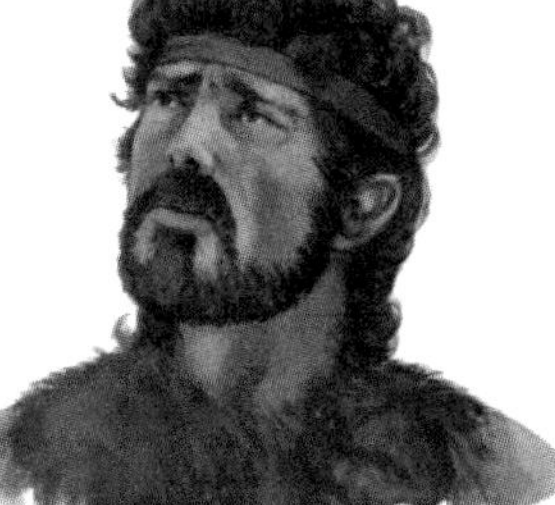

Cain

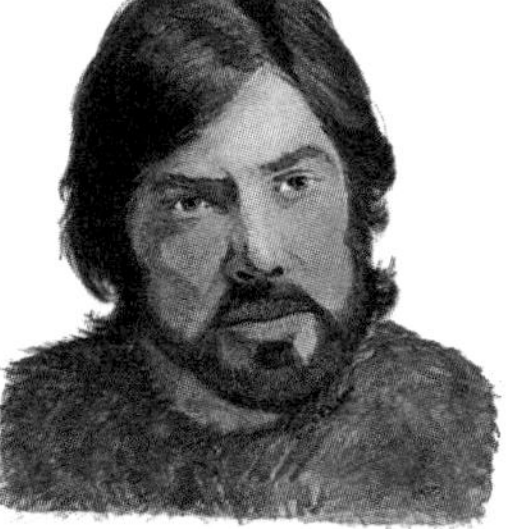

Abel

I trusted my brother and went into the field with him. ◯

My punishment seemed too great to bear, but God was merciful. ◯

My offering was not acceptable to God. ◯

God asked my brother where I was. ◯

I offered the fruits of the soil to the Lord. ◯

God does not expect His people to guess how to please Him; His Word shows them.

Complete the sentences to show some of the ways God is pleased. You may use your Bible for help.

1. God is pleased when His people praise Him with ______________ and give Him ______________ (Ps. 69:30-31).
2. A ______________ controlled by the Holy Spirit pleases God (Rom. 8:6-9).
3. Doing ______________ and sharing with others pleases God (Heb. 13:16).
4. Children who ______________ their parents please God (Col. 3:20).
5. Without ______________ it is impossible to please God (Heb. 11:5-6).

Role Models

Name ______________________

Many hundreds of years after Cain and Abel, the apostle John used Cain as an example of how *not* to treat someone.

Read I John 3:11-16. Write a question for each answer given. You may want to work with a partner.

1. **Question:** ______________________

   Answer: Love one another.

2. **Question:** ______________________

   Answer: from the beginning

3. **Question:** ______________________

   Answer: His own actions were evil, and his brother's actions were righteous.

4. **Question:** ______________________

   Answer: a murderer

5. **Question:** ______________________

   Answer: Jesus Christ laid down His life for us.

Think of a Christian you know who is Christlike in his/her relationships with other people. Write a one-word description of that person on each cross.

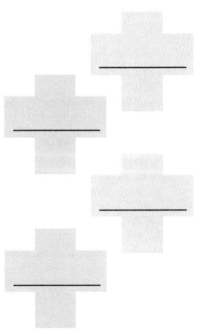

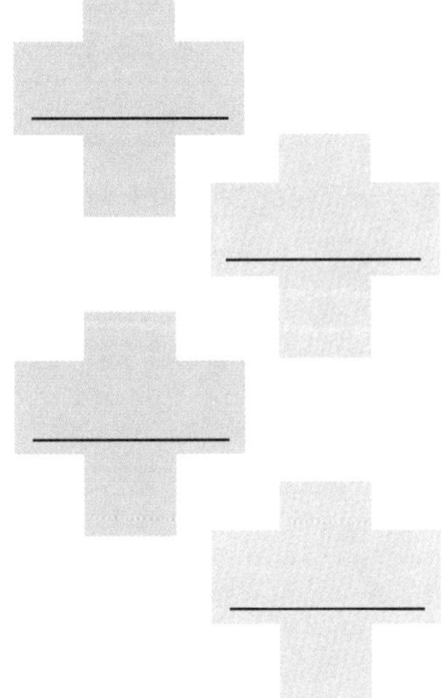

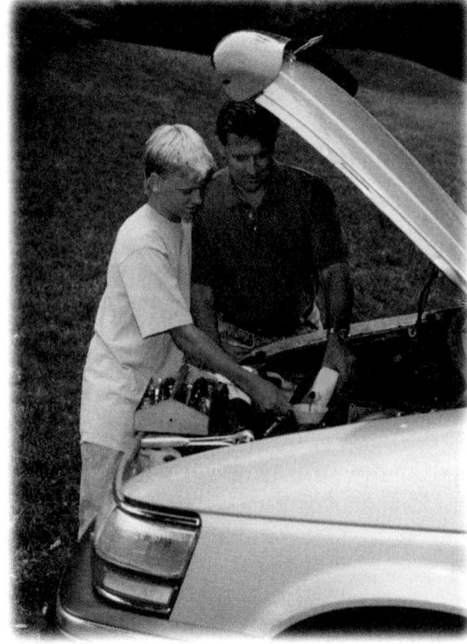

Adam's Line

Genesis 5

Name ______________________

After Abel's death and Cain's banishment, Adam and Eve had other sons and daughters.

Write the names to complete the genealogy of Adam to Noah. Circle the name of the man who went directly to be with God without dying. You may refer to Genesis 5:3-29.

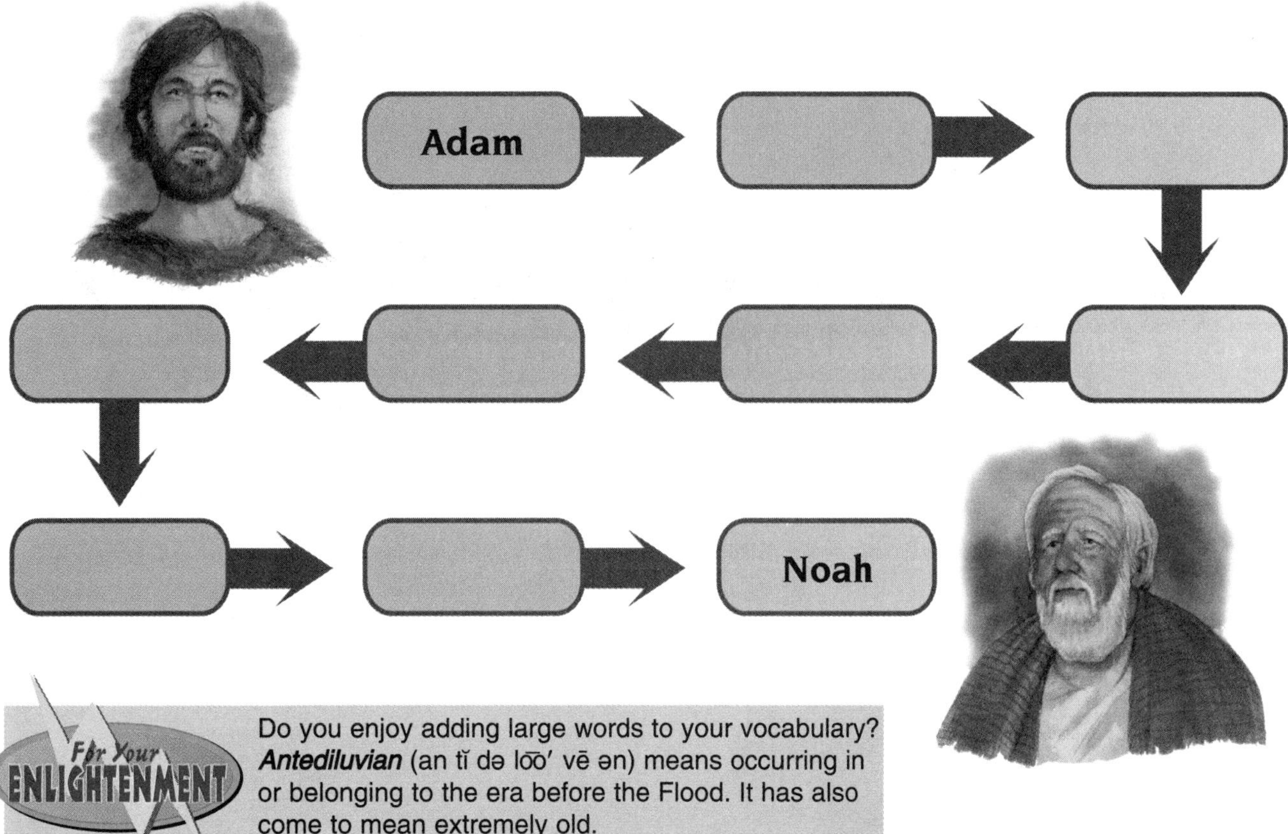
Adam
Noah

For Your ENLIGHTENMENT

Do you enjoy adding large words to your vocabulary? ***Antediluvian*** (an tĭ də lo͞o′ vē ən) means occurring in or belonging to the era before the Flood. It has also come to mean extremely old.

What was life like in the antediluvian period (from Adam to Noah)?

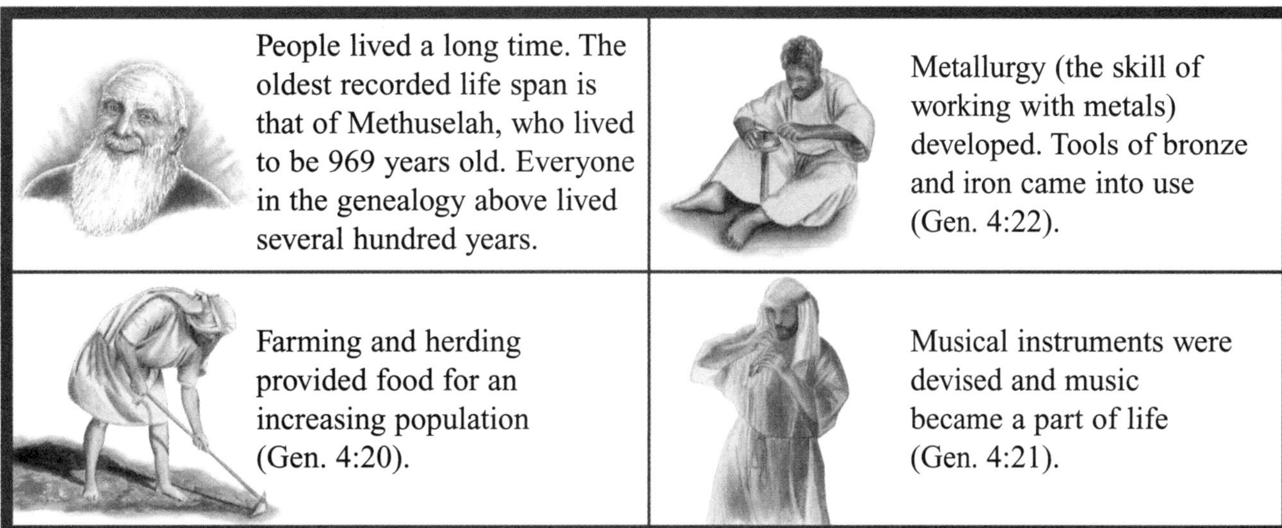

People lived a long time. The oldest recorded life span is that of Methuselah, who lived to be 969 years old. Everyone in the genealogy above lived several hundred years.

Metallurgy (the skill of working with metals) developed. Tools of bronze and iron came into use (Gen. 4:22).

Farming and herding provided food for an increasing population (Gen. 4:20).

Musical instruments were devised and music became a part of life (Gen. 4:21).

Walking with God

Genesis 5:21-24

Name ______________________

Enoch stood alone among the people as wickedness increased. The Scripture says that Enoch walked with God, and God took him to heaven. Each of the other men named in Genesis 5 has a statement of his age and death. Only Enoch's age is stated because God took him from the earth without death. This is not the only exceptional thing about Enoch. He was unique because he walked with God when others did not.

Your *walk* is your lifestyle—how you live, what you do, what is important to you. What will your *walk* be like if you are walking with God?

Answer the questions. You may use your Bible to help.

1. How will you live? (Gal. 2:20)

____

____

2. What will you do? (Eph. 2:10)

____

____

3. What will you love and what will you hate? (Amos 5:15)

____

____

4. What will you think about? (Phil. 4:8)

____

____

____

____

5. What will be missing from your life? (Col. 3:8)

____

____

____

6. What should you do if you fail to walk as you should? (I John 1:9)

____

____

What Does God Say About My Attitude?

Name ______________________________

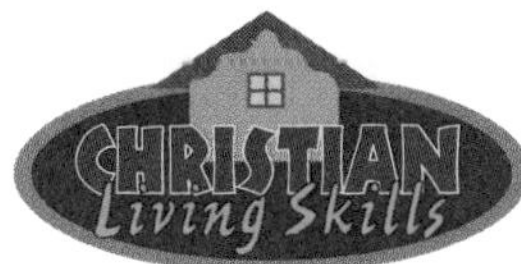
CHRISTIAN
Living Skills

When you confess your sin and accept salvation through Christ, your life changes entirely. The Bible teaches that your heart is the center of your will and emotions.

Read Proverbs 4:23 and tell why it is important that you guard your heart.

____

The condition of your heart determines your attitude toward everything in your life. Your **attitude** can be defined as the outward demonstration of what is in your heart. Every choice you make about your friends, how you do your assignments, and how you react to your parents is a result of what is in your heart.

Read Philippians 2:5-8 and answer the questions.

1. Whose example should you follow when it comes to your attitude? ______________
2. What kind of attitude did Jesus demonstrate when He became a man so that He could save us? ______________

Read Galatians 5:22-25. Write the attitudes that result when Jesus is in the center of your heart.

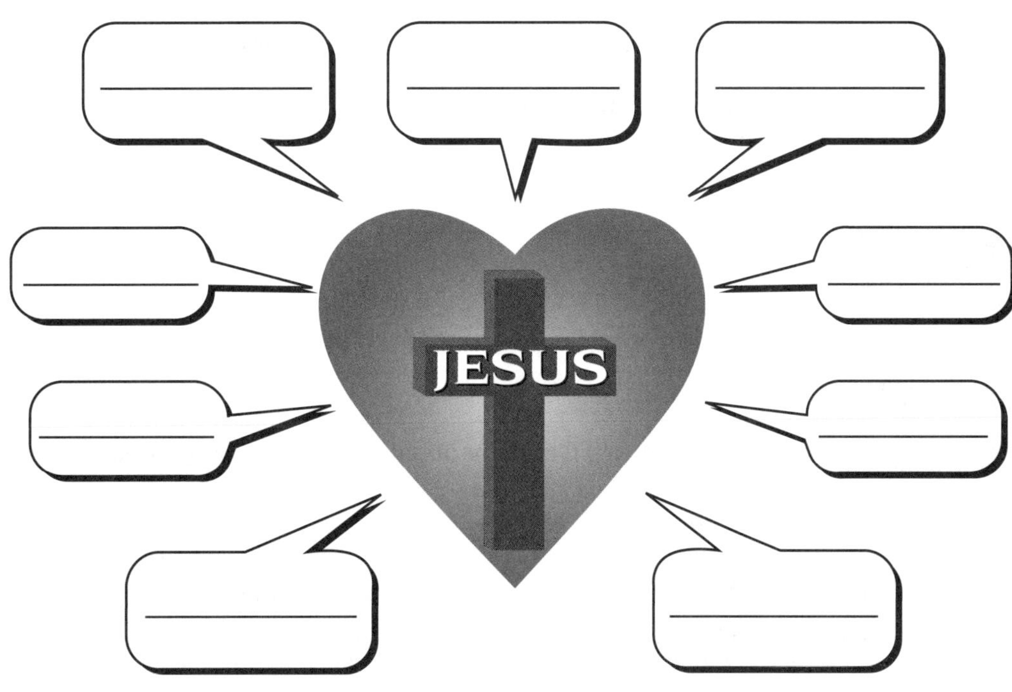
JESUS

Something to Think About

My Attitude

Name ____________________

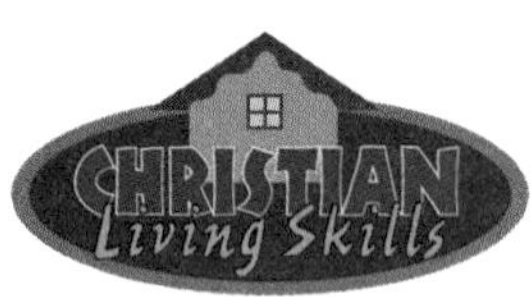
CHRISTIAN
Living Skills

God alone can see the condition of your heart. However, everyone around you can observe what is in your heart by the external "clues" that you give them.

Read the verses and tell how you give others clues about what is in your heart.

- **Proverbs 15:13** ____________________
- **Proverbs 15:28** ____________________
- **Jeremiah 17:23** ____________________
- **Proverbs 6:12-14** ____________________

Your ***attitude*** shows in your responses to circumstances, how you deal with your feelings about those circumstances, your beliefs about God, and the choices you make between pleasing yourself and pleasing God.

Read the situations and decide what your attitude would be if you wanted to please yourself. Then read the references and write a description of the attitude that would be pleasing to God in that situation.

Situation	Pleasing Myself	Pleasing God
You are hot and thirsty. Someone cuts in front of you at the water fountain.		Philippians 2:3
Your mom tells you to clean your room before you go outside. Your friends are waiting for you.		Ephesians 6:1-3
You find out that your friend told a lie about you. Some of your other friends believe the lie.		Romans 12:21

What About Me?

Take time at home to think about your attitude. Carefully consider the following questions.

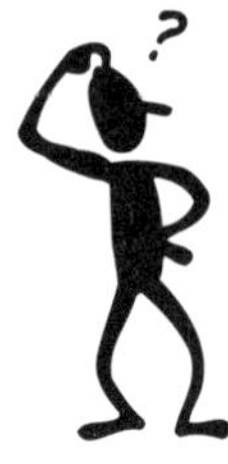
?

Is Jesus Christ at the center of my heart?
Am I pleasing God with the attitude that I display to others?
Would my parents say that I am pleasing God with my attitude?
Would my friends say that I have the attitude of Christ?
What attitudes do I need to change to become more like Christ?

Safe in the Ark

Name ______________________

Many accounts in the Old Testament show **types** (pictures) of salvation in Jesus Christ. The building and launching of the ark is one such account.

Cross out the pairs of letters. Write the remaining letters to spell the missing words. Then show how the idea has a parallel in (is similar to) salvation. You may use your Bible for help.

1. In the days of Noah, God waited patiently for mankind to ______________________.

W	W	R	X	X	E	T	T	U	U	P	B	B	E	K	K	R	R	N	V	V	Q	Q	T

Parallel: II Peter 3:9

____

2. The ark was the only way to ______________________ for Noah and his family.

O	O	V	V	S	I	I	A	E	E	C	C	F	M	M	E	L	L	H	H	T	Y	J	J

Parallel: John 14:6

____

3. After God shut the ark, nothing could ______________________ Noah and his family from its safety.

N	N	T	T	R	G	G	E	S	S	F	F	M	Y	Y	O	D	D	I	I	V	S	S	E

Parallel: John 10:28-29

____

4. The flood waters ______________________ all that was old so that Noah and his family began a new life in a world washed clean of sin.

D	P	P	E	W	W	S	O	O	T	R	N	N	O	Q	Q	Y	E	L	L	D	A	A

Parallel: I Peter 3:20*b*-21

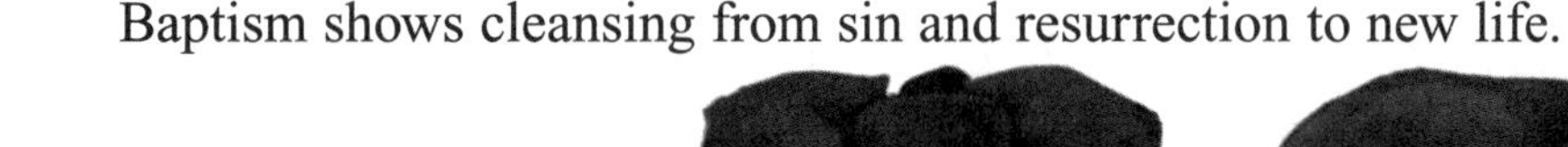

Baptism shows cleansing from sin and resurrection to new life.

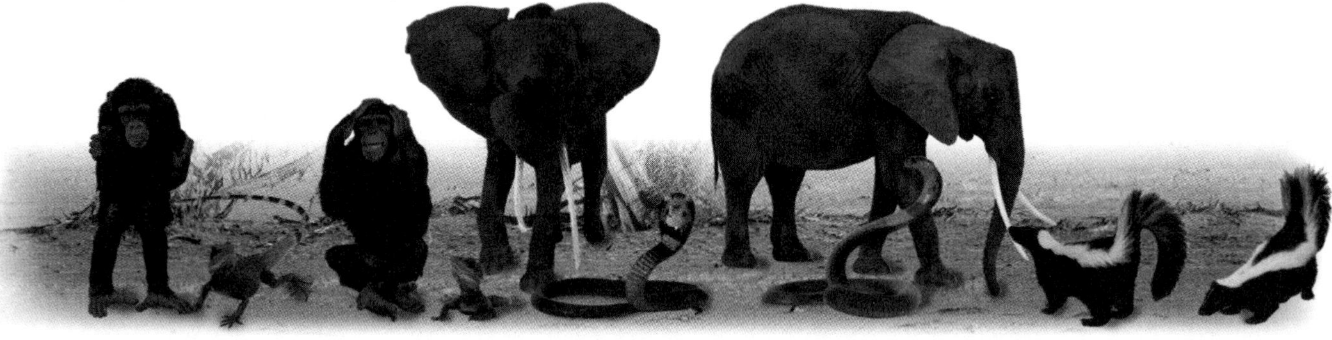

Building Plans for the Ark

Genesis 6-7

Name ______________________

Complete the information organizer. You may use your Bible for help.

Reason for the project (Gen. 6:17-18)

____

____

____

Materials list (Gen. 6:14)

Basic material: ______________________

Waterproofing material: ______________________

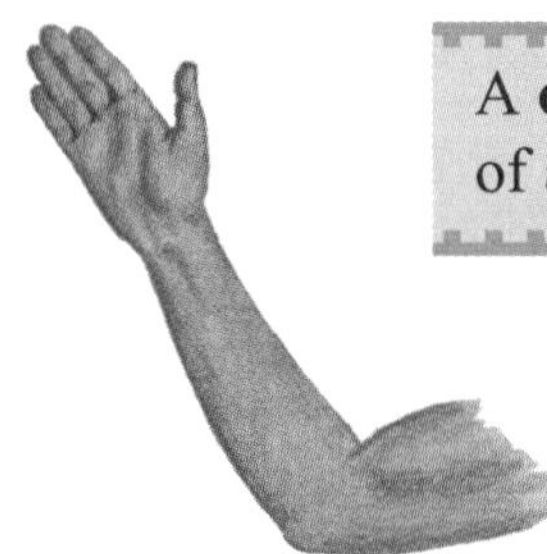

A **cubit** was linear measure determined by the length from the point of a man's elbow to the end of the middle finger (approx. 18 inches).

1 cubit = approx. 1.5 feet = approx. 0.455 meters

Specifications (Gen. 6:15)

Rename cubits as feet and cubits as meters. (Your teacher may allow you to use a calculator.)

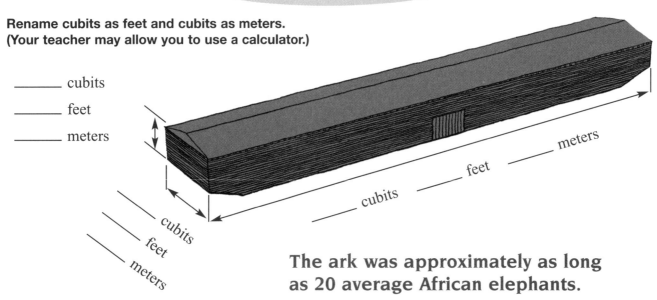

_____ cubits

_____ feet

_____ meters

_____ cubits

_____ feet

_____ meters

_____ cubits

_____ feet

_____ meters

The ark was approximately as long as 20 average African elephants.

Features (Gen. 6:16)

_____ window(s)

_____ door(s)

_____ deck(s) or floor(s)

Passenger List (Gen. 7:13)

__________ and his wife,

__________, __________,

__________, and their wives

How many in all? _____

Animals (Gen. 7:2)

_____ pairs of each kind of clean animal

_____ of each kind of unclean animal

What Does God Say About Making Choices?

Name ______________________________

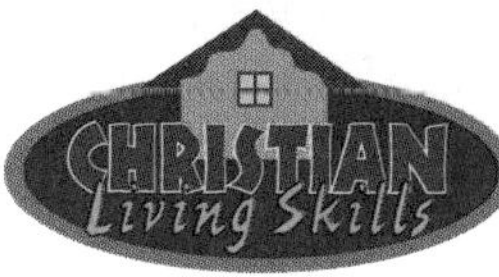
CHRISTIAN
Living Skills

You make many choices every day. Some choices seem more important than others. God's Word gives you instructions for making every decision. These instructions are called principles. A **principle** from God's Word is a basic truth upon which you can build wise decisions and right conduct before God. When you obey the principles of God's Word, you receive God's blessings. When you ignore or disobey the principles of God's Word, you will always receive negative consequences.

Read Matthew 7:24-27 and answer the question.

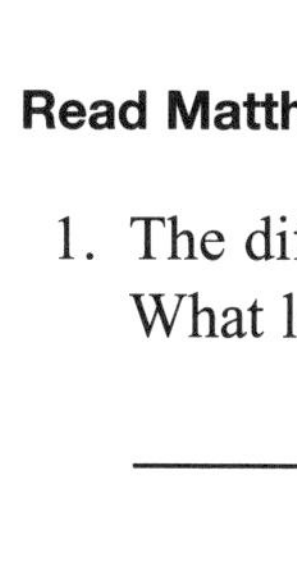

1. The difference between the two houses is that they were built on different foundations. What lesson do you think Jesus wants you to learn from this parable?

____

____

Sometimes people build weak foundations. They make a decision because of how they feel, what they want, or because of their circumstances. This always leads to WRONG CHOICES that do not please God.

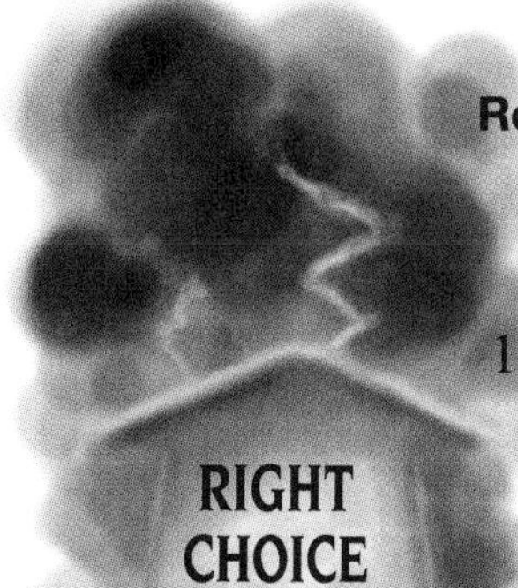
RIGHT
CHOICE

Principle from God's Word

Read the verses and answer the questions.

Jeremiah 17:9 Proverbs 14:12

1. Why is it never a good idea to make a choice based on how you feel or what you want?

____

2. Why should you never make a choice based only upon what YOU think you should do?

____

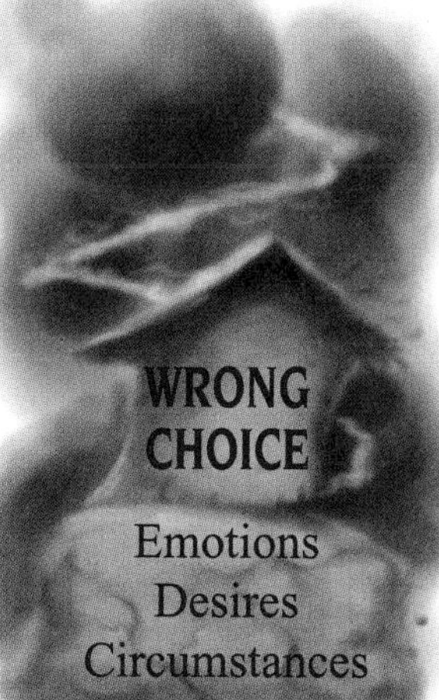
WRONG
CHOICE
Emotions
Desires
Circumstances

What does God say about how to make choices?

Using each verse, write a question that you could ask yourself when trying to make a right choice. The first one has been completed for you.

1. I Corinthians 10:31 Will this choice bring glory to God?
2. Romans 14:13 ______________________________
3. Colossians 3:20 ______________________________
4. I Timothy 4:12 ______________________________

Something to Think About

Making Choices

Name ______________________

Making choices based on God's Word brings joy and security. God's Word provides a solid foundation upon which to make decisions. In the Book of Psalms, David describes God's Word for God's children—it is sweeter than fresh honey from a honeycomb.

Read Psalm 19:7-11. Write adjectives that describe the sweetness of God's Word.

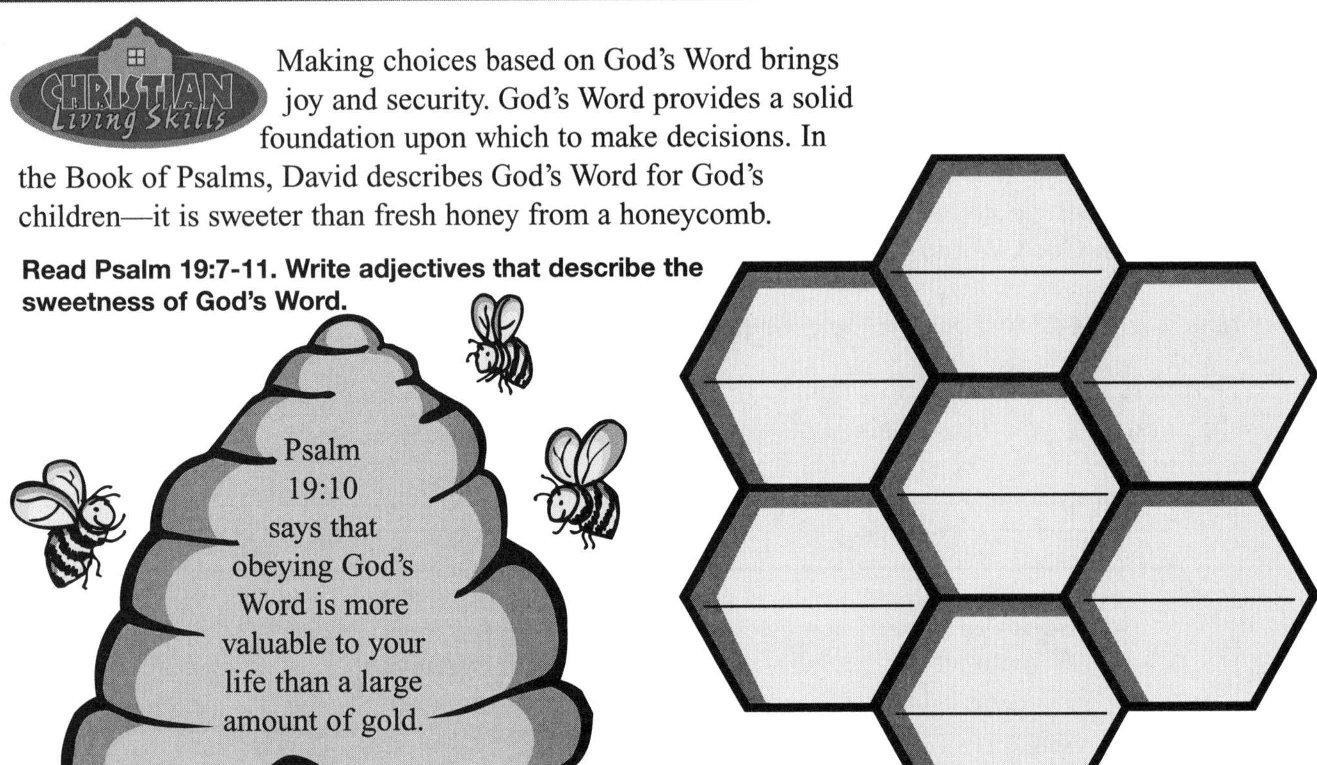
CHRISTIAN
Living Skills
Psalm 19:10 says that obeying God's Word is more valuable to your life than a large amount of gold.

Read Psalm 19:7-8, 11 and complete the sentences that list six valuable things God's Word will do for you.

1. God's Word will restore my ______________.
2. God's Word will give me ______________.
3. God's Word will bring joy to my ______________.
4. God's Word will give light to my ______________.
5. God's Word promises great ______________ if I obey.

What About Me?

Take time at home to think about the choices you make. Carefully consider the following questions.

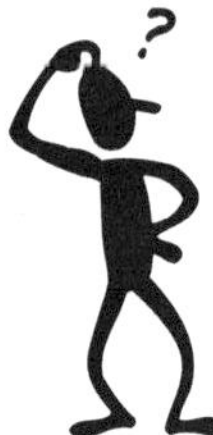

Do I want to please God when I make choices?
Do I ever make choices so that I can get what I want?
Do I ever make choices because I feel angry about the situation?
Do I ever make choices because I want my friends to accept me?
Do I find out what God says about choices before I make them?

Noah Is Blessed

Genesis 8:1–9:17

Name ______________________

Unscramble the word on the first dove and write it on the second dove. Look up the word in the glossary and write the definition.

God's purpose is to show His **carge** to individuals and to all mankind.

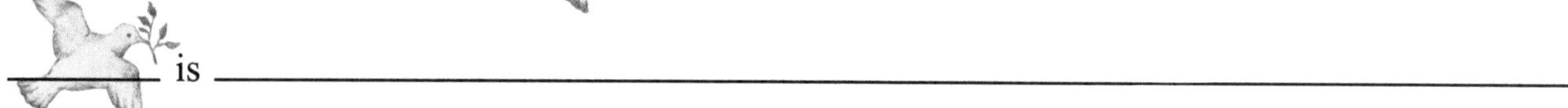

__________ is ____.

Complete the sentences. You may use your Bible for help.

1. To show his thanks and dedication to God, Noah ______________ and sacrificed burnt offerings as soon as he and his family exited the ark (Gen. 8:20).

God's promises after the Flood were made to all mankind, even to the wicked who do not acknowledge Him.

God promised that—

2. He will never again ____________ the earth with a ____________ (Gen. 9:11).
3. As long as the earth remains, there will be ______________ and harvest, cold and heat, summer and winter, day and ____________ (Gen. 8:22).
4. God told Noah that the fear of man will be upon all animals, because the killing of animals is permitted for ______________ (Gen. 9:2-3).
5. God told Noah that everyone who takes the life of a human being is accountable to God and will be punished because man was made in the __________ of God (Gen. 9:5-6).

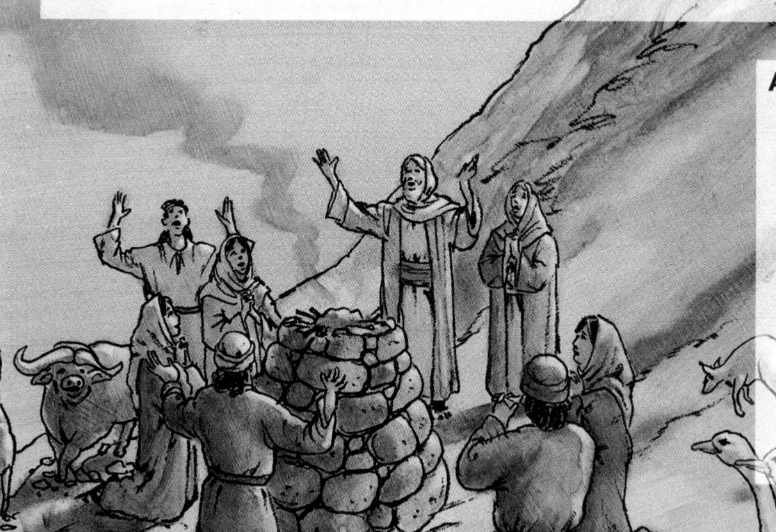

Answer the question.

6. Because God found Noah righteous, God saved Noah and his family. Since the Flood, mankind has descended from Noah. Which descendant of Noah became a servant who will someday rule the world?

____

Singing with Understanding

"O God, Our Help in Ages Past" (vv. 2-4)

Name ______________________

Read verses 2-4 of the hymn on page 311. Answer the questions.

1. Who wrote this hymn? ______________________
2. On what psalm did he base this hymn? ______________________
3. Read Psalm 90:1-4. Which words and phrases in the psalm remind you of the hymn?

   ____

4. Some Bibles include the name of the person inspired by God to write each psalm. Who wrote Psalm 90? (You may need to check other Bibles for this answer.) ______________________

Numbering Your Days

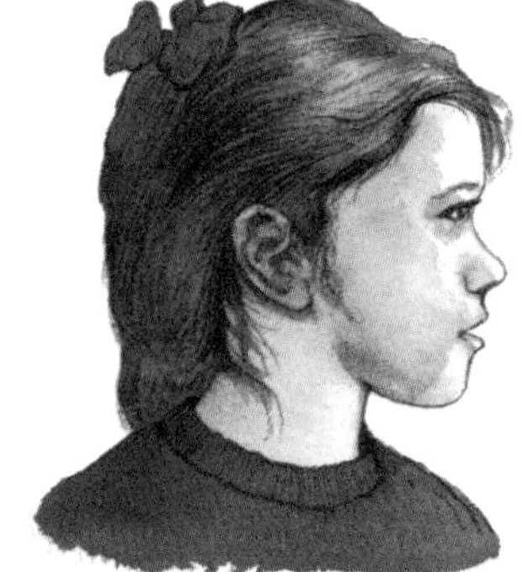

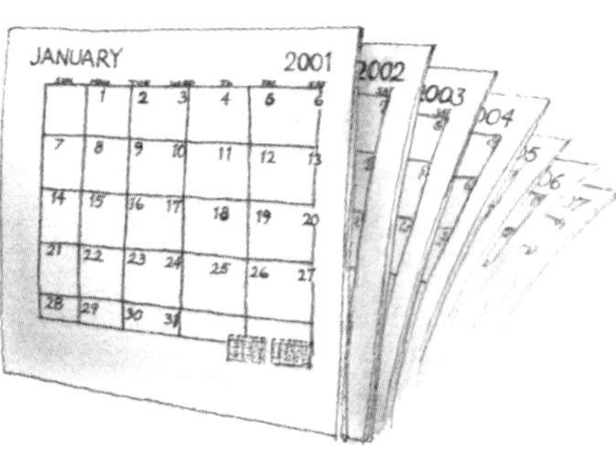
JANUARY
2001
2002
2003
2004

Read Psalm 90:12.

After meditating on God's anger toward sin and the shortness of human life, the psalmist asks God to teach him to number his days—make each day count in service for the Lord. When you are young, it is easy to think, "I've got my whole life ahead of me. Why should I be in any hurry to get serious about the Lord?" No one knows how long he has to live. After life on earth comes eternity. Only the things you do for the Lord will last. How can you serve the Lord this year? Consider taking some of these ideas as your goals.

Place a check mark beside three or four ideas; if desired, write in some goals of your own.

- ❑ Read through Psalms and Proverbs.
- ❑ Read through the Gospels.
- ❑ Memorize a psalm.
- ❑ Memorize a hymn.
- ❑ Pray for your pastor every day.
- ❑ Pray for a missionary every day.
- ❑ Pray for an unsaved relative or friend every day.
- ❑ Give out a gospel tract each week.
- ❑ Bring an unsaved friend to Sunday school or church.
- ❑ Volunteer to help your Sunday school teacher with class projects.
- ❑ Read a Christian biography.
- ❑ ______________________
- ❑ ______________________

After the Flood

Name ______________________________

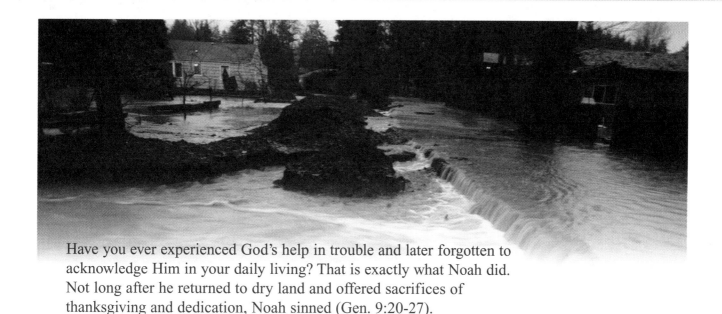

Have you ever experienced God's help in trouble and later forgotten to acknowledge Him in your daily living? That is exactly what Noah did. Not long after he returned to dry land and offered sacrifices of thanksgiving and dedication, Noah sinned (Gen. 9:20-27).

Find out how a Christian can walk with God in times of crisis and in daily living. Use the grid to decode the words that complete each sentence.

▲	A	C	G	Q	Z
●	E	F	H	L	K
■	I	N	M	R	P
✦	O	S	J	D	B
★	U	T	W	X	Y
	❍	❏	☆	✧	➪

(✧●)(❍■)(☆▲)(☆●)(❏★)

1. Keep a right relationship with Christ and others: walk in the ___ ___ ___ ___ ___ (I John 1:7).

(❏▲)(❍▲)(✧■)(❍●)(❏●)(❍★)(✧●)(✧●)(➪★)

2. Walk ___ ___ ___ ___ ___ ___ ___ ___ ___, not foolishly (Eph. 5:15).

(✧✦)(❍●)(❍▲)(✧✦)

3. Remember that you are ___ ___ ___ ___ to sin and alive in Christ (Rom. 8:1).

(❍●)(✧★)(❍▲)(☆■)(➪■)(✧●)(❍●)

4. Have Christ as your ___ ___ ___ ___ ___ ___ ___ (I John 2:6).

(➪■)(✧■)(❍▲)(➪★)

5. ___ ___ ___ ___ all the time, not just when you are in trouble (I Thess. 5:17).

(❍✦)(➪✦)(❍●)(➪★)

6. Know and ___ ___ ___ ___ the Word of God (Ps. 119:11, 60).

(❏★)(☆●)(❍■)(❏■)(➪●)

7. ___ ___ ___ ___ ___ about the right things (Phil. 4:8).

Using Cross-References and Marginal Notes

Name ____________________

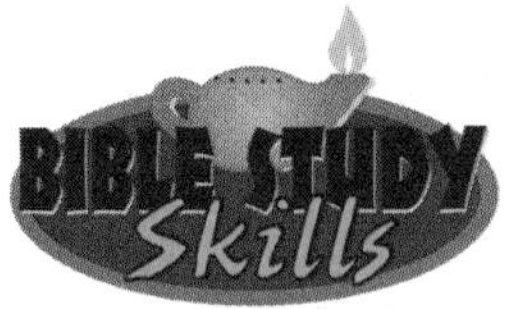
BIBLE STUDY
Skills

Many Bibles have **cross-references,** Scripture references that tell where the same ideas or stories may be found elsewhere in the Bible. Cross-references are usually found down the center or the sides of the page.

THE EPISTLE TO THE

EPHESIANS

Author: Paul   *Theme:* The Church, Christ's Body   *Date of writing:* c. A.D. 60

a See 2 Pet.3:18, *note*. *Grace:* vv. 2,6; Eph. 1:7. (Jn. 1:14; Jn. 1:17, *note*)
b *Election* (corporate): v. 4; Col.3:12. (Dt.7:6; 1 Pet. 5:13)
c Gk. *kosmos*
d *Sanctification* (N.T.): v. 4; Eph. 2:21. (Mt. 4:5; Rev. 22:11)

Introduction (1:1–2)

1 PAUL, an apostle of Jesus
Christ by the will of God, to
the [1]saints who are at Ephesus,
and to the faithful [2]in Christ
Jesus:
2 [a]Grace *be* to you, and peace,
from God, our Father, and *from*
the Lord Jesus Christ.

I. The Believer's Standing in Grace, 1:1–3:21

(1) The believer in Christ in the heavenlies

3 ¶ Blessed *be* the God and Father of our Lord Jesus Christ,
who hath blessed us with all
spiritual blessings [3]in heavenly
places in Christ,
4 According as he hath [b]chosen
us in him before the foundation
of the [c]world, that we should be
[d]holy and without blame before
him, in love
5 Having [e]predestinated us unto
the [4][f]adoption of [g]|sons| by Jesus
Christ to himself, according to
the good pleasure of his will,
6 To the praise of the glory of
his [a]grace, through which he
hath made us accepted in the Beloved;
7 In whom we have [h]redemption
through his [i]blood, the [j]forgive-

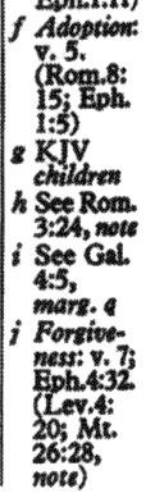
e *Predestination:* v. 5; Eph.1:11. (Rom. 8:29; Eph.1:11)
f *Adoption:* v. 5. (Rom.8:15; Eph. 1:5)
g KJV *children*
h See Rom. 3:24, *note*
i See Gal. 4:5, *marg. a*
j *Forgiveness:* v. 7; Eph.4:32. (Lev.4:20; Mt. 26:28, *note*)

Marginal notes give many kinds of supplementary information about a Scripture passage. They are usually found at the top or bottom of a page. Sometimes a cross-reference indicates that there is a marginal note accompanying that reference which will help you to better understand the first Scripture.

3:13   ROMANS   3:25

a vv. 13–18; Ps.5:9; 10:7; 36:1; 140:3; Isa.59:7–8
b See Rom. 2:18, *marg. a*
c Cp. Ezek. 16:63
d i.e. *to be under the judicial sentence of God*
e Ps.143:2; Gal.2:16
f See Rom. 3:4, *marg. w*
g See v. 23, *note*
h KJV *without*
i See v. 21, *note*

that doeth good, no, not one.
13 [a]Their throat *is* an open sepulcher; with their tongues they
have used deceit; the poison of
asps *is* under their lips;
14 Whose mouth *is* full of curs-
ing and bitterness.
15 Their feet *are* swift to shed
blood;
16 Destruction and misery *are*
in their ways;
17 And the way of peace have
they not known.
18 There is no fear of God
before their eyes.
19 ¶ Now we know that whatever
things the [b]law saith, it saith to
them who are under the law,
that every mouth may be [c]stopped,
and all the world may [d]become
guilty before God.
20 Therefore, by the deeds of
the law [e]there shall no flesh be
[f]justified in his sight; for by the
[b]law *is* the knowledge of [g]sin.

II. Justification by Faith in Christ, 3:21–5:21

(1) Justification defined

21 ¶ But now the [1]righteousness
of God [h]|apart from| the law is
manifested, being witnessed by
the [b]law and the prophets,
22 Even the [i]righteousness of
God *which is* by faith [j]of Jesus
Christ unto all and upon all them
that [k]believe; for there is no difference.
23 For all have [2]sinned, and
come short of the glory of God,
24 Being [f]justified [l]freely by his
[m]grace through the [3]redemption
that is in Christ Jesus,
25 Whom God hath [n]set forth *to
be* a [4]propitiation through [k]faith in
his blood, to declare his [i]right-
eousness for the [o]remission of

j Lit. *in*
k *Faith:* vv. 22,25; Rom.3:26. (Gen. 3:20; Heb.11:39, *note*)
l i.e. *as a gift*
m *Grace:* v. 24; Rom. 4:4. (Jn. 1:14; Jn. 1:17, *note*)
n *Sacrifice* (of Christ): v. 25; Rom.4:25. (Gen. 3:15; Heb.10:18, *note*)
o Lit. *the passing over of sins done formerly*, i.e. *since Adam*. Cp. Heb. 9:15

[1](3:21) The righteousness of God is all that God demands and approves, and is ultimately found in Christ Himself, who fully met in our stead every requirement of the law. Through imputation Christ is "made unto us . . . righteousness" (1 Cor.1:30; cp. Lev.25:47–52; Rom.3:26; 4:6; 10:4; 2 Cor.5:21; Phil.3:9; Jas.2:23).

[2](3:23) Sin, Summary: The literal meanings of the Hebrew and Greek words variously rendered "sin," "sinner," etc. disclose the true nature of sin in its manifold manifestations. Sin is (1) transgression, an overstepping of the law, the divine boundary between good and evil (Ps.51:1; Rom.2:23); (2) iniquity, an act inherently wrong, whether expressly forbidden or not (Rom.1:21–23); (3) error, a departure from right (Rom.1:18; 1 Jn.3:4); (4) missing the mark, a failure to meet the divine standard (Rom.3:23); (5) trespass, the intrusion of self-will into the sphere of divine authority (Eph.2:1); (6) lawlessness, or spiritual anarchy (1 Tim.1:9); and (7) unbelief, or an insult to the divine veracity (Jn.16:9). Sin (1) originated with Satan (Isa.14:12–14); (2) entered the world through Adam (Rom.5:12); (3) was, and is, universal, Christ alone excepted (Rom.3:23; 1 Pet.2:22); (4) incurs the penalties of spiritual and physical death (Gen.2:17; 3:19; Ezek.18:4,20; Rom.6:23); and (5) has no remedy but in the sacrificial death of Christ (Acts 4:12; Heb.9:26) availed of by faith (Acts 13:38–39). Sin may be summarized as threefold: (1) an act, the violation of, or want of obedience to, the revealed will of God; (2) a state, absence of righteousness; and (3) a nature, enmity toward God.

[3](3:24) "Redemption" means *to deliver by paying a price*. The work of Christ fulfilling the O.T. types and prophecies of redemption is set forth in three principal Greek words: (1) *Agorazō, to buy in the market* (from *agora, market*). Man is viewed as a slave "sold under sin" (Rom.7:14) and under sentence of death (Ezek.18:4; Jn.3:18–19, Rom.6:23) but subject to redemption by the purchase price of the blood of the Redeemer (1 Cor.6:20; 7:23; 2 Pet.2:1; Rev.5:9; 14:3–4). (2) *Exagorazō, to buy out of the market*, i.e. to purchase and remove from further sale (Gal.3:13; 4:5; Eph.5:16; Col.4:5), speaking of the finality of the work of redemption. And (3) *lutroō, to loose or set free* (Lk.24:21; Ti.2:14; 1 Pet.1:18), noun form, *lutrōsis* (Lk.2:38; Heb.9:12). Compare also "redeemed" (lit. *to make redemption*, Gk. *epoiēsen lutrōsin*, Lk.1:68), and "deliverance" (intensive form, *apolutrōsis*) used commonly to indicate release of a slave (Lk.21:28; Rom.3:24; 8:23; 1 Cor. 1:30; Eph.1:7,14; 4:30; Col.1:14; Heb.9:15; 11:35). Redemption is by sacrifice and by power (Ex. 14:30, *note*); Christ paid the price, the Holy Spirit makes deliverance actual in experience (Rom. 8:2). See Ex.14:30, *note*; Isa.59:20, *note* 1; Rom.1:16, *note*.

Answer the questions.

1. Look at Ephesians 1:7. Write the reference that has an accompanying marginal note that will help you to better understand the word *redemption* as it is used in this verse.

   ____

2. Look at that verse and its marginal note. Write the definition of *redemption* that is found there.

   ____

   ____

   ____

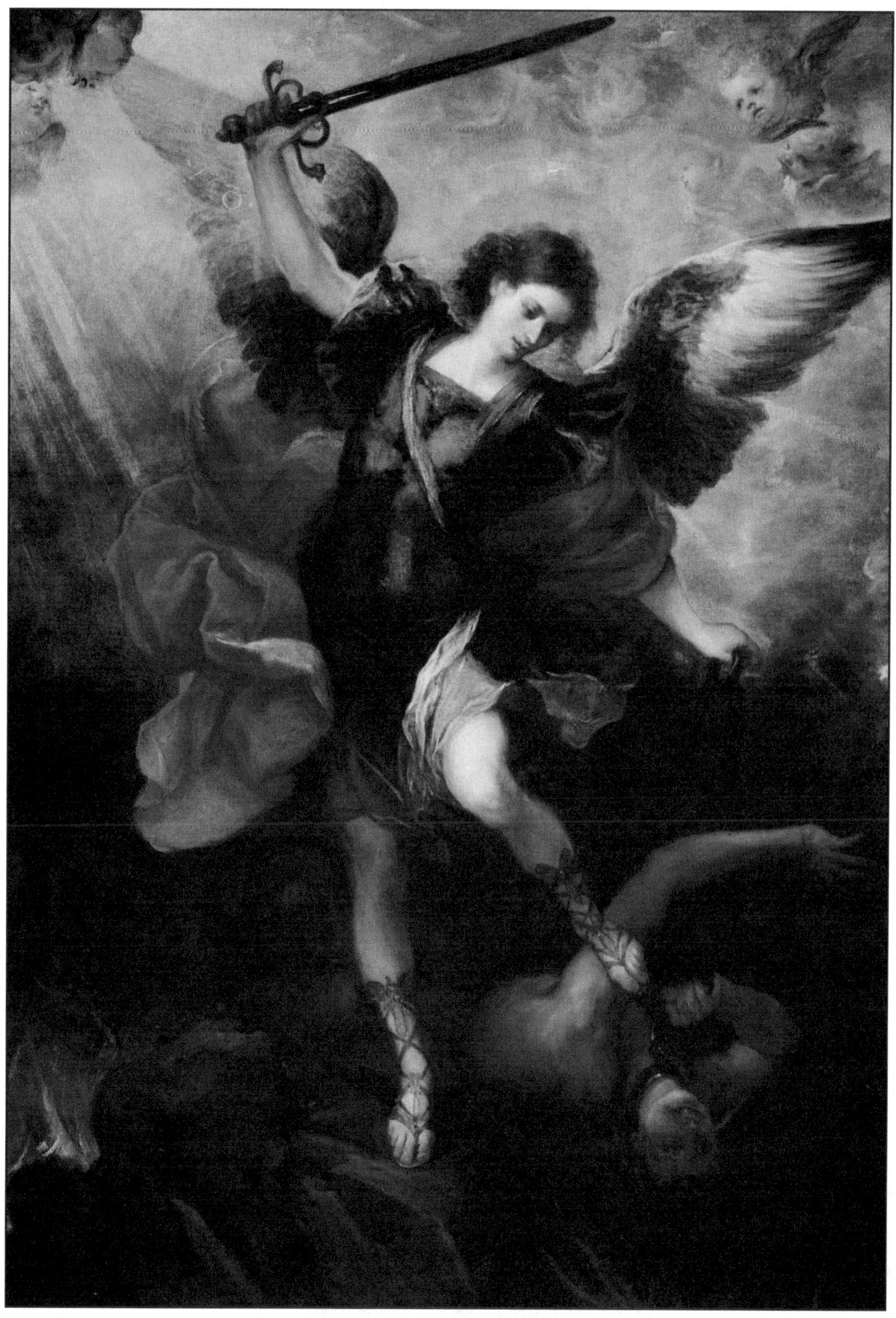

Michael Overcoming Satan

Jose Antolinez

Bob Jones University Museum & Gallery, Inc.

Name ______________________________

Michael Overcoming Satan

by Jose Antolinez (1635-1675)

Jose Antolinez (Hō sā′ An tō lē′nĕth) lived all of his life in the capital city of Spain. Though he never visited Rome, Venice, or the Flemish colonies, he knew about the art styles of their artists through the paintings the king had purchased.

During Antolinez's career, a new style of painting became popular in Madrid which made human figures elegant, beautiful, and athletic. Artists blended colors to achieve soft edges so that it looked as if light were shining right out of the painting.

This picture is full of contrasts. One of the most obvious is the contrast between the archangel Michael and Satan. Michael is young and elegant, seemingly weightless and effortless in his control. Satan, on the other hand, is homely, weak, and awkward. He looks like he is trying to stop the blow about to come from the uplifted sword, but the archangel is stepping on Satan's arm, robbing him of his power.

There is another contrast: light and darkness. The artist has divided the painting in half, placing the light at the top and the dark at the bottom. The light is full of faces of little cherubs looking on from heaven and protecting the archangel; some of the light even seems to glow from Michael himself. At the bottom of the painting, everything is dark and unclear. Though a fire is burning, it is not giving out much light. The lower part of Satan's body seems to be coiling like an enormous snake (Rev. 12:9). The artist leaves just enough light to reveal the form. The void in front of Satan seems to be a bottomless pit, undefined except for flames which do not allow enough light to see clearly.

This conflict is based on Revelation 12:7-9 and 20:1-3.

Know the Enemy

Name ______________________

Satan is the declared enemy of God and His people. It is wise for Christians to know who he is and what he is like.

Spell the answers by matching the Arabic numeral with the Roman numeral to find the correct letter.

I	II	III	IV	V	VI	VII	VIII	IX	X	XI	XII	XIII	XIV	XV	XVI	XVII	XVIII	XIX
A	N	V	G	M	O	W	B	H	R	T	U	C	E	I	D	Y	L	S

Names

19 1 11 1 2

"___ ___ ___ ___ ___" is from the Hebrew word for *adversary* or *opponent.*

16 14 3 15 18

"___ ___ ___ ___ ___" is from the Greek word for *slanderer.* He is also called the dragon, the evil one, the prince of the power of the air, the ruler (or god) of this world, Apollyon, Abaddon, Belial, and Beelzebub.

Origin, Nature, and Characteristics

13 10 14 1 11 14 16

Satan is not eternal. He was ___ ___ ___ ___ ___ ___ ___ by God at a point in time (Ezek. 28:15). Like all creatures, he is accountable to his Creator. As an angel in the order called

13 9 14 10 12 8 15 5

___ ___ ___ ___ ___ ___ ___ ___, he stood in the presence of God's holiness (Ezek. 28:14).

7 15 19 16 6 5

He was unparalleled in ___ ___ ___ ___ ___ ___

8 14 1 12 11 17

and ___ ___ ___ ___ ___ ___ (Ezek. 28:12).

Before he rebelled against God, Satan was

8 18 1 5 14 18 14 19 19

___ ___ ___ ___ ___ ___ ___ ___ ___ (morally upright) in his ways (Ezek. 28:15).

Sin

1 10 10 6 4 1 2 13 14

Satan's sin was ___ ___ ___ ___ ___ ___ ___ ___ ___ and pride (I Tim. 3:6).

Isaiah 14:12-14 is a record of what Satan said:

9 14 1 3 14 2

I will ascend to ___ ___ ___ ___ ___ ___.

11 9 10 6 2 14

I will make my ___ ___ ___ ___ ___ ___ higher than the stars of God.

5 6 12 2 11 1 15 2

I will be enthroned on the sacred ___ ___ ___ ___ ___ ___ ___ ___.

13 18 6 12 16 19

I will rise above the highest ___ ___ ___ ___ ___ ___.

5 6 19 11 9 15 4 9

I will make myself like the ___ ___ ___ ___ ___ ___ ___ ___.

Already Defeated

Name ______________________

Long before Satan rebelled against God, long before Adam and Eve yielded to his temptation, God's perfect plan had made provision for Satan's defeat. As an enemy, however, he and his armies are not to be underestimated. Satan's repeated assaults on God's people are subtle, often mimicking God's purposes and activities. God's Word likens them to fiery darts (Eph. 6:16).

Complete the sentences that tell some of Satan's activities against God's people. You may use your Bible for help.

sin	good	vain
stopped	wrong	boast

1. Satan tries to get God's people to be ______________ by circumstances (I Thess. 2:18).
2. Satan tries to get God's people to give in to their ______________ desires (James 1:14).
3. Satan tries to distract God's people from God's purposes, and to discredit their testimony so that their work is in __________ (I Cor. 15:58).
4. Satan tries to get God's people to ______________ about their own abilities and accomplishments instead of boasting in Jesus Christ. (I Cor. 1:30-31).
5. Satan tries to keep God's people from doing the __________ things they know they should do (James 4:17).
6. Satan tries to make God's people think that they are still slaves to ________ (Rom. 6:6-7).

Even though Satan has already been defeated by the work of Jesus Christ, individuals have no chance of victory without the armor God has provided for spiritual warfare.

Write a label for each piece of equipment listed in Ephesians 6:13-17. You may use your Bible for help.

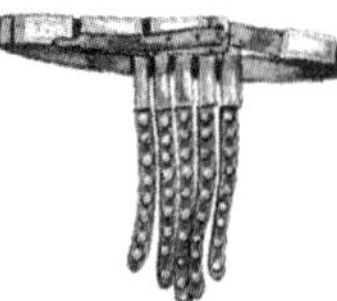

The belt of ______________

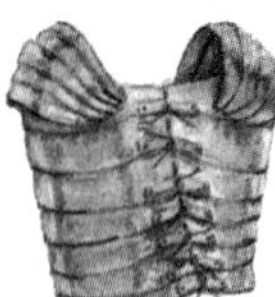

The breastplate of ______________

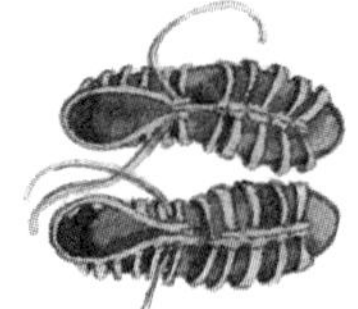

Shoes that are in the readiness of the ______________

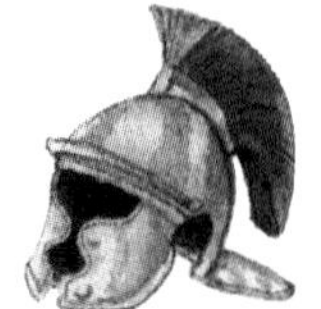

The helmet of ______________

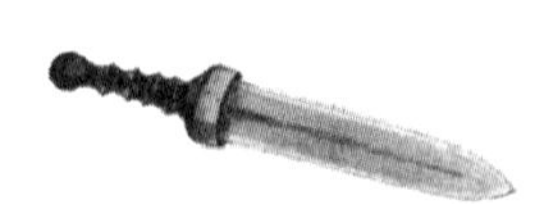

The sword of the ____________, which is the ______________

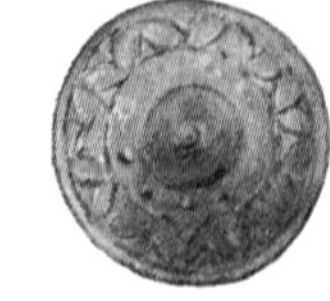

The shield of ______________

One Head

Ephesians 1:3-10

Name ______________________

The New Testament church is a living organism, not a building or organization. Members are to be supporters and encouragers of one another, working together as the parts of the body work together. Leaders in the church are not to be regarded as superiors of higher rank whose job is to control other believers. The body has only one head, Jesus Christ. God's ultimate purpose is to bring all things in heaven and on earth together in Him.

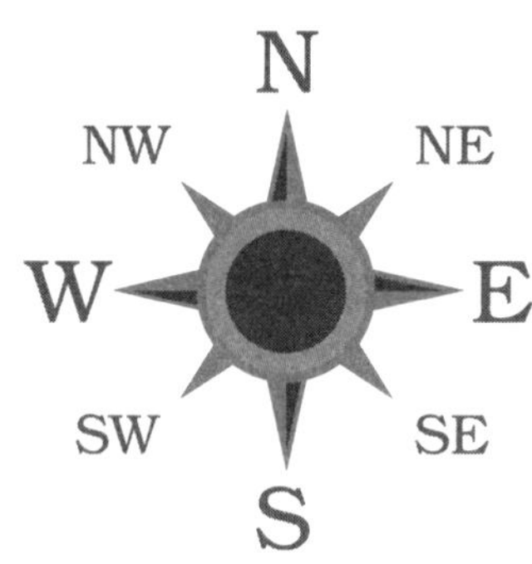

N
NW
NE
W
E
SW
SE
S

Start with the letter on the matching colored cell. Write the adjoining letter that is indicated by each compass direction from the previous letter.

In Jesus Christ, God has given believers—

1. Spiritual (B) ___ ___ ___ ___ ___ ___ ___ ___
   NE S SW S S NE N NW

2. (H) ___ ___ ___ ___ ___ ___ ___
   S NW NW SW S SE S

3. (P) ___ ___ ___ ___ ___ or blamelessness
   NW SW NW SW NW

4. (L) ___ ___ ___
   SE S NW

5. (A) ___ ___ ___ ___ ___ ___ ___ into His family
   N SE N NW NE N SE

6. (G) ___ ___ ___ ___
   SE SE SE N

7. (R) ___ ___ ___ ___ ___ ___ ___ ___ ___
   NE SE SE SW SE SW S NE S

8. (F) ___ ___ ___ ___ ___ ___ ___ ___ ___ ___
   S SW NW SW N NE NW NW NE SE

9. (W) ___ ___ ___ ___ ___ and understanding
   S SW S SE SE

10. (U) ___ ___ ___ ___ in Christ
    NW SW SW NW

O I H T O E
A N L P J R D
I B O M N W E
T E E H S T M
P S V E S I P
D F G F N S T
O S R E E F O
A B N A V D I
Y I U C G O N
T R P I R M

Singing with Understanding

"O God, Our Help in Ages Past" (v. 5)

Name ______________________________

Read Hebrews 13:8 and answer the question.

How long will Jesus stay the same? ____________________

Think about God's ability to help believers. Complete each list with your own examples.

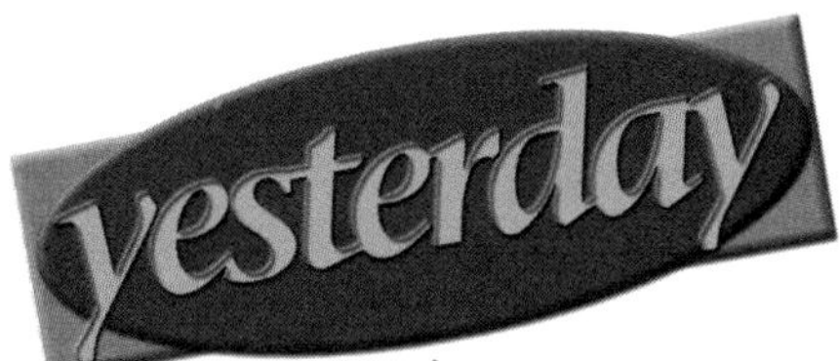
yesterday

All through history, God has been the help of those who trust Him.

- He helped the Israelites cross the Red Sea.
- He helped Gideon defeat the Midianites.
- He delivered Daniel from the lions' den.
- ____
- ____

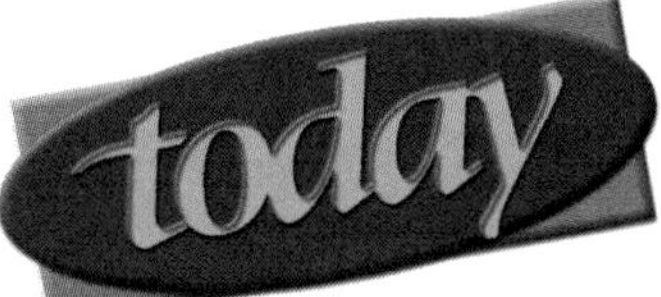
today

Today, God helps believers in every aspect of daily life.

- He helps them obey at home and at school.
- He gives them opportunities and courage to witness to unsaved friends.
- He comforts them when they are sad or discouraged.
- He protects them as they travel from place to place.
- ____
- ____

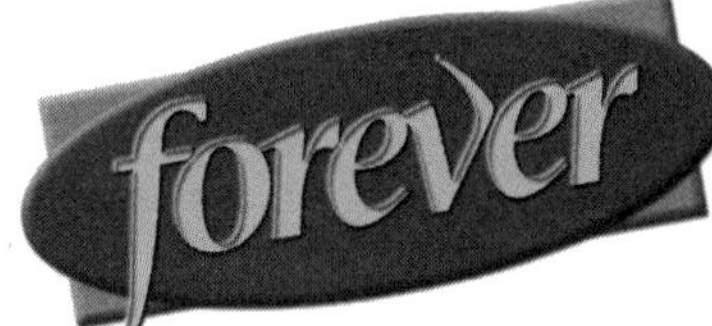
forever

God will continue to help believers in the future and throughout eternity.

- He will stay beside them in times of poor health.
- He will give them wisdom about what careers they should pursue.
- He will provide for their needs when finances are tight.
- He will encourage them when they are elderly and feeble.
- ____
- ____

Plans and Purposes

Genesis 11:1-9

Name ______________________

Fill in the circle beside every answer that will complete a true sentence.

1. In the beginning civilization in Shinar after the Flood, people had a common __________.
   - ○ plan
   - ○ language
   - ○ house

2. The people who settled in Shinar made plans to build a __________.
   - ○ fortress
   - ○ tower
   - ○ city

3. A purpose they had for their building project was __________.
   - ○ to gain fame (a name)
   - ○ to escape future floods
   - ○ to keep from being scattered

4. God prevented their plans and purposes by __________.
   - ○ causing them to be unable to understand each other's language
   - ○ scattering them over the whole earth
   - ○ sending fire from heaven on them

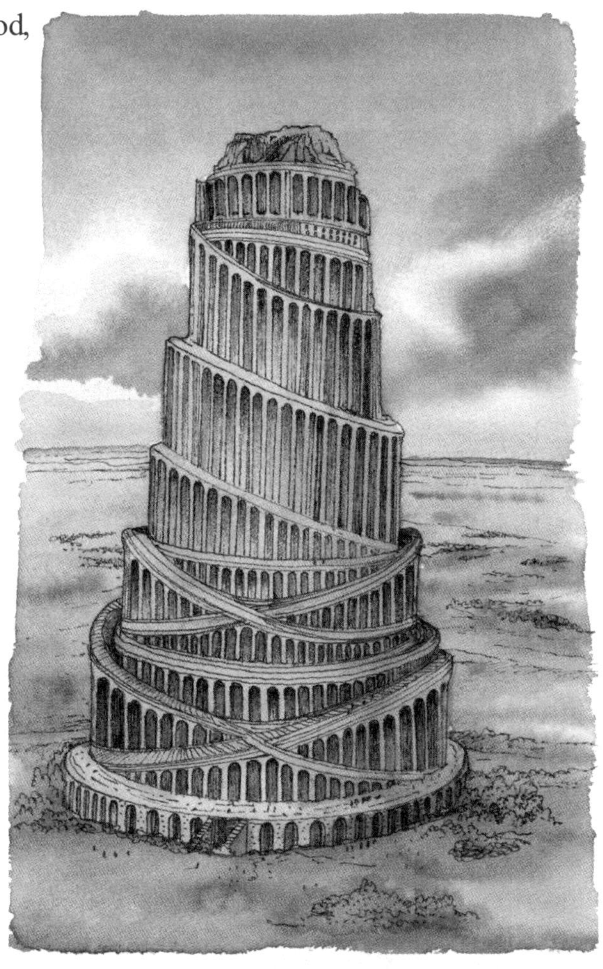

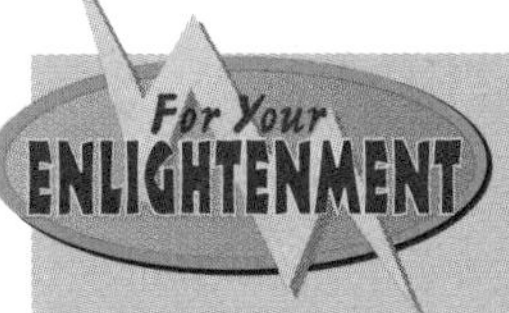
For Your
ENLIGHTENMENT

For years, there has been interest in having one language spoken throughout the world. Some people believe that such a language would promote understanding, strengthen cultural ties, facilitate business transactions, and simplify communication among the nations. It has been suggested that an existing language be adopted or that a new language be developed. Although several universal languages have been proposed, **Esperanto** (ĕs′ pĕ răn′ tō) has proven the most popular. It was created by a Polish doctor in 1887, and has gained a few million supporters. The base for Esperanto is mainly root words that are common to Indo-European languages, and all nouns end in ***o.*** For example, *astronaut* is *astronauto.*

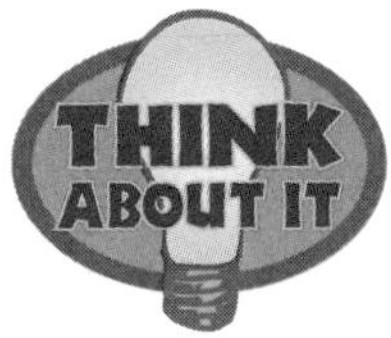
THINK
ABOUT IT

Do you think that it would ever be possible to have a worldwide universal language? Why or why not?

____

____

A Mystery of Love and Grace

Name ______________________

God did not keep His plan and purpose a secret from mankind. He gave glimpses of it during Old Testament times, but it could not be fully understood until Jesus Christ came. God's plan will not be perfectly revealed until He comes to gather all believers to be with Him forever.

Write a word to complete each sentence. You may use your Bible for help.

Abraham David Eve Judah Shem	1. God promised that although the offspring of __________ would be made to suffer by Satan, Satan would ultimately be defeated by Him (Gen. 3:15, 20). 2. After the Flood, God singled out the descendants of __________ (the Semitic nations) as the people through whom the Messiah would come (Gen. 9:26). 3. With the promise to __________, God narrowed the promise to the Jews (Gen. 26:4-5). 4. When Jacob blessed his family before he died, he prophesied that the Messiah would be a king from __________, a specific tribe of the Hebrew nation (Gen. 49:10). 5. Almost 1,000 years later, God told __________ that the Messiah would come from David's line and would rule from his throne forever (II Sam. 7:8, 12-14).

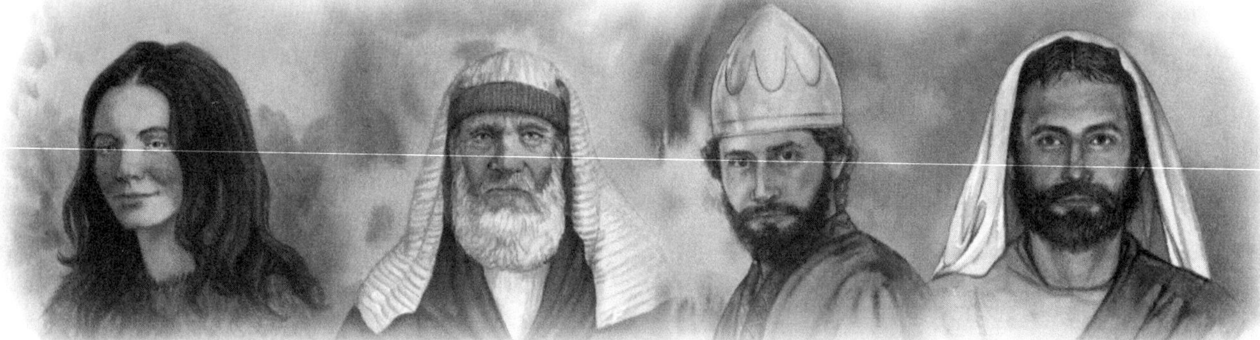

Write a word to complete each sentence. You may use your Bible for help.

effects glory heaven known salvation	1. In the future, God will reveal a new __________ and a new earth (Rev. 21:1). 2. God will welcome His people to a new city where they will see His __________ revealed (Rev. 21:10-11). 3. God's people will know as they are __________ (I Cor. 13:12). 4. God's people will know what it is like to live without sin and its __________: death, sorrow, tears, and pain (Rev. 21:4). 5. __________ will at last be perfectly revealed in every believer (I Pet. 1:5).

What Does God Say About Pride?

Name ____________________

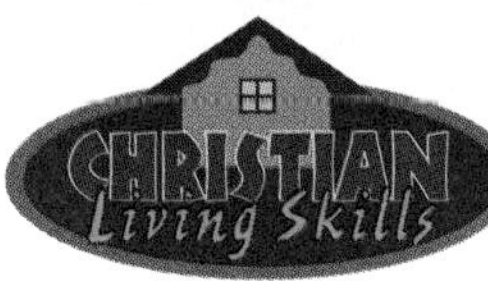

Christian
Living Skills

When God talks about your **heart** in His Word, He is usually not referring to the organ that pumps blood throughout your body. He is most often talking about the innermost center of your thoughts and emotions. Just as a healthy physical heart is necessary to have a healthy physical body, so a healthy spiritual heart is necessary to live a healthy Christian life. It is the condition of your **spiritual heart** that determines what you say and do.

Read Matthew 15:18-19 and fill in the blanks to describe what comes out of the heart of an unsaved person.

When you are saved, your sinful heart is transformed, and you are given the Holy Spirit to help you resist the temptations of sin. One of these temptations you must resist is the sin of pride. If you choose to allow pride to control your heart, every other area of your life will also be affected.

Using the code, discover biblical words that describe someone who is proud.

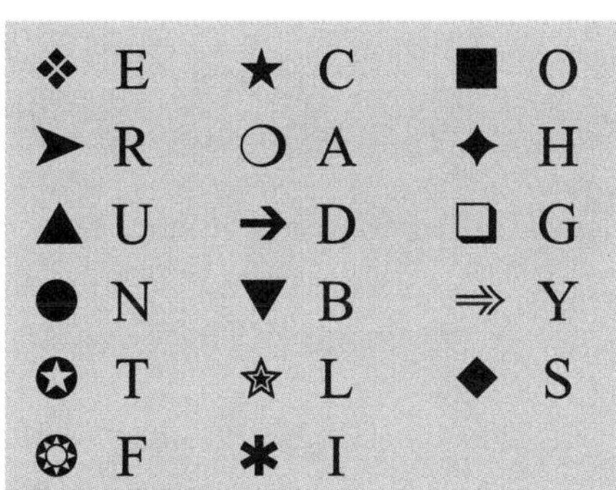

❖	E	★	C	■	O
➤	R	❍	A	✦	H
▲	U	➔	D	❑	G
●	N	▼	B	⇛	Y
✪	T	☆	L	◆	S
❂	F	✱	I		

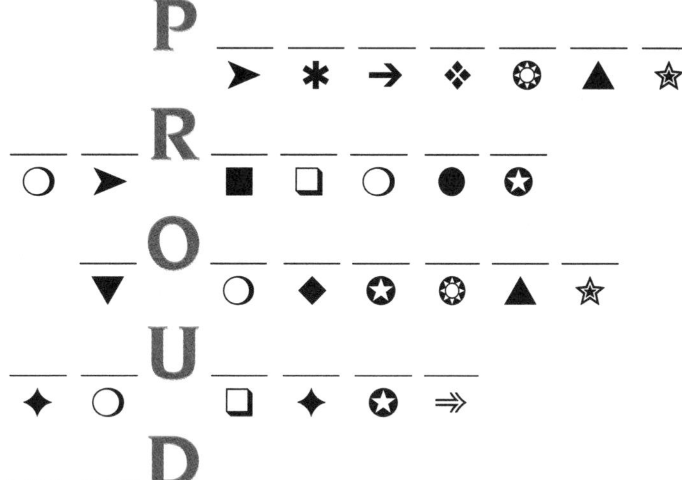

P ___ ___ ___ ___ ___ ___ ___
➤ ✱ ➔ ❖ ❂ ▲ ☆
___ ___ R ___ ___ ___ ___ ___
❍ ➤ ■ ❑ ❍ ● ✪
___ O ___ ___ ___ ___ ___ ___
▼ ❍ ◆ ✪ ❂ ▲ ☆
___ ___ U ___ ___ ___ ___
✦ ❍ ❑ ✦ ✪ ⇛
___ ___ ___ ___ ___ ___ ___ ___ D
★ ■ ● ★ ❖ ✱ ✪ ❖

God calls pride a sin and warns against allowing pride to control you.

Read the verses and match the references to the correct warnings.

1. ______ Pride leads to destruction in your life. A. Proverbs 13:10
2. ______ A proud heart will bring shame and disgrace to you. B. Proverbs 8:13
3. ______ Quarrels and contention are caused by pride. C. Proverbs 16:18
4. ______ God hates pride and arrogance. D. Proverbs 11:2

Read James 4:6 and I Peter 5:5 to complete the sentences.

God __________________ proud people. God __________________ humble people.

Something to Think About

Pride

Name ______________________________

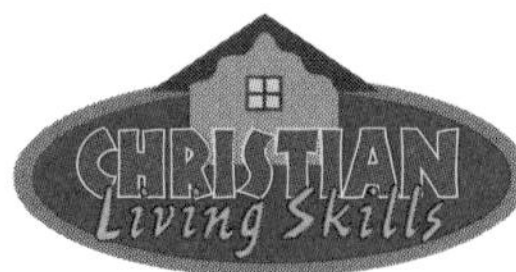
CHRISTIAN
Living Skills

Pride is shown in many ways. It can be seen on your face, heard in your speech, and observed in your actions. You deceive yourself when you think more highly of yourself than you should. God sees pride in your heart even when no one else can.

Read Micah 6:8 and complete the sentence.

The three things God requires of me are

______________________, ______________________, and ______________________.

Read the scenarios. Match the responses of pride to the correct scenario.

A. Your soccer team has been practicing for the big game. Your neighbor is on the other team. When you pass him on the street, you yell, "Your team stinks! You might as well give up!"	B. You and your friend study diligently for a science test. When the tests are returned, you receive an A. Your friend receives a B. You comment, "I'm just so smart. I can't help making good grades."
C. Roy got in trouble with the teacher again. He is always talking without permission. You think, *What is his problem? I never get in trouble.*	D. The pastor talked about having devotions. You didn't bother to pay attention because you already read your Bible regularly. You even helped your mom last night without being asked. You're sure that God is impressed by how good you've been lately.

Responses:

1. _____ Looking down on someone else in your private thoughts
2. _____ Being proud of your "spirituality"
3. _____ Cutting down someone else to make yourself look better
4. _____ Bragging about your God-given abilities

What About Me?

Take time at home to think about pride in your life. List several areas in which you believe God has blessed you (sports, academics, music, drama, appearance, etc.).

1. ______________________ 2. ______________________ 3. ______________________

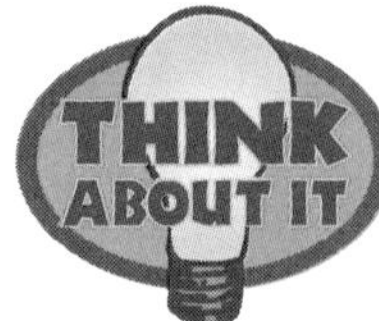
THINK
ABOUT IT

Look back to the Responses. Think about two areas in which you are tempted to be proud and what your response should be.

CAUTION!

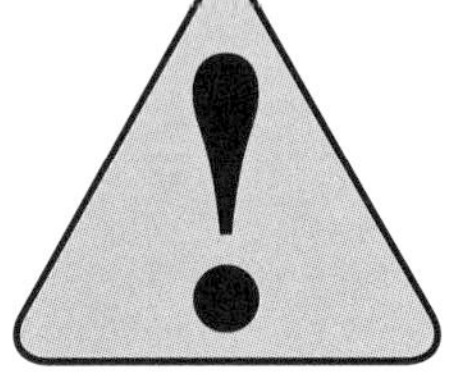

The areas in which you have confidence are prime targets for the attack of pride! Be on guard! If you recognize pride in your heart, confess this sin and ask God for help in fighting it!

Get the Bible Reading H.A.B.I.T.

Name ______________________

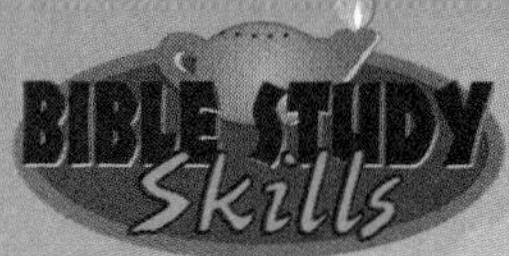

Have a special time set aside each day to read your Bible. If possible, make it the same time every day.

Ask God to teach you from His Word. Remember to thank Him for helping you to understand and apply it.

Be still and give your attention to what you are reading.

Investigate the Scripture by asking yourself questions about it.

Take time to look up words and ideas you do not understand.

As you read the Scripture for each day, write the date in the box.

Abraham was justified by his faith, not his works. **Romans 4:1-5**	It is a blessing to have God count believers righteous apart from their works. **Romans 4:6-12**	Abraham believed God's promises. **Romans 4:13-18**	Abraham's faith in God's promises never wavered, but grew stronger. **Romans 4:19-21**	Believers also are counted righteous if they have faith in Christ. **Romans 4:22-25**
Those who are justified by faith are Abraham's children. **Galatians 3:6-9**	Those who are justified by faith are God's children. **Galatians 3:26-29**	Melchizedek can be compared to Christ in many ways. **Hebrews 7:1-3**	Christ learned obedience by suffering, and Christians should obey Him. **Hebrews 5:5-10**	Abraham offered Isaac, believing God could raise him from the dead. **Hebrews 11:17-19**
Christians should diligently serve each other out of love. **Hebrews 6:10-12**	When God makes a promise, He cannot lie. **Hebrews 6:13-18**	The hope Christians have in Christ is a sure promise to anchor their souls. **Hebrews 6:19-20**	God chose Jacob over Esau because of His mercy. **Romans 9:10-16**	We should not be like Esau, who did not receive God's blessing. **Hebrews 12:14-17**
God is faithful to deliver Christians from temptation. **I Corinthians 10:12-13**	Christians glorify God when they suffer patiently for doing right. **I Peter 2:18-20**	Christ is our example of patient suffering. **I Peter 2:21-25**	Joseph prospered in Egypt because God was with him. **Acts 7:9-10**	Christians must not be bitter, but kind and forgiving to others. **Ephesians 4:30-32**

Bible Study Methods

Synthetic

Name ____________________

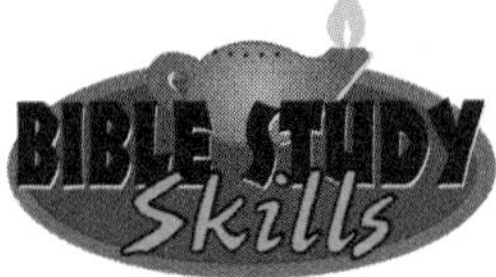

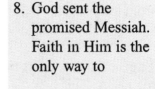

BIBLE STUDY
Skills

The synthetic or survey method of Bible study provides a "bird's eye view" of Scripture much like an aerial view. Specific books or passages are considered in the light of the overall teaching of the Bible. For example, the Bible as a whole teaches that God has always sought to bring man into right fellowship with Himself. This type of Bible study points to the consistency and timelessness of God's Word. Some useful tools for synthetic study are cross-references, commentaries, and parallel passage Bibles.

Complete each sentence with the words from the word bank.

come	nation	Savior	judges	rule	slavery	king	salvation

1. The sin of the first people pointed to the need of a ______________.

2. God chose Abraham to establish a ______________ that would demonstrate His love and power.

3. God led His people out of ______________ and established them in a land flowing with milk and honey.

4. God blessed His people and gave them ______________ to lead them in His ways.

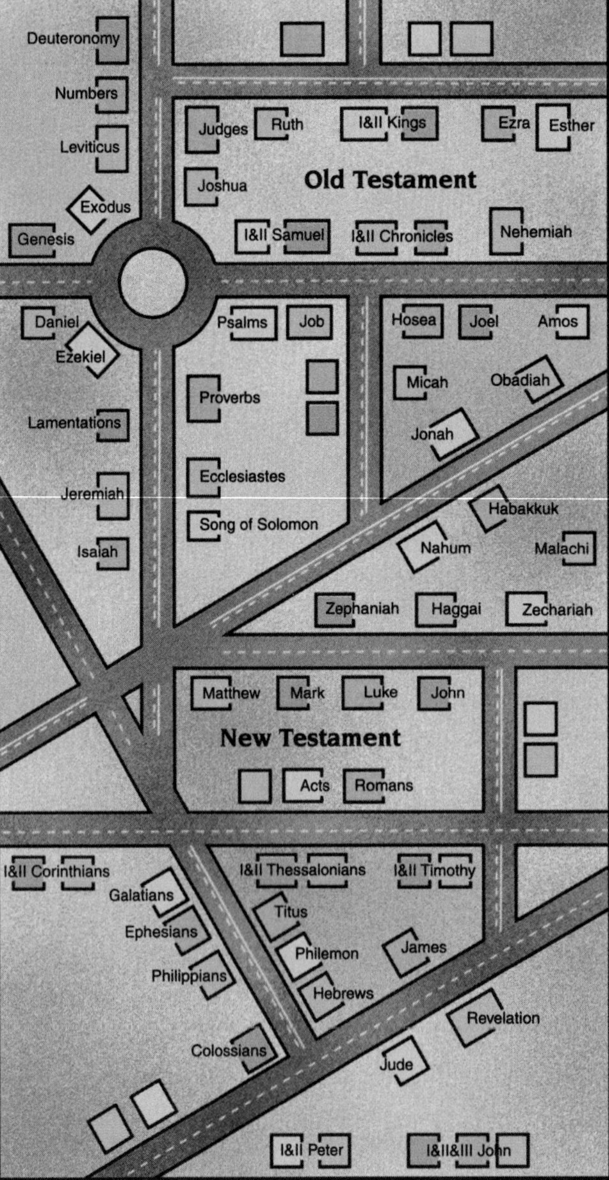

Old Testament
Genesis
Exodus
Leviticus
Numbers
Deuteronomy
Joshua
Judges
Ruth
I&II Samuel
I&II Kings
I&II Chronicles
Ezra
Nehemiah
Esther
Job
Psalms
Proverbs
Ecclesiastes
Song of Solomon
Isaiah
Jeremiah
Lamentations
Ezekiel
Daniel
Hosea
Joel
Amos
Obadiah
Jonah
Micah
Nahum
Habakkuk
Zephaniah
Haggai
Zechariah
Malachi
New Testament
Matthew
Mark
Luke
John
Acts
Romans
I&II Corinthians
Galatians
Ephesians
Philippians
Colossians
I&II Thessalonians
I&II Timothy
Titus
Philemon
Hebrews
James
I&II Peter
I&II&III John
Jude
Revelation

5. God established a ______________ from whose line would come the Savior.

6. God allowed His people to suffer captivity under foreign ______________ that they might see their need of Him.

7. The Old Testament ended with the promise that a Savior would ______________.

8. God sent the promised Messiah. Faith in Him is the only way to ______________.

Broken Communication

Genesis 12

Name ______________________

A strong relationship takes communication. God and Abram had to communicate to stay in proper fellowship with each other.

Make an *X* in the box of each event that occurred at each place. You may use your Bible for help.

Locations	God spoke to Abram.	Abram built an altar to God.	Abram called on God.
Haran (Gen. 12:4)			
Shechem (Gen. 12:6-7)			
Bethel (Gen. 12:8)			
Egypt (Gen. 12:10-13)			

Refer to the chart as you answer the questions.

1. How did God communicate with Abram?

   ____

2. What did Abram build as part of his communication with God?

   ____

3. Does it seem that Abram communicated with God as he traveled into Egypt?

   ____

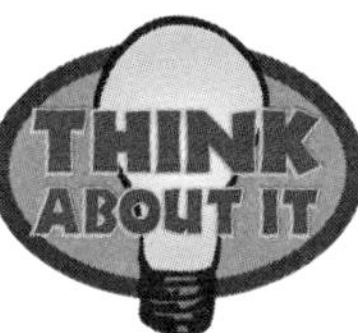
THINK
ABOUT IT

Abram deceived Pharaoh about Sarai's being his wife. The Scriptures do not record Abram communicating with God until after he left Egypt.

Do you desire to read your Bible and pray when you are in sin?

____

How is broken communication with God restored?

____

____

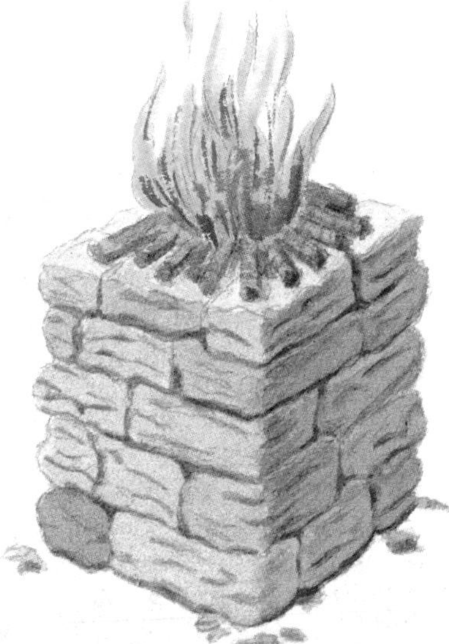

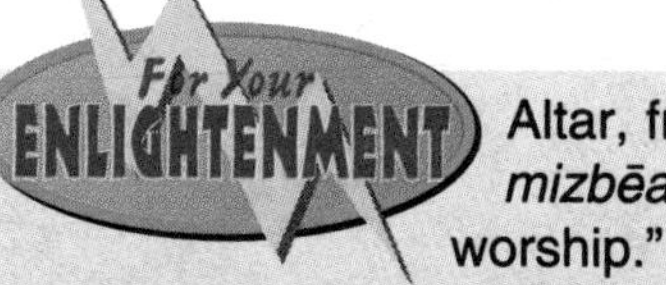
For Your
ENLIGHTENMENT

Altar, from the Hebrew *mizbēah,* means "place of worship." There are several reasons altars were used in worship to God. Noah built an altar to thank and praise God for bringing his family safely through the Flood. God established the use of altars in the tabernacle and temple for atonement from sin. Isaac built an altar to show his trust in the promise that God had given to Abraham. Elijah used an altar to demonstrate God's power to the prophets of Baal. Altar sacrifices were eliminated when Christ's death and resurrection provided the final sacrifice for the sin of all men.

Famine, Lies, and Plagues

Genesis 12

Name ______________________

Number the events in order. The first one is done for you.

_____ Abram took his family into Egypt because there was a famine in the land.

_____ God smote Pharaoh and his family with plagues because of Abram's lie.

__1__ Abram was in Haran when God told him to move his family. God led Abram to Canaan.

_____ Pharaoh commanded Abram to leave Egypt.

_____ Abram told Sarai to say that she was his sister rather than his wife.

_____ Pharaoh confronted Abram with his lie.

_____ Pharaoh took Sarai into his household.

Write the letter of the reference that matches each statement.

_____ Others should be able to learn truth about God by watching the lives of believers.

_____ Something gotten by lying does not bring much joy.

_____ A liar can become snared or trapped in his lies.

_____ Christ is the example of grace and truth to Christians.

A. John 1:14

B. I Peter 2:12

C. Proverbs 12:13-17

D. Proverbs 20:17

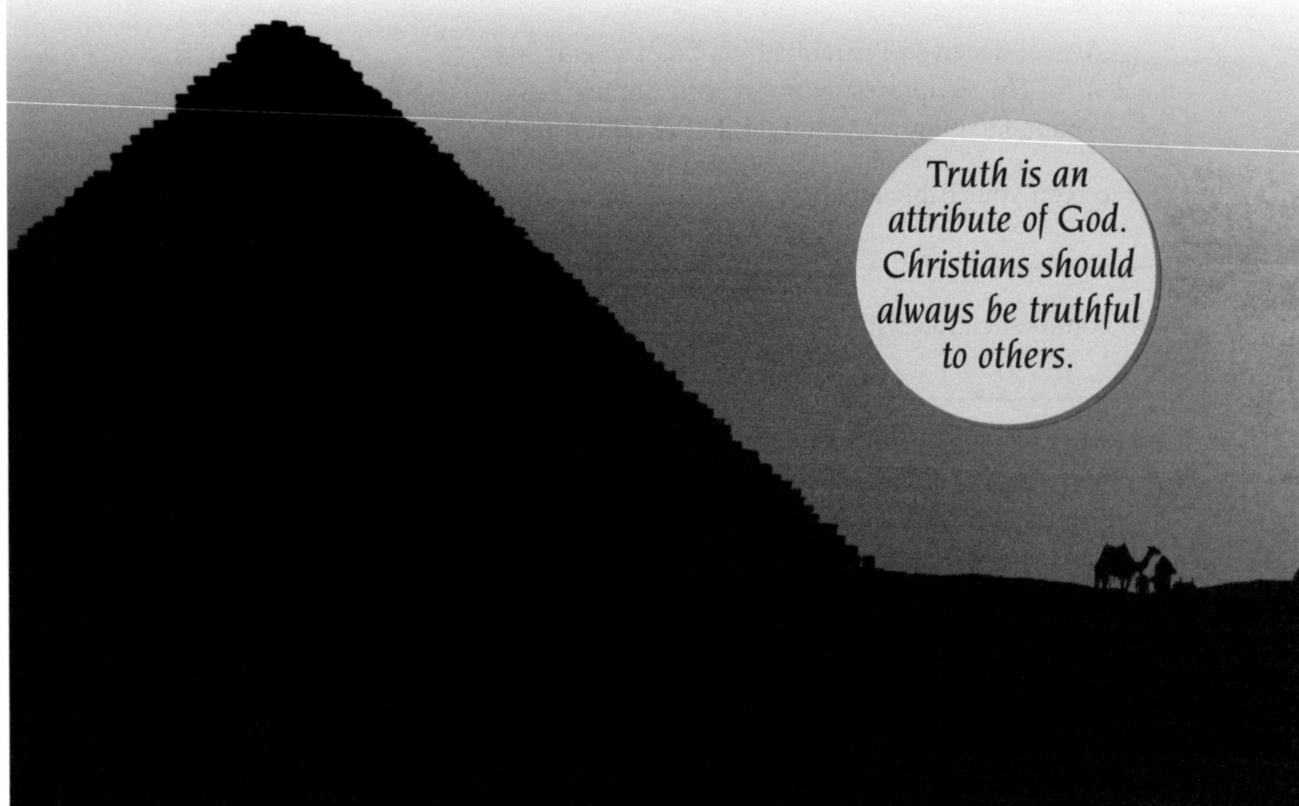
Truth is an attribute of God. Christians should always be truthful to others.

Following God

Name ______________________

Complete each sentence about Abram's following God's leading. You may use your Bible for help.

1. Abram left his father's home in ______________ (Gen. 12:4).
2. Abram, Sarai, and Lot traveled to the land of ______________ (Gen. 12:5).
3. At ______________________, God promised the land to Abram and his descendants (Gen. 12:6-7).
4. Abram then went to a mountain between ______________ and ______________ (Gen. 12:8).
5. As he continued traveling south, Abram finally came to the land of ______________ (Gen. 12:10).
6. Abram, Sarai, and Lot returned to the place between ______________ and ______________ (Gen. 13:3).
7. Lot chose land in the plain of the Jordan River near ______________ and Gomorrah (Gen. 13:11-12).
8. Abram moved his tents to the plain of Mamre in ______________ (Gen. 13:18).

Draw a red line for Abram's route of travel

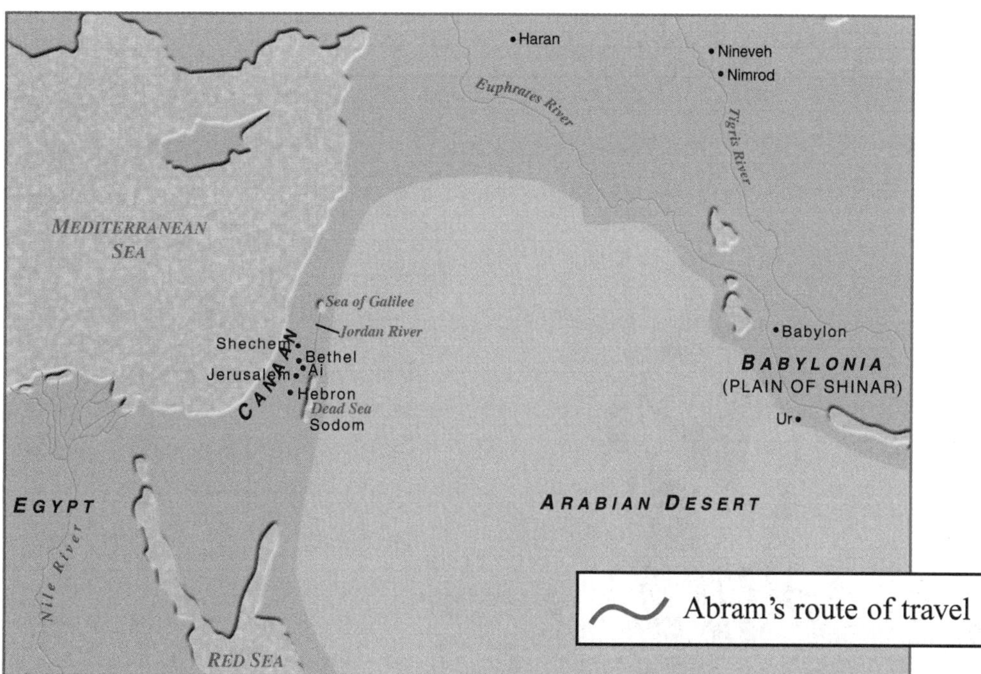

Haran
Nineveh
Nimrod
Euphrates River
Tigris River
MEDITERRANEAN SEA
Sea of Galilee
Jordan River
Shechem
Bethel
Ai
Jerusalem
CANAAN
Hebron
Dead Sea
Sodom
Babylon
BABYLONIA (PLAIN OF SHINAR)
Ur
EGYPT
Nile River
ARABIAN DESERT
RED SEA
Abram's route of travel

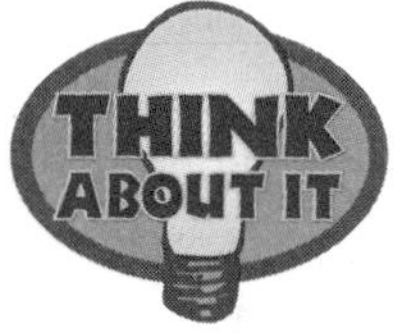

THINK ABOUT IT

There was not enough land for Abram and Lot to share to feed their flocks and herds. To avoid further strife between their herdsmen, Abram suggested that they each choose a part of the land.

Conflicts can not always be avoided. What can you learn from the example of Abram to help you avoid a continuing conflict with a friend or family member?

____

A Divine Covenant

Genesis 13:14-18

Name ______________________

Each chain link is made of two or three words that share letters. The last letter of one word will be the first letter of the next word in that link. Use the words to complete the sentences about the two parts of the covenant God made with Abram.

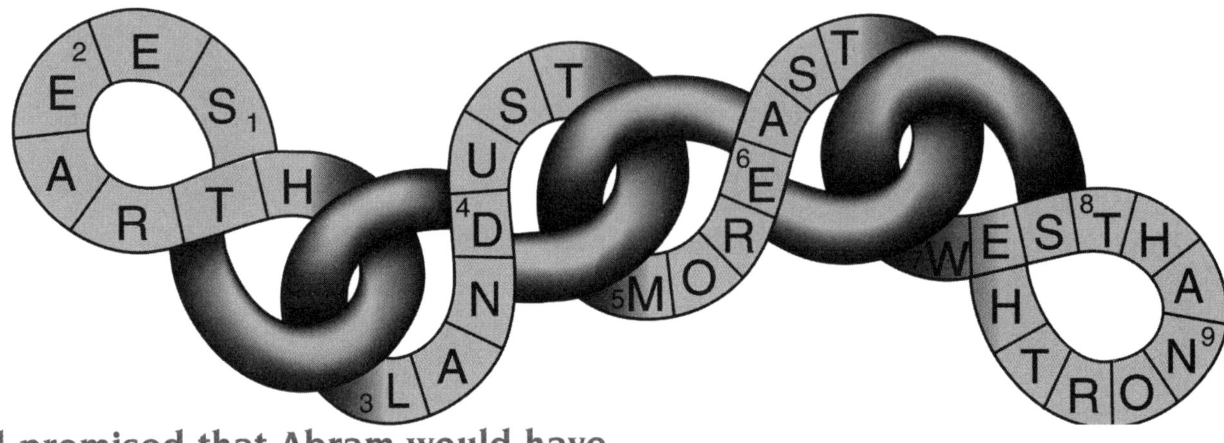

God promised that Abram would have . . .

all the (3) ___ ___ ___ ___ he could (1) ___ ___ ___ to the (9) ___ ___ ___ ___ ___,

south, (6) ___ ___ ___ ___, and (7) ___ ___ ___ ___.

(5) ___ ___ ___ ___ descendants (8) ___ ___ ___ ___ the (4) ___ ___ ___ ___ of

the (2) ___ ___ ___ ___ ___.

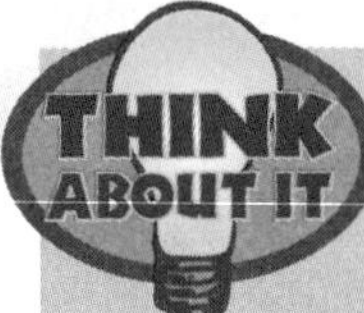
THINK
ABOUT IT

In Genesis 12, God told Abram to follow Him, and He would make him a great nation.

In Genesis 13, after Abram followed God's leading, God gave Abram land and promised that he would have more descendants than could be numbered.

God gave Abram only the information that he needed at the time. As Abram was obedient, God guided him further and gave him more details.

Today as Christians remain obedient to God's Word, He reveals His will to them. Are you obedient to the tasks God has for you today?

What Does God Say About How to Be Happy?

Name ______________________________

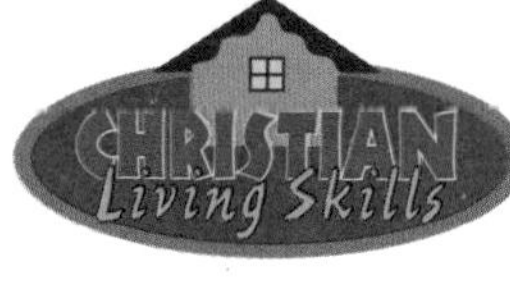
CHRISTIAN
Living Skills

Everyone wants happiness. People seek happiness in a variety of ways. Some people look for happiness in money, sports, or friendships. What about you?

List several things that bring YOU happiness.

______________________ ______________________ ______________________

Are you satisfied that God has given you everything you need? Are you thankful for what He has given you? If you aren't, you may be falling for the false belief that getting more things will make you happy. This is called **materialism.** When you choose to have this attitude, you start focusing on trying to get more and more things to please yourself. However, it is always impossible to find happiness when you try to please yourself and not God. Most likely, you will become discouraged and depressed. God's Word warns you against believing that more things will make you happy.

Read the verses. Match the warning and key to happiness with the correct reference.

WARNINGS		Verses		KEYS TO HAPPINESS
A. Do not love money.	_____	Luke 12:15	_____	E. Live a godly and righteous life.
B. Say no to sin and ungodly choices.	_____	I Timothy 6:10-11	_____	F. Be content with the food and clothing God provides.
C. Guard against becoming coveteous or greedy.	_____	I Timothy 6:8-9	_____	G. Seek to develop faith, love, and righteousness in your life.
D. Do not desire to be rich.	_____	Titus 2:11-12	_____	H. Realize that a person's value does not come from what he owns.

Read Matthew 6:25, 28-33. Using these verses, complete the sentences to give advice to a friend who thinks that to be happy he must have the latest style of clothes.

Your life is more important than ______________________________

Don't worry about ______________________________

God takes care of ______________________________

You are worth more than ______________________________

Seek first ______________________________

Name ______________________

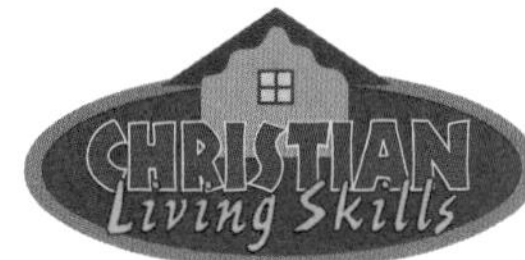
CHRISTIAN
Living Skills

In their quest to be happy, many people make the wrong choices. Every time you make a decision, you have only two choices. It is simple. Either you can please God, or you can please yourself.

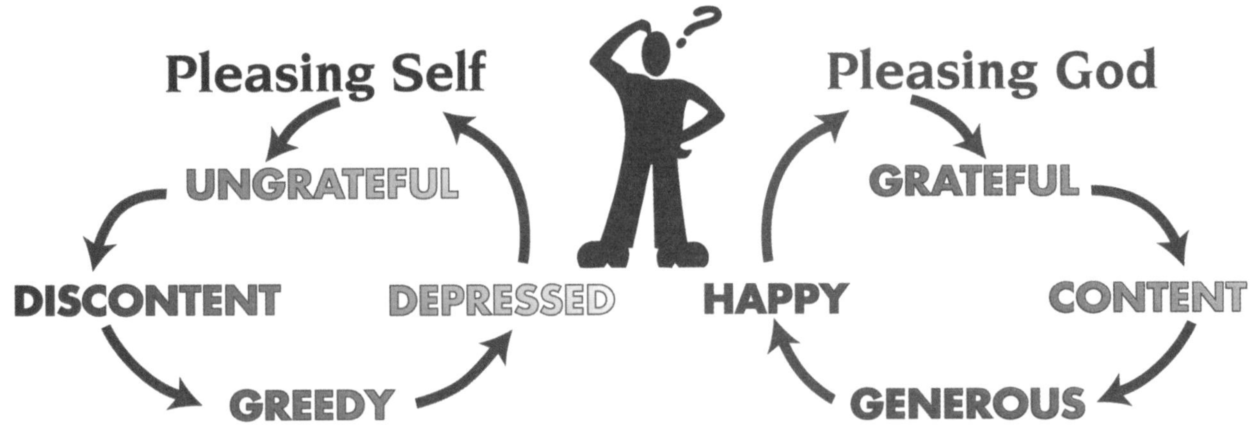
Pleasing Self
UNGRATEFUL
DISCONTENT
DEPRESSED
GREEDY
Pleasing God
GRATEFUL
HAPPY
CONTENT
GENEROUS

Study the cycles and think about the cause and effect of each attitude. Use the cycles to complete the chart.

Situation	Attitude in the cycle	CAUSE of attitude	EFFECT of attitude	Choice pleases self?	Choice pleases God?
Tim is not thankful for the allowance he receives.	Ungrateful	Pleasing self			
Alena shares her candy with her younger brother and sister.		Content	Happy		
Megan wants to impress her friends by having many pairs of shoes.	Greedy		Depressed		
J.R. is thankful for his new soccer ball given to him although it wasn't the one he had wanted.	Grateful				

What About Me?

Take time at home to think about your attitude toward material things. Carefully consider the following questions.

Am I grateful for what God has provided for me?
Am I fully satisfied and content with what I have?
Am I generous to those around me?
Do I believe that my worth does not come from what I own?
Do I encourage my friends to be content with what they have?
Do I express my gratitude to my parents for what they do for me?

Promises Kept

Name ______________________

God's covenant with Abraham was also with his descendants. By faith Abraham followed God's leading to the land of promise. Throughout the Bible, the people of God remembered Abraham's obedience and God's promise to him.

Write the letter of the reference that correctly matches the statement about God and His covenant with Abraham.

A. Exodus 33:1

B. Numbers 32:11-13

C. Deuteronomy 1:1-8

D. I Chronicles 16:1-2, 7-18

E. II Chronicles 20:1-9

F. Acts 6:9, 7:1-5

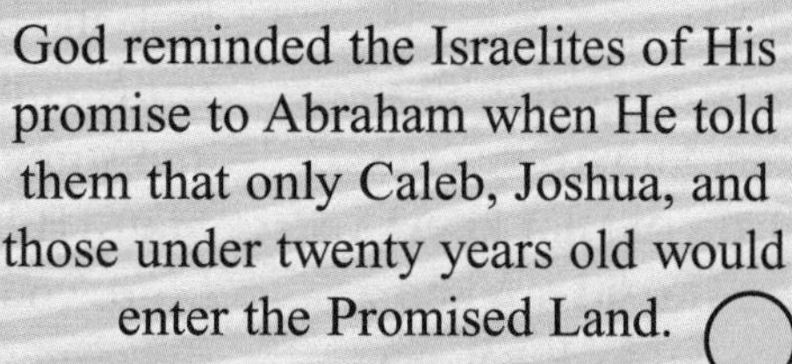

God reminded the Israelites of His promise to Abraham when He told them that only Caleb, Joshua, and those under twenty years old would enter the Promised Land. ◯

When the ark of the covenant was brought into Jerusalem, David reminded the Israelites how God had kept His promise to Abraham. ◯

Jehoshaphat claimed God's promise to Abraham as he prayed for God's deliverance against the enemy. ◯

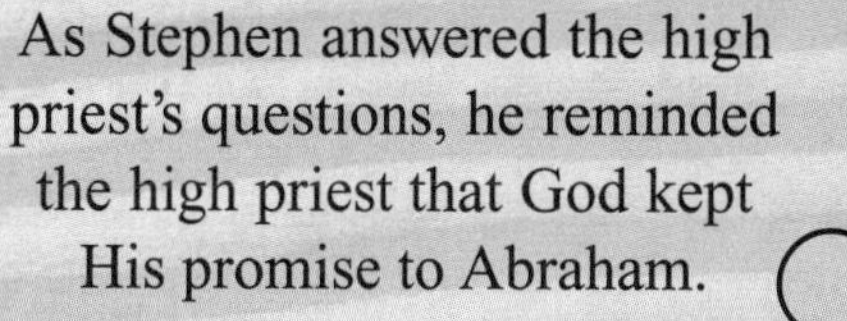

As Stephen answered the high priest's questions, he reminded the high priest that God kept His promise to Abraham. ◯

Moses reminded the Israelites of God's promise as they prepared to cross the Jordan River and enter the land promised to Abraham. ◯

◯ God reminded Moses of His promise to Abraham.

In Hebrews 6:9-18, the believers are reminded of God's faithfulness to Abraham. God does not lie. God is faithful to give Christians hope of eternal salvation. Later, in Hebrews 11, the example of Abraham's faith in following God's leading is used to illustrate the meaning of faith.

Have you accepted God's promise of salvation?

Name two other promises of God in which Christians can trust.

____

____

Destination Unknown

Hebrews 11:8

Name ______________________

Bible Study Skills

Have you ever helped plan a vacation or trip? There are many preparations to make. Before the trip begins, decisions are made about destinations, transportation, lodging, and time schedules. In today's society, people like to know the details as soon as possible.

Imagine how it was for Abraham. God told Abraham to take his family and go to the promised inheritance. Abraham did not know where God was sending him. He did not know how long the trip would take. All he knew was that God wanted him to go. Through faith, Abraham willingly obeyed God's command to follow Him.

Abraham *knew* to obey God. We can *know* for certain everything the Bible tells us about God and the Christian life. A concordance is a useful help in finding verses with the word *know.* A **concordance** is an alphabetical list of key words and some references where they may be found. Many Bibles have a small concordance included. More complete concordances are available in separate volumes or computer programs.

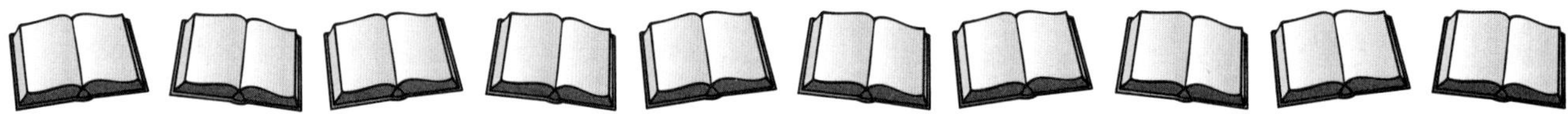

Each **entry word** is followed by a list of references where the word may be found. A portion of the verse is included to show the word in context. In these portions, the entry word is abbreviated with its first letter.

The title of a Bible book is usually written once, followed by all the references in that book.

The references under each entry word are listed in the same order in which they are found in the Bible.

KNEW, Gen.28:16, the Lord is in this place, and I *k* it not
Jer.1:5, before I formed thee I *k* thee
Mt.7:23, I never *k* you, depart
Jn.4:10, if thou *k* the gift of God
2 Cor.5:21, who *k* no sin
KNOW, 1 Sam.3:7, Samuel did not yet *k* the Lord
1 Chr.28:9, *k* thou the God of thy father
Job 5:27, *k* thou it for thy good
8:9, we are but of yesterday, and *k* nothing
13:23, make me to *k* my transgression
19:25, I *k* that my redeemer liveth
Job 22:13; Ps.73:11, how doth God *k*
Ps.39:4, make me to *k* mine end
46:10, be still, and *k* that I am God
56:9, this I *k*, for God is for me
103:14, he *k* our frame
139:23, *k* my heart
Eccl.9:5, the living *k* they shall die
11:9, *k* that for all these things
Isa.1:3, the ox *k* his owner
Jer.17:9, the heart is deceitful, who can *k* it
31:34; Heb.8:11, *k* the Lord, for all shall *k* me
Ezek.2:5; 33:33, *k* there hath been a prophet
Hos.2:20, thou shalt *k* the Lord
7:9, yet he *k* it not
Mt.6:3, let not thy left hand *k*
13:11; Mk.4:11; Lk.8:10, given to you to *k*
25:12, I *k* you not
Mk.1:24; Lk.4:34, I *k* thee, who thou art
Lk.19:42, if thou hadst *k*
22:57,60, I *k* him not
Jn.7:17, he shall *k* of the doctrine
10:14, I *k* my sheep, and am *k* of mine
13:7, *k* not now, but shalt *k* hereafter
17, if ye *k* these things
35, by this shall all men *k* ye are my disciples
Acts 1:7, it is not for you to *k*
Rom.8:28, we *k* that all things work
1 Cor.2:14, neither can he *k* them
13:9,12, we *k* in part
Eph.3:19, and to *k* the love of Christ
2 Tim.1:12, I *k* whom I have believed
3:15, thou hast *k* the scriptures
1 Jn.2:4, he that saith, I *k* him
3:2, we *k* that when he shall appear
Rev.2:2,9,13,19; 3:1,8, I *k* thy works
KNOWLEDGE, 2 Chr.1:10,11,12, give me *k*
Job 21:14, we desire not *k* of thy ways
Ps.94:10, he that teacheth man *k*
139:6, such *k* is too wonderful
144:3, that thou takest *k* of him
Prov.10:14, wise men lay up *k*
14:6, *k* is easy to him that understandeth
17:27, he that hath *k* spareth words
24:5, a man of *k* increaseth strength
30:3, nor have the *k* of the holy
Eccl.1:18, increaseth *k* increaseth sorrow
9:10, nor *k* nor wisdom in sheol
Isa.11:2, the spirit of *k*
40:14, who taught him *k*
53:11, by his *k* justify many
Dan.1:17, God gave them *k*
12:4, *k* shall be increased
Hos.4:6, destroyed for lack of *k*

Answer the questions.

1. Find the entry for *know.* Which verse from Psalms tells you that you can know who God is?

   ____

2. Which Old Testament verse tells you that Christ, the Redeemer, lives?

   ____

3. What New Testament verse lets you know some of the details about when Christ will come again and appear to Christians?

   ____

4. List two other passages you will look at on your own.

   ____

   ____

To the Rescue

Genesis 14:5-24

Name ____________________

In the following report, there are a number of errors to be corrected.

- **Put a ~ on each word that does not belong.**
- **Insert the missing words in the blanks: *goods, gift, battle, Chedorlaomer***
- **Write the correct word above the underlined words: *king, Abram, Melchizedek, rich, 318***

The kings near Abram and Lot and Jacob joined in battle against the kings of Sodom and Gomorrah. They plundered and took the residents captive—including Lot and his family. God gave Abram's <u>3,380</u> men victory over ____________ and the other kings. Abram returned with the captives and their belongings. The king of Sodom and Melchizedek, a priest of God, brought food and drink and money for <u>Lot</u> and his men. Melchizedek blessed Abram for serving God and recognized that God had delivered the enemy into the hand of Abram. In thankfulness to God, Abram gave <u>the king of Sodom</u> a tithe of all the goods from the ____________. The king of Sodom wanted to honor Abram; he did not recognize that God had made Abram victorious. The <u>queen</u> of Sodom wanted Abram to keep the ____________ for himself. All that Abram would take was what the soldiers had eaten and what was rightfully theirs. Abram believed that if he were to take a ____________, the king of Sodom might someday say that he had made Abram <u>poor</u>.

Write the letter of the correct king to complete each statement.

_______ recognized God's leading in the victory.

_______ wanted to reward Abram with the goods from battle.

_______ received Abram's tithe offering to God.

_______ blessed Abram as a servant of God.

_______ did not see God's working through Abram.

A. Melchizedek
B. King of Sodom

The Right Choice

Name ______________________

Abram glorified God in the way he battled the enemy. The Book of Deuteronomy was not written by Moses until hundreds of years after Abram went to battle. But Abram followed the principles of war laid out by God in Deuteronomy 20.

Mark an *X* next to the principles that Abram followed in war.

_____ 1. Do not be afraid of the size of the enemy (Deut. 20:1-3).

_____ 2. Trust that God will fight for you (Deut. 20:4).

_____ 3. If the enemy wants peace, they should surrender and become your servants (Deut. 20:10-11).

_____ 4. All the males of a defeated city should be killed (Deut. 20:12-13).

_____ 5. Your army may take the spoils of the defeated city (Deut. 20:14-15).

Answer the questions.

6. What did Abram do in response to the news about Lot's capture? (Gen. 14:14)

____

7. How many men did Abram take to battle the enemy kings? (Gen. 14:14) ____________

8. Who else was victorious when he took only 300 men into battle? (Judg. 7:7) ____________

Abram loved God and this love showed in his relationship with Lot. Abram's generosity and kindness toward Lot benefited many. Abram could have used events in Lot's life as reasons not to come to his rescue.

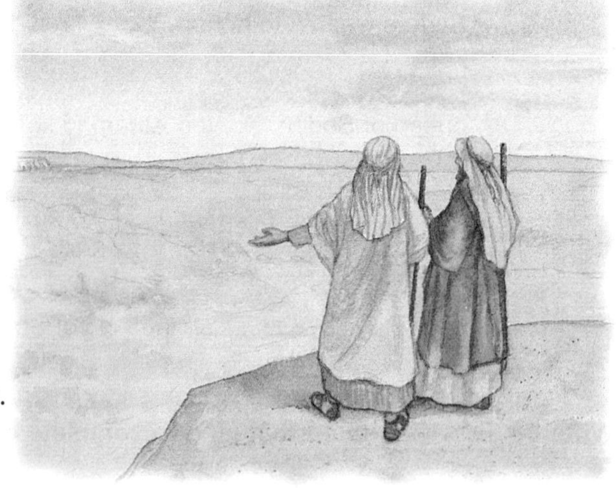

Color the circle next to two faults Abram could have used against Lot.

- ○ Lot was Abram's nephew.
- ○ Lot took the best land for his herds.
- ○ Lot chose to move into the wicked city of Sodom.
- ○ Lot traveled with Abram to the land of Canaan.

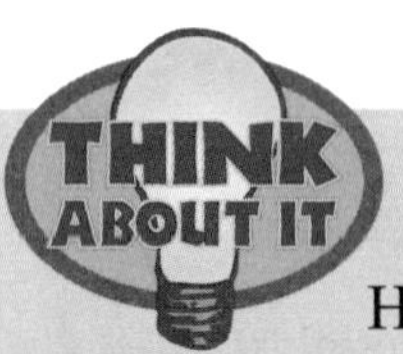
THINK
ABOUT IT

Do you let previous events influence your willingness to help a friend? Do you let them influence your willingness to witness to neighbors? How should you act toward others who have mistreated you?

____

____

Stranger in the Land

Name ______________________

Read Hebrews 11:9-10. Answer the questions.

1. What are some problems that Abraham faced after leaving his home in Haran?

____

2. What word describes Abraham once he arrived at the place he received as an inheritance?

____

3. Abraham was living in the land of promise, but he did not act like a permanent resident. He was looking forward to living somewhere else. How is this place described in verse 10?

____

4. What is the name of the city referred to in verse 10 that Abraham was looking forward to living in? (If you need help, read Heb. 11:16, 12:22, and Rev. 3:12.)

____

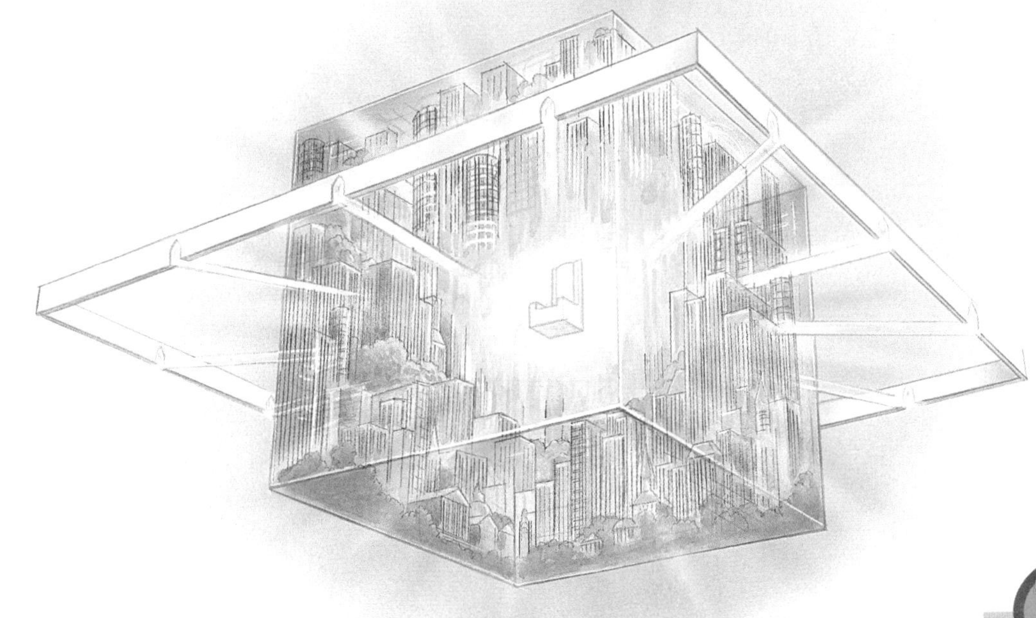

THINK ABOUT IT

What problems or difficulties are you experiencing in your life at this time? Remember, no matter how difficult it seems now, this problem is temporary.

5. What is another name for this place? ______________________

6. Are Christians today permanent residents on earth? ______________________

7. What types of problems do Christians today face while living on earth?

____

____

Name ______________________________

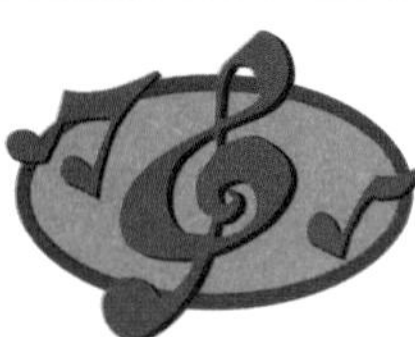

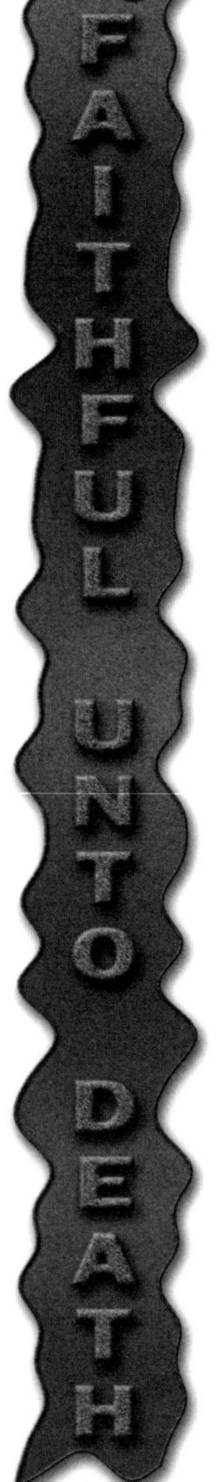

FAITHFUL UNTO DEATH

Polycarp

He was burned at the stake for refusing to give up his faith in Christ. "Fourscore and six years have I continued serving him," he said, "and he hath never wronged me at all; how then can I blaspheme my King and my Savior?"

Stephen

He was stoned to death because of his faith in Christ. As he died, he called upon Jesus to receive his spirit. Then he prayed for his persecutors: "Lord, lay not this sin to their charge."

Perpetua

She was imprisoned because of her faith in Christ. Later she was gored by a wild steer in a Roman arena and eventually beheaded. Before her death, she wrote from prison: "Can one call anything by any other name than what it is? So neither can I call myself anything else than what I am, a Christian."

Read verses 1-2 of the hymn on page 312.

1. What do you think Christians should do when they are persecuted because of their faith in Christ?

____

____

2. What can you do when someone makes fun of you for being a Christian?

____

____

Most Christians are not called upon by God to die as these martyrs did, but they are commanded to be true to Christ in spite of what others say and do to them.

Write a prayer asking the Lord's help to be true to Christ—even if you suffer for your faith.

____

____

____

____

____

____

Renewed Covenant

Genesis 17

Name ______________________

Answer the questions. You may use your Bible for help.

Abram was faithful to follow God's Word. God was faithful to keep His Word and fulfill His covenant with Abram. When God renewed and explained His covenant to Abram, He changed Abram's name.

1. What did Abram's new name, Abraham, mean? (Gen. 17:5)

   ____

2. How did this new name describe Abraham better? ______________

   ____

   ____

   ____

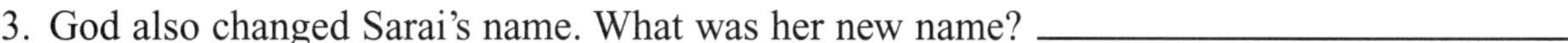

3. God also changed Sarai's name. What was her new name? ____________________

4. God promised that Abraham and Sarah would have a son together. What were Abraham and Sarah to name their son? (Gen. 17:19) ____________________

5. Abraham had tried to help God fulfill His promise by having a child with Sarai's servant, Hagar. The son born to Hagar was named Ishmael. With which son did God promise to establish His covenant? (Gen. 17:20-21) ____________________

Vol. 12

CANAAN TIMES

There is a reason everything has a name.

In Bible times, the names of people and places were important. Many places were named for a special event that happened at that spot. Names of some people had prophetic meanings, such as those of Abraham and Sarah.

In John 13:35, Christ called those who followed Him ____________________. After the death and resurrection of Christ, Acts 11:25-26 records another name, ____________________, given to identify those who believed in Christ and followed His teachings.

A Willing Sacrifice

Genesis 22:1-18

Name ______________________________

Abraham and Sarah desired a child for many years. God seemed to have closed that door until they were far past the years people can have children. Late in their lives God miraculously gave Abraham and Sarah a son as part of the fulfillment of the promised covenant.

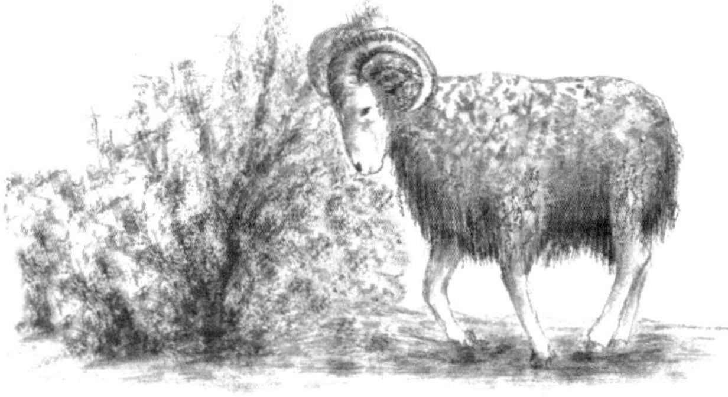

Years later, God called Abraham and instructed him to offer Isaac as a sacrifice. Obediently Abraham followed God's command.

Answer the questions in your own words.

1. How did Abraham respond to God's command? ______________________
2. What did Isaac ask that makes you think he had probably helped his father offer sacrifices before? ______________________
3. What was Abraham's response? ______________________
4. What was Isaac's attitude about carrying the wood? ______________________
5. How did Isaac demonstrate that he also trusted God? ______________________

God had given Abraham several promises since he left Haran.

6. What is one promise that God kept? ______________________
7. God promised that Abraham would have descendants as numerous as the sand and the stars. God said this promise would be fulfilled through Isaac. With this in mind, why do you think Abraham was willing to offer Isaac?

   Explain your answer. ______________________

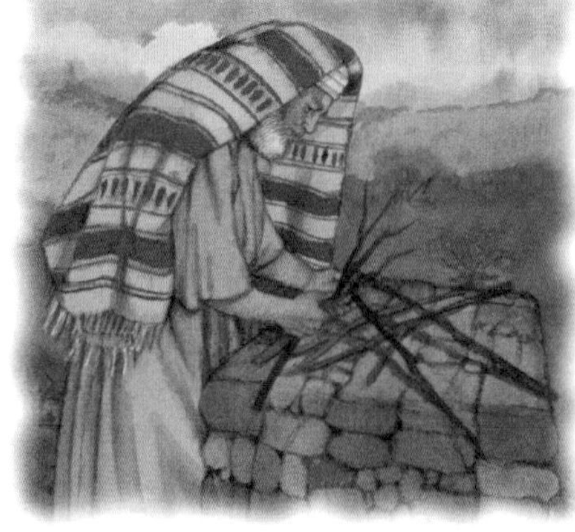

THINK ABOUT IT God does not ask more of a person than He is able to bear. Do you have a problem that seems too great to handle? At such a time, read I Corinthians 10:13 and claim God's promise of help.

What Does God Say About My Parents?

Honor and Obey

Name ______________________

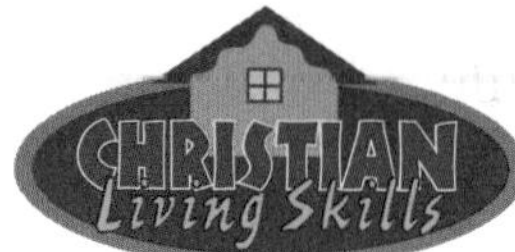
CHRISTIAN
Living Skills

Your parents' responsibilities include providing food for you to eat, a place to live, clothes to wear, protection from harm, and medicine when you are sick. A very important responsibility your parents have is to prepare you to live a life that is pleasing to God. Have you ever thought about the commands that God gives to your parents?

Read the verses. In your own words, write the commands God gives to your parents.

Proverbs 22:6 ______________________

Proverbs 19:18 ______________________

You have probably been told at one time or another that you should honor and obey your parents. **Obedience** is simply doing what you're told.

Read Exodus 20:12, Colossians 3:20, or Ephesians 6:1-3.
In your own words, write the commands God gives to you.

____

Obedience to your parents isn't the only command given to you. God also commands you to show your parents honor. If you want to have God's blessing on your life, it is important that you follow both commands.

Using the glossary, define the verb form of *honor.* ______________________

Solve the puzzle to discover six ways you can honor your parents. Every time three letters are together as they are in the alphabet, cross them out. Write the remaining words on the lines.

abcobeymyauthoritiesdeftakeresponsibilityformyworkghishow
gratefulnesstomyparentsjklchoosegoodfriendsmnomakewise
decisionspqrnevertalkbadlyaboutmyparentsortomyparentsstu

1. ______________________
2. ______________________
3. ______________________
4. ______________________
5. ______________________
6. ______________________

____

Something to Think About

Honoring and Obeying My Parents

Name ______________________________

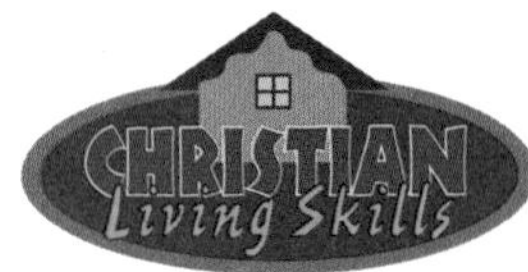
CHRISTIAN
Living Skills

Obedience to God's Word will bring God's blessing on your life. Disobedience will bring God's judgment. God makes special promises to children who obey their parents. He also speaks strong words about those who don't.

Match the verses to the correct summary. Underline the three blessings of obedience.

_______ 1. You will be called a fool.

_______ 2. Your lamp will be put out.

_______ 3. You will live a successful life.

_______ 4. You will be unstable like the wind.

_______ 5. You will bring joy to your parents.

_______ 6. You will please God.

_______ 7. You will be friends with people who are known for destroying others.

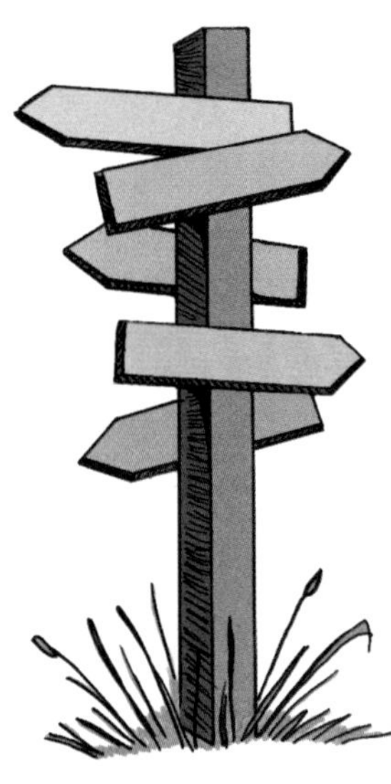

A. Proverbs 20:20

B. Proverbs 28:24

C. Ephesians 6:1-3

D. Proverbs 23:24

E. Colossians 3:20

F. Proverbs 11:29

G. Proverbs 15:5

Read each scenario and write a response that pleases God.

Scenario	A Response That Pleases God Is...
Kai tells the guys that his parents are mean because they won't let him see the new action movie. Some of the other guys start complaining about their parents. Your parents won't let you see the movie either.	
You have several friends over to work on homework. One of them wants to copy the answers instead of doing the work herself. After they leave, your mom talks to you about the kind of friends you have and suggests that you be careful.	
You receive an allowance for doing chores at home. You're pleased with the amount and are saving up for a new bike. Then you find out that your friend gets an allowance without doing any chores and that he has just gotten a new bike.	

What About Me?

Take time at home to think about your attitude toward obeying your parents.

Do you look for ways to bring them honor?

What two things can you do that would bring joy to your parents?

______________________________ ______________________________

For the Camels Also

Genesis 24

Name ______________________________

God's covenant with Abraham included that he would have a multitude of descendants. The time came for Isaac to get married. To remain separate from the ungodly people and false religions around Canaan and according to tradition, Isaac's wife was to come from the family of a relative.

Complete each sentence.

1. Abraham instructed his eldest ________________ to return to the family's homeland to find a wife for Isaac.
2. The servant ________________ for God to lead him to the right person.
3. The servant asked God to have the right woman offer a ________________ to him and his camels.
4. When the servant ________________ the woman about her family, he found out that she was a relative of Abraham.
5. The servant prayed and ________________ the name of the Lord for leading him to this woman.
6. Taking ________________ as his wife was a comfort to Isaac after the death of his mother.

List some of the godly characteristics of the servant and Rebekah.

Abraham's Servant

1. ______________________________
2. ______________________________
3. ______________________________

Rebekah

1. ______________________________
2. ______________________________
3. ______________________________

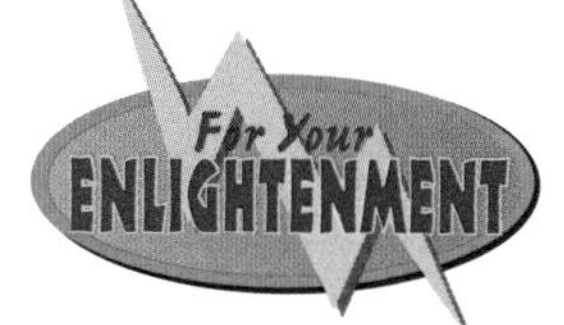
For Your
ENLIGHTENMENT

Since camels do not sweat much, the water in their bodies lasts longer than in most other animals. Still, a hot, thirsty camel can drink over fifty gallons of water at once.

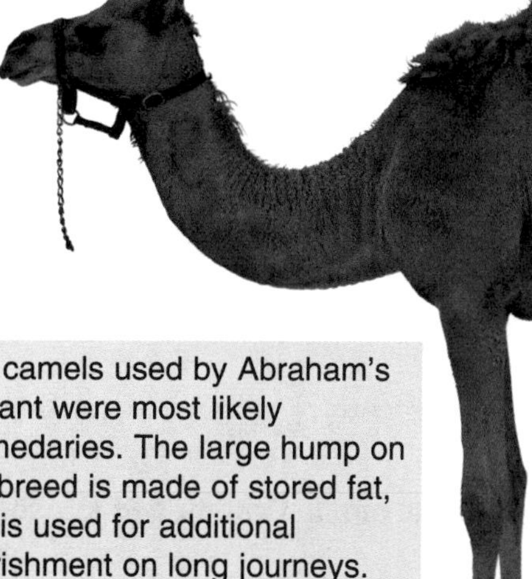

The camels used by Abraham's servant were most likely dromedaries. The large hump on this breed is made of stored fat, and is used for additional nourishment on long journeys.

Camels can comfortably carry about 400 pounds. Their large padded feet prevent them from sinking into sand.

Not Too Old

Name ______________________

Read Hebrews 11:11-12 and answer the questions.

1. Did Sarah and Abraham have the strength in themselves to have a child? ____________
2. Who gave them the ability to have a son? ________________
3. Who was born to Abraham and Sarah in fulfillment of God's promise? ____________________
4. What attributes of God are you reminded of in verse 11?

____

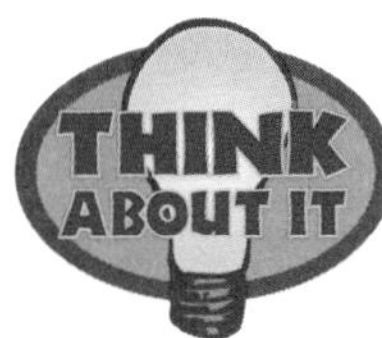
THINK
ABOUT IT

Truthfulness and faithfulness are attributes of God that Christians should also display in their lives. Have you been truthful and faithful to your word this week?

Remember that a **simile** is a comparison between unlike things using *like* or *as.* The author of Hebrews uses similes to help you understand his description of Abraham's descendants.

Read Hebrews 11:12. Write the two similes and explain their meaning.

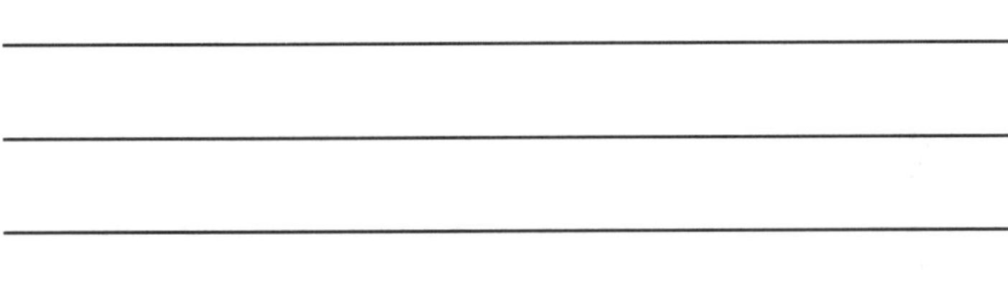

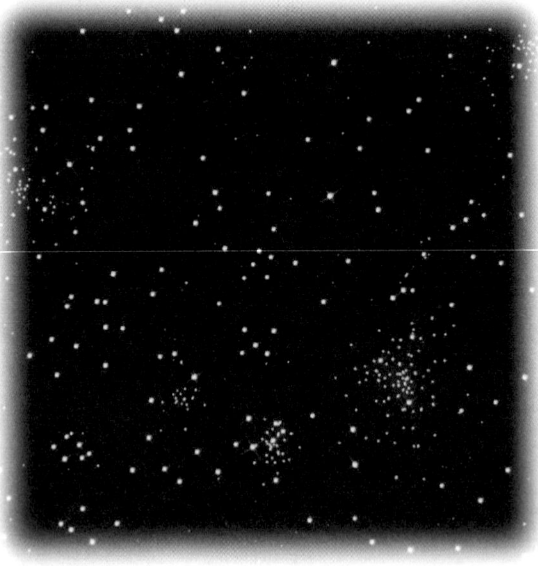

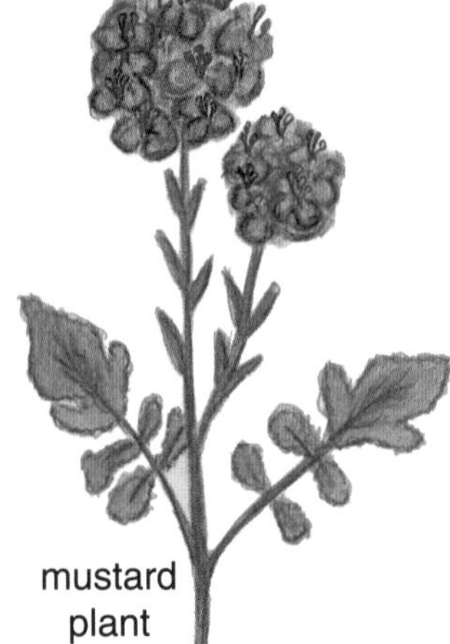

mustard plant

Christ used many similes when teaching the disciples.

Write the simile Christ used in each passage.

Matthew 17:20 ______________________________

Matthew 18:3 ______________________________

Luke 12:27 ______________________________

Singing with Understanding

"Faith of Our Fathers" (v. 3)

Name ______________________

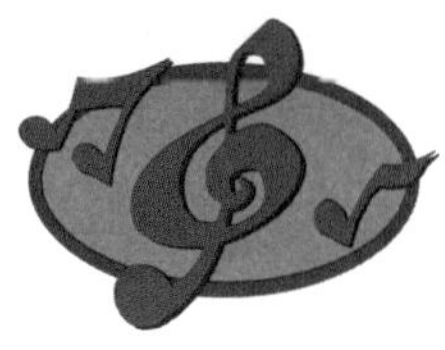

Faith of our fathers, we will strive
To win all nations unto thee,
And through the truth that comes from God
Mankind shall then be truly free.

Read Matthew 28:19-20 and answer the questions.

1. Are these verses teaching that God calls everyone to go to foreign countries as missionaries? ______________
2. What does God expect everyone to do?

____

3. What are some ways you can help win all nations to Christ?

____

____

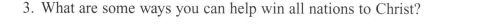

Perhaps some day the Lord will call you to go to another country and proclaim the truth of God's Word. But whether you serve Him at home or overseas, you should develop an interest in foreign missions right now!

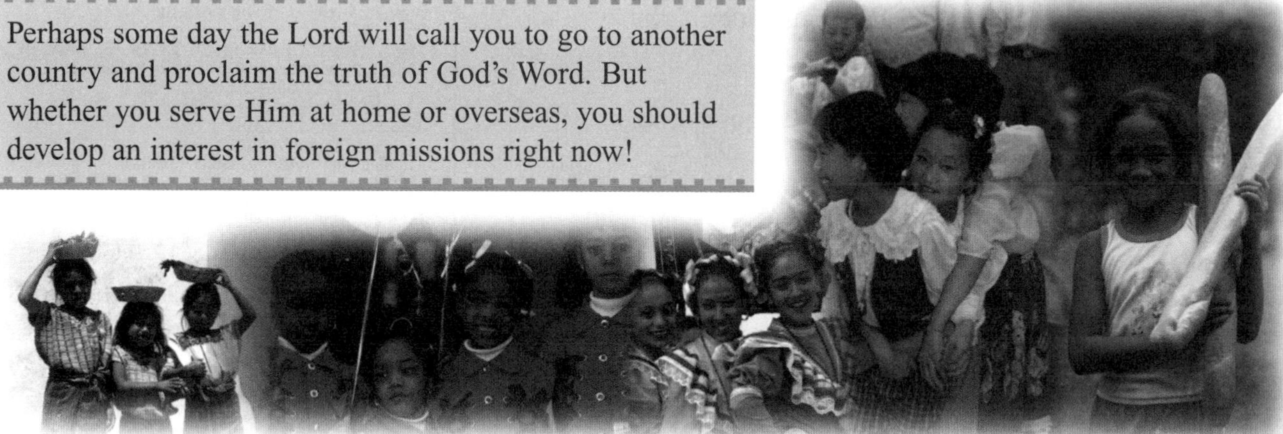

Circle the ideas below that interest you most.

Read missionary prayer letters and pray for their requests.

Write to missionaries.

Learn about the geography, people, and customs of other countries.

Give part of your money to missions.

Learn a foreign language.

Try international foods.

Send care packages to missionary children.

Read missionary biographies.

Talk to the missionaries who come to your church.

Finding Promises in the Word

Concordance

Name ______________________

Bible Study Skills Josh's family was planning to go on a mission trip with a group from church. To prepare, they had attended team meetings and special Bible studies and had read missionary biographies. The family prayed that all the details would be worked out, and especially that they would get enough money for the trip.

As each request was answered, it was clear to them that God wanted them to go. Before the trip was planned, Josh could not find any neighbors willing to hire him to cut their lawns. But in the last two months, three neighbors asked him to come cut their grass. Josh and his parents kept praying for money to pay for the trip, and they knew God would provide.

Answer the questions.

What request was Josh's family waiting for God to answer?

____

Josh used his concordance to find some verses to help his family claim the promise that God would supply the needed money.

Use the concordance entry to answer the questions.

Some entries list a short description of the main subject followed by the reference(s) where that topic is found.

1. **Look at the first entry for *prayer.* Write one reference that encourages you to pray often.**

____

Josh wanted even more verses, so he looked at the second entry for *prayer.* This entry lists specific headings about prayer.

2. **Write three headings that Josh could use to find verses to help encourage his family.**

____

____

____

PRAY, Gen.20:7, a prophet and shall *p* for thee
1 Sam.7:5, I will *p* for you to the Lord
12:23, sin in ceasing to *p* for you
2 Chr.7:14, if my people shall *p*
Ezra 6:10, *p* for the life of the king
Job 21:15, what profit if we *p* to him
Ps.5:2, to thee will I *p*
55:17, evening, morning, and at noon will I *p*
122:6, *p* for the peace of Jerusalem
Isa.45:20, *p* to a god that cannot save
Jer.7:16; 11:14; 14:11, *p* not for this people
37:3; 42:2,20, *p* now to the Lord for us
Zech.7:2, they sent men to *p*
Mt.5:44, and *p* for them who despitefully use you
6:5, they love to *p* standing
14:23; Mk.6:46; Lk.6:12; 9:28, to mountain to *p*
26:36; Mk.14:32, while I *p* yonder
Mk.11:25, and when ye stand *p*, forgive
Lk.11:1, Lord, teach us to *p*
18:1, men ought always to *p*
Jn.14:16; 16:26, I will *p* the Father
17:9, I *p* for them, I *p* not for the world
20, neither *p* I for these alone
Acts 9:11, behold he *p*
Rom.8:26, know not what we should *p* for
1 Cor.14:15, I will *p* with the spirit, and *p* with understanding also
Eph.6:18, *p* always with all prayer
1 Th.5:17, *p* without ceasing
1 Tim.2:8, that men *p* everywhere
Jas.5:13, is any afflicted? Let him *p*
16, *p* one for another
1 Jn.5:16, I do not say he shall *p* for it
PRAYER, 2 Chr.7:15, ears shall be attentive to the *p*
Ps.65:2, thou that hearest *p*
72:15, *p* shall be made continually
109:4, I give myself to *p*
Prov.15:8, the *p* of the upright
Isa.1:15, when ye make many *p*
56:7; Mt.21:13; Mk.11:17; Lk.19:46, house of *p*
Mt.21:22, whatever ye ask in *p*, believing
23:14; Mk.12:40; Lk.20:47, long *p*
Lk.6:12, all night in *p* to God
Acts 3:1, the hour of *p*
6:4, give ourselves continually to *p*
12:5, *p* was made without ceasing
16:13, where *p* was accustomed to be made
Phil.4:6, in everything by *p*
Jas.5:15, *p* of faith shall save the sick
16, effectual fervent *p* of a righteous man
1 Pet.4:7, watch unto *p*
Rev.5:8; 8:3, the *p* of the saints
PRAYER, occasions, objects, examples of. 1 Chr. 16:35; Job 33:26; Ps.122:6; Mt.5:44; 9:38; 26:41; Lk.18:3,38; Rom.15:30; 1 Cor.7:5; Jas.5:13; 1 Pet. 3:7; 4:7
commanded. Isa.55:6; Mt.7:7; 26:41; Lk.18:1; 21:36; Eph.6:18; Phil.4:6; Col.4:2; 1 Th.5:17,25; 1 Tim.2:1,8
encouragements to. Job 33:26; Ps.6:9; 32:6; 66:19; Isa.65:24; Zech.13:9; Mt.18:19; 21:22; Mk.11:24; Lk.11:9; Rom.10:13; Jas.1:5
God hears and answers. Ps.10:17; 65:2; 99:6; Isa.58:9; Jn.11:42
how to be offered. Ps.145:18; Prov.15:29; Eccl. 5:2; Mt.6:5,7; 21:22; Mk.11:24; Lk.11:5; 18:1; Jn.9:31; 15:7; Rom.12:12; Eph.6:18; Col.4:2; 1 Tim.2:8; 5:5; Heb.11:6; Jas.1:6; 4:8
through Christ. Eph.2:18; Heb.10:19
in the name of Christ. Jn.16:26
promises for. Isa.65:24; Amos 5:4; Zech.13:9; Mt.6:6; Lk.11:9; Jn.14:13
posture for. Num.16:22; Josh.5:14; 1 Ki.8:22; 1 Chr.21:16; 2 Chr.6:13; Ps.28:2; 95:6; Isa.1:15; Lam.2:19; Mt.26:39; Mk.11:25; Lk.22:41; Acts 20:36; 1 Tim.2:8

3. **Write the reference to one verse and explain how Josh could use that verse to help claim the promise that God supplies our needs and answers prayer.**

____

____

Decided Before Birth

Bible Study: Genesis 25–27

Name ____________________

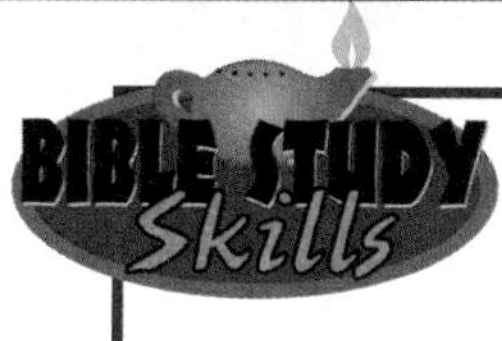

Read Genesis 25:19-23 

1. What did Isaac pray for?

2. When the babies seemed to be fighting inside her, what did Rebekah do?

3. The Lord answered that the babies would become the leaders of two different nations. Write the two prophecies that God made about these nations.

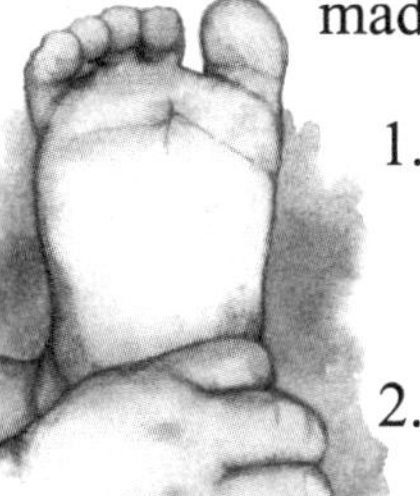

1. ____________________

2. ____________________

Read Genesis 25:24-28  

1. How is the newborn Esau described?

2. What is said about the newborn Jacob?

3. As the boys got older, what traits did each have?

Esau ____________________

Jacob ____________________

Jacob's holding Esau's heel in birth was a sign that Jacob's descendants would later rule over Esau's descendants.

Read Genesis 25:29-34. 

1. What had Jacob made?

2. Esau was so tired he thought he would die. What was he willing to give up in order to have food immediately?

3. Write about a time you chose to give in to your immediate desires instead of waiting.

Read Genesis 27:6-17, 27-29, 41. 

1. What was Isaac planning to give Esau?

2. Who gave Jacob the idea to pretend he was Esau?

3. Isaac gave Jacob the blessing for the firstborn of the family. Who did he say would be bowing down to Jacob?

4. How did Esau react to Jacob's receiving the blessing?

Departure and Return

Bible Study: Genesis 27-32

Name ______________________

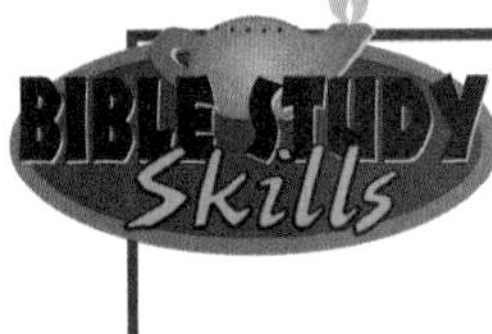

1

Read Genesis 27:42–28:5.

1. What did Rebekah hear?

____

2. When Rebekah went to Isaac, she
   - ○ wanted Isaac to handle the situation, so she told him that Esau wanted to kill Jacob.
   - ○ told Isaac that since she didn't like the women in the area, she wanted Jacob to go to Laban's family to find a wife.

3. What did Isaac do before Jacob left that lets you think Isaac was no longer angry with Jacob? ______________________

____

2

Read Genesis 28:11-21.

One night on Jacob's trip to Laban's home, God gave him a dream of a heavenly ladder.

1. What four promises did God give to Jacob?

____

____

____

____

2. After Jacob awoke, what promise did he make? ______________________

____

____

____

3

Laban was dishonest when dealing with Jacob about his wages and livestock. Jacob, his wives, and his herds left secretly to return to Jacob's homeland. Laban caught up with them and met with Jacob.

Read Genesis 31:41-45, 48-49, 54-55.

Evidently, Laban and Jacob resolved their differences. Laban suggested they make a covenant together.

1. What did they ask in their agreement as they worshiped God together?

____

2. Why did Jacob need to return to his homeland so that God's covenant with Abraham could be fulfilled through Jacob?

____

____

4

Read Genesis 32:6-12, 24-30.

1. How did Jacob react when he received the report that Esau was coming with four hundred men? ______________________

2. In addition to taking action to prevent harm to his family, what did Jacob do? __________

3. What were two permanent results from the night God came to Jacob?

____

____

When you become distressed, do you pray for God to help guide you?

What Does God Say About Jealousy?

Name ______________________

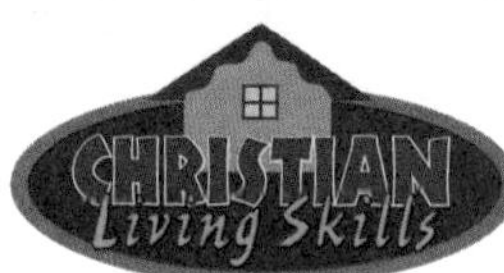
CHRISTIAN
Living Skills

Selfishness is a deadly trap. When you focus on pleasing yourself, you will become **envious** or **jealous.** Both words mean about the same thing. **Jealousy,** or **envy,** is simply wanting what someone else has. This temptation comes from dissatisfaction with yourself and your possessions.

Read II Corinthians 10:12 and answer the questions.

1. What does this verse say about people who compare themselves to others?

   ____

2. Why do you think it is not wise to compare yourself with others?

   ____

When you choose to compare yourself to others, you will either start thinking that you are better than others or you will grow discontent with what you have. When you think that you are better than others, you are guilty of the sin of pride. When you become discontent with what you have, you are guilty of jealousy (envy), also the result of pride. You will start to think that you deserve better than what you have been given. Your deceitful heart will begin to whisper questions to your mind that will cause you to doubt God's goodness to you.

Read Titus 3:3-5 and answer the questions.

1. Describe the lifestyle of a person who does not have Jesus Christ as his Savior.

   ____

   ____

2. Who enables a person to have victory over the sin of jealousy? ______________________

Satan loves to deceive you. He likes to make it seem like wicked people are having all the fun. When you become discontent with God's provisions for you, you may become envious and jealous of other people—even of wicked people who appear to be successful in this life. God warns you against this temptation by reminding you of His coming judgment on the wicked.

Happiness comes from having a grateful heart!

Match the verses to the correct reason for not being envious of wicked people.

1. ________ Psalm 37:1-2
2. ________ Proverbs 24:1-2
3. ________ Proverbs 3:31-32
4. ________ Proverbs 24:19-20

A. God detests a perverse or froward person but loves righteousness.
B. Wicked people will soon wither away like the grass and herbs.
C. Wicked people have no future. Their candle will be put out.
D. The wicked plot violence and talk about mischief.

Something to Think About

Jealousy

Name ______________________

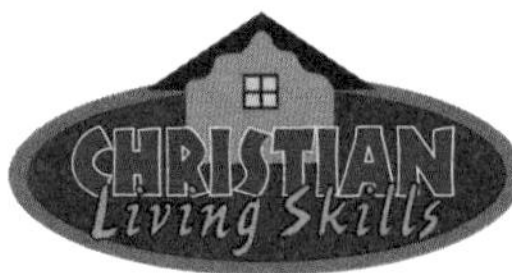
CHRISTIAN
Living Skills

Read each scenario below and answer the questions.

Scenario	Why was this person tempted to feel sorry for himself?	Why did this person feel jealous?
Kim and her family recently moved. Kim's sister, Anna, immediately became friends with girls down the street, but Kim couldn't seem to make any friends. When Anna's friends came over, they invited Kim to play a game with them. Kim refused, went to her room, and slammed the door.		
Josh studied diligently for his exam. Stacy, a classmate, commented that she hadn't even studied. When they received their grades, Josh had received a C. He was happy with his grade until he heard Stacy say that she had received a B.		
Kevin found out that Eric's dad had purchased tickets for their family to go to the state championship game. Kevin has always wanted to go to that game, but his family couldn't afford extra expenses like that.		
Carol noticed that Amy was wearing a new dress today at church. Carol didn't get new dresses. Her clothes were passed down to her when her older sister outgrew them.		

The opposite of jealousy is **unselfishness**, the sincere happiness you choose to have for the blessings or success of someone else, no matter what has happened to you.

Choose two of the scenarios and write how the person could have been happy for someone else.

1. ______________________________

2. ______________________________

What About Me?

Take time at home to think about some of your feelings. Carefully complete the statements.

I feel discontented and sorry for myself when ______________________.

Instead of feeling sorry for myself, I should ______________________.

I feel jealous when ______________________.

The next time I am tempted to be jealous I will ______________________.

I know that God is pleased when I ______________________.

Seeking Heavenly Things

Name ______________________

In Hebrews 11:8-14, the author shows how Abraham followed God's leading to the land of promise. Once he arrived, Abraham lived as a stranger. Although Abraham, Isaac, and Jacob each lived in the Promised Land of Caanan, they looked forward to the promise of a heavenly home. They never built homes, but lived in tents. The Israelites did not live in houses and cities until after they came out of Egypt.

God has promised all Christians a home in heaven. Believers' words and actions should display that they are looking to their heavenly home.

Becca pushed her elbow in front of Linda's backpack as they hurried into the classroom. They were to have a new seating arrangement, and Becca wanted to be the first to find her seat. She hoped the teacher had noticed the expensive clothes she wore each day. *Miss Williams might place me in the front to see my pretty clothes instead of some of the dull outfits those other girls wear,* Becca thought to herself. She was also certain that she would be seated in the front since she usually knew the answers during discussion times. As Becca hurried to beat Linda and Meredith to see the seating chart, her sweater caught the vine of a plant on the bookcase. Bang! Crash! What a mess! Becca turned to look at the broken pottery and soil as Miss Williams walked toward her. Now she would be the last to find her new seat, especially if she helped Miss Williams clean the floor.

Answer the questions.

1. What was occupying Becca's thoughts?

____

____

2. What are some things Becca should have been caring about?

____

____

____

3. What did Becca's actions show she was living for: earth or heaven? ____________

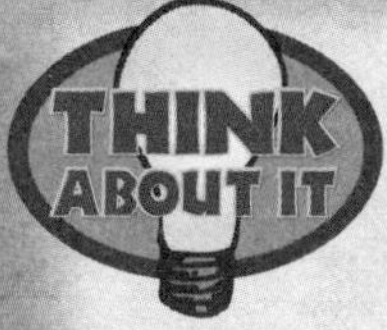
THINK ABOUT IT

How about you? Are you looking forward to a home in heaven, or are you seeking the riches of an earthly home? Write some things you can do to let others see your focus on a heavenly home.

____

____

Name ____________________

Read verse 4 of the hymn on page 312.

What is one of the most powerful ways to "preach" our faith?

____
____
____
____
____
____
____

These men are known as the **patriarchs,** or fathers, of the Israelites. Can you think of ways they showed their faith?

Choose one man and write about his example of faith.

____
____
____
____
____

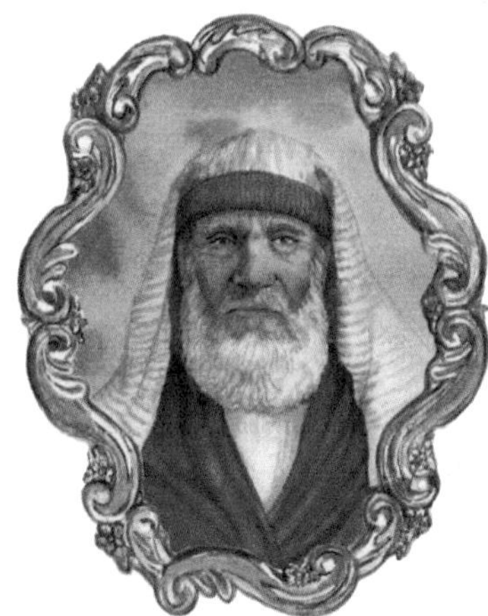

Abraham

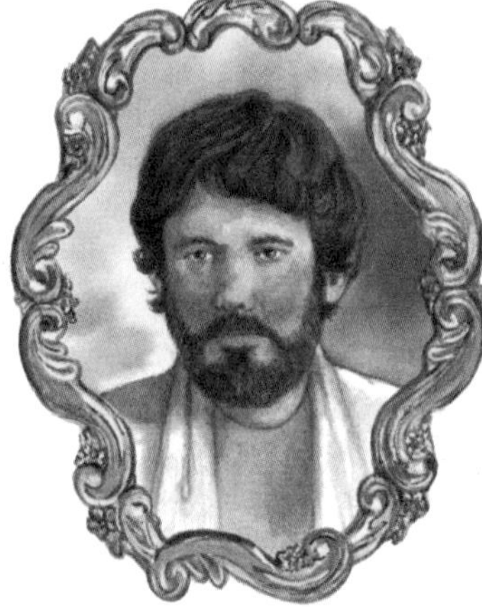

Isaac

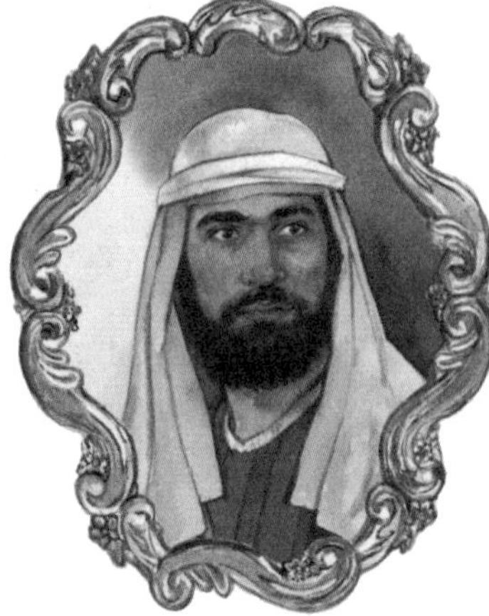

Jacob

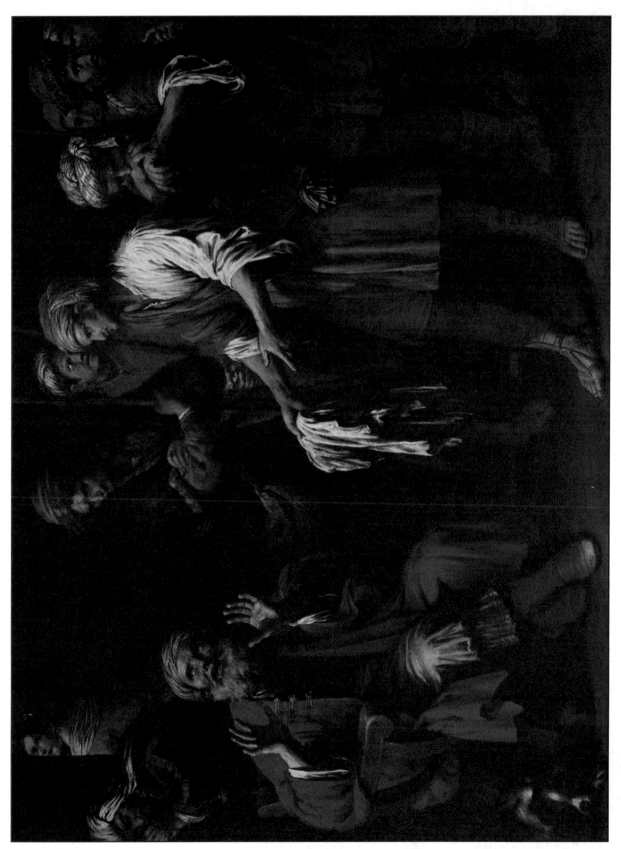

Jacob Shown the Coat of Joseph
Giovanni Battista Carlone

Bob Jones University Museum & Gallery, Inc.

Name ______________________

Jacob Shown the Coat of Joseph

by Giovanni Battista Carlone (1603-1677)

Giovanni Battista Carlone (Jē ə vä´nē Bä tēs´ tä Kâr lō´nā) was from a family of artists beginning in the late fifteenth century and extending on into the early nineteenth century. Giovanni was the best in this family of artists.

Giovanni Battista Carlone was born in Genoa, Italy and lived most of his life there, but he spent time in Florence and Rome, studying art under the masters. Carlone's best work was done in series—several paintings that each portrayed one scene of a story.

The painting you are looking at was one of a series about the life of Joseph, a popular subject because of the detail given in Genesis and because of the story's drama. In addition to this scene described in Genesis 37:26-35, Carlone also painted scenes of Joseph interpreting Pharaoh's dream, the discovery of Joseph's cup in Benjamin's sack, Reuben and Benjamin presenting Joseph with gifts, and Jacob blessing Joseph's two sons.

Carlone's painting style was quite **naturalistic,** meaning that he tried to imitate as closely as possible the details of how things really look. He used a lot of brown and tan colors and contrasted them with bright red. Brown and tan were among colors called **earth tones** since they are made from pigments that occur naturally in soil. Other earth tones include mustard yellow, red-brown, and grey-brown. Earth tones were the easiest and least expensive for a painter to obtain.

Like many artists of his day who studied in Rome, Carlone used dark spaces that were lighted by a sort of spotlight with which he could highlight any character that he wanted the viewer to look upon. Carlone's main highlights are on Jacob and the brother extending the coat. Other "spotlights" shine on a brother sympathetically shielding his face and another one standing defiantly looking on. Notice that most of the brothers are looking at each other rather than at Jacob. Notice also the girl with a horrified look, running from the room, probably to tell the news to others.

What Does God Say About Being Honest?

Name ______________________

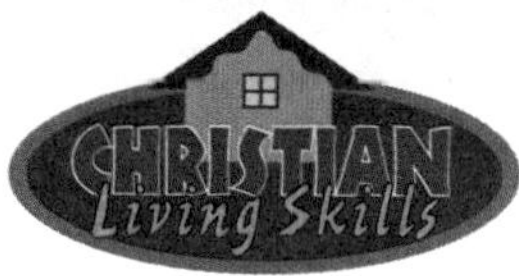
CHRISTIAN
Living Skills

Growing in Christlikeness means that you are becoming more like Christ each day. You seek to know Him and to imitate His character. To become like Christ, you must love what God loves and hate what God hates.

Read Proverbs 6:16-19 and list seven things that God hates. Circle the action that is mentioned twice in this list.

- ______________________
- ______________________
- ______________________
- ______________________
- ______________________
- ______________________
- ______________________

Notice that dishonesty is mentioned twice in a list of things which God hates. God's enemy, the devil, loves to lie and has tempted humans with lies since the Garden of Eden.

Read John 8:44 and answer the questions.

1. What does Jesus call the devil? ______________________
2. What does the devil not have in him? ______________________

Study the causes and effects in the chart.

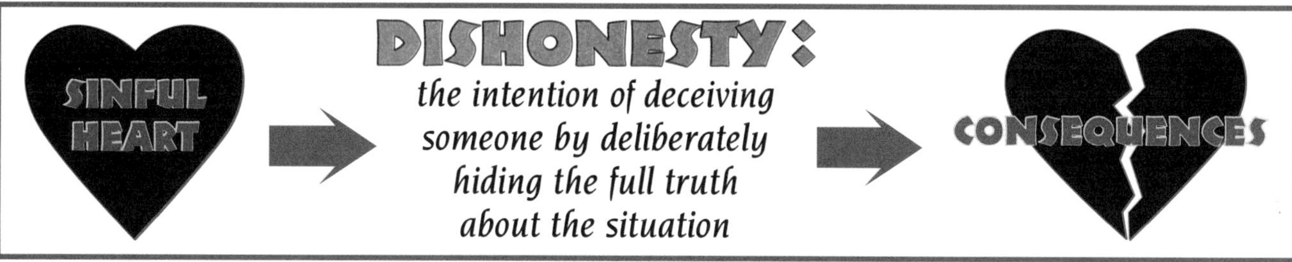
SINFUL HEART
DISHONESTY:
the intention of deceiving someone by deliberately hiding the full truth about the situation
CONSEQUENCES

Dishonesty comes out of a sinful heart. When you deceive someone, you choose to imitate the devil instead of Christ. As with every sin, God promises negative consequences to those who choose to disobey Him.

Read the verses and write in your own words what God says about those who are dishonest.

Proverbs 19:9 ______________________

Proverbs 12:22 ______________________

If you love God and desire to grow in Christlike character, you will have the same attitude toward dishonesty that God does. You will hate it. Instead of lying, you will make a habit of telling the full truth in every situation.

Something to Think About

Honesty

Name ______________________

CHRISTIAN Living Skills

Remember that **dishonesty** is more than just telling a lie. It is having the intention of deceiving someone by deliberately hiding the full truth.

Read the scenarios and describe the deception taking place. Then write an honest response that could have been given.

Scenario	How was each one deceitful?	What should have been said to be honest?
When Kodie's mom asked if she had cleaned her room, Kodie said that she had, but she didn't explain that she had cleaned the room by stuffing everything under the bed.		
Rebecca was invited to a slumber party. She knew that her parents would not approve the video the girls were renting. When asked about the activities, she didn't mention the video so that her parents would give her permission to attend.		
Chris threw the football to his sister in the living room. She missed the ball and it shattered a flower vase. When their mom came home, Chris said he didn't know about it and suggested that maybe the dog had broken it.		

What About Me?

Take time at home to think about your attitude toward being honest in all that you say and do. Carefully consider the following questions.

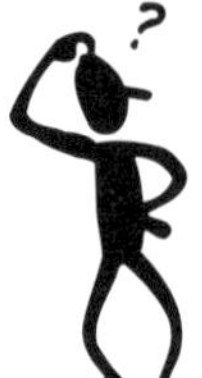

Do I have a reputation for telling the truth?
Have I ever told a lie to try to stay out of trouble?
Have I ever deceived my parents by not telling them the whole truth?
Have I ever falsely accused someone else to make myself look good?
Is God pleased with the way I imitate Christ in telling the truth?

It's not too late! If you have a habit of dishonesty, confess this sin and ask God for His forgiveness. Then ask Him to help you to become a person who always tells the truth.

Trust Brings Blessing

Genesis 37-41

Name ____________________

Write the letter of the effect next to the correct cause in the events in the life of Joseph.

CAUSE

_______ 1. Joseph was Jacob's favorite son.

_______ 2. Joseph's brothers let their hatred control them.

_______ 3. God helped Joseph resist the temptation to sin with Potiphar's wife.

_______ 4. Potiphar's wife lied to Potiphar about Joseph.

_______ 5. In jail, Joseph had a godly response to his circumstances and was obedient.

_______ 6. God helped Joseph correctly interpret the dreams of the baker and butler.

_______ 7. God helped Joseph correctly interpret Pharoah's dreams and give wise counsel.

_______ 8. God gave Joseph wisdom about raising and storing food.

EFFECT

A. Joseph was brought to interpret Pharoah's dreams.

B. Potiphar's wife became angry and lied about Joseph.

C. Joseph was placed over the other prisoners.

D. Joseph's brothers became jealous and hated him.

E. Egypt had plenty during the time of famine.

F. They sold Joseph into slavery.

G. Joseph was sent to jail.

H. Joseph was promoted to second in command in Egypt.

An Honoring Response

Name ______________________________

Joseph's brothers did not like the favoritism shown by their father toward Joseph. They chose not to see Joseph's dreams as prophecy from God about their future. They demonstrated their bad feelings and distrust by mistreating Joseph. Joseph experienced many ups and downs in his life, yet his responses were always honorable.

Sequence the events in the life of Joseph. Write the letter in the correct circle on the diagram.

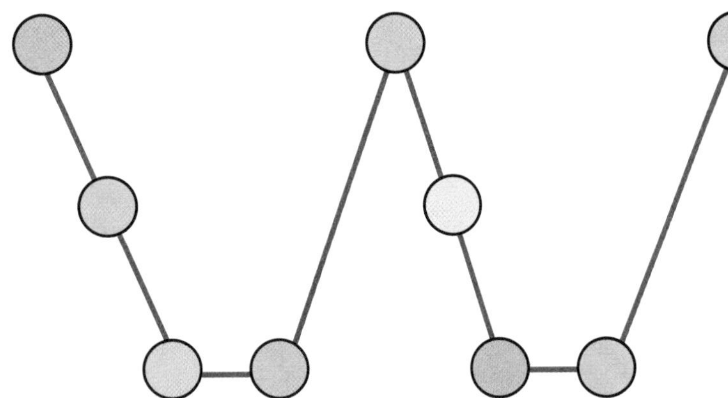

A. falsely accused
B. sold into slavery
C. forgotten by the butler
D. placed in a pit
E. wrongly imprisoned
F. coat taken
G. command of Potiphar's household
H. favored son
I. second in command over Egypt

Remember Rebekah's response when she saw that the camels needed water? She could have ignored the camels and given water only to Abraham's servant. But she saw the need and knew the right action to take. Look at how the Lord blessed her response! Throughout the Bible God gives examples of those who accepted their circumstances and responded properly.

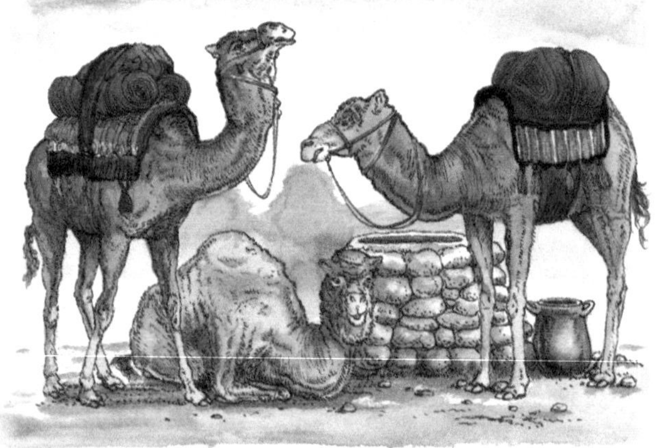

Read the verses. Write the response that each person gave that honored God.

Genesis 14:21-23 **Abraham** ______________________________

I Samuel 3:10 **Samuel** ______________________________

Daniel 6:10 **Daniel** ______________________________

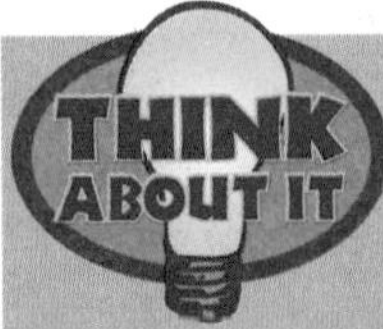
THINK
ABOUT IT

God controls all circumstances and is pleased with proper responses. When things don't go as you planned, perhaps God is trying to teach you to have the proper response in that situation.

Have you ever been in a situation where you have been wronged? ____________

What did you do? ______________________________

What would have been a better response? ______________________________

Reunited

Genesis 42-50

Name ______________________

When accused of being spies, Joseph's brothers immediately remembered their sin of selling Joseph. At this time they did not know that it was Joseph speaking to them, but they still carried the guilt from their actions years before.

God desires every sinner to seek forgiveness. Sin carries guilt. Guilt can show itself in a variety of ways. One way is to make the sinner suspicious of the thoughts and actions of others. A guilty person interprets the events in his life as being punishment for sin.

Answer the questions. You may use your Bible for help.

1. Joseph saw his brothers' sin as the instrument of God to place him in Egypt. When did Joseph finally reveal himself to his brothers? (Gen. 45:1-12)

   ____

2. Did the brothers ask forgiveness at this time? ______________

3. What did Pharaoh do when he heard that Joseph's brothers had come? (Gen. 45:16-19)

   ____

4. Jacob lived in Egypt for seventeen years before he died. After his burial in Canaan, what were the brothers' thoughts about Joseph? (Gen. 50:14-18)

   ____

5. Did Joseph's brothers ask forgiveness at this time? ______________

6. What did Joseph tell his brothers about their actions? (Gen. 50:19-20)

   ____

   ____

   ____

THINK ABOUT IT

Have you committed a sin that keeps coming to mind? Does thinking about that sin cause you to act differently toward God and others? Perhaps you should be asking God's forgiveness and that of someone you may have wronged.

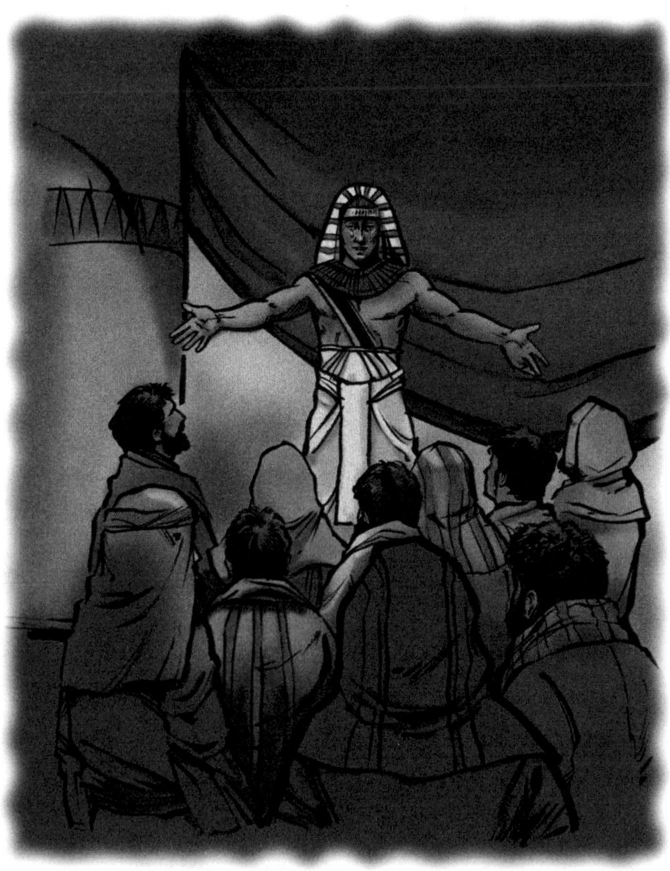

Covenant Review
Abraham Through Joseph

Name ____________________

Many times throughout Scripture, God is called the God of Abraham, Isaac, and Jacob. The covenant is often identified with these three names. Once the children of Israel returned to occupy the Promised Land, the inheritance was divided among the twelve sons of Jacob (Gen. 49). Since Levi's descendents were made the priests and keepers of the tabernacle, they did not receive an inheritance of land. Because of the blessing given them by Jacob (Gen. 48:5), Joseph's inheritance was divided between his two sons, Ephraim and Manasseh.

Write *T* if the sentences are true and *F* if the sentences are not true about God's covenant with Abraham and his descendants.

______ 1. God included Lot in the covenant as Abraham's son.

______ 2. Ishmael was included in God's covenant with Abraham.

______ 3. God fulfilled His covenant with Abraham through Isaac.

______ 4. God promised to make Abraham a great nation.

______ 5. God led Abraham to a land of promise.

______ 6. Abraham lived a sinless life and always did as God wanted.

______ 7. God planned for Esau to be the son of Isaac included in the covenant.

______ 8. God planned for Jacob to receive the blessing as part of the covenant.

______ 9. Through Joseph, God provided for Abraham's descendants in time of famine.

______ 10. Both Abraham and Christians today share the same faith to believe God's promises.

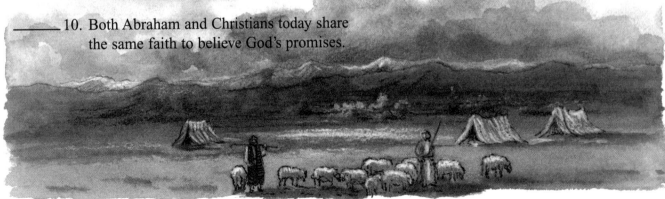

Locate and circle the twelve tribes on the map.

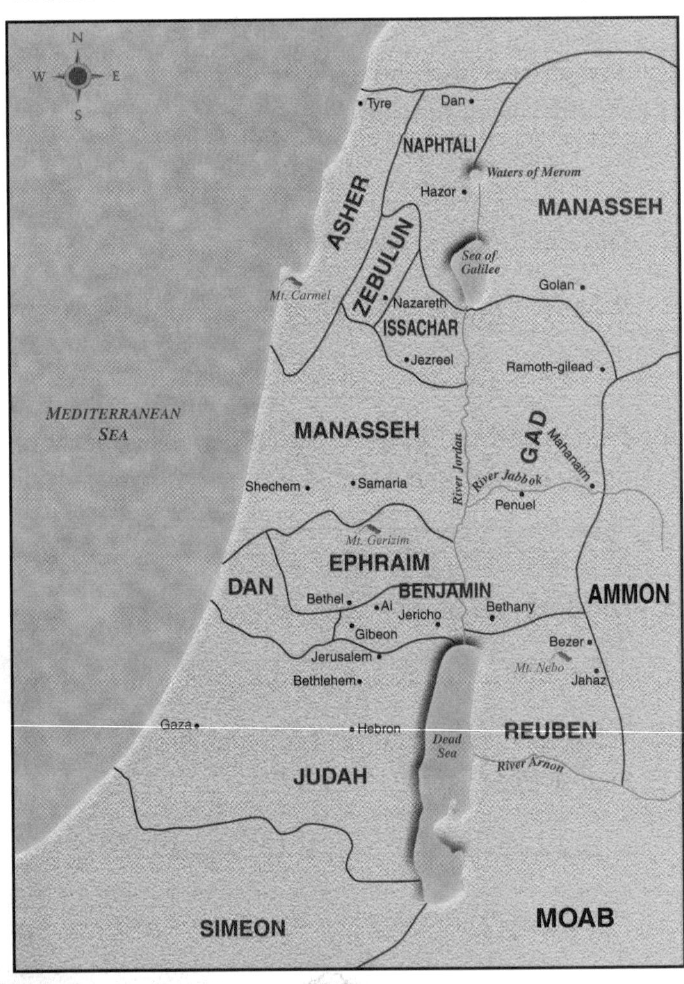

N
W
E
S
Tyre
Dan
NAPHTALI
Waters of Merom
Hazor
MANASSEH
ASHER
ZEBULUN
Sea of Galilee
Golan
Mt. Carmel
Nazareth
ISSACHAR
Jezreel
Ramoth-gilead
MEDITERRANEAN SEA
MANASSEH
GAD
Mahanaim
River Jordan
River Jabbok
Shechem
Samaria
Penuel
Mt. Gerizim
EPHRAIM
DAN
BENJAMIN
AMMON
Bethel
Ai
Jericho
Bethany
Gibeon
Bezer
Jerusalem
Mt. Nebo
Bethlehem
Jahaz
Gaza
Hebron
Dead Sea
REUBEN
River Arnon
JUDAH
SIMEON
MOAB

Get the Bible Reading H.A.B.I.T.

Name ____________________

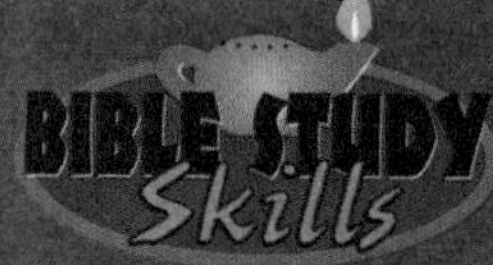

BIBLE STUDY
Skills

As you read the Scripture for each day, write the date in the box.

Have a special time set aside each day to read your Bible. If possible, make it the same time every day.

Ask God to teach you from His Word. Remember to thank Him for helping you to understand and apply it.

Be still and give your attention to what you are reading.

Investigate the Scripture by asking yourself questions about it.

Take time to look up words and ideas you do not understand.

God has chosen the weak to show His strength. **I Corinthians 1:26-31**	God can show His power through a weak and fearful speaker. **I Corinthians 2:1-5**	God's strength is made perfect when we are weak. **II Corinthians 12:9-10**	God has not given us a spirit of fear, but of boldness and love. **II Timothy 1:7-10**	Love for others gives believers boldness to testify of Christ. **I John 4:10-18**
Now is the best time to receive God's salvation. **II Corinthians 6:1-2**	God hardened Pharaoh's heart to display His power. **Romans 9:17-18**	Man should not harden his heart to Christ through unbelief. **Hebrews 3:12-15**	A hard, unrepentant heart will receive God's wrath one day. **Romans 2:5-8**	If you are justified by Christ's blood, you will be saved from wrath. **Romans 5:9-11**
With the law comes the knowledge that all have sinned. **Romans 3:20-23**	Christians are justified freely by grace, not by keeping the law. **Romans 3:24-28**	Faith in Christ justifies sinners; the works of the law do not. **Galatians 2:16-18**	Christians are crucified with Christ, and now His righteousness lives in them. **Galatians 2:19-21**	Christians are expected to obey God's laws. **James 2:10-12**
Jesus understands how Christians feel and offers mercy. **Hebrews 4:14-16**	Jesus is our High Priest forever by the oath of God. **Hebrews 7:17-21**	Because Jesus is a permanent High Priest, He is able to save us. **Hebrews 7:22-25**	Jesus is a perfect High Priest who needed to offer only one sacrifice. **Hebrews 7:26-28**	Jesus, our High Priest, sits at God's right hand, serving in His tabernacle. **Hebrews 8:1-2**

Praying with Purity

Name ______________________

Many Christians wonder why God does not seem to answer their prayers. One of the reasons is that unconfessed and unforgiven sin in a believer's life hinders prayer (Ps. 66:18). As you pray, ask yourself the following questions, and ask the Holy Spirit to point out any sins that you need to confess.

Use the verses to help you unscramble the words.

1. Have you **deiesyodb** God? (Mic. 3:4)

   ___ ___ ___ ___ ___ ___ ___ ___ ___

2. Have you failed to do things **Gwoydas**? (Prov. 1:28-30)

   ___ ___ ___' ___ ___ ___ ___

3. Have you been proud and **hhayutg**? (James 4:6)

   ___ ___ ___ ___ ___ ___ ___

4. Have you said one thing and done **ahnroet**? (Ezek. 33:31)

   ___ ___ ___ ___ ___ ___ ___

5. Have you prayed in self-righteousness and not in **hlutmiiy**? (Luke 18:9-14)

   ___ ___ ___ ___ ___ ___ ___ ___

6. Have you failed to **fioervg** those who have done wrong to you? (Mark 11:25)

   ___ ___ ___ ___ ___ ___ ___

REMEMBER!

God does not answer *yes* to every prayer, even if it is made from a pure heart. Sometimes He answers *no* or *wait*, but a Christian who prays purely can always be assured that God will hear and give the answer that is best.

Safe in the Ark

Exodus 2

Name ____________________

Moses' mother, Jochebed, hid her son in a basket, or ark, to keep him safe. She trusted God to protect her baby when she set him afloat in the Nile River. Noah trusted God to protect him and his family as they were adrift in the ark God told him to build. These arks are pictures of salvation in Jesus Christ.

Read Hebrews 11:7, 23. What did Noah and Jochebed need to have? Shade all shapes with two dots.

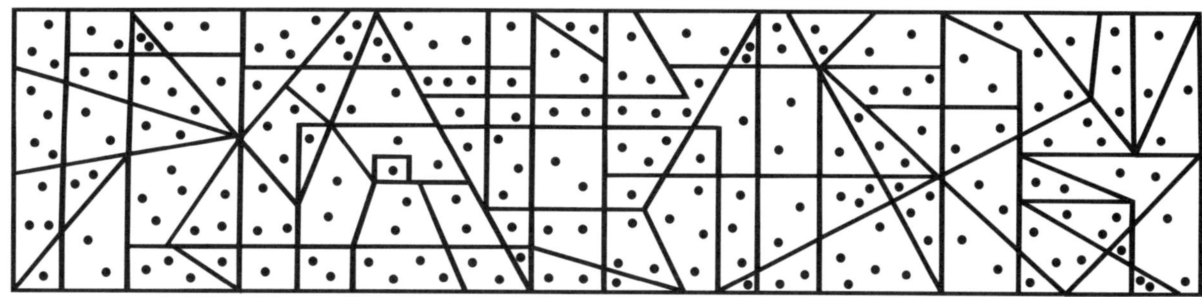

Answer the questions. You may use your Bible for help.

1. What do you need to have to be safe in Jesus Christ? ____________________

2. What happened to those who did not believe and come into the ark? (Gen. 7:23)

   ________ ______________ _____ __________________ ________ ________

3. Pharaoh made a decree concerning the baby boys of the Hebrews. What did he tell the people to do with the baby boys? (Exod. 1:22)

   ________________ ____ ______________________________

Complete the sentences.

4. These two accounts show us that those who have ____________________ in Christ will live.

5. Those who do not put their faith in Jesus Christ for salvation will ____________________

   __________ __________ ___ ________ ________ ______________.

Have you put your faith in Jesus Christ for salvation from sin and death? Trust Him today!

For Your ENLIGHTENMENT

Papyrus, a water plant, grew along the Nile River and in areas of Palestine. Ancient Egyptians used papyrus to construct boats. These boats were lightweight, but sturdy. Papyrus reeds were tied together, and the cracks were sealed with mineral pitch or asphalt. Deposits of pitch (asphalt) were located along the Dead Sea, the Euphrates River above Babylon, and other places. Pitch was used to waterproof Noah's ark (Gen. 6:14) and Moses' basket (Exod. 2:3).

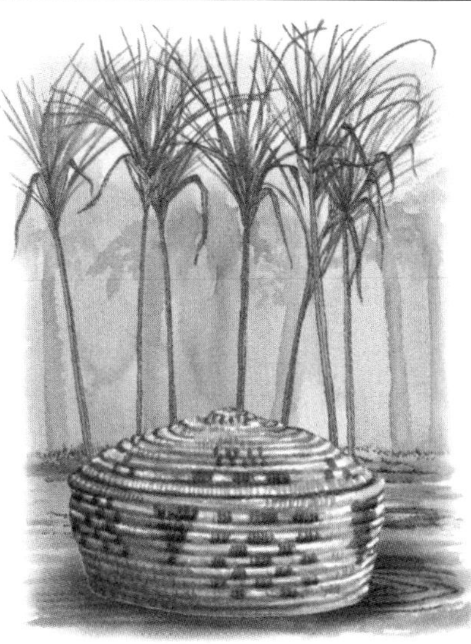

Burned, but Not Consumed

Exodus 3:2

Name ____________________

Use the code on the burning bush to find out how God strengthened and prepared Moses to lead the Israelites.

1. Moses, an Israelite, grew up in [6 3 1 6 1 5 3 6] household.
2. Moses was sensitive to the [4 7 6 2 5 8 6] of the Israelites.
3. In vengeance, Moses [1 1 4 4 5 2] an Egyptian.
4. Moses was afraid and fled to [7 1 2 1 1 8] to escape the wrath of Pharaoh.
5. Moses was sensitive to the needs of Jethro's [2 1 7 8 3 4 5 6 6].
6. Moses was afraid to look upon [8 5 2].
7. Moses [2 5 7 4 4 5 2] his abilities to be a leader.
8. God [6 6 5 7 1 6 5 2] that He would be with Moses.

Y 2 I H 1 U 3 C F E 8 5 O M 7 T 4 S 3 R 5 4 G 6 1 6 W 3 4 5 J 8 B V L 2 D 1 A X 6 P 8 N K 2 7 4

God has given Christians many wonderful promises to be with them during times of trial and testing. Finish the riddle. You may use your Bible for help.

Sometimes God allows Christians to go through times of testing to strengthen them, to draw them closer to Him, or to bring others to Himself. Many people of the Bible went through these "fires" of testing.

Into the furnace the three men were cast.
The king called these Hebrews to come out at last.
No sign of a burn from the head to the toe

On brave ____________________,

____________________, and ____________________. (Dan. 3:26-28)

God in His wisdom may give or may take.
He knows my way, and He makes no mistake.
"When tested by Him I shall come forth as gold,"

Said ______________, who later gained riches untold. (Job 23:10; 42:10)

THINK ABOUT IT

What fears do you have? Are you trusting God? God may someday allow you to go through a time of testing. Will you be ready?

Read Isaiah 43:1-2. What promise does God give that should comfort you during times of testing? ______________________________

Right or Wrong?

Exodus 2

Name ______________________

Moses encountered two situations where someone was being mistreated. Both times he stopped the mistreatment—once God's way, and once his own way.

Read the passages and answer the questions.

Exodus 2:11-15 1. How did Moses react? ______________________

Exodus 2:15-19 2. How did Moses react? ______________________

3. In which situation did Moses respond properly? ______________________

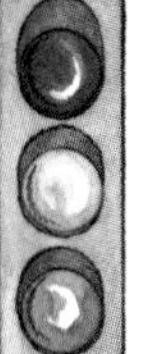

Color the light green if the person's reaction is right, and red if the person's reaction is wrong.

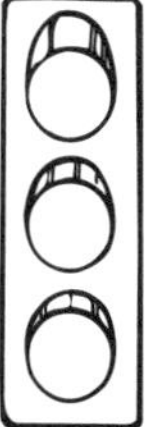

Jose hears his brother making fun of their little sister. He tells his brother to stop, and then tells a parent about the problem.

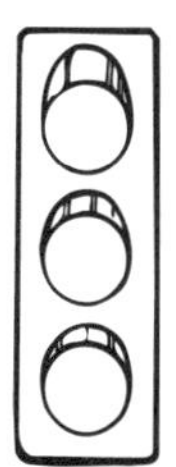

Jose hears his brother making fun of their little sister. He punches his brother in the nose.

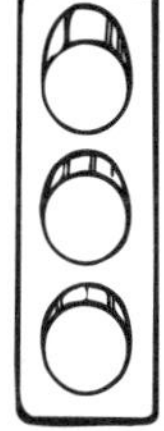

The most popular girl in the class has been making fun of Rachel at recess, so Rachel makes insulting remarks back to her.

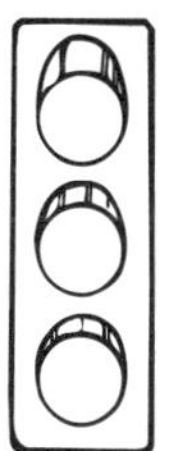

The most popular girl in the class has been making fun of Rachel at recess, but Rachel doesn't return insults. Instead she prays for her.

Read the following situation. Think about how Rhett can respond in the right way, and then write your advice to Rhett.

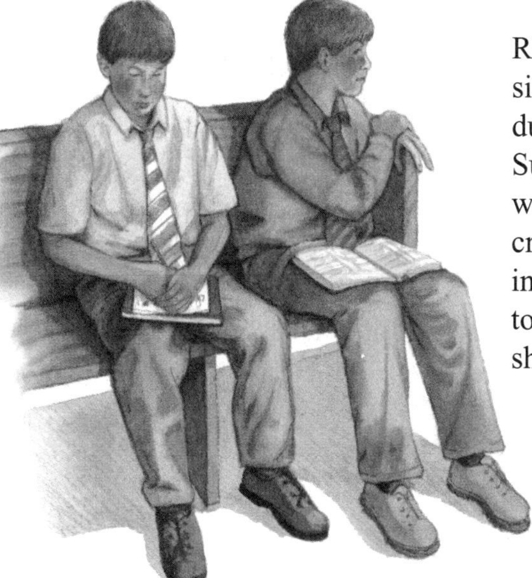

Rhett is allowed to sit with Bryan during church. One Sunday, Bryan worked on a crossword puzzle instead of listening to the sermon. What should Rhett do?

Using a Bible Dictionary

Name ______________________

BIBLE STUDY Skills

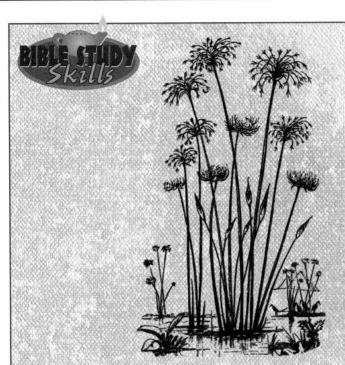
Papyrus plant

Papyrus. The papyrus is a water plant that grew luxuriantly in ancient times in Egypt and certain sections of Palestine. In ancient times papyrus writing material was made by cutting the pith of the papyrus plant into thin strips, criss-crossing them, and pressing them into sheets. These pale yellow sheets were frequently combined to form rolls from ten to thirty feet long and about nine and one-half inches high. Egyptians sometimes had huge papyrus rolls, such as the 123-foot-long Papyrus Harris. Use of papyrus for writing materials goes back to the Old Kingdom in Egypt, probably before 2700 B.C. The dry Egyptian climate was favorable to the preservation of papyri and some extant copies go back to the third millennium. In antiquity Egypt was a source of supply for ancient paper. Gebal on the Mediterranean coast received papyrus from Egypt, and this center of the paper trade was later called Byblos, meaning "papyrus" or "book" by the Greeks. Our modern word *Bible* through Gk. and Lat. goes back to this source. Leather was used early, and parchment also came into use later. Papyrus reeds tied together to form boats were used in ancient Egypt. Isaiah refers to Ethiopians dispatching messengers by the sea "in papyrus vessels" (18:2). In Egyptian art the papyrus growing in the marshes of the Delta symbolized Lower Egypt. The lotus, on the other hand, stood for Upper Egypt. For further discussion, *see also* Papyrus in the general listing.

M.F.U.; H.F.V.

Read the article. Write *T* if the statement is true and *F* if the statement is false.

_____ 1. Papyrus writing material was made from the pith or stem of the plant.

_____ 2. Papyrus sheets were placed in books.

_____ 3. A papyrus roll could be 30 feet long and 9 1/2 inches high.

_____ 4. The dry climate made preservation of the fragile material impossible.

_____ 5. The modern word *Bible* comes from the word *byblos* which in Greek meant "papyrus" or "book."

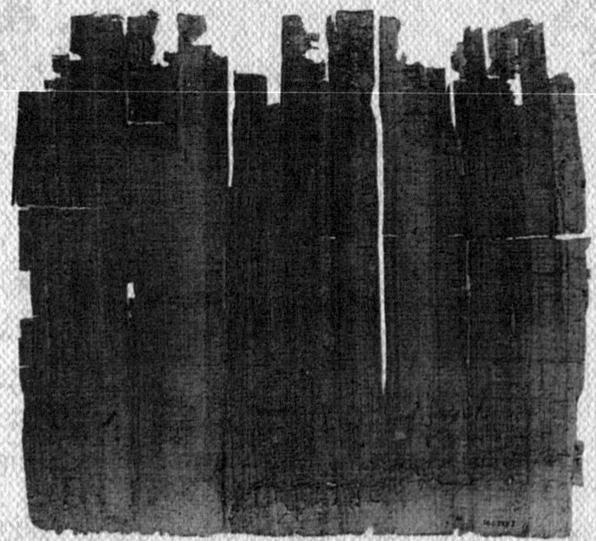
Egyptian papyrus paper

What Does God Say About Getting Even?

Revenge vs. Forgiveness

Name ____________________

CHRISTIAN
Living Skills

The desire for revenge is powerful and is the theme of much of popular "entertainment." If someone hurts you, the world teaches you that you should make them pay for what they have done to you. The world says that you should want revenge. The world is wrong. God speaks directly to His children about seeking revenge.

Read Romans 12:17-21 and answer the questions.

1. What is God's command to you in verse 17 about getting even?

   ____

2. What should you make every effort to do according to verse 18?

   ____

3. According to verse 19, why should you never seek revenge when someone wrongs you?

   ____

4. What command does God give to you in verse 20? ____________________

   ____

5. According to verse 21, with what should I overcome evil?

   ____

God is the only one who is qualified to judge anyone. He alone has authority to repay people for their sin. When you seek revenge, you are not trusting that God knows what He is doing and you are acting like you are equal with God. **Revenge** is a sin of pride. What should you do when people sin against you? It **will** happen. Someone **will** say things that hurt you. Someone **will** lie about you. Someone **will** mistreat you. How should YOU respond?

Read the verses and complete the sentences.

Luke 6:35	____________ your enemies.
Ephesians 4:32	Be ____________ to each other.
Leviticus 19:17	Do not ____________ your brother.
Luke 6:36	Be ____________.
Ephesians 4:31	Get rid of bitterness and ____________.

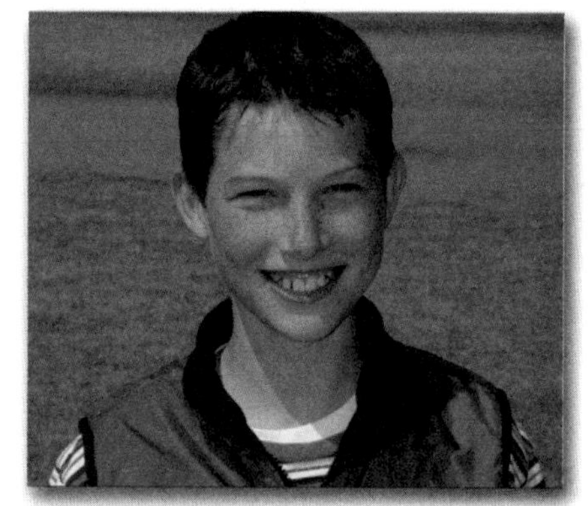

Something to Think About

Revenge vs. Forgiveness

Name ______________________

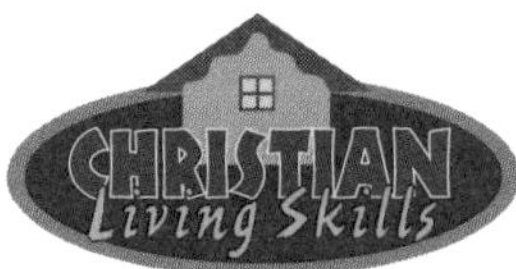
CHRISTIAN
Living Skills

Forgiving someone is the opposite of seeking revenge against him. You must get the big picture of forgiveness if you are to understand why you *must* forgive others. Remember: YOU have sinned against God and yet God has shown His love and mercy to YOU by providing a way of salvation through His Son, Jesus Christ. In other words, God is your supreme example of forgiveness because He was willing to forgive you.

Forgiveness is granting pardon to someone who has sinned against you without holding any grudge or resentment against him.

Read Colossians 3:13 and fill in the blanks.

I must ______________________ others just as Jesus Christ also ______________________ me.

Pretend that you are involved in each scenario. Make a ✔ in the box marking whether you were wronged by someone else or whether you were the one who was wrong. Write a response that would please God.

Scenario	Were you wronged?	Were you wrong?	What should you do to please God in this situation?
You enter the bike race at your church and are looking forward to the close competition between you and another boy. During the race, he purposely runs you off the road so that he wins.			
Your parents go to a meeting at church and leave you in charge at home. They don't allow you to watch TV while they are gone. After putting your younger sister to bed, you quietly turn on the TV. The next morning, your little sister tells your parents what you did.			
You really want to make a good grade on the math test. You know all the answers on the test except for the last one. Sara, who sits in front of you, always makes good grades in math. You lean forward and pretend like you're stretching to see what Sara has written down. Tim notices and tells the teacher.			

What About Me?

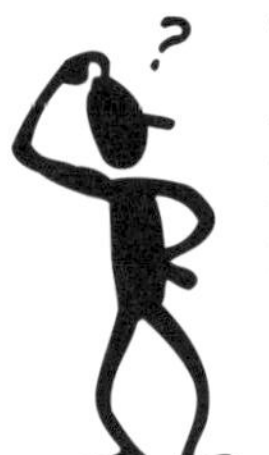

Take time at home to think about the following questions.

Do you want to get even with someone for something he did to you?
Do you need to apologize to someone for being angry with him for doing right?
Do you forgive others as Christ forgave you?
Have you been trying to be equal with God by planning revenge on someone?
Have you completely forgiven everyone who has wronged you in your life?

From Shepherd to Spokesman

Exodus 4:10-12

Name ____________________

When God called Moses to be His spokesperson before Pharaoh, Moses made excuses.

Read Exodus 4:10 and answer the questions.

1. What was Moses' first excuse? ____________________
2. What was Moses' second excuse? ____________________

Read Exodus 4:11-12. Complete the questions God asked Moses.

3. Who made man's ____________?
4. Who made the mute or the ____________?
5. Who made those who see and those who are ____________?

Have you ever felt tongue-tied or awkward when speaking in front of people? Many people feel uncomfortable when speaking in public. Moses felt this way too.

The Lord made man's mouth. He made the mute, the deaf, the seeing, and the blind. The God who created man's senses can also control them.

God used this same method of asking questions to make the point to Job that God is in control of every circumstance that comes in life. He knows what is best for us.

Read Job 42:1-2 and Exodus 4:12 and answer the questions.

6. What did Job say when he understood what God told him?

   ____

   ____

7. Why is it wrong to fail to trust God for help when He gives you a task to do?

   ____

   ____

8. What promise did God make to Moses when He asked Moses to speak to Pharaoh?

   ____

   ____

9. If God wants you to speak to someone for Him, will He enable you to do it? ____________

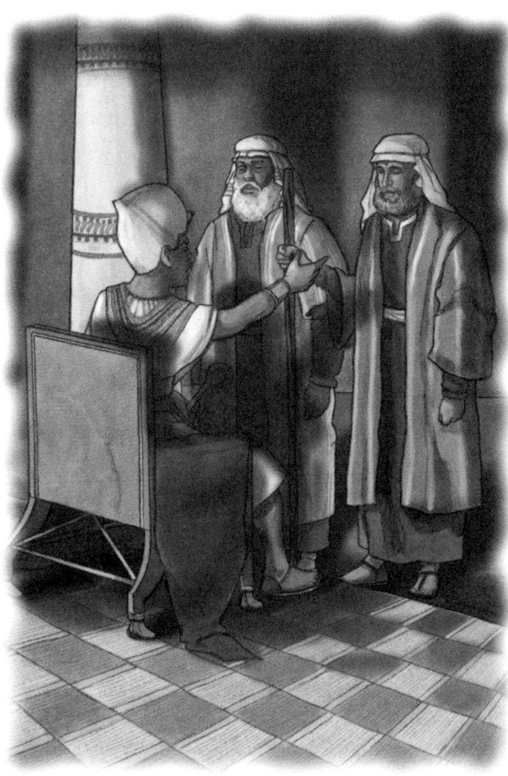

No Excuses!

Name ______________________

Just as God was with Moses and promised to help him, so God continues to guide His children today.

Read each of the situations below and write a promise from God's Word to answer each excuse. You may want to memorize one of these verses to help you when you are tempted to make excuses to God.

John 14:26 **Psalm 28:7** **Hebrews 13:6**

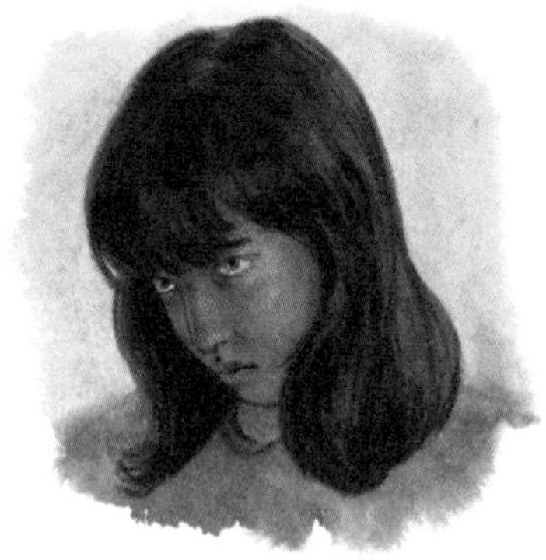

1. Juanita's Sunday school class is going door-to-door to hand out Bible Club invitations. Juanita has never gone door-to-door inviting people to church before. She is afraid people might laugh at her or slam the door in her face. Which verse might her mother share with her to help her not use fear as an excuse for failing to invite others to church?

____

____

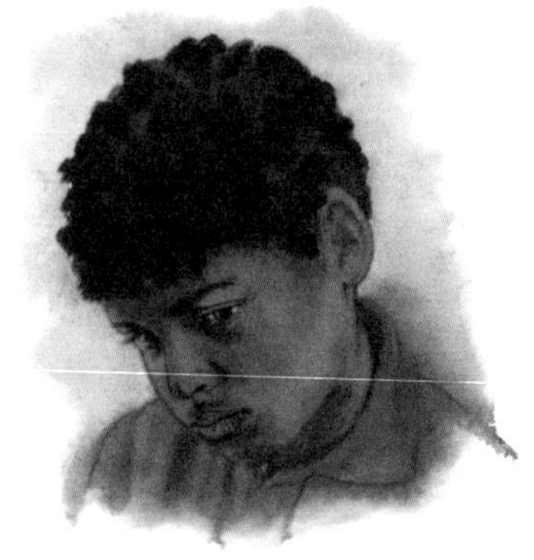

2. Timothy has been dreading the sixth grade trip to a nursing home for a Christmas program. After the program each student is supposed to find a resident to talk with for fifteen minutes while refreshments are being set up. The whole class has memorized some verses on salvation to share, but Timothy is sure his mind will go blank. Timothy is afraid he won't be able to think of anything to say or that he will feel awkward talking to a total stranger. What verse might Timothy's teacher share with him to keep him from using his fear of forgetfulness as an excuse for not serving God and others?

____

____

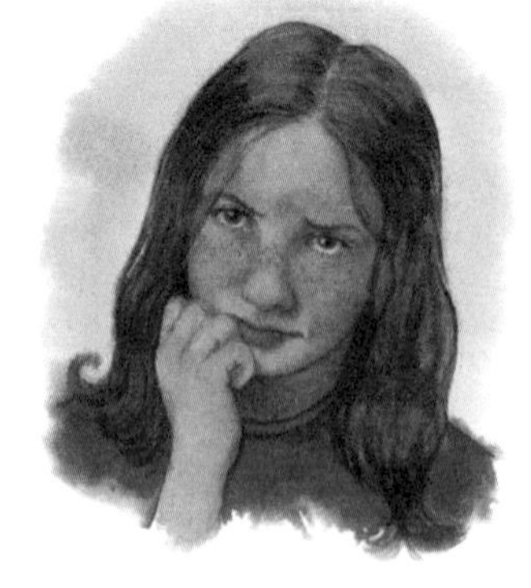

3. Angela has been asked to sing a solo for youth night at church. She has sung in the youth choir and performed duets with her older sister, but she has never sung alone. Even though she has done these things she has always gotten very nervous and felt shaky and scared. She is afraid if she sings alone she might get so scared that she'll forget the words or her voice will crack. What verse could her sister share with her to remind her not to use her fear of failure as an excuse for not serving God or praising Him with her voice?

____

____

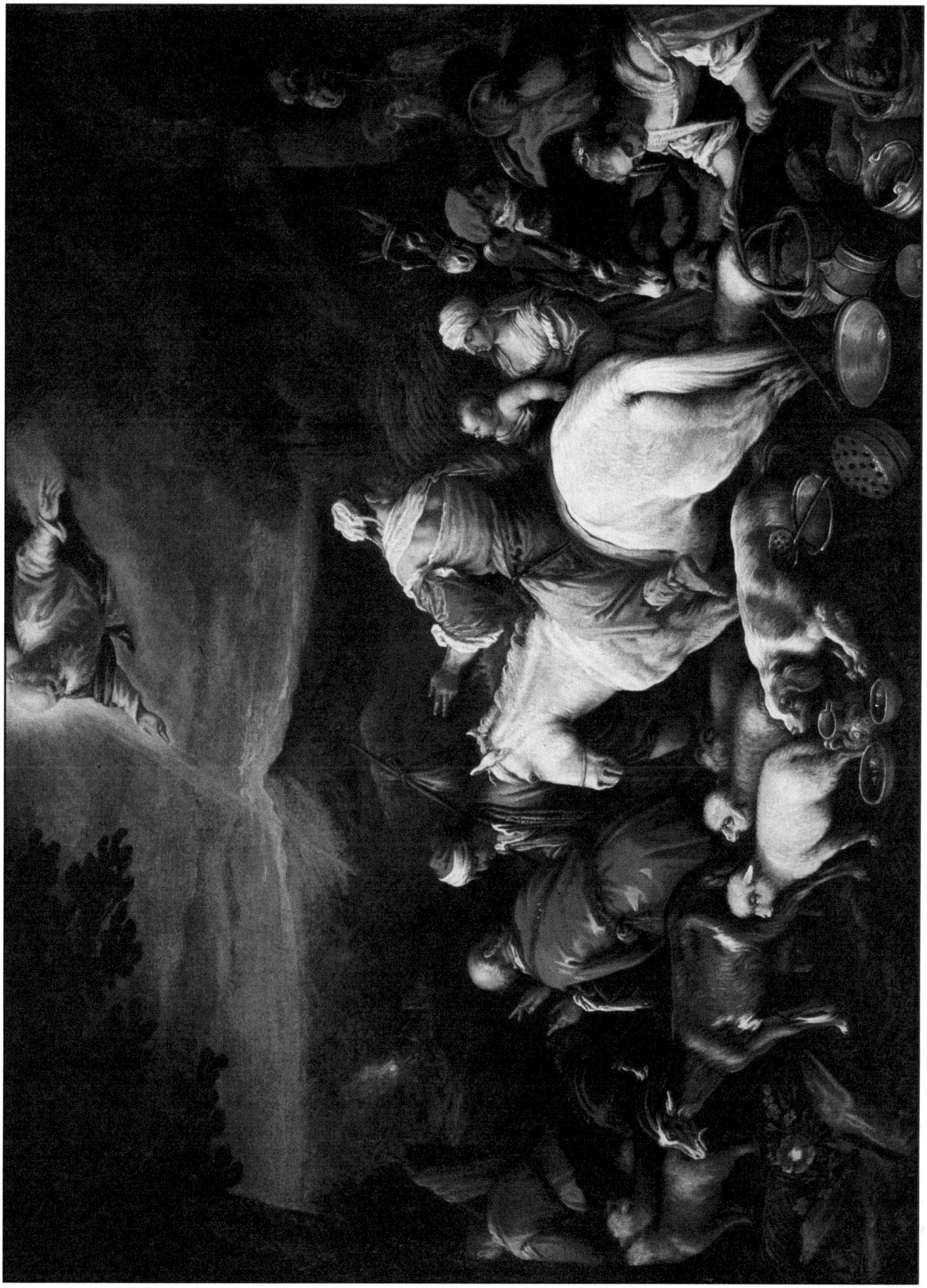

Preparing to Depart for Canaan

Leandro Bassano

Bob Jones University Museum & Gallery, Inc.

Name ______________________

Preparing to Depart for Canaan

by Leandro Bassano (1557-1622)

Leandro Bassano (Lā än′drō Bä sä′nō) was another artist from a family of artists. He and his brothers worked and studied with their father, Jacopo, who also studied with *his* father. When one of the brothers died suddenly, Leandro was left to complete several of his brother's paintings. By that time, Leandro was living in Venice, where it was easy to get commissions to paint portraits. Historical records show that Leandro Bassano was a member of an artist's guild in Venice in 1588. He painted portraits and worked for the doge, the ruler of Venice, who knighted Bassano in 1595.

In several ways, Leandro Bassano's paintings have the rustic style of his father's paintings. Jacopo painted a picture very similar to this one that Leandro copied at least twice. There are at least three other paintings almost identical to *Preparing to Depart for Canaan:* the original signed by Jacopo and his son Francesco; a copy made by an unknown artist, possibly another brother; and another version by Leandro. In each case, there are little variations in the details of the foreground, but the arrangement of the picture is almost identical.

Notice God in the sky, pointing the direction He wants the people to go.

There are at least six kinds of animals in the picture. Apparently Bassano was familiar with dogs, sheep, goats, and chickens, because he painted them realistically. He may even have had a goat in his studio to pose! No doubt he was familiar with horses too, but he apparently tried to draw the horse's head without looking at a real horse. Probably Bassano had never seen a camel and did not know exactly what one looked like, so he placed the camel in the far right of the picture, partially hidden by the edge of the painting.

The Ten Plagues of Egypt

Exodus 7-12

Name ______________________

> Many of the plagues showed God's power over the Egyptians' false gods.

Match the name of the plague with its description.

A. hail	B. boils	C. frogs	D. Nile turned to blood	E. darkness
F. lice or gnats	G. locusts	H. disease on cattle	I. death of firstborn	J. flies

_____ 1. The second plague was directed at Heqit, the Egyptian god of resurrection, sometimes pictured as a particular amphibian.

_____ 2. The ninth plague showed God's power over Ra, the Egyptian god of the sun and creation.

_____ 3. The fifth plague destroyed much of Egypt's livestock. It was possibly a judgment on the Egyptians for worship of Mnevis, one of several sacred bulls.

_____ 4. The seventh plague was a judgment against Min, the god of harvest.

_____ 5. The eighth plague was a judgment against Seth, protector of crops.

_____ 6. The first plague showed Hapi, god of the Nile, to be powerless.

_____ 7. This was the third plague and was the first one that could not be copied by the magicians of Egypt.

_____ 8. The sixth plague showed that Imhotep, the god of medicine, was powerless against the God of Israel.

_____ 9. The fourth plague fell on only the Egyptians.

_____ 10. The tenth and final plague showed God's power over Osiris, the ruler of the dead and granter of life.

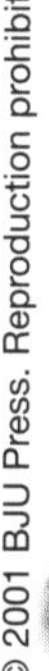

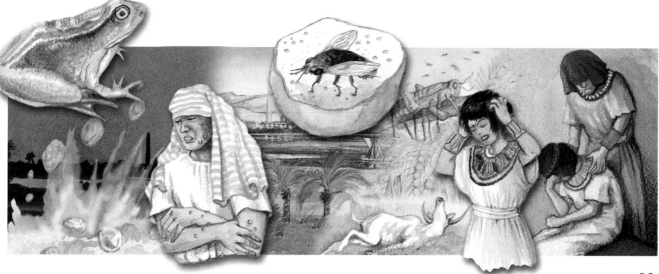

Under the Blood

Exodus 11:1–12:37

Name ______________________

When I See the Blood

Christ our Redeemer died on the cross,
Died for the sinner, paid all his due;
Sprinkle your soul with the blood of the Lamb,
And I will pass, will pass over you.

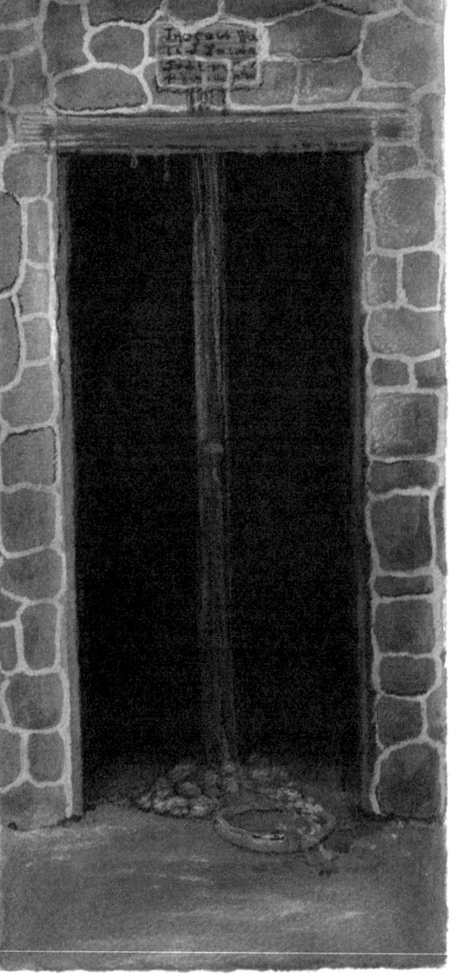

Complete the sentences. You may use your Bible for help.

1. The final plague would occur at ______________ (Ex. 11:4).
2. The people of Israel prepared for the plague by selecting a lamb and applying the blood to the door with a bunch of ______________ (Ex. 12:22).
3. If blood covered the doorway, the ______________ would pass over the house (Ex. 12:23).
4. When the tenth plague was over, every unbelieving house in Egypt had at least one ______________ (Ex. 12:30).
5. The special meal of roasted lamb and unleavened bread is in celebration of the Lord's ______________ (Ex. 12:11).
6. The death of the firstborn was God's ______________ on Egypt (Ex. 12:12).
7. When the Israelites left Egypt there were ________ hundred thousand men plus women and children (Ex. 12:37).

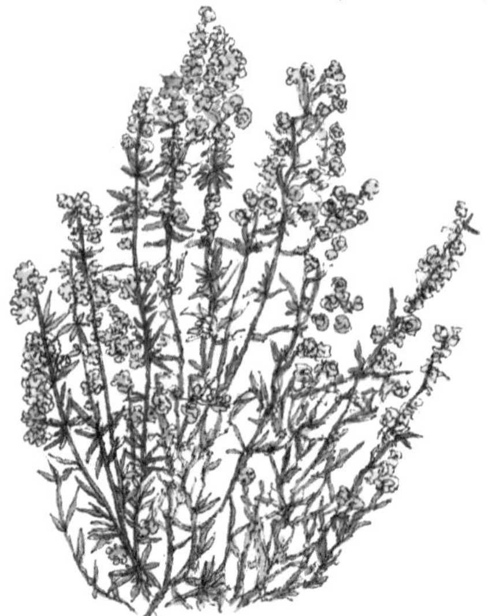

For Your ENLIGHTENMENT

The **hyssop** is a small, bushy plant that grew out of walls. Its clusters of tiny flowers made it a natural brush. It was used to sprinkle blood on the doorposts before the final plague on Egypt. It was also used in the purification ceremony from leprosy and other uncleanness. Hyssop showed that a covenant would be kept or that something was set apart to God.

What Does God Say About My Speech?

Name ____________________

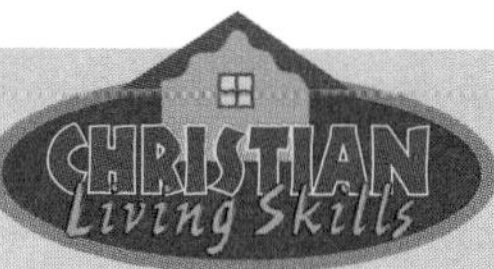
CHRISTIAN
Living Skills

The ability to speak is a wonderful gift from God. He designed our throats to produce sound when air passes over our vocal chords. Since we are uniquely created to speak to others, we are responsible to use this gift wisely. Christians should please God with this gift of speech.

King David wanted to please the Lord with the words of his mouth and with the meditations of his heart. God created you with the ability to communicate to others what is in your heart. What you *say* is a powerful tool that can be used for good or evil (Prov. 18:21).

Read the verses and match the references to the types of speech that displease God.

_____ 1. whispering or gossiping — A. Proverbs 10:18

_____ 2. harsh or angry words — B. Proverbs 11:13

_____ 3. lying lips and slander — C. Proverbs 15:1

_____ 4. talebearing or revealing secrets — D. Proverbs 16:28

Because of the many ways to misuse your gift of speech,
God gives instructions about how to control what you say.

Read the verses and write God's commands to you about controlling your speech.

Proverbs 17:27 ____________________

Proverbs 15:28 ____________________

I Corinthians 10:31 ____________________

Ephesians 4:15 ____________________

God gave us the gift of speech for many reasons. When we use our speech to glorify God, we receive God's blessing on our lives and give joy to others.

Read the verses and match the references to ways you can use your speech to please God.

1. _____ to pray without ceasing — A. Psalm 106:1
2. _____ to give thanks to God — B. Ephesians 4:29
3. _____ to tell people about Jesus — C. Acts 5:42
4. _____ to always tell the truth — D. I Thessalonians 5:17
5. _____ to edify and build up others — E. Ephesians 4:25

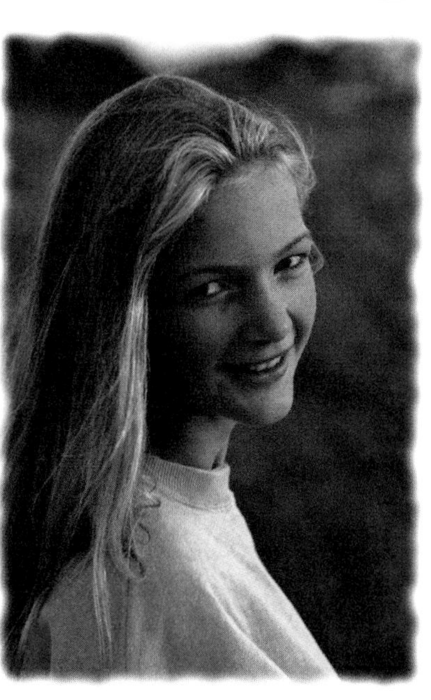

Something to Think About

My Speech

Name ______________________

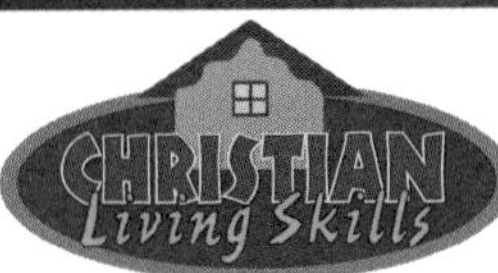
CHRISTIAN
Living Skills

Read the verses and write the reference of the verse that tells you what to do in each situation.

James 4:11 | Proverbs 12:25 | Ephesians 5:4

Scenario	Which verse applies?
Bobby has noticed that his dad seems worried about some problems at work. What can he do?	
When Janella walked into the room, several of the girls were talking about the strange clothes that Sharon wears. Then another girl mentioned the way Sharon fixes her hair. Everyone burst out laughing. What should Janella remember?	
Ben recently joined the soccer league and wants to fit in with the guys on the team, but they have a habit of telling dirty jokes and using bad words. What should Ben remember?	

What About Me?

Take time at home to think about your habits of speech. Answer each question by rating yourself on the scale.

Questions for Thought	Never ⟷			Always
1. Do I make it a habit to say things that are uplifting?	1	2	3	4
2. Do I know how to keep my mouth shut when I should?	1	2	3	4
3. Do I express appreciation for what other people do for me?	1	2	3	4
4. Do I always tell the truth no matter what?	1	2	3	4
5. Do I avoid gossiping about others?	1	2	3	4
6. Do I make only positive comments and avoid complaining?	1	2	3	4
7. Are the words I say and the jokes I tell pure and wholesome?	1	2	3	4
8. Do I speak kindly, even if I am frustrated about something?	1	2	3	4
9. Do I speak respectfully to my authorities?	1	2	3	4
10. Do I faithfully talk about the goodness of God with others?	1	2	3	4

Evaluate the words you have spoken today as you think about these questions.

Have I thanked God today for His goodness to me?

Would my parents say that God is pleased with the way I use my speech?

Do my friends know that I love God because of the words I spoke today?

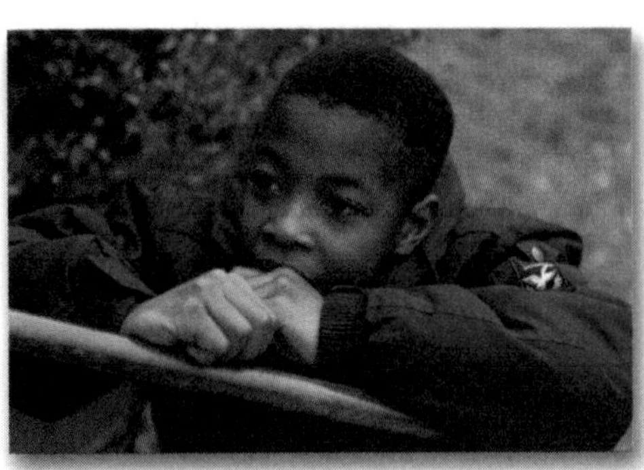

The Ten Commandments

Exodus 20:3-17

Name ______________________

Number the commandments in the order God gave them to Moses. (Remember that some commandments deal with man's attitudes and actions toward God and others deal with man's attitudes and actions toward other people.) Match each commandment to its teaching. You may use pages 383-385 for help.

Commandment	Teaches	
____	____	Remember the sabbath day, to keep it holy.
____	____	Thou shalt have no other gods before me.
____	____	Thou shalt not make unto thee any graven image, or any likeness of any thing that is in heaven above, or that is in the earth beneath, or that is in the water under the earth.
____	____	Thou shalt not commit adultery.
____	____	Honour thy father and thy mother: that thy days may be long upon the land which the Lord thy God giveth thee.
____	____	Thou shalt not covet thy neighbor's house, thou shalt not covet thy neighbor's wife, nor his manservant, nor his maidservant, nor his ox, nor his ass, nor any thing that is thy neighbor's.
____	____	Thou shalt not take the name of the Lord thy God in vain; for the Lord will not hold him guiltless that taketh his name in vain.
____	____	Thou shalt not kill.
____	____	Thou shalt not bear false witness against thy neighbor.
____	____	Thou shalt not steal.

A. Worship God in a proper manner and avoid idolatry.

B. Tell the truth.

C. Respect the property of others and be honest and industrious.

D. One day of the week is God's special day.

E. Avoid anger and injury to others.

F. Be pure in heart, language, and conduct.

G. Be content with what you have.

H. Worship God alone.

I. Reverence God's name, Word, and works.

J. God blesses those who love and obey their parents.

What name for the Ten Commandments means "Ten Words?"

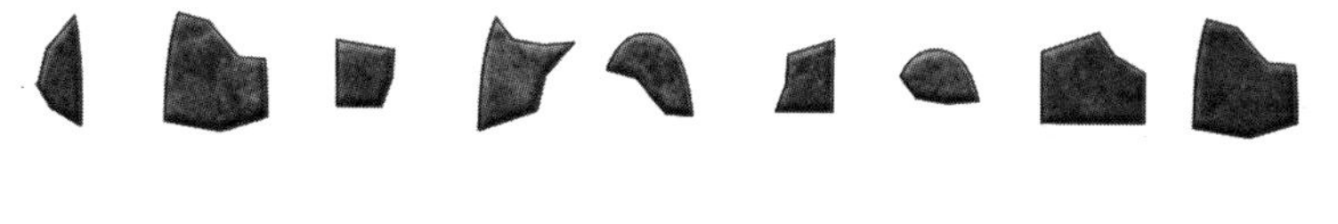

___ ___ ___ ___ ___ ___ ___ ___ ___

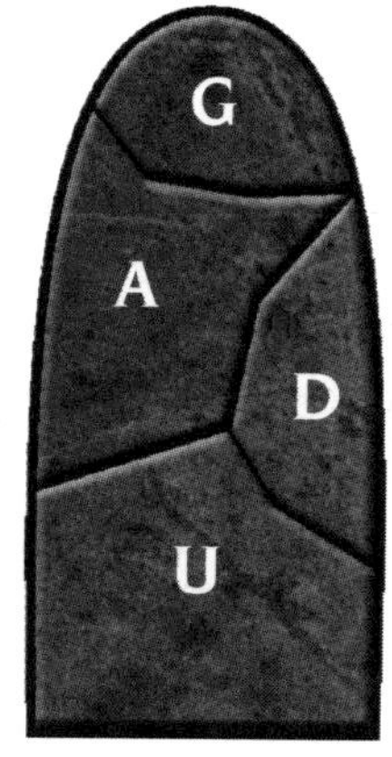
G
A
D
U

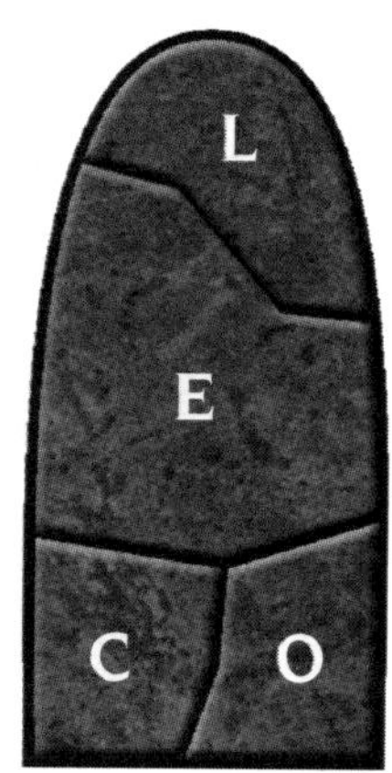
L
E
C
O

The Greatest Commandment

Name ____________________

Read Matthew 22:36-40; then complete the statements so that the equations are true.

1. Love God with all your ____________, ____________, and ____________ = the first and greatest commandment.
2. Love God > love your ____________________ as yourself.

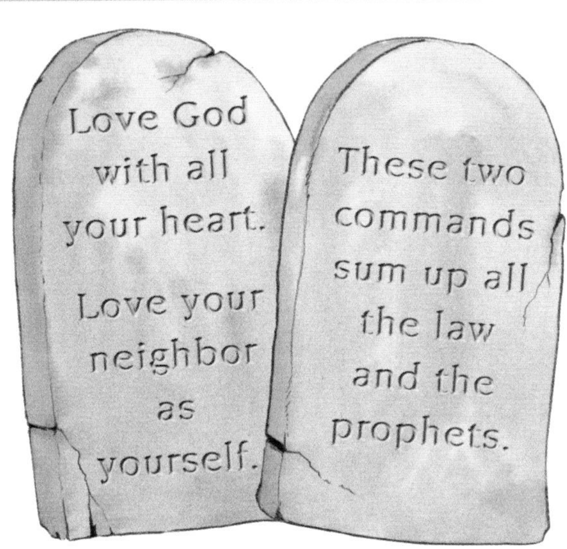
Love God with all your heart.
Love your neighbor as yourself.
These two commands sum up all the law and the prophets.

Read Romans 13:9-10; then complete the statement so that the equation is true.

3. Loving your neighbor as yourself =

   not ____________________ + not committing murder + not ____________ + not ____________ + not bearing false witness.

Shade the heart that answers the question.

	yes	no
4. If you love God with all your heart, will you worship idols?	♡	♡
5. If you love God with all your heart, will you use His name carelessly?	♡	♡
6. If you love your neighbor as God wants you to, will you covet?	♡	♡
7. If you love your neighbor as God wants you to, will you steal?	♡	♡
8. If you love your neighbor as God wants you to, will you murder?	♡	♡

9. How does loving God and loving your neighbor sum up all the other commandments?

   ____

   ____

10. How can you show love to God and others today?

   ____

   ____

A New Covenant

Name ______________________________

Covenant—A *promise or an agreement between two or more persons.*
Divine Covenant—A *promise between God and man.*

Match the description with the correct covenant.

A. Davidic
B. Adamic
C. New Testament
D. Mosaic
E. Abrahamic
F. Noachian

_____ 1. Moses was a picture of Christ's work of salvation. The Law reveals the conditions Christ would fulfill, and its ceremonies and sacrifices reveal what Christ would do in presenting Himself as an offering for sin (Exod. 34:10-27).

_____ 2. God made a covenant with David that God's promised Son would come from David's royal line of succession (Ps. 89:3-4).

_____ 3. This covenant was made between God and Adam when Adam was driven from the garden of Eden. God promised to send a Redeemer (Gen. 3:15; I Cor. 15:45-47).

_____ 4. God promised Noah that He would never again destroy the earth with a flood (Gen. 9:8-17).

_____ 5. God promised to make Abraham's descendants a great nation. These would be God's chosen people. The Messiah would be born of this nation. God also promised to give them the land of Canaan (Gen. 12:1-3; 17:1-8).

_____ 6. This is the new covenant. The Old Testament covenants foreshadowed what was to come. The birth of the Messiah, His death on the cross, and His resurrection from the tomb fulfilled the Old Testament covenants, bringing about the end of the law and the beginning of grace (Acts 4:12; I Cor. 11:23-26).

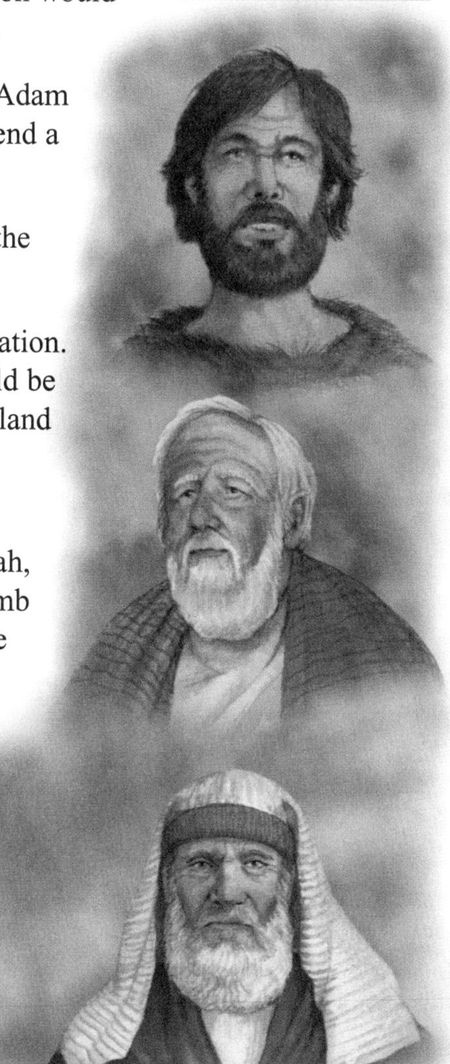

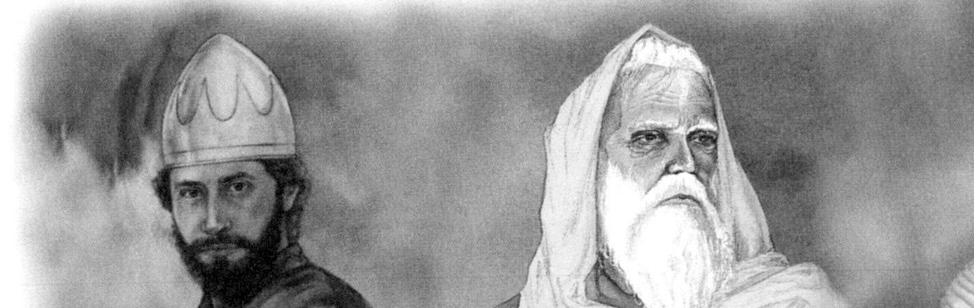

Read Romans 6:14 and complete the sentence.

7. Since Christ's death and resurrection, man is no longer obligated to keep ceremonial law, which was fulfilled by Christ. Instead man

receives God's ______________________ .

The Law Brings Us to Christ

Name ______________________

Complete the sentences. You may use your Bible for help.

1. How do we know what sin is? The __________ teaches us to recognize sin (Rom. 7:7).
2. A lawbreaker has to break only __________ law (James 2:10).
3. In Old Testament times, people offered sacrifices to show their faith. It was a picture of the sacrifice for sins that Jesus would make of Himself. These Old Testament sacrifices had no power to take away __________ (Heb. 10:4).
4. The law could not set us free from sin, but God sent His own __________ who could set us free from sin and death (Rom. 8:1-3).
5. Rather than admit their sinfulness and helplessness, some go about trying to prove their own ________________ instead of accepting the righteousness of God through Christ, who fulfilled the law (Rom. 10:3-4).
6. While we cannot keep the law to save ourselves, we can become the children of __________ by faith in Jesus, who can give us His righteousness (John 1:12, 17).

Read Galatians 3:24. Circle the word that best tells the purpose of the law.

The law is our ________________ to lead us to ________________

teacher friend doctor heaven Christ church

that we might be justified by ________________.

good deeds faith the law

Read each situation below. If the person is trying to establish his own righteousness, draw a frowning face in the circle. If the person is showing his salvation by his works of righteousness, draw a smiling face.

Richard donates his old clothes to a local charity organization at the beginning of each school year. The charity also receives his old toys each Christmas. Richard carefully inspects each item he donates to make sure it is in good condition. It makes Richard feel good to know that children will have nice things because of his generosity. Richard's neighbor Ken has asked him to come hear the special speaker at summer Bible school, but Richard doesn't feel like going. "I'm already a good kid like Ken. I don't need to go to church more than usual," reasons Richard. ◯

Mr. Adams is a mechanic and owns a small auto repair shop. Last month he repaired the church bus so that it ran smoothly during vacation Bible school. He is faithful to check the oil and make sure the bus is running properly for Sunday School outings and trips to camp. Although Mr. Adams's shop isn't open on Sundays, he has helped many families in the church with emergencies. Last Sunday, he repaired Mrs. Reed's flat tire while she was in choir practice. "Helping people get to and from church to share or hear the Word of God is just a small way I can serve God," says Mr. Adams. ◯

What Does God Say About Being Patient?

Name ______________________________

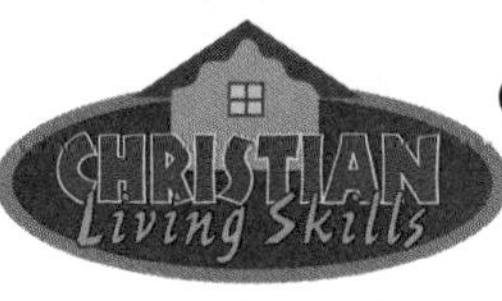
CHRISTIAN
Living Skills

Our world moves at a fast pace. God has allowed us to discover the technology to communicate instantly with people around the globe. While advances in technology give us more independence and control of our time, God is still ultimately in charge of every event in our lives. His timetable can not and will not be rushed or manipulated by human technology. He is our Creator. We are the workmanship of His hands.

As we become accustomed to instant answers from the Internet, we must guard against being tempted to demand instant answers from God.

God reminds us over and over again in His Word that true joy comes from trusting in His care, believing in His promises, resting in His presence, and waiting for His answers. When you begin to understand the unchangeable character of God, you will realize that God will always keep His promises on time.

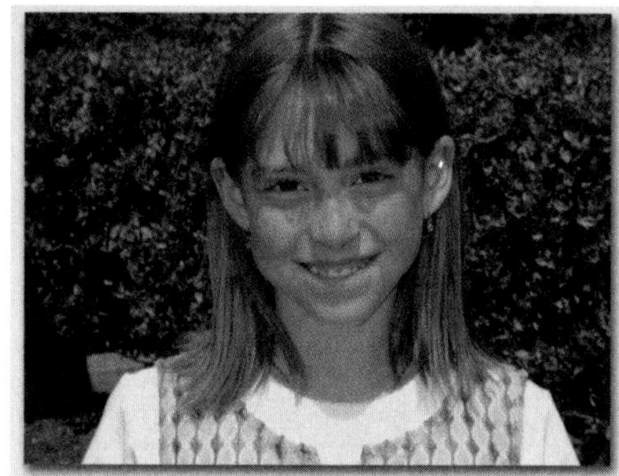

Read the verses and write the promises God gives to His children.

Philippians 1:6 ______________________________

I Peter 5:7 ______________________________

I Peter 3:12 ______________________________

Psalm 29:11 ______________________________

Fighting the temptation to be impatient is a common battle among God's children. God's Word is filled with encouragement to us about waiting patiently on God and His timing.

Match each verse with its correct summary.

_____ Galatians 6:9

_____ Psalm 27:14

_____ Hosea 12:6

A. Wait on the Lord; He will give strength to your heart.
B. Don't get weary in doing what is good; God will reward you.
C. Turn to God; love justice; wait on God continually.

PATIENCE

Something to Think About

Being Patient

Name ______________________

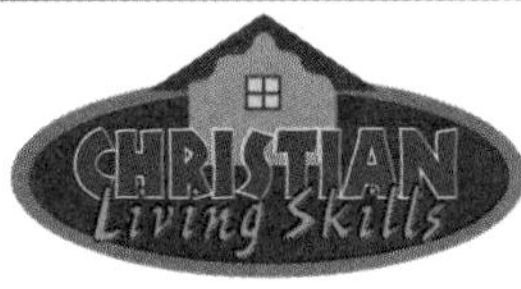
CHRISTIAN
Living Skills

When things do not go as you planned and you have to wait for something you want, you will be tempted to become impatient. Be careful to recognize impatience for what it is and ask God for help in fighting this temptation.

Read and compare each step of the definitions. Use the chart to answer the questions.

Impatience is . . .	Patience is . . .
1. the frustration of not getting what I want.	1. the calm reaction to delay, hardship, or trouble.
2. making my plans more important than the plans of others—even God's.	2. realizing that God's plans are perfect and superior to my own.
3. my sinful heart trying to control what is not mine to control.	3. my heart fully surrendered to the fact that God is in control and I'm not.
4. the irritation that comes from trying to be in control of my own life.	4. the joy of recognizing my position beneath the control of God.

Questions for Thought

1. What do you think is meant by *impatience?*

____

2. Why is it unwise to place my plans ahead of God's plans for me?

____

What About Me?

When are you most tempted to be impatient? Is it waiting on your mom to fix your dinner? Is it when you wait in line for something? Is it waiting on God to answer a specific prayer? Your sinful heart deceives you into blaming others for not giving you what you want when you want.

BEWARE!

Put a warning flag up when you feel yourself becoming irritated with someone else because you are being required to wait. Confess your selfish attitude, submit to God's timetable, and adjust your thinking. **Remember: Learning to be patient will bring you great joy!**

Take time at home to think about your reactions. Complete the following statements.

I am most tempted to be impatient when ______________________________.

One thing I can do to become more patient is ______________________________.

The next time I am tempted to be impatient, I will ______________________________.

The Place of Dwelling

Exodus 25-30

Name ______________________

The tabernacle was God's dwelling place while the Israelites were in the wilderness and later while they were in Canaan until the temple was built. God gave very specific instructions for how the tabernacle was to be built and furnished. The priests were required to be clean inwardly and outwardly according to God's laws when they came into God's presence.

Match each picture to what it symbolizes.

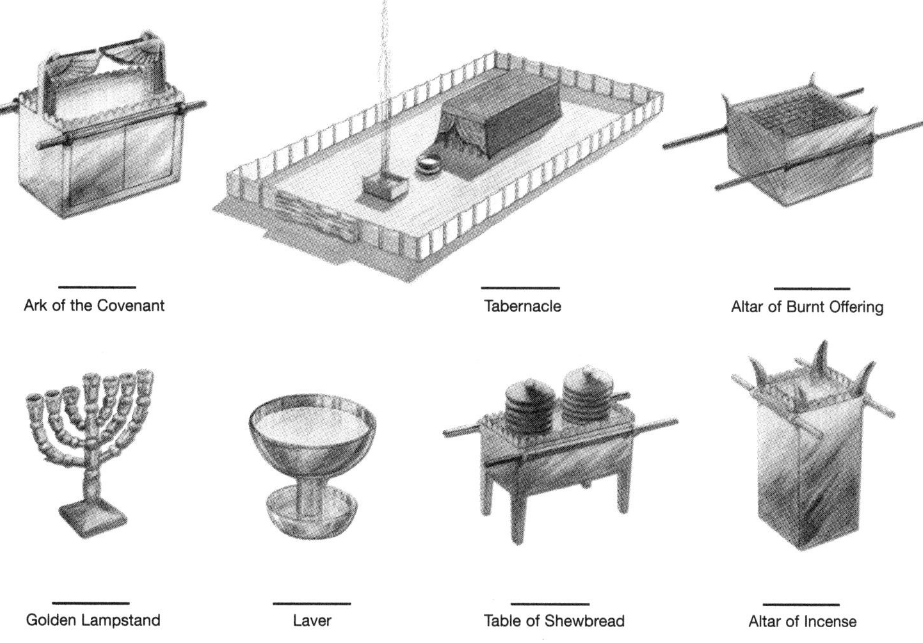

____ Ark of the Covenant

____ Tabernacle

____ Altar of Burnt Offering

____ Golden Lampstand

____ Laver

____ Table of Shewbread

____ Altar of Incense

A. Christ is the true light.

B. Christ, the Bread of Life, supplies all their needs.

C. Christ can wash away their sins.

D. God hears their prayers.

E. God promises His covenant to Israel.

F. God dwells with them.

G. Christ, the Lamb of God, is the final sacrifice.

Since there is no longer a tabernacle in which God dwells, where is His place of dwelling now?

Read the verses and complete the sentences.

I Corinthians 3:16 Christians are the ______________________ of God, and His ______________________ dwells in them.

I Peter 1:15-16 God is holy, and He expects Christians to be ______________________.

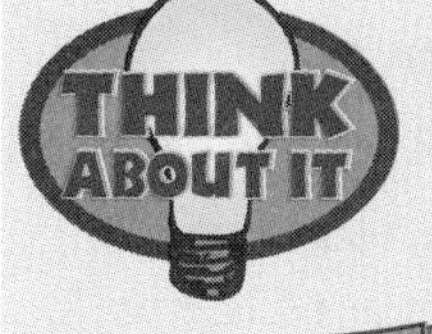
THINK
ABOUT IT

IF your body is God's temple, and

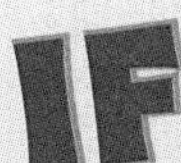
IF

the Spirit of God dwells in you, and

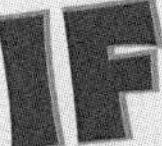
IF

Jesus bought you with His own blood,

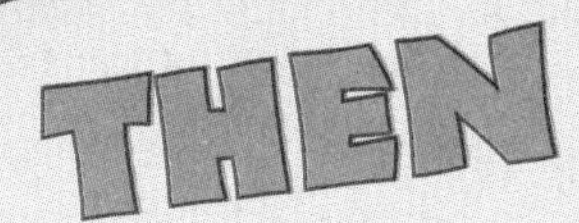
THEN

the only reasonable thing to do is to glorify and honor God with your body by holy living. It is only reasonable to serve and worship the Lord as a living sacrifice for Him (Rom. 12:1).

Our High Priest

Hebrews 2-10

Name ______________________

The Levites were set apart to be the priestly tribe. Aaron was appointed by God as the first high priest. Aaron's descendants were to be the spiritual leaders of the Israelites. They maintained the tabernacle and its furnishings. Christ, the only High Priest without sin, offered the only perfect sacrifice to atone for the sins of all mankind.

If the statement agrees with Scripture, color the jewel in the *True* column. If the statement does not agree with Scripture, color the jewel in the *False* column.

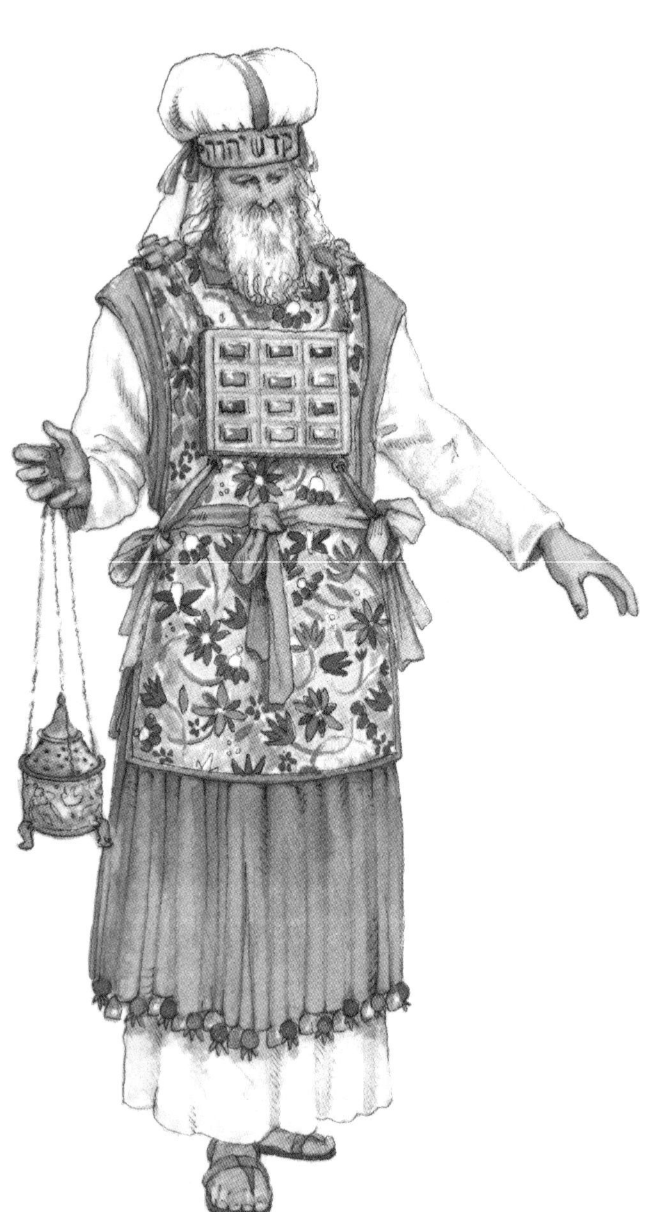

True	False	
◇	◇	1. Our High Priest is merciful and faithful (Heb. 2:17).
◇	◇	2. Jesus is our High Priest (Heb. 3:1).
◇	◇	3. Our High Priest is here on earth (Heb. 4:14).
◇	◇	4. Our High Priest was never tempted to sin (Heb. 4:15).
◇	◇	5. Our High Priest was tempted just as we are (Heb. 4:15).
◇	◇	6. Jesus' priesthood is a permanent position because He will never die (Heb. 7:23-25).
◇	◇	7. It wasn't necessary for Jesus to offer Himself as a sacrifice (Heb. 8:3).
◇	◇	8. Our High Priest is in heaven in the presence of God (Heb. 9:24).
◇	◇	9. Our High Priest made only one sacrifice (Heb. 9:25-28).
◇	◇	10. Our High Priest's sacrifice is able to take away sins (Heb. 10:11-12,14).
◇	◇	11. We can approach God directly because of the way provided by Jesus (Heb. 10:18-22).

What Does God Say About My Temple?

Honoring God in My Body

Name ______________________________

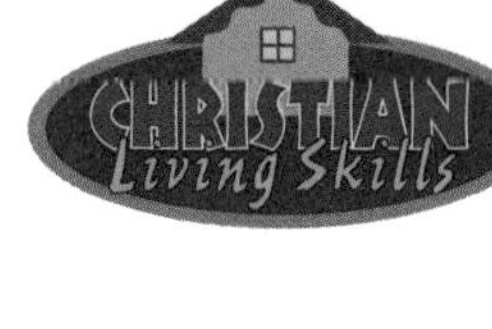

CHRISTIAN
Living Skills

Genesis 1 records the order and perfect design of creation. God spoke this world into existence and then pronounced it good. However, God had a special plan in creating men and women. He wants us to have personal fellowship with Him. This close fellowship with God is a gift that plants and animals have not been given. God created mankind with the ability and desire to communicate with Him.

Read Genesis 1:26-27 and answer the questions.

1. In whose image was man created? ______________________________
2. List five areas of creation over which God gave man authority.

   a. ______________________ b. ______________________

   c. ______________________ d. ______________________

   e. ______________________________

3. What do you think it means to be created in the image of God?

   ____

   ____

When Adam and Eve sinned by rebelling against God, the close fellowship they had with God was destroyed. Thankfully, God sent His Son, Jesus Christ, to pay the penalty for our sins so that we could once again have fellowship with Him. After Jesus' death, burial, resurrection, and ascension, God sent His Holy Spirit to dwell in the hearts of all who believe in Him.

Read I Corinthians 6:19-20 and fill in the blanks.

My ______________ is the temple of the ____________ ____________.

I am not my ______________. I have been ______________ with a price.

Therefore, I must ______________ God in the way I take care of my body.

List several ways you can take good care of your temple. Keep in mind that you are created in the image of God.

1. ______________________________
2. ______________________________
3. ______________________________

Something to Think About

Honoring God in My Body

Name ______________________

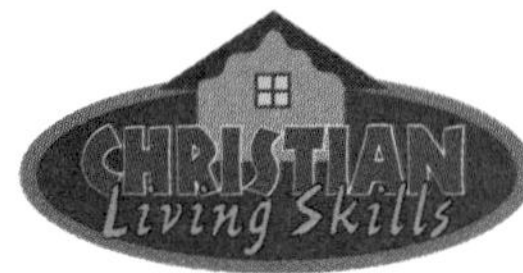
CHRISTIAN
Living Skills

As a Christian, your body is not your own. You are the caretaker of the temple of the Holy Spirit. This means you hold a serious responsibility of protecting and maintaining the health of your body. This responsibility also means that you must keep your body in the best possible condition so that you are free to be an active and useful servant for Christ.

Read Romans 12:1. Fill in the blanks.

I should present or offer my body to ____________ as a living ______________.

My body should be ____________ and ______________________________________ to God.

Several keys to developing and maintaining a healthy body include receiving the proper amount of sleep, getting the proper amount of exercise, and eating the proper amount of healthy food. The Bible teaches us about these three key areas, but also gives warnings for anyone who lacks **self-discipline.**

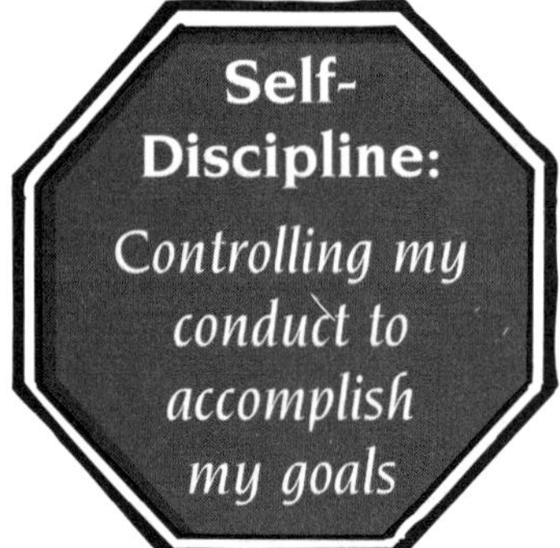
Self-Discipline:
Controlling my conduct to accomplish my goals

Read the verses. Write the sin to which a lack of self-discipline in each issue will lead.

Health Issue	Reference	A Lack of Self-Discipline Will Lead to …
Eating the right types and amount of food	Proverbs 23:19-21	
Receiving the right amount of sleep	Proverbs 20:13; 6:9-11	

WARNING:

Going to the extreme in any area is usually harmful to your body. Too much exercise is dangerous and can cause your focus to be on yourself instead of on glorifying God.

What About Me?

Take the time at home to evaluate the health habits you have established.

- ✔ Am I making healthy choices about what I eat?
- ✔ Am I getting enough sleep each night so that I can concentrate on my work each day?
- ✔ Do I spend time exercising to increase my energy?
- ✔ Is God pleased with the current condition of my body?
- ✔ Do I treat my body like it is a true temple of the Holy Spirit?

Choose one area in which you need to develop self-discipline. Complete the statements by writing out your commitment to God to work on this area.

I need to develop self-discipline in ______________________________________.

To do this, I will ______________________________________.

Tithes and Offerings

I Chronicles 16:29

Name ______________________

Put the phrases in order to write I Chronicles 16:29. Not all the coins will be used.

and in

Give unto the Lord

the beauty of holiness

bring an offering

holiness

a tithe

and come before Him

unto His name

the glory due

unto God

holy array.

worship the Lord in

the splendor of his

His name

Ascribe to the Lord

____

____

Read Psalm 96:8-9*a* and answer the questions.

1. What do you notice about these two passages? ______________________
2. Is worshiping the Lord with tithes and offerings important in service to God? ________

Read each verse and circle the correct answer.

Proverbs 3:9

1. When Christians give to God of their wealth and material possessions, they give Him _____.
   riches honor blessings
2. Christians should give God their offering _______.
   first after their needs are met whenever they have money left over

Genesis 28:22

3. This example of giving a tithe to the Lord is a _______.
   token tenth trade

II Corinthians 9:7

4. Giving should be _______.
   a public show only during prosperity purposed in a Christian's heart
5. Christians should give because _______.
   it's expected they love and obey God they expect to gain something

Giving to God

Name ____________________

Answer the questions. You may use your Bible for help.

Genesis 14:18-20
1. Which priest did Abraham give a tithe to? ____________________

Hebrews 7:1-2
2. How much did Abraham give to him? ____________________

Mark 12:42-44
3. Why did Jesus say the widow's offering was greater than that of the rich?

____

II Corinthians 9:7
4. Is God more concerned with how much is given or with the attitude of the giver?

____

Read each problem and determine the amount that each person should tithe.

Kendra's dad gives her a \$5.00 allowance every payday. She plans to put her tithe in the offering plate on Sunday morning. What is Kendra's tithe?

0.1 × \$5.00 = \$________

A **tithe** *is a tenth of someone's total income.*

To find 1/10 *of a number, multiply by* 0.1.

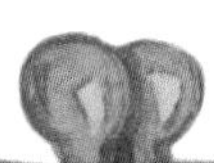

Every Tuesday during the summer, from 9:00-10:00, Carly's mother has a Bible study with the ladies of the neighborhood. Carly watches the smaller children in the backyard and plays games with them. Her mother pays her \$0.50 for each child. Last Tuesday she watched three children. What is Carly's tithe?

0.1 × \$________ **= \$**________

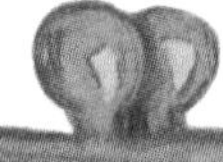

Devon earned \$15.00 for mowing and trimming the neighbor's lawn. He also earned \$5.00 for watering the lawn and picking up the mail while she was out of town. Devon plans to save half of the money he earned for summer Bible camp. What is Devon's tithe?

0.1 × \$________ **= \$**________

Singing with Understanding

"When I See the Blood" (vv. 1-4)

Name ______________________

The Passover as a Symbol

The Passover was a symbol of Christ's work on the cross. Just as the Passover brought the Israelites deliverance from bondage in Egypt, so Christ's work on the cross brings deliverance from sin and its penalty. The hymn "When I See the Blood" draws several parallels between the cross and the Passover.

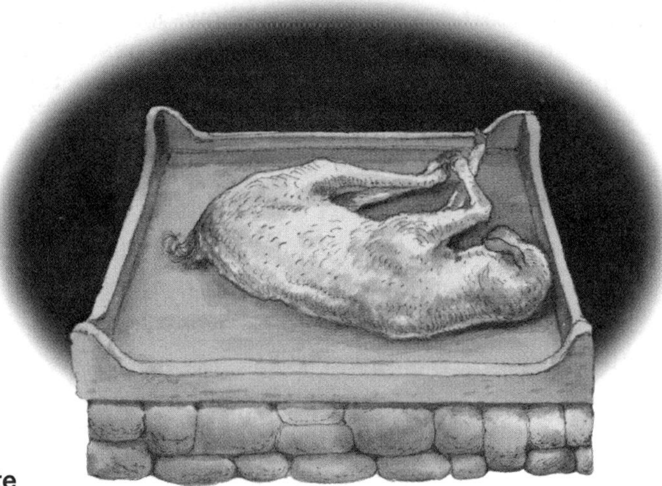

Use verses 1-3 of the hymn on page 313 to complete the sentences about Christ's work on the cross.

The Passover	Christ's Work on the Cross
An unblemished lamb had to die before the Passover meal could be eaten.	Christ, the unblemished ______________, had to die to accomplish our redemption.
When the Passover lamb died, its blood was sprinkled on the top and side doorposts of the house.	______________'s blood is sprinkled on the soul of a sinner who calls on Him for salvation.
When judgment time came, God passed over the homes that had the blood on them.	When ______________ comes, God will pass over the souls that have had Christ's blood applied to them by faith.
During the Passover, the Israelites could "hide" behind the blood and be saved from the terrible tenth plague.	We too can ______________ in the sin-cleansing blood of Christ and be saved from a terrible eternity in hell.

Read verse 4 of the hymn on page 313 and notice the qualities of God. Read the Scripture passages and draw a line matching them to the correct quality.

Psalm 36:7	Compassion or Mercy
Psalm 145:8	Faithfulness and Truth
Ephesians 2:14	Peace
Revelation 19:11	Lovingkindness or Love

My Body, God's Temple

I Corinthians 6:19-20

Name ____________________

Color the heart red if the action shows someone who is honoring God with their body and protecting their heart. Write the reference of the verse that might help him overcome this temptation.

Dominic just moved to a new neighborhood and made friends with Tyler, who lives down the street. Dominic and Tyler both like soccer and baseball, and they both enjoy playing computer games. Tyler's computer has Internet access, and he wants Dominic to come over to surf the Net with him. Dominic knows he's only allowed to get on the Internet with his parents because their computer has an Internet filter. Dominic also knows Tyler's computer doesn't have a filter and that Tyler has found Internet sites that don't please Jesus. "Come surf the Net at my house," Dominic says. "My parents can help us find some good sites on our computer."

Is Dominic being careful to guard his heart? What verse might help Dominic?

____

Gina's aunt and uncle invited her for a visit. Gina's cousins don't know the Lord, and Gina's parents want her to be a good testimony to them. When Gina last stayed with her relatives, she discovered that her oldest cousin had started smoking. Gina has worried about what to say if Stacy offers to let her try one. She wants her cousins to think she's cool, but she knows smoking cigarettes is harmful to her lungs. After asking God for the courage to do the right thing, Gina decides to say "no" if Stacy asks her to try a cigarette.

Is Gina trying to honor God with her body? What verse might help Gina?

____

Daniel 1:8*a* Isaiah 42:5-6 Psalm 101:3 I Timothy 4:12

Maria's mom let her spend Saturday afternoon at Melissa's house with several girls. Melissa's older sister let them make pizza for lunch. As Maria was getting the cheese out for the pizza, she noticed several bottles of beer on the bottom shelf. Later, when the pizzas were ready and her sister wasn't around, Melissa opened a bottle of beer, took a sip, and dared the other girls to try it. Maria knows that alcohol can have a harmful effect on the body and that damaging her body would not please God. Maria decided to call her mom to come pick her up.

Is Maria trying to honor God with her body? What verse might help Maria?

____

Daryl is spending the night at Rick's house. Rick's parents had to take a neighbor lady to the hospital, so Rick's high-school brother Phil is in charge while the adults are gone. Phil and Rick want to watch a program on TV that Daryl knows his parents don't approve of. Daryl doesn't want his friend to think he's a baby, so he watches the program with them. Although what he is seeing and hearing is offensive and bothers him, he doesn't say anything because they might laugh at him. Maybe Rick won't even invite him back if he says something. "I'll just keep quiet," Daryl thinks. "As long as I don't watch it all the time I'll be okay."

Is Daryl being careful to guard his heart? What verse might help Daryl?

____

Name ______________________

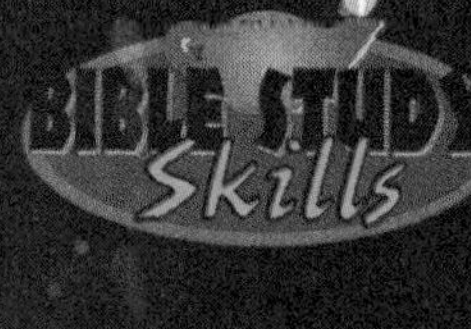
BIBLE STUDY
Skills

As you read the Scripture for each day, write the date in the box.

Have a special time each day set aside to read your Bible. If possible, make it the same time every day.

Ask God to teach you from His Word. Remember to thank Him for helping you to understand and apply it.

Be still and give your attention to what you are reading.

Investigate the Scripture by asking yourself questions about it.

Take time to look up words and ideas you do not understand.

CHRIST, the Promised One

☐ Jesus is the exact image of God the Father's nature and glory. **Hebrews 1:1-3**

☐ Jesus is above the angels because He is God's Son. **Hebrews 1:4-5**

☐ At Jesus' birth, God commanded the angels to worship Him. **Hebrews 1:6-7**

☐ God sent Jesus to redeem us that we might be adopted as His sons. **Galatians 4:4-5**

☐ He gave us His Spirit to testify that we are His sons and heirs. **Galatians 4:6-7**

CHRIST, the Key to the Prophecies

☐ All Scripture is inspired by God and teaches us. **II Timothy 3:16-17**

☐ All true Christians confess that Jesus Christ has come in the flesh. **I John 4:1-3**

☐ Jesus' coming fulfilled the inspired words of the prophets. **II Peter 1:19-21**

☐ Jesus came that we might know the true God and have eternal life. **I John 5:18-20**

☐ God manifested His love by sending His only Son into the world for us. **I John 4:7-9**

Bible Study Methods

Analysis

Name ______________________

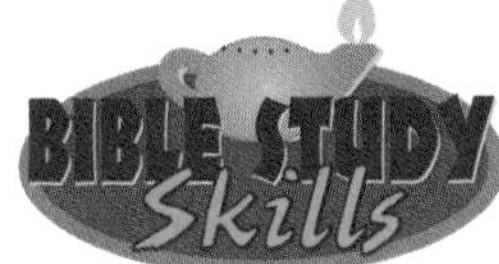

While the *synthetic* method of Bible study looks at the Bible as a whole, *analytical* Bible study closely examines everything possible about a book, passage, or chapter. Commentaries, cross-references, concordances, Bible dictionaries, and Bible encyclopedias are useful tools for analytical Bible study.

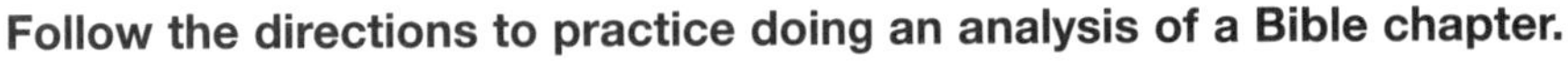

Follow the directions to practice doing an analysis of a Bible chapter.

1. Choose a chapter in the New Testament. Write the reference.

   ____

2. Read questions 3-9, and then read the chapter several times. Put an X here for each time you read it.

   ___ ___ ___ ___ ___

3. Briefly state the main idea of the chapter.

   ____

4. What subjects or doctrines are stated/explained in the chapter? ______________________________

   ____

   ____

   ____

5. Whom did the Holy Spirit inspire to write the chapter? ______________________________

6. Where and when was it written? ______________________________

7. What people are mentioned? ______________________________

8. What places are mentioned? ______________________________

   ____

9. Write any unfamiliar words and find their meanings. ______________________________

   ____

   ____

Royal Heritage

Matthew 1:1-17; Luke 3:23-38

Name ____________________________

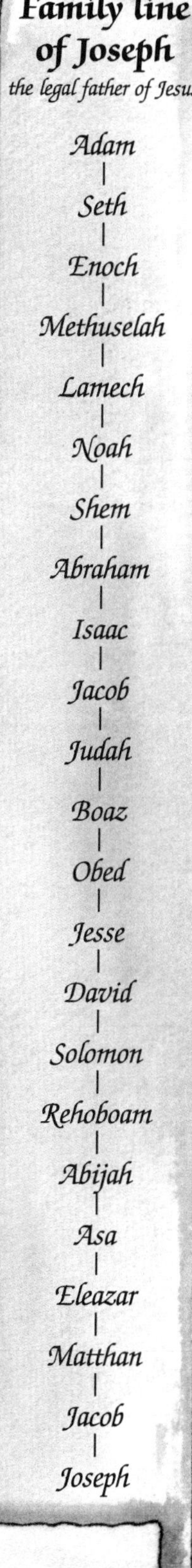

Family line of Joseph
the legal father of Jesus
Adam
Seth
Enoch
Methuselah
Lamech
Noah
Shem
Abraham
Isaac
Jacob
Judah
Boaz
Obed
Jesse
David
Solomon
Rehoboam
Abijah
Asa
Eleazar
Matthan
Jacob
Joseph

Family and heritage have always been important to the Jewish people. A clear family line was necessary to prove that a person was a descendant of Abraham. As a descendant of Abraham, the person could claim to be part of the covenant God made with Abraham.

Both Matthew and Luke record the lineage of Christ to show that He was a true descendant of Abraham and David. Joseph was Christ's legal father. Matthew shows the royal ancestry of Christ, proving Him a descendant of both Abraham and David. Luke gives the line of relationships through Mary's family background to Adam. By doing this, Luke showed the Jews and the Gentiles that Christ came to earth for all men.

Throughout history, God made promises that only the true Messiah could fulfill.

Use the family lines of Jesus' parents to complete the sentences. (*Note:* Not all generations are included in the lists.)

1. At the Fall of man in the Garden of Eden, God promised ____________________ that his seed would have victory over Satan (Gen. 3:15).

2. Christ is a descendant of ____________________, which shows us that God kept His promise of never again destroying the earth with a flood (Gen. 9:8-17).

3. God promised ____________________ that Sarah would have a son, and a great nation would be established through whom all nations would be blessed (Gen. 17:15-19).

4. Through a prophet, God told ________________ that the throne of his kingdom would be established through his descendants forever. Christ, the King of Kings, will reign forever. As a descendant of David, Christ fulfills this prophecy (II Sam. 7:12-16).

5. The family lines differ at ____________________ and ____________________, both sons of David.

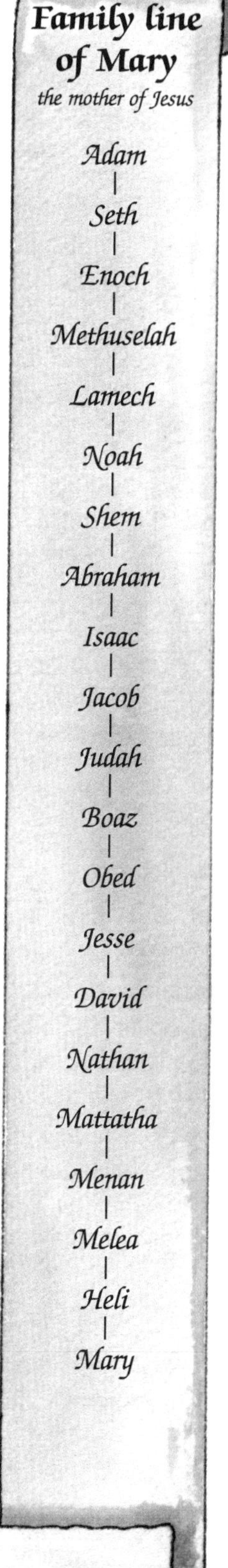

Family line of Mary
the mother of Jesus
Adam
Seth
Enoch
Methuselah
Lamech
Noah
Shem
Abraham
Isaac
Jacob
Judah
Boaz
Obed
Jesse
David
Nathan
Mattatha
Menan
Melea
Heli
Mary

Prepared for the Promise

Luke 1:26-35, Matthew 1:18-25

Name ____________________

Imagine Mary's surprise when Gabriel appeared to her. Using Old Testament prophecies, Gabriel described the Son that would be born to her (Luke 1:32-33). During and after Christ's ministry, these prophecies were fulfilled as Christ was recognized by these same descriptions.

Answer the questions. You may use your Bible for help.

1. What was Mary's reaction to Gabriel? (Luke 1:29)

____

2. How did Gabriel comfort Mary? (Luke 1:30)

____

Write the letter of the reference next to the description given to Mary by Gabriel.

	Old Testament Prophecy	Gabriel's description of Christ	Fulfilled Prophecy	
A. Daniel 7:13-14, 27		He will be great.		D. Acts 2:29-32
B. Malachi 1:11		He will have the throne of David.		E. Hebrews 1:8
C. Isaiah 9:6-7		His kingdom will never end.		F. Titus 2:13

A *betrothal* or engagement was a legal contract that could only be broken by divorce. Once the wedding took place the couple could live together. For Mary and Joseph, the betrothal agreement had already been made. Soon it was evident to Joseph that Mary was expecting a baby. It looked as if she had sinned and deserved the law's penalty, stoning. The only ways to avoid the stoning were for Joseph to divorce Mary or make her his wife.

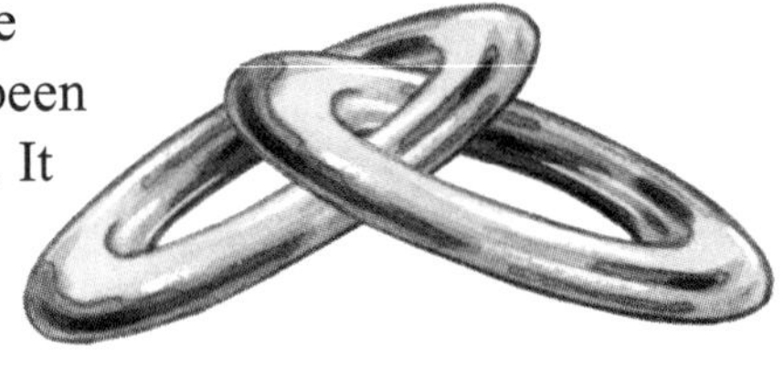

Complete the sentences. You may use your Bible for help.

1. God sent an ______________ in a dream to tell Joseph the truth about Mary (Matt. 1:20).
2. Joseph was told that Mary's child was of the ______________ Ghost (Matt. 1:20).
3. The child born of Mary would ______________ what the Lord had said through a prophet (Matt. 1:22).
4. The prophet had said a virgin would have a Son and His name would be

   ______________________ (Matt. 1:23).
5. Joseph obeyed the angel's command and took Mary home as his ______________ (Matt. 1:24).

Message from the Lord

Isaiah 7:14-16

Name ______________________

Some messages of prophecy had a meaning for thc distant future as well as the immediate future. God gave Isaiah a message to deliver to King Ahaz, the king of Judah, as the king prepared for battle. The meaning for the immediate future was that the two enemy kings would be defeated before Isaiah's newborn son would be old enough to discern good and evil. Unwisely, King Ahaz refused to listen to God. Years later this decision would contribute to the captivity of Judah by the Assyrians.

Isaiah's message to King Ahaz was also a prophecy for the distant future.

Read Isaiah 7:14. Complete the three prophecies about the promised Messiah in this verse.

1. The mother will be a ______________________.
2. The baby will be a ______________________.
3. His name will be ______________________.

Answer the questions.

4. Ahaz did not accept the message God sent through Isaiah. In the New Testament, which people rejected Christ as the promised Messiah?

   ____

   ____

5. Did keeping the laws of Moses provide salvation for these people? ________
6. Does keeping the laws of Moses and doing good provide salvation for people today? ________

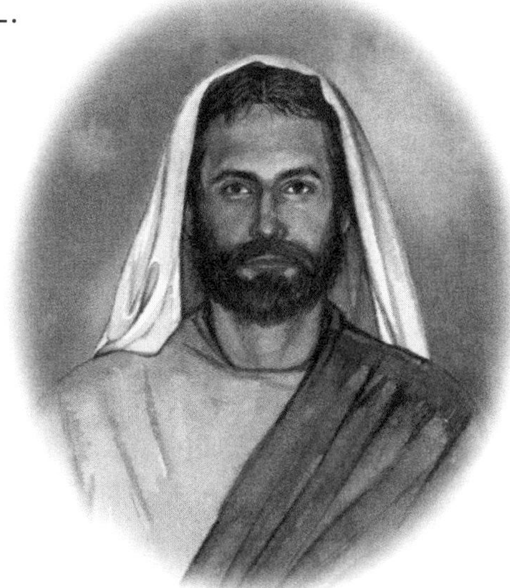

God gave His people a variety of pictures through which He revealed His plan of salvation before the coming of Christ. Obedience to the law did not bring salvation.

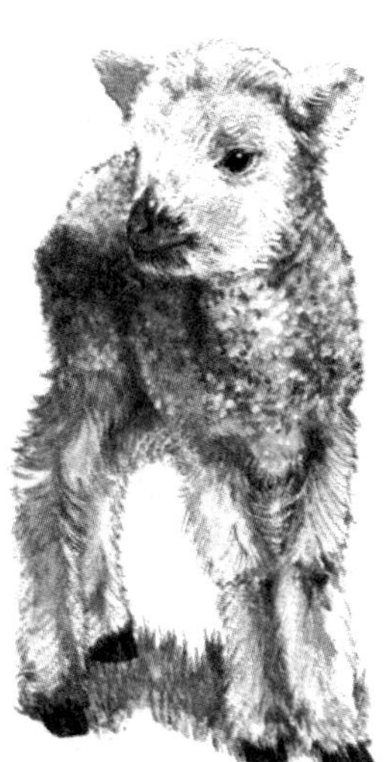

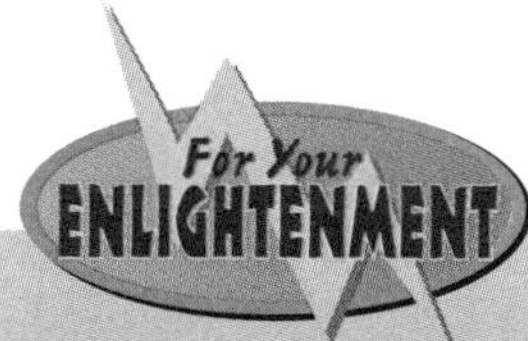
For Your
ENLIGHTENMENT

Sacrifices to God were offered upon altars to show *faith* in a Savior to come. The Old Testament sacrifices represented Christ, the Lamb of God, who was to die for sinners.

How would you explain salvation to someone who was trusting in his obedience to the law and good works for salvation?

____

____

____

____

____

Scripture-Filled Music

Name ______________________

The Book of Psalms is the hymnbook of the Israelites. Each hymn was set to a particular tune and sung during worship, feasts, and times of rejoicing. Many choruses and hymns that we sing today have words that come directly from Scripture.

A popular Christmas oratorio is Handel's *Messiah*. George Frederick Handel used Scripture as he composed this famous work in 1741.

Each music note contains a section of text from the oratorio *The Messiah.* Write the Scripture reference used for each text.

I Corinthians 15:57

Isaiah 53:6

John 1:29

Isaiah 40:1-2

Luke 2:14

Comfort ye, comfort ye my people, saith your God. Speak ye comfortably to Jerusalem, and cry unto her, that her warfare is accomplished, that her iniquity is pardoned.

Glory to God in the highest, and peace on earth, good will toward men.

Behold the Lamb of God, that taketh away the sins of the world.

All we like sheep have gone astray; we have turned every one to his own way; and the Lord hath laid on him the iniquity of us all.

But thanks be to God, who giveth us the victory through our Lord Jesus Christ.

What Does God Say About Music?

Name ____________________

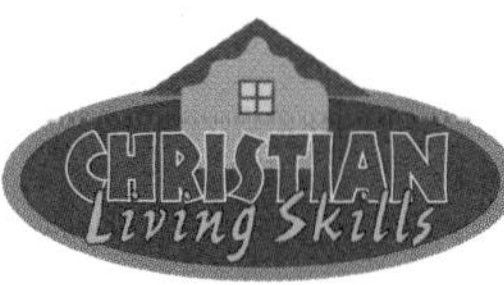
CHRISTIAN
Living Skills

Music is powerful. It can make you feel happy or sad, sleepy or energetic, safe or fearful. It has the power to influence you. Composers and performers know this is true, and they seek to attract interest in their music or style of performance.

What about Christians? What does God say about music? Does He care about what kind of music you listen to? **Absolutely.** Music was created by God before He created the world. The Bible teaches that the angels use music in heaven to worship God for His holiness. Because music was created by God, it is important to Him.

God has given people the gift of music for the purpose of glorifying Him.

Read Psalm 149:1. Write the command given to God's people in these verses.

____

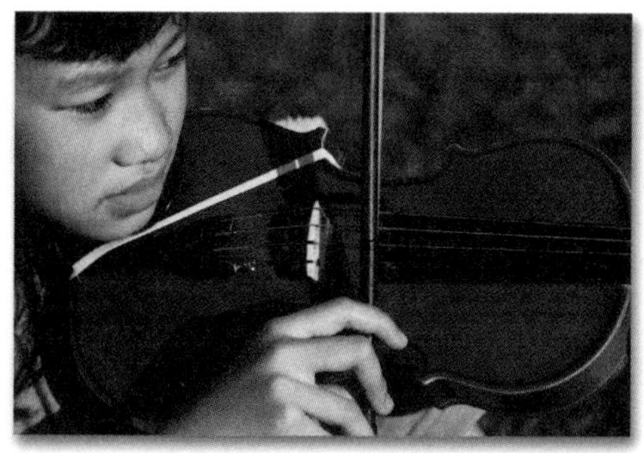

Music can be good or evil. Satan has taken something that God created to be beautiful and has twisted it to accomplish his own wicked purposes. How can a Christian choose between music that pleases God and music that pleases Satan?

Read the verses and fill in the blanks to discover what God says about making choices to please Him.

What God Says	Principles to Live By
I Peter 1:15-16 God is ______________.	Because God is holy, I must be ______________.
I Thessalonians 5:21-22 I must ______________________ everything to see whether or not it pleases God.	I must hold on to __________ things and avoid every kind of __________ thing.
I John 5:2-3 Because I ______________ God, I cannot ______________ worldly things.	If I ______________ worldly things, then the ______________ of God is not in me.

For Your ENLIGHTENMENT Both historical and contemporary musical scholars agree that all music is a combination of three types of sounds: **melody, harmony, and rhythm.** The **melody** is the most obvious arrangement of sounds by which you recognize a song. The **harmony** adds variety to the melody, and the **rhythm** is the background support of the main melody. Music sounds different when different aspects are emphasized. Classical music emphasizes melody. Rock music emphasizes rhythm. *When words are added to musical sounds, the melody must be emphasized for the words to be clearly understood.*

Name ____________________

What about Christian music?

Christian Living Skills

Does the kind of music we use to worship God matter to Him? **Absolutely.** When God tells His children to do something, He wants it done in a way that pleases Him. Since the Bible tells us it is good for Christians to use music to worship the Lord, Christians must worship God with music that pleases Him.

While the Bible does not name a certain style of music that is pleasing to God, Christians can use their God-given ability to discern God-honoring music from Satan-honoring music. When a Christian desires to please God, he will get serious about choosing God's music.

What Is Christian Music?

Christian music is that music in which text, music, performers, and the performance reflect the holiness of Christ.

Read the verses and answer the questions.

I John 5:14-15 If you want to know what kind of music pleases God, what should you do?

____

Colossians 1:16 Who created music, and why did He create it?

____

BEWARE!

You cannot mix God's holiness with the sinful things of this world. He hates sin. He hates the world's music. Don't be deceived.

God is not pleased when people sing words that praise Him to music that dishonors Him.

What About Me?

Ask yourself these questions to choose worship music that pleases God.

What kind of thoughts does this music bring to my mind?
What kind of physical reaction do I have to this music?
Is the message of God's holiness clear in this music?
Do the words of the song clearly point my thoughts to Jesus Christ?
Does the performer's life reflect the values he is singing about?
Does the music emphasize the rhythm or the melody?
Can I clearly hear the words over the music?

Promised Redemption

Galatians 4:4-5

Name ______________________

The Jews had waited centuries for the promised Messiah to come. Their salvation rested in their faith that God would one day send a Savior to redeem them from sin. God established the laws of offering sacrifices not to provide salvation, but to reveal the sinfulness of man. Christ, as the perfect sacrifice, fulfilled every requirement set by God and provided redemption for man's sin.

A	B	D	E	F	I	L	M	N	O	P	R	S	T	U	W
2	10	4	3	6	7	8	9	12	18	14	15	16	5	20	21

Use the math code to find words to complete each sentence.

1. In Paul's letter to the Galatians, he wrote that God planned to send His Son when

   the ____ ____ ____ ____ ____ ____ ____ ____ of ____ ____ ____ ____ had come.
   A×E B+B O−B T+E E×D O÷F D×D U−D   A+E D+E E×E F÷A

2. For Christ to live as a human, He had to be ____ ____ ____ ____ of a
   U÷A M×A T×E F×A

   ____ ____ ____ ____ ____. This woman was Mary.
   I×E F×E O÷A U÷B O−F

3. As a man, Christ had to live ____ ____ ____ ____ ____ the ____ ____ ____
   T×D B+A S÷D R−N N+E   S÷A U−O E×I

   of Moses. God had established these laws to show man his sin. Christ kept all of these laws.

4. As the perfect Lamb of God, Christ gave Himself to ____ ____ ____ ____ ____ ____
   B+T I−D A+A W−O T−A F+E

   man from his sins.

5. God is the heavenly Father of all believers. Christians are ____ ____ ____ ____ ____ ____ ____
   N÷F A×A M+M I×A U÷D M−F U÷T

   as ____ ____ ____ ____ into the family of God.
   A×L N+F L+D I+M

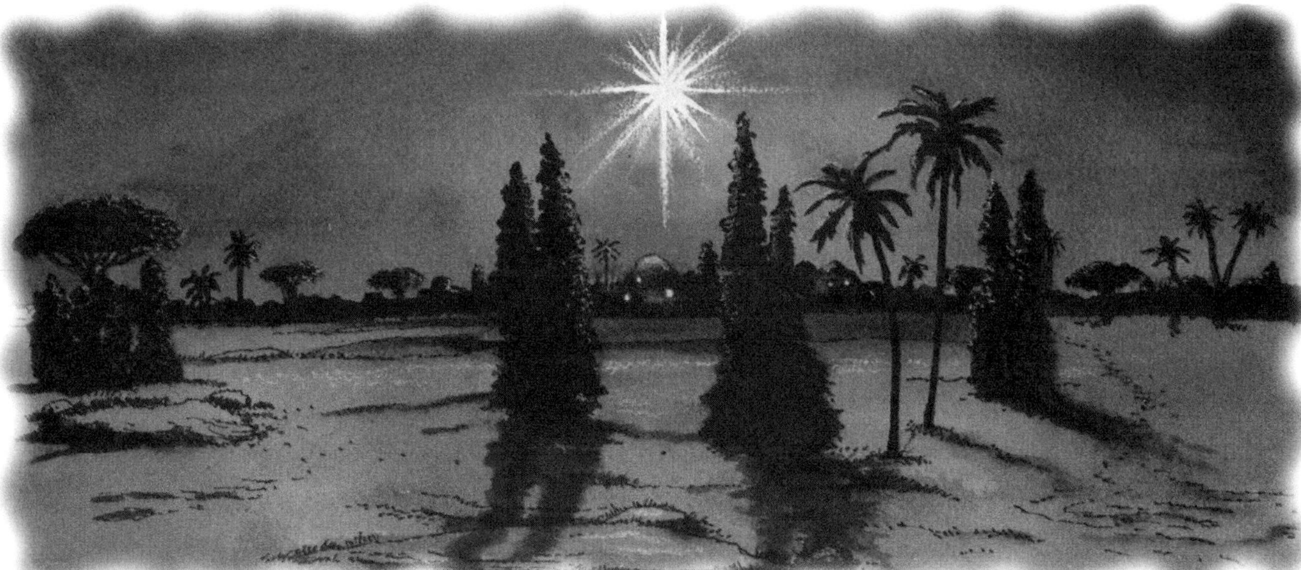

Prophecy Fulfilled

Using Cross-References

Name ______________________

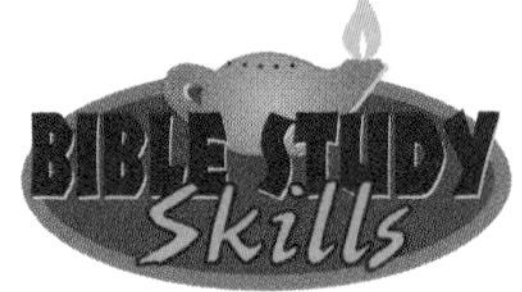

BIBLE STUDY
Skills

Cross-references are useful when studying prophecies in Scripture. A passage fulfilling a prophecy will have a cross-reference to the verses stating the prophecy.

1:66 LUKE 2:15

dwelt round about them; and all
these sayings were noised abroad
throughout all the hill country of
Judæa.
66 And all they that heard *them*
laid *them* up in their [a]hearts, saying, What manner of child shall
this be! And the hand of the
Lord was with him.

Zacharias' "Benedictus"

67 ¶ And his father, Zacharī'as,
was [b]filled with the Holy [c]|Spirit|,
and prophesied, saying,
68 [d]Blessed *be* the Lord God of
Israel; for he hath [e]visited and
[f]redeemed his [g]people,
69 And hath raised up an [h]horn
of [i]salvation for us in the house of
his servant, David;
70 [j]As he [k]spoke by the mouth of
his [l]holy prophets, who have
been [m]since the [n]|ages| began;
71 That we should be saved
from our enemies, and from the
hand of all that hate us;
72 To perform the mercy *promised* to our fathers, and to remember his [l]holy [o]covenant;
73 The [p]oath which he swore to
our father, Abraham,
74 That he would grant unto
us that we, being delivered out of
the hand of our enemies, might
serve him without fear,
75 In [l]holiness and [q]righteousness
before him, all the days of our life.
76 And thou, child, shalt be
called the [r]prophet of the Highest;
for thou [s]shalt go before the face
of the Lord to prepare his ways;
77 To give [t]knowledge of [u]salva-
tion unto his people by the remission of their [v]sins,
78 Through the tender mercy of
our God; whereby the [w]dayspring
from on high hath visited us,
79 To give [x]light to them that sit
in darkness and *in* the shadow of
death, to [y]guide our feet into the
way of peace.
80 And the [z]child grew, and
[aa]|became| strong in spirit, and
was in the deserts till the day of
his showing unto Israel.

Jesus is born in Bethlehem
(Mt.1:18–25; 2:1; cp. Jn.1:14)

2 AND it came to pass, in those
days, that there went out a
decree from Cæsar Augustus, that
all the [1]world should be [bb]|regis-
tered|.
2 (*And* this |[cc]registration| was
first made when Quirin'ius was
governor of Syria.)
3 And all went to be [bb]|regis-
tered|, everyone into his own
city.
4 And Joseph also went up from
Galilee, out of the city of Nazareth, into Judæa, unto the city
of David, which is called [dd]Beth-
lehem (because he was of the
[ee]house and lineage of David),
5 To be [bb]|registered| with Mary,
his espoused wife, being great
with child.
6 And so it was that, while they
were there, the days were accomplished that she should be delivered.
7 [ff]And she [gg]brought forth her
first-born son, and wrapped him
in swaddling clothes, and laid
him in a manger, because there
was no room for them in the inn.

Angelic announcement
of Jesus' birth

8 ¶ And there were in the same
country shepherds abiding in the
field, keeping watch over their
flock by night.
9 And, lo, [hh]|an| [ii]angel of the
Lord came upon them, and the
glory of the Lord shone round
about them; and they were [jj]|very
much| afraid.
10 And the angel said unto
them, [kk]Fear not; for, behold, I
bring you good [ll]tidings of great
joy, which shall be to [mm]all people.
11 For unto you is born this day
in the city of David a [i]Savior,
who is Christ the Lord.
12 And this *shall be* a sign unto
you: Ye shall find the babe
wrapped in swaddling clothes,
lying in a manger.
13 And suddenly there was with
the angel a multitude of the heavenly host, praising God, and
saying,
14 Glory to God in the highest,
and on earth [nn]peace, good will
toward men.

Shepherds visit the baby, Jesus

15 ¶ And it came to pass, as the

c 5 B.C., 2:7
a Lk.2:19
b v. 41
c KJV *Ghost. Holy Spirit* (N.T.): v. 67; Lk.2:25. (Mt.1: 18; Acts 2:4, *note*)
d 1 Ki.1: 48; Ps. 106:48
e Cp. Lk. 2:27–32
f See Ex. 6:6 and Rom.3: 24, *notes*
g *Israel* (history): vv. 68–79; Lk. 13:35. (Gen.12: 2; Rom. 11:26)
h 2 Sam. 22:3; see Dt. 33:17, *note*
i See Rom.1: 16, *note*
j Rom.1:2
k *Inspiration*: vv. 70–79; Lk.3:4. (Ex.4: 15; 2 Tim. 3:16)
l *Sanctification* (N.T.): vv. 70, 72,75; Lk.2:23. (Mt.4:5; Rev.22: 11)
m Acts 3:21
n KJV *world.* Gk. *aiōn.* See Mk. 10:30, *note*
o See Gen. 12:2, *note*
p Gen.22: 16–18
q Eph.4: 24; see Rom.10: 10, *note*
r Mt.11:9
s v. 17; Lk.7:27
t Mk.1:4
u See Rom.1: 16, *note*
v See Rom.3: 23, *note*
w Or *sun-rising.* Cp. Mal. 4:2; 2 Pet. 1:19
x Isa.9:2; Acts 26: 18
y Jn.10:4
z Cp. Lk. 2:40
aa KJV *waxed*
bb KJV *taxed.* Acts 5:37
cc KJV *taxing*
dd Mic.5:2
ee See Mt. 1:1, *note*
ff c. 5 B.C.
gg *Christ* (first advent): vv. 1–7; Lk.2:26. (Gen.3: 15; Acts 1:11)
hh KJV *the*
ii See Heb.1:4, *note*; cp. Jud.2: 1, *note*
jj KJV *sore*
kk Lk.1: 13,30
ll *Gospel*: vv. 10–11; Lk. 4:18. (Gen. 12:3; Rev. 14:6)
mm Gen. 12:3; Isa. 49:6
nn See Mt. 10:34, *note*

[1](2:1) The "world" (Gk. *oikoumenē*, signifying *the inhabited earth*) throughout the N.T. has reference politically to the Roman Empire or the Roman world.

1. Look at the first cross-reference for Luke 2:4. What reference is referred to?

    ____

2. What prophecy from that verse was fulfilled in Luke 2:4?

    ____

    ____

3. What two Old Testament references referred to in Luke 2:10 are prophecies about the Savior coming for all people—Jews and Gentiles?

    ____

    ____

4. What word in Luke 2:1 has a number before it?

    ____

5. In this verse, what does *world* mean?

    ____

6. According to the footnote, who ruled over the known inhabited earth at the time of Christ's birth?

    ____

Sometimes there are numbers that refer to footnotes. Footnotes are longer notes printed at the 'foot' or bottom of a page.

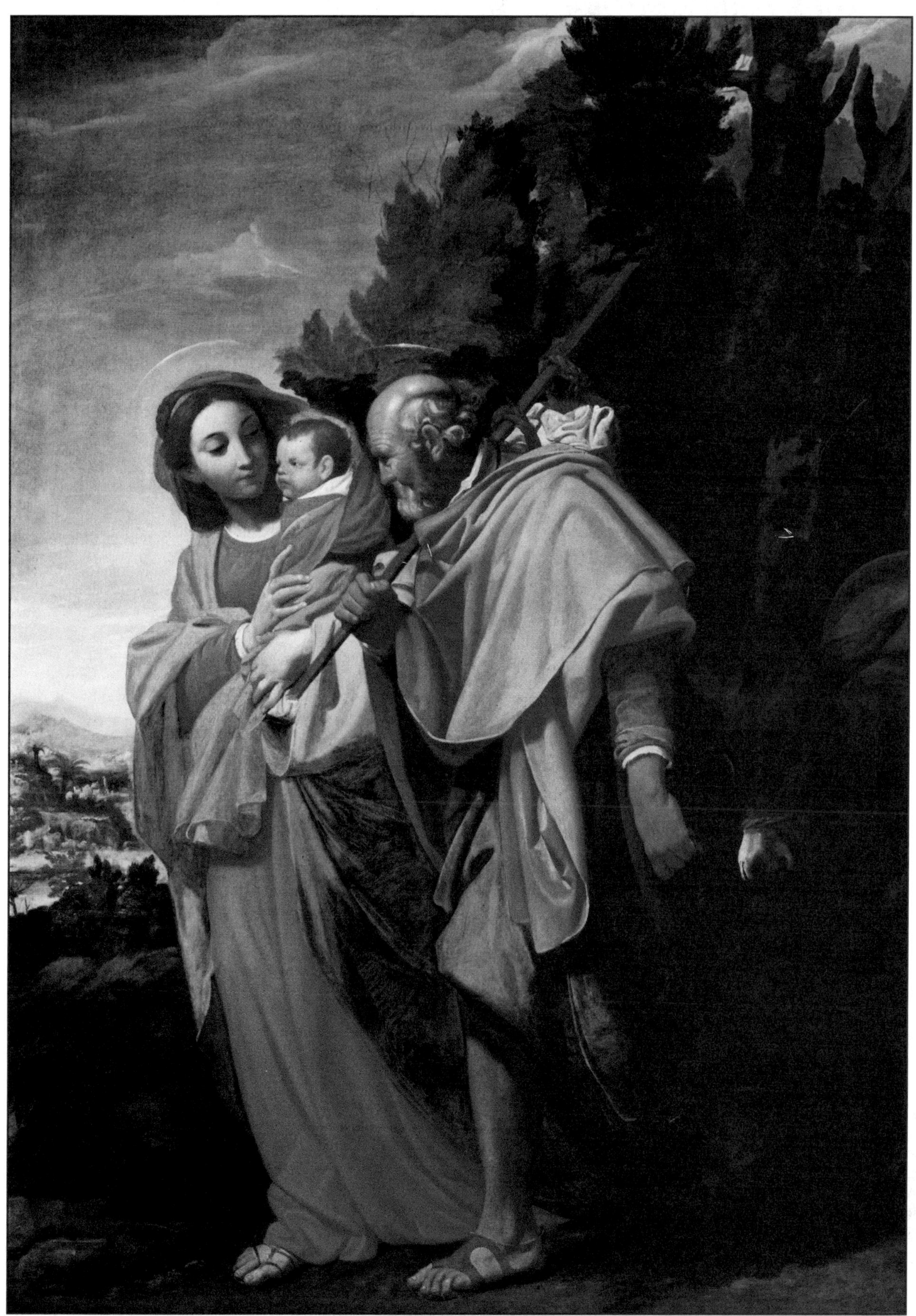

The Flight into Egypt

Domenico Fiasella

Bob Jones University Museum & Gallery, Inc.

Name ____________________

The Flight into Egypt

by Domenico Fiasella (1589-1669)

Domenico Fiasella (Də mĕn ē´ko Fē ə sĕl´ə) began his art training with his father, a goldsmith who made jewelry and decorative ornaments for wealthy patrons. Young Domenico moved to Rome in 1607 to study a variety of artistic styles with many masters. Domenico learned many things and combined them in his own work without making his paintings look like anyone else's. His style was calm, three-dimensional, and colorful, with a strong contrast of light and dark.

The event depicted in this painting is recorded in Matthew 2:13-15, where God warned Joseph to take the baby to Egypt to protect Him from King Herod. There are no details given about how they traveled, but we suppose that they got there the same way that they journeyed from Nazareth to Bethlehem—by donkey. Artists had usually shown Mary sitting on the donkey with the baby in her arms and Joseph leading. Shortly before Fiasella was born, artists began to show Mary walking beside Joseph to emphasize their family unity.

In comparing the head of Joseph to Mary's face, we see that Joseph is much more detailed and realistic. Mary is generalized and ideally beautiful, but she doesn't look like a real person. Joseph is traditionally shown as much older than Mary. Because many people believed that Mary was sinless and would therefore not age or wrinkle as normal people, she is usually shown ideally beautiful and young.

Artists were instructed by the Catholic Church how to represent holy subjects from the Scriptures. In this way, they tried to ensure that no holy subjects were presented in a disrespectful way and that people would readily identify who was being depicted. To represent the family of Christ, Fiasella painted their halos as transparent glass edged with gold rims. Color was also used to represent biblical characters. Mary and Joseph both wear red and blue robes—blue representing heaven and red representing the blood of Christ.

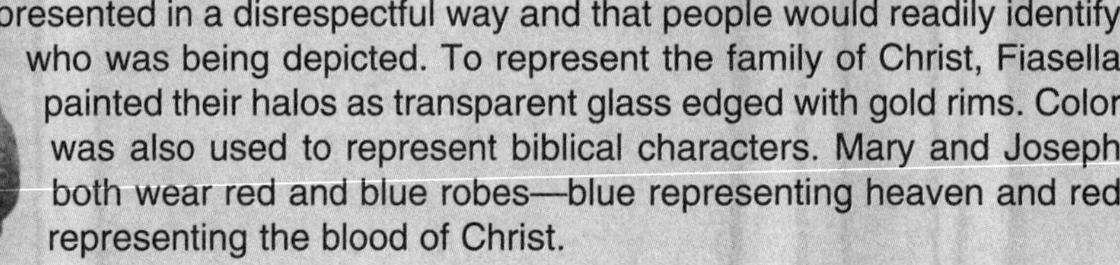

Though Mary and Joseph are fleeing for their baby's life, the mood of the painting is very calm. The landscape behind them doesn't resemble Israel or Egypt but looks like a place near Rome where Fiasella was living when he painted this picture. Notice that there is a hint of trouble behind Mary and Joseph in the woods from which they have just come. The trees are crowded together, and it is very dark. Mary and Joseph are leaving the darkness of the forest and coming out into a peaceful little clearing.

All in God's Plan

Matthew 2:1-23; Luke 2:9-23

Name ____________________

Often we think that God directs the lives of Christians only. In Colossians, Paul reminds us that God created all things, including governments and rulers. That which God created He continues to maintain. It is through God that all things consist or continue. God is omniscient. He knows all things, including the actions of unbelievers.

God used believers, the ungodly, and a miraculous event of nature to fulfill prophecies about the coming Messiah.

Write the name of the person or thing that is speaking.

Bethlehem

Although I didn't know it, God used me to make a decree that brought Mary and Joseph to Bethlehem.

____

I lovingly wrapped my new Son and laid Him in a manger to sleep.

____

We stopped in Jerusalem as we traveled to worship the King of the Jews.

____

I and others like me came to the shepherds to announce the birth of the Savior.

____

God directed me to take my family into Egypt for protection, then later to Nazareth to live.

____

I led the wise men to the young Savior as they traveled from the East.

____

After talking with my counselors about the prophesied King of the Jews, I sent men to kill all the young boys in Bethlehem.

____

Harmony of the Gospels

Parallel Accounts of Christ's Birth

Name ______________________

BIBLE STUDY *Skills* Since each of the Gospels was written through inspiration by a different man, they all agree, but the details and accounts are from differing human perspectives. Reading about an event from two or more authors helps bring the details together for a well-rounded picture. The similarity of the Gospels and their "bringing together" of details in the life of Christ has come to be called the harmony of the Gospels.

Event	Matthew wrote of Jesus as the promised King.	Mark wrote of Jesus as the obedient Servant.	Luke wrote of Jesus as the perfect Man.	John wrote of Jesus as the divine Son.
1. Gabriel announces the Messiah's coming birth to Mary.			Luke 1:26-35	
2. Mary visits Elizabeth.			Luke 1:39-56	
3. An angel tells Joseph of the coming birth of the Messiah.	Matt. 1:18-23			
4. The genealogy is given of the earthly ancestry of Jesus.	Matt. 1:1-17		Luke 3:23-38	
5. Jesus is born in Bethlehem.	Matt. 2:1		Luke 2:1-7	
6. Angels announce the Messiah's birth to the shepherds.			Luke 2:8-20	
7. Jesus is dedicated in the temple.			Luke 2:22-39	
8. Wise men seek the Messiah in Jerusalem.	Matt. 2:1-12			
9. Wise men come to Bethlehem to worship Jesus.	Matt. 2:8-11			
10. Joseph, Mary, and Jesus flee to Egypt.	Matt. 2:13-15			
11. King Herod orders all the male infants in Bethlehem killed.	Matt. 2:16			
12. An angel instructs Joseph to return to Israel.	Matt. 2:19-21			
13. Joseph, Mary, and Jesus settle in Nazareth.	Matt. 2:21-23			

Use the chart to answer the questions.

1. Where would you look to read about
   - Mary being told about the Messiah's birth? ______________________
   - Joseph being told about the Messiah's birth? ______________________
   - the shepherds being told about the Messiah's birth? ______________________
   - the fulfillment of the prophecy that the Messiah would be from Nazareth? ______________________
2. What events are recorded in two of the gospels? ______________________

   ____
3. Which gospels do not record events about the birth of Jesus? ______________________

Name ______________________

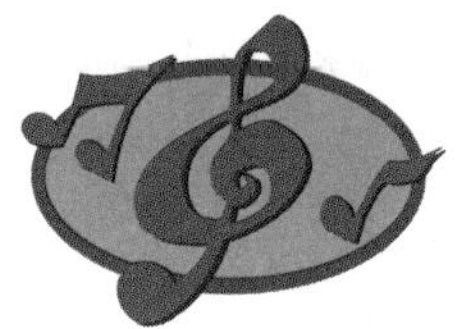

EMMANUEL

Emmanuel means "God with us." Isaiah called the coming Messiah by this name in Isaiah 7:14. Jesus Christ was God with us, living as a man for all to observe.

In Luke 1:78-79, Zacharias, the father of John the Baptist, referred to Christ as the dayspring or rising sun who would give light to all who sit in darkness.

Dayspring

Rod of Jesse

In Isaiah 11:1-2, the Messiah is called a rod, or shoot, out of the stem of Jesse. Christ was a descendant of David, Jesse's son, and in the royal line.

In Isaiah 22:22, "the key of the house of David" refers to royal authority. This verse is applied to Jesus Christ by John in Revelation 3:7.

Key of David

Old Testament prophecies include many names and descriptions of the coming Messiah. Each name describes a different aspect of Christ's person and work. There are many names and descriptions of believers.

Read Acts 11:26 and answer the questions.

1. What other name were the believers called? ______________________
2. Why do you think believers of Christ were called by this name? ______________________

____

Read Matthew 5:13 and answer the questions.

3. How does Jesus describe believers? ______________________
4. What effect does salt have on food if it doesn't taste salty? ______________________
5. What effect does a believer have on others if his actions are not Christlike? ______________________
6. If a believer does not act like a Christian, what will non-believers assume?

____

____

Sent to Be the Savior

Name ______________________

Many people talk about the birth of Christ during the Christmas season. This provides opportunities for you to share the gospel message with unbelievers.

Here are some truths about Christ and His salvation that you can share with others.

Read each Scripture passage. Write what you would say about each passage as you share it with an unbeliever.

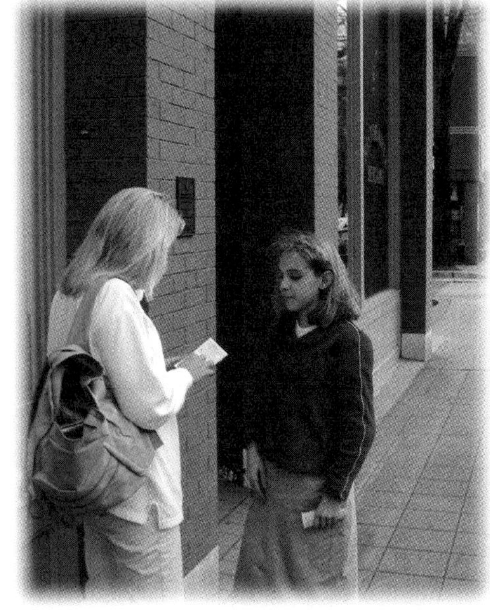

Matthew 3:16-17

____

____

____

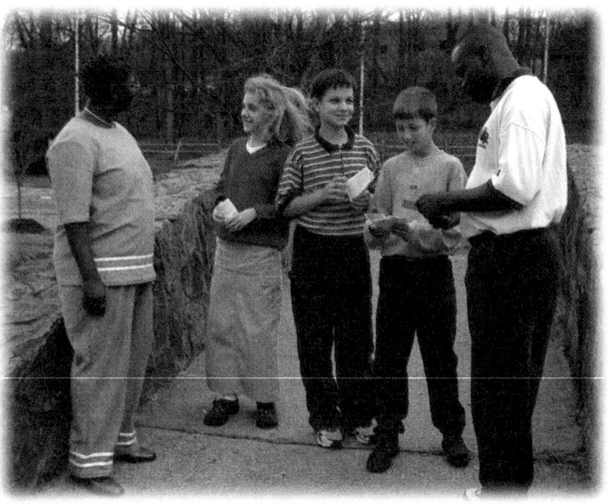

I John 4:14

____

____

____

I Corinthians 15:3-4

____

____

____

John 20:31

____

____

____

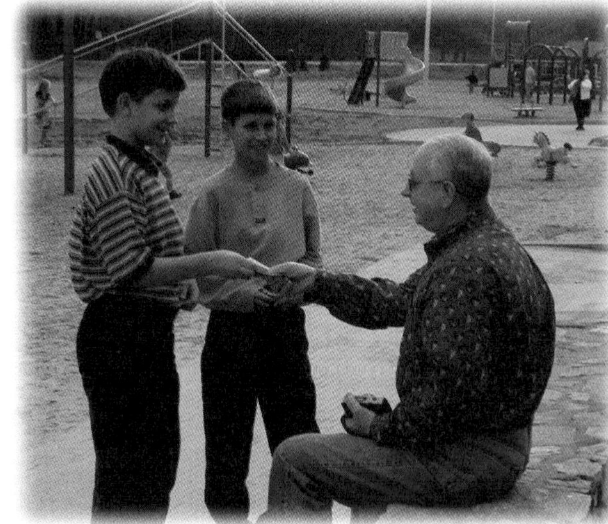

I John 5:11-12

____

____

____

What Does God Say About Serving Others?

Name ____________________

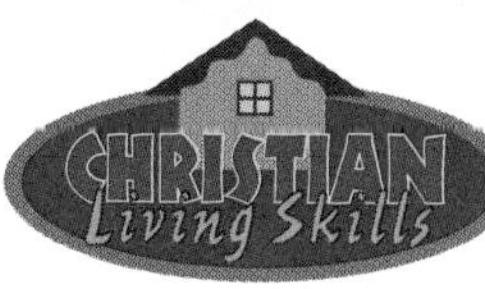
CHRISTIAN
Living Skills

You live in a "me first" world. Many around you say that you should please yourself. Being selfish is a temptation you will face every day of your life. However, **selfishness is sin** and will lead you only to an empty, lonely life.

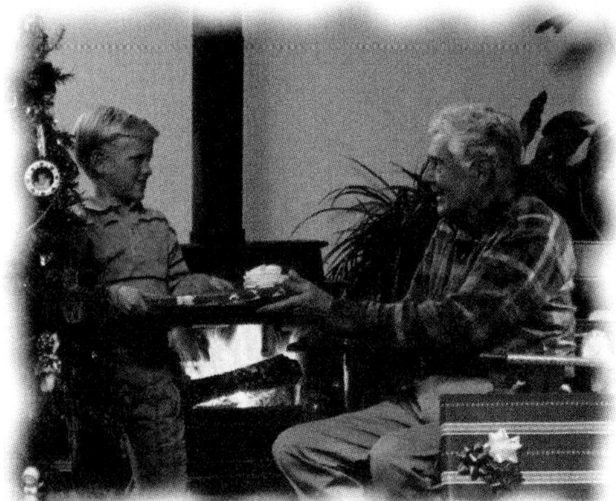

You may have heard of a person becoming **depressed.** This means that a person has an attitude of unhappiness that comes from hopelessly focusing on himself. God's Word gives us the remedy for this kind of depression: living to please God by becoming a humble servant to others.

Look up *humble, humility,* and *servant* in the glossary. Combine the definitions to write a description of a servant who would be pleasing to God.

____

____

The Bible gives you a perfect example of a humble servant. Jesus willingly gave up His exalted position in heaven to become a human being who experienced hunger, thirst, and pain because He loves you.

Read Philippians 2:5-11 and number the statements in the correct order from 1-7.

_____ 1. God exalted Jesus above everything else.

_____ 2. Jesus became a human and a humble servant.

__1__ 3. My attitude should imitate Christ's attitude.

_____ 4. Jesus was in the very form and nature of God.

__7__ 5. Everyone will confess that Jesus is Lord.

_____ 6. Jesus obeyed His Father and died on the cross for you.

_____ 7. Everyone will bow before Jesus.

Where should your focus be? Focusing on yourself is a dead end. Focusing on pleasing God by serving others is a key to true joy. Ask God to give you the same attitude that Christ had.

Read the verses and write the references under the correct statement about serving others.

Galatians 6:2	I Peter 5:5-6	Galatians 6:10	Philippians 2:3-4

God wants me to be submissive to others by clothing myself with a humble attitude of service.	I will fulfill the law of Christ when I find ways to serve others.	I should look for ways to help others because I consider them to be more important than myself.	Every time I have the opportunity, I should look for ways to serve others—especially other Christians.
________	________	________	________

Something to Think About

Being a Servant

Name ____________________

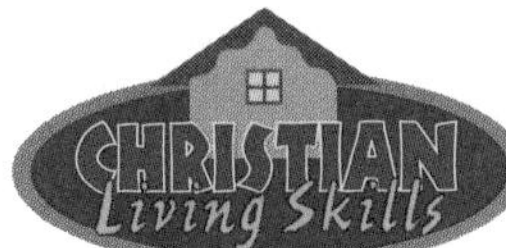
CHRISTIAN
Living Skills

Being a humble servant is a full-time job. It means consistently placing the needs of other people above your own. It requires personal sacrifice.

For a Christian, a servant is not one who just does nice things for others. Rather, **servanthood** is a condition of your heart. It is a genuine desire to please God by ministering to others.

Read each scenario. Describe how you could be a servant in each situation.

Scenario	How could YOU be a servant in this situation?
At church, you notice that the new girl looks a little lost. She doesn't seem to know where to go after Sunday school, and she has a worried expression on her face.	
It is your little sister's turn to do the dishes after supper. You know that she's not feeling well and that she has a major project for school to finish tonight.	
After recess, it is the responsibility of your class to pick up the recreational equipment used during recess. Everyone is hot and tired after recess and wants to be the first in line to get a drink at the water fountain.	

What About Me?

Take time at home and think about the condition of your heart.

What is your reputation? Are you self-centered? Or do you look for ways to show that you think more highly of others than yourself? Your actions tell others what is in your heart.

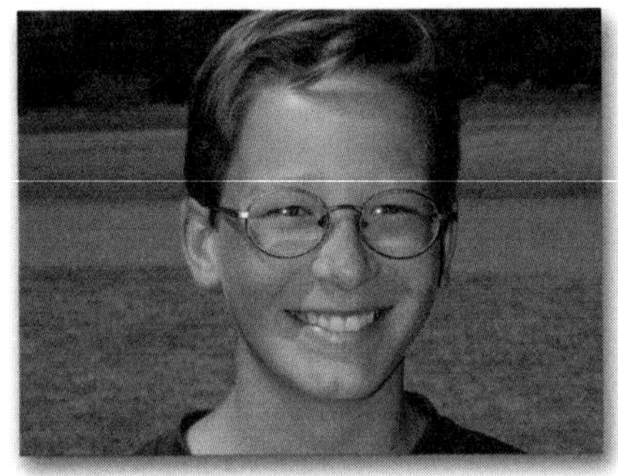

Write Proverbs 20:11.

____

____

List the names of three people that you will see today. Write one way that you can please God by serving them. Then look for an opportunity today to do it!

Name	How can I please God by serving this person today?

Get the Bible Reading H.A.B.I.T.

Name ______________________

BIBLE STUDY Skills

As you read the Scripture for each day, write the date in the box.

Have a special time set aside each day to read your Bible. If possible, make it the same time every day.

Ask God to teach you from His Word. Remember to thank Him for helping you to understand and apply it.

Be still and give your attention to what you are reading.

Investigate the Scripture by asking yourself questions about it.

Take time to look up words and ideas you do not understand.

God's Word can discern a person's thoughts and motives. **Hebrews 4:12-13**	If you confess your sins, God is faithful to forgive and cleanse you. **I John 1:7-10**	Even if you do not believe, God remains faithful. **II Timothy 2:11-13**	God is faithful to continue His good work in the lives of Christians. **Philippians 1:3-6**	God is faithful to fulfill all of His promises. **II Corinthians 1:18-20**
It is right to obey and honor your parents. **Ephesians 6:1-3**	It pleases the Lord when children obey their parents as they obey Him. **Colossians 3:20-23**	The wisdom of this world is not meek, but unspiritual and devilish. **James 3:13-16**	God's wisdom is pure, peaceable, gentle, merciful, good, and sincere. **James 3:17-18**	The wisdom of the world is foolishness in God's sight. **I Corinthians 3:18-20**
Christians should boast only in the Lord, not in themselves. **II Corinthians 10:17-18**	True faith shows itself in works of goodness and mercy. **James 2:13-17**	Believers must not have close relationships with unbelievers. **II Corinthians 6:14-16**	God wants Christians to be a separated people for Himself. **II Corinthians 6:17-18**	Obey those who have spiritual authority over you. **Hebrews 13:17**
Continue in the truth you have been taught from God's Word. **II Timothy 3:14-15**	God is not to be worshiped with images man has made. **Acts 17:24-29**	Idolaters will be judged for perverting the glory of God. **Romans 1:22-25**	The prayer of a righteous man accomplishes much. **James 5:14-18**	The Holy Spirit intercedes for Christians when they pray. **Romans 8:26-27**

Two Sides of the Coin

Name ________________________

God speaks to the believer

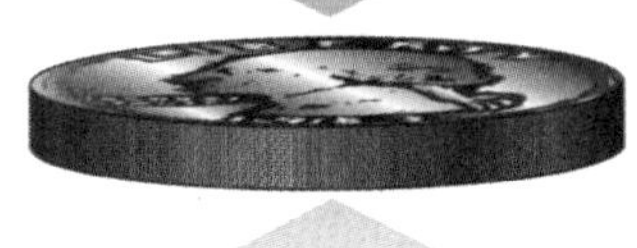
The Word of God
Prayer

In the devotional life of a Christian, prayer and Bible study cannot be separated. They are like two sides of the same coin. Neither should be neglected because both are important parts of personal communication.

The believer speaks to God

Read Psalm 5:1-8. Complete the following statements about this prayer of David, a man after God's heart. Match the number and the side of the coin to find each letter.

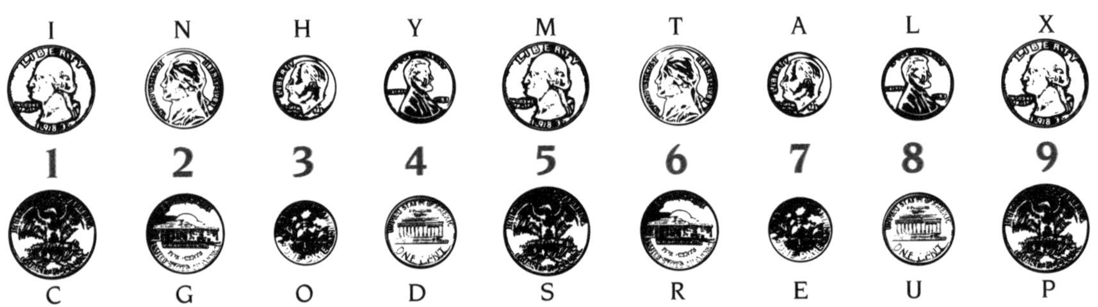
I N H Y M T A L X
1 2 3 4 5 6 7 8 9
C G O D S R E U P

Verses 1-2 David believed that when he prayed, God was giving him His careful ________.

7 heads	6 heads	6 heads	7 tails	2 heads	6 heads	1 heads	3 tails	2 heads

Verse 3 David had a special time of day for ________ with God.

1 tails	3 tails	5 heads	5 heads	8 tails	2 heads	1 heads	1 tails	7 heads	6 heads	1 heads	2 heads	2 tails

Verses 4-6 David knew that God should be ________ in righteousness, humility, and truth.

7 heads	9 tails	9 tails	6 tails	3 tails	7 heads	1 tails	3 heads	7 tails	4 tails

Verse 7a David came to God trusting in His ________.

5 heads	7 tails	6 tails	1 tails	4 heads

Verse 7b David came to God recognizing His ________.

3 heads	3 tails	8 heads	1 heads	2 heads	7 tails	5 tails	5 tails

Verse 8 David sought God's ________.

2 tails	8 tails	1 heads	4 tails	7 heads	2 heads	1 tails	7 tails

God's Plan for Ruth

Ruth 1-4

Name ______________________

Complete each sentence. You may use your Bible for help.

Ruth willingly left her family, her homeland, and her religion. She selflessly joined her mother-in-law and moved to Bethlehem. Ruth desired to become like an Israelite and worship the God of Israel.

1. Ruth married a son of ______________________, an Israelite living in her homeland of Moab (Ruth 1:2-4).
2. After her husband died, Ruth chose to return to Israel with her mother-in-law, __________ (Ruth 1:8, 16-18).
3. Ruth assured Naomi of her decision to stay with her by telling Naomi that wherever Naomi was going Ruth would ________, and Naomi's people would become her ______________, and Naomi's God would be her ________.

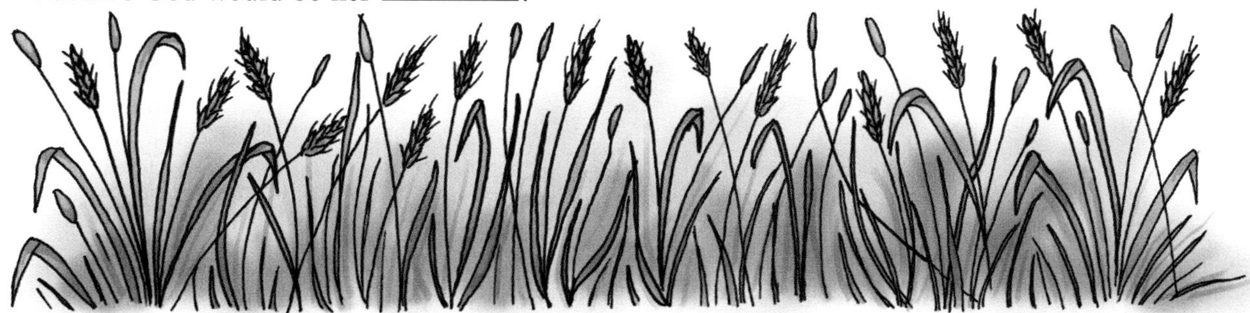

4. In Ruth 2:6, Ruth was described by the field workers as the Moabite woman that came back with Naomi. By this description, does it seem Ruth was accepted into the community or treated as a foreigner?

____

5. In Ruth 3:11, Ruth is known as a virtuous woman—noble in character, excellent, and brave. By this description, does it seem Ruth was accepted into the community or treated as a foreigner?

____

6. Ruth was the great grandmother of King David. What significance does that have as you remember promises by God about the Messiah?

____

____

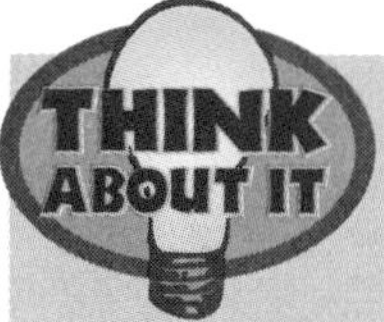
THINK
ABOUT IT

What character traits might your neighbors report about you?

____

Are there any traits you may need to change? ______________

List one trait you would like to improve on. ______________________________

Christ, Our Kinsman-Redeemer

Using a Bible Commentary

Name ______________________

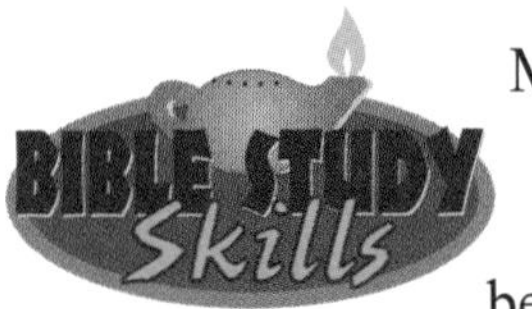
BIBLE STUDY
Skills

Many people see the account of Boaz and Ruth as an illustration of the relationship between Christ and believers. Bible scholars often write their thoughts and comments in Bible commentaries.

For Your ENLIGHTENMENT

A Bible commentary contains *comments* on and explanations of Scripture. Bible commentaries vary in organization. Some commentaries are for only one book of the Bible, while others may be for either the Old or New Testaments. A commentary that is for both the Old and New Testaments is usually called a *complete* Bible commentary.

Use the commentary section of Ruth 4 to answer the questions.

1. What did Ruth find it good to do until Boaz returned? ______________
2. What New Testament book does the commentator use to contrast two principles about eternal life and righteousness as they relate to the story of Ruth and Boaz?

   ____
3. What did Ruth receive by "sitting still"?

   ____

   ____
4. What are some Christians doing rather than "sitting still" and waiting on God?

   ____
5. Who is the Divine Kinsman? ______________
6. What does the author use to illustrate Ruth's becoming an Israelite? ______________

   ____
7. Boaz's redemption of Ruth to make her an Israelite shows that Gentiles could receive the same promises of God's covenant with whom?

   ____

137 RUTH 4

RUTH IV.—Ruth found it to be good to " sit still " and let Boaz do everything. When there is anything important to be done the person interested cannot " sit still " unless assured that the successful execution of the matter rests in hands that are competent, and faithful. Herein lies the principle of salvation by faith. The second chapter of Galatians contrasts two principles for the obtaining of life and righteousness—the one principle: works of law, i.e., religious ceremonies and personal moral efforts; the other principle: the hearing of faith, i.e., " sitting still." The Holy Spirit teaches in that chapter that nothing can be had upon the first principle, but everything upon the second. So Ruth " sat still," wholly trusted Boaz, and, as a result, obtained what her heart had never conceived of when leaving Moab. From the position of a pauper she was, in one day, raised to the dignity of a princess. The love of an husband, the joy of motherhood, and the dignity of a palace were the fruits of " sitting still." This is all a lovely picture of the satisfying joys that fill the hearts of those who give up trying to save themselves, and who rest wholly in the hands of a Redeemer and Kinsman, greater than Boaz, but typified by him, who has already accomplished the entire work of redemption.

In the Christian life there is a great need of this " sitting still." Christian people are too restless. They do not wait sufficiently upon God and for God. Saul was willing to wait " upon God " but not " for God " and so lost the Kingdom (1 Sam. xiii). There is usually an abundance of thinking, planning, and scheming, and a neglect of prayer and sitting still and permitting God to act and plan, and the result is trouble and spiritual loss.

Boaz had to purchase Ruth from a kinsman who had a prior claim, but who declared that he could not redeem her (v. 6). The Law has a prior claim to sinners, but it cannot redeem them. Christ, the Divine Kinsman, became Man in order to redeem. It cost Boaz nothing to redeem Ruth, beyond the setting aside of himself and his own interests, but it cost Christ everything to redeem sinners.

Thus Ruth, a " wild olive tree," was grafted into, and became a partaker of, " the root and fatness of the olive tree, i.e., Israel; but she could not boast that this was due to any commanding personal claim, all she could say was " Why have I found grace in thine eyes (ch. ii. 10) seeing I am a Gentile."

This is a beautiful fore-picture of that future day when the Redeemer shall bring the Gentile nations into the Covenant made with Abraham.

The Job of a King

Name ______________________

Most kings today grow up as princes in royal families. Princes enjoy the many privileges associated with this elite class of citizens. David's father was not a king, so David did not benefit from growing up as a prince. David served others through various jobs before he became king.

Write the letter of how David served next to each passage.

_____ 1. I Samuel 16:11-13

_____ 2. I Samuel 16:16-19

_____ 3. I Samuel 16:21

_____ 4. I Samuel 18:5

A. Harp player

B. Armor bearer

C. Keeper of sheep

D. Leader in Saul's army

David sought to follow God's leading. He looked to God for guidance throughout his life. God's plan included David's learning different jobs. God taught David things he would use later as he ruled over Israel.

Mark each job that might have helped prepare David for being king of Israel.

As king, David would—	Keeper of Sheep	Harp Player	Armor Bearer	Leader in Saul's Army
write psalms to praise and worship God.				
fight enemy nations.				
lead God's people.				
meet the needs of others.				

THINK ABOUT IT

Have you ever said, "Why do I have to learn this? I'm not going to do this the rest of my life."

Think about one thing you are "enduring." Write some ways it may be preparing you for your future service to God.

____

____

____

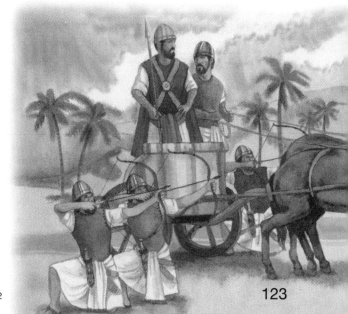

Do you need an attitude adjustment? Choose today to accept this training as part of God's preparation for your future service to Him.

Where and When?

II Samuel 2-15

Name ______________________________

Complete each sentence with words from the verses.

1. David was anointed king over Judah in his capital city of ______________________ (II Sam. 2:1-4).
2. David reigned as king over Israel in Hebron, and then he moved to ______________________ where he reigned over Israel and Judah (II Sam. 5:5).
3. Jerusalem was known as Zion and as the city of ______________________ (II Sam. 5:6-7).
4. David and thirty thousand men brought the ark of the covenant from ______________________ and eventually to the tabernacle in Jerusalem (II Sam. 6:1-4, 17).

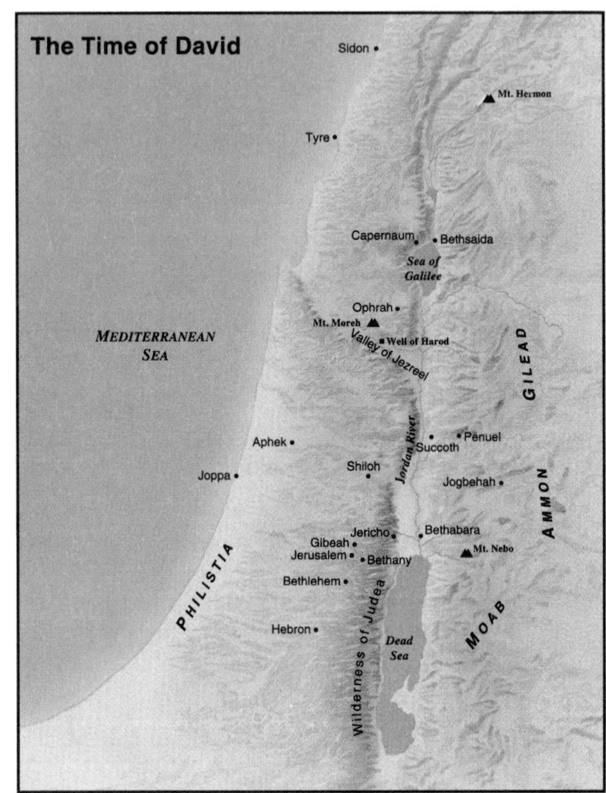
The Time of David
Sidon
Mt. Hermon
Tyre
Capernaum
Bethsaida
Sea of Galilee
Ophrah
Mt. Moreh
Well of Harod
Valley of Jezreel
MEDITERRANEAN SEA
GILEAD
Aphek
Penuel
Succoth
Jordan River
Shiloh
Joppa
Jogbehah
AMMON
Jericho
Bethabara
Gibeah
Jerusalem
Bethany
Mt. Nebo
PHILISTIA
Bethlehem
MOAB
Hebron
Dead Sea
Wilderness of Judea

Number the events in the life of King David in order (1-10).

_____ David is anointed king over Israel.

__1__ David is anointed king over Judah.

_____ David brings the ark of the covenant into Jerusalem.

_____ Ishbosheth, Saul's son, is murdered.

_____ David moves to Jerusalem, making it the capital city.

_____ David has Uriah killed so he can marry Bathsheba.

_____ Absalom tries to overthrow David's rule.

_____ Nathan addresses David's sin, and David repents to God.

__6__ David chooses to stay at home instead of going with his army into war.

_____ David chooses to please himself by sinning with Bathsheba.

What Does God Say About Being a Good Citizen?

Name ______________________________

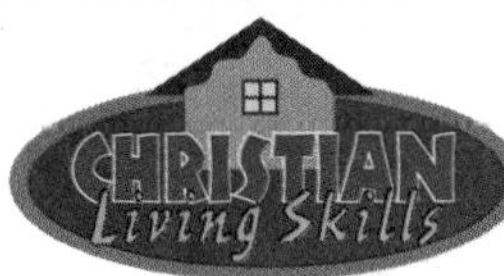
Christian
Living Skills

You are a citizen of a country. You became a citizen of the country you were born in. If you move to a different country, you can become a citizen there by following their rules for becoming part of their nation. There are specific rights and privileges you have because you are a citizen of a particular country. Along with these privileges, you also have responsibilities. God's Word has much to say about being a good citizen.

Read the verses and write the correct references under the responsibilities and privileges of citizens.

Titus 3:1	I Timothy 2:1-3	Proverbs 14:34
Luke 20:22-25	Philippians 2:14-15	I Peter 2:13-17

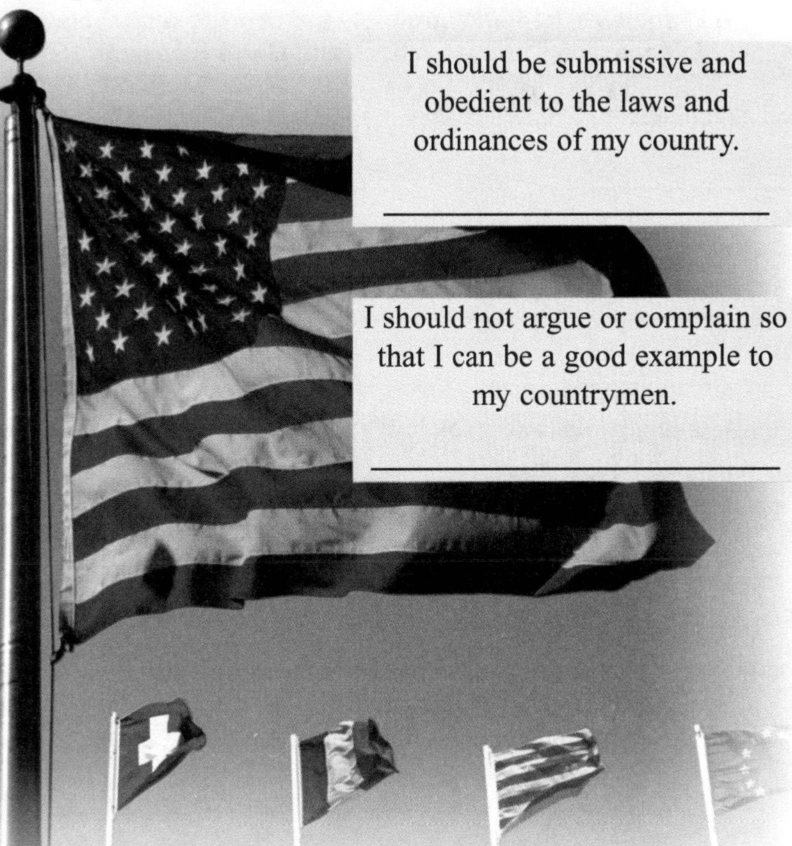

I should pay the taxes required by the government of my country.

____

I should pray for the authorities and rulers of my country.

____

I should honor my country by making righteous decisions.

____

I should be subject and obedient to the rulers of my country.

____

I should be submissive and obedient to the laws and ordinances of my country.

____

I should not argue or complain so that I can be a good example to my countrymen.

____

What should you do if the government of your country forbids you to worship God? If your government threatens to persecute you if you continue to please God, what should you do? Some books of the Bible such as II Timothy and I Peter were written to Christians in this situation. When it comes down to the question of choosing between obedience to God and obedience to your government, Christians should choose to obey God. In doing so, they should also be willing to suffer whatever consequences may come as a result of their disobedience to their government.

Read Acts 5:17-29. Write verse 29 to record Peter's and the apostles' attitude when they had to choose between obeying God or the government.

____

____

Something to Think About

Good Citizenship

Name ______________________

CHRISTIAN *Living Skills*

As a citizen, you have the civil responsibility to obey the laws of your country.

As a Christian, you have the responsibility to pray for your country and its leaders.

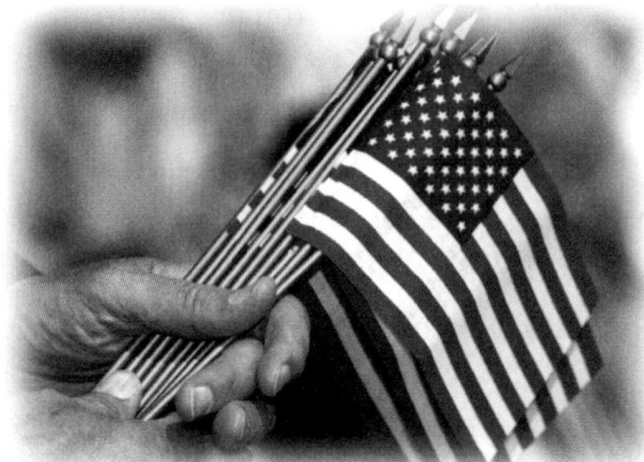

Read II Chronicles 7:14 and complete the chart to learn your responsibilities as a Christian citizen and God's blessings for obedience.

If My People Will…	Then Will I…
1.	1.
2.	2.
3.	3.
4.	

Read Psalm 33:12*a* and explain what it means in your own words.

____

____

What About Me?

Think about the country in which God has placed you. Follow the instructions.

Of what country are you a citizen? ______________________

What is the title of the highest office of authority in your country? ______________________

What is the name of the highest ruling official in your country? ______________________

List four responsibilities or obligations you have as a citizen of your country.

1. ______________________ 2. ______________________

3. ______________________ 4. ______________________

List two responsibilities you have as a **Christian** citizen in your country.

1. ______________________ 2. ______________________

List two governing officials for whom you should pray.

1. ______________________ 2. ______________________

Take time at home to pray for your country and your governing officials!

Prophet Focus

Zephaniah (ministered 640-608 B.C.)

Name ____________________

Throughout the Old Testament, God used prophets to deliver messages to His people. The prophet Zephaniah lived during the time King Josiah ruled Judah. Zephaniah's message included God's desire for Judah to remain true to Him. Zephaniah warned that destruction would come if the people did not turn away from the gods and religions of other nations and worship the one true God. God wanted the people to return to Him.

God brought to remembrance the cities of Sodom and Gomorrah and the judgment that fell on them because of their sin. Through Zephaniah, God condemned those who worshiped idols and the stars, those who tried to include God in their worship along with other gods, and those who had never sought God.

Zephaniah's message was delivered to the nation of Judah. It also mentioned the destruction of both Nineveh and Jerusalem. Nineveh was the capital of the mighty Assyrian Empire. The people of Nineveh repented in the time of Jonah, but a hundred years later they had forgotten God and had returned to the sin of the world. God said that the destruction of Jerusalem, the capital of Judah, would come as a result of the people turning away from Him and to other gods.

History records show that by 600 B.C., just a few years after Zephaniah delivered God's message, the Babylonians conquered both Nineveh and Jerusalem.

Use words from the paragraphs to complete each sentence. Write your answers in the boxes below.

1. God used the cities of Sodom and ______ as an example of His judgment of sin.
2. Zephaniah was warning the people in ______, the capital of Judah, to leave their sin and worship God.
3. God condemned the people who chose to ______ idols, stars, or other gods.
4. The Assyrian capital of ______ had once followed God, but had returned to sin.
5. ______ was the ruler of Judah at the time Zephaniah delivered God's message.
6. Zephaniah's message was for the people to ______ to God.

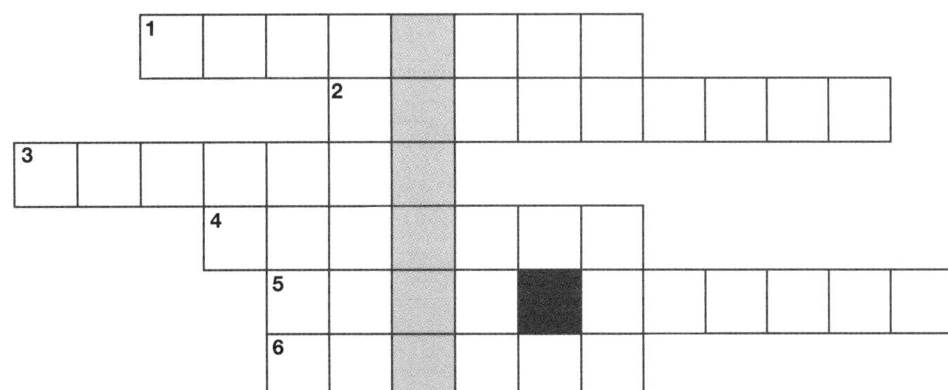

1
2
3
4
5
6

Use the letters from the shaded boxes to complete the sentence.

Through the message delivered by Zephaniah, God wanted the people to

___ ___ ___ ___ ___ ___ of their sin.

The Way of Blessing

Name ______________________

In the Bible, God gives Christians guidelines for their lives—not to make the lives of Christians difficult, but as a way to strengthen and equip believers to resist temptations of this world and to witness for Him.

It is easy to look in the Bible and find people who followed God and were blessed. What is not seen are the daily choices these people made to stand for God despite attitudes, actions, and comments of others.

Use words from Psalm 119:1-4 to complete the sentences and answer the questions.

1. God blesses those who ______________ in the law of the Lord (Ps. 119:1).
2. Since God doesn't intend for believers to step in their Bibles, what does He mean when He says to "walk" in the law? ____

   ____
3. God does not want believers to follow His Word only when it's convenient. He wants them to obey and keep His law with their whole ______________ (Ps. 119:2).

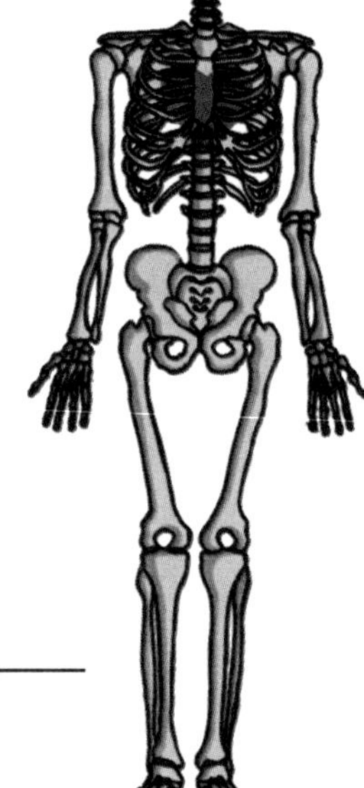

4. Which phrase could best be substituted for *heart* in the previous sentence?
   - ○ an organ for pumping blood
   - ○ the center, as in the phrase "the heart of the matter"
   - ○ feelings, emotions, or desires
5. As Christians seek to maintain a clean and undefiled walk with God, they are commanded to diligently keep and obey the ______________ of God (Ps. 119:3-4).
6. According to the glossary, what is a *precept* of God?

   ____
7. What are some precepts that God wants you to follow? (List three.)

   ____

   ____

   ____

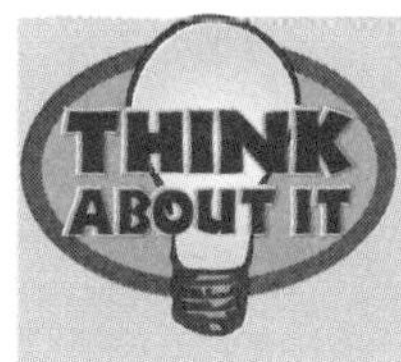
THINK
ABOUT IT

As you read the Bible, do you look for ways to strengthen your walk with God? Do you try to stay within the guidelines given by God's law, or do you regularly push against them and go a different way?

Royal Petitions

I Kings 3

Name ____________________

When God asked King Solomon what he desired, King Solomon made a humble request of God. Solomon loved the Lord and sought to follow Him and rule Israel as David his father had.

Answer the questions. You may use your Bible for help.

1. What did Solomon desire from God? (I Kings 3:9) ____________________

2. How did God answer this request? (I Kings 3:12-14) ____________________

By this request Solomon showed that he was not trusting in himself. He was relying on God as He ruled the people of Israel. Other leaders in the Bible also trusted God for guidance and help.

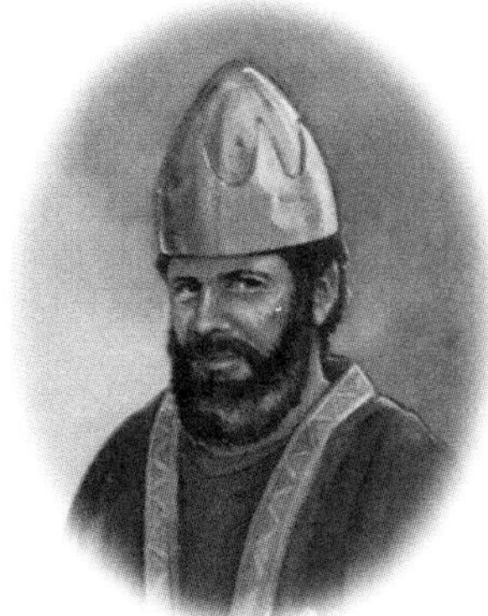

Complete the chart by writing the name of the person who prayed and the type of prayer.

Prayer for the country **Prayer for help from God**
Prayer for leaders **Prayer to show God to unbelievers**

Person	Reference	Prayer	Type of Prayer
	I Samuel 15:10-11	He prayed all night for King Saul, who had disobeyed God.	
	Daniel 9:1-11	He prayed for the nation of Israel, asking God to forgive them of sin.	
	I Kings 18:36-39	He prayed that God would send fire to show the power of God to Israel.	
	II Chronicles 20:5, 10-12	He prayed for God's help as they faced an enemy in battle.	

Just like these leaders who are mentioned in the Bible, you can take your requests to God.

Choose one type of prayer from the chart above and write your request. Then pray and ask God to answer your request.

____

____

God's House

I Kings 5-8

Name ________________________

Answer the questions. You may use your Bible for help.

1. Why had Solomon chosen this time to begin building the temple? (I Kings 5:3-4)

   ____

2. What prophecy was fulfilled by Solomon's building the temple? (I Kings 5:5) ______________

   ____

3. What promise did God make to Solomon as the temple was being built? (I Kings 6:11-13)

   ____

   ____

4. Solomon saw that the best craftsmen came and prepared the furnishings for use in the temple. What things came from the tabernacle without being changed? (I Kings 8:4)

   ____

5. What had Moses placed in the ark of the covenant that was still in it? (I Kings 8:9)

   ____

6. How long had it been since the Israelites left Egypt? (I Kings 6:1) ______________ years.

7. What did the appearance of the cloud mean when it filled the holy place? (I Kings 8:10-11)

   ____

8. During the dedication of the temple, Solomon praised God and blessed the people. How did Solomon and the people show honor to God? (I Kings 8:62-64)

   ____

THINK ABOUT IT

After the dedication and sacrifice, Solomon declared a time of feasting that lasted fourteen days. The whole country was rejoicing that God's house was complete and that the people now had a beautiful place to worship God.

What is your attitude toward worship? Do you think you could spend two weeks thinking only about God and worshiping Him?

I Kings 7:23
molten sea

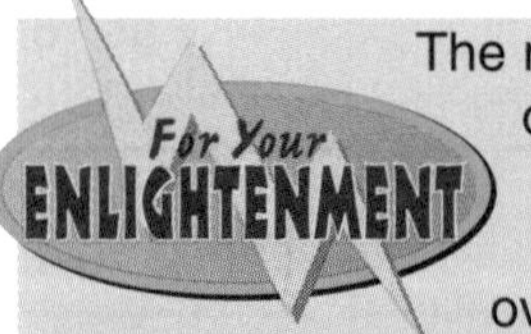
For Your
ENLIGHTENMENT

The months of the Hebrew calendar overlap those of the Gregorian calendar we use today. Each Jewish month starts in the middle of one of our months.

The new year of the Hebrew calendar starts in the spring. The months of the Hebrew calendar closely follow the cycle of the moon. A full moon marks the first of each month.

Many Men

I Kings 5

Name ______________________

Hiram, the king of Tyre, agreed to provide cedar and fir for the temple. Many of King Solomon's men joined King Hiram's men in Lebanon to cut and prepare the trees to be floated in the sea to Jerusalem.

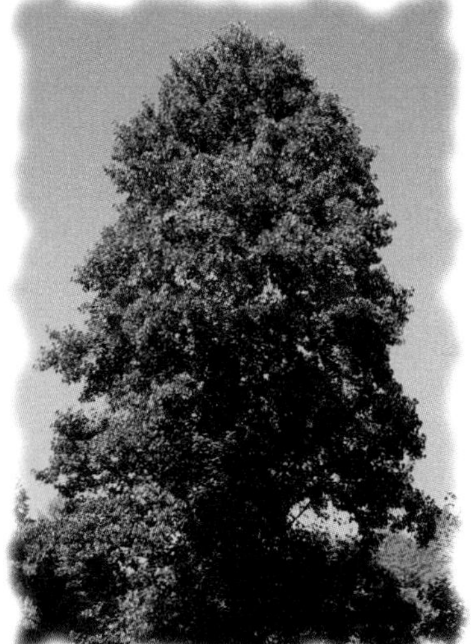

cedar tree

Many men were needed to prepare the wood and rock and the site before construction could begin. It took about seven years to build the temple. The Bible records the number of men Solomon used for this preparation.

Sidon
Mt. Lebanon
Mt. Hermon
Tyre
Capernaum
Bethsaida
Sea of Galilee
Ophrah
Mt. Moreh
Well of Harod
Valley of Jezreel
MEDITERRANEAN SEA
GILEAD
Aphek
Penuel
Succoth
Joppa
Shiloh
Jordan River
Jogbehah
AMMON
Jericho
Bethabara
Gibeah
Jerusalem
Bethany
Mt. Nebo
Bethlehem
PHILISTIA
Hebron
Wilderness of Judea
Dead Sea
MOAB

Rewrite each number word form in standard form on the chart.

1. **Three thousand three hundred** men were used as supervisors over the other workers.	men
2. **Thirty thousand** men went to cut and prepare wood with King Hiram's men.	men
3. **Fourscore thousand** men went to the mountains to cut and shape rock for the foundation. (*Hint:* A score is a group of twenty. Fourscore = 4 × 20.)	men
4. **Threescore and ten thousand** men carried the prepared materials to Jerusalem.	+ men
Total	**183,300** men

Use the chart to answer the questions.

5. Which group had the least men?

____

6. Which group had the most men?

____

7. Why do you think this group needed more men than the others? ______________________

____

____

THINK ABOUT IT

Solomon's workmen treated the house of God with respect. They worked quietly as the temple was being built. Is there a difference in your behavior and actions when you enter church for a service? Do you act as if you are prepared to listen to God's Word and learn from Him?

The Sure Way

Name ______________________

Read Psalm 119:5-8. Use words from the passage to complete the sentences.

1. The psalmist recognizes that only God is able to direct and establish the ____________ of a believer as he seeks to follow God's Word (Ps. 119:5).
2. Through obedience to God's Word, a Christian will not be ______________________ by the truth he sees as he reads the Bible (Ps. 119:6).
3. Consider the reverse of this truth. If a Christian is in sin, what will happen when he reads the truth of God's Word?

   ____

4. God knows Christians have difficulty staying on the right path and following His Word. Once the Word of God reveals sin and the believer asks forgiveness,

   he is able to praise God and thank Him for the ______________ judgments and laws found in the Bible (Ps. 119:7).

Put an *X* in the box for the best word(s) to complete each sentence.

		Ashamed	Not Ashamed
Acts 2:36-37	Peter shared with a group of Jews the truth about Christ's death and resurrection and the part they had played in God's plan. This truth caused the people to be ______.		
Romans 1:14-18	Paul was ready to preach the gospel to the Jews and Gentiles. He was ______ of the truth of God's Word.		
Psalm 38:1-6	As David realized his sin, he was ______, and asked God for forgiveness and mercy.		

THINK ABOUT IT Do you take comfort in reading the Word of God, or do you feel ashamed and guilty each time you open your Bible? As God reminds you of sin, take time to repent and ask forgiveness. Only then will you be able to truly praise God and thank Him for the truth found in His Word.

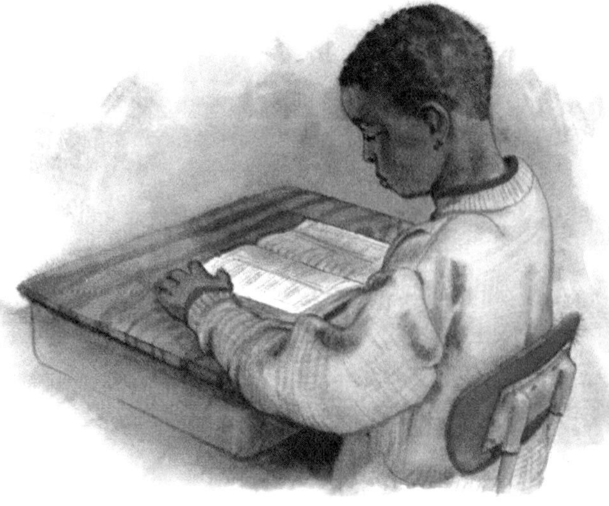

What Does God Say About My Worship?

Name ______________________

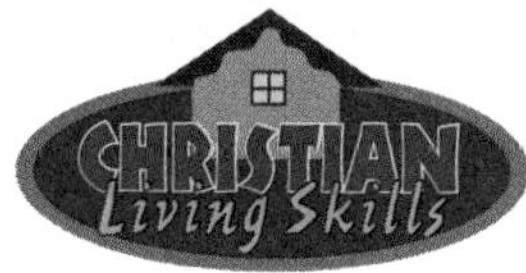
CHRISTIAN
Living Skills

What is **worship?** You hear about it in Sunday school and read about it in the Bible. You may have even participated in a worship service at your church. Many people think that worship is just something that you do on Sunday. However, you can worship God every day of the week. True worship is in the heart. The Bible teaches that expressing your sincere gratefulness to God for His love and mercy is a natural response for a Christian.

Using the glossary, write the definition of *worship*.

Worship means ____.

Read the verses and match them to the correct statement. Write who in the passage was worshiping God.

_____ 1. He built an altar, giving thanks to God for the safety of his family. ____________________

_____ 2. They willingly gave of their money and possessions to build God's tabernacle. ____________________

_____ 3. They spoke praises to God and gave glory to Him for sending His Son to earth. ____________________

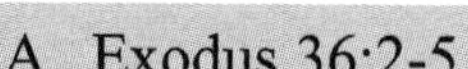

A. Exodus 36:2-5

B. Genesis 8:15-20

C. Luke 2:13-14

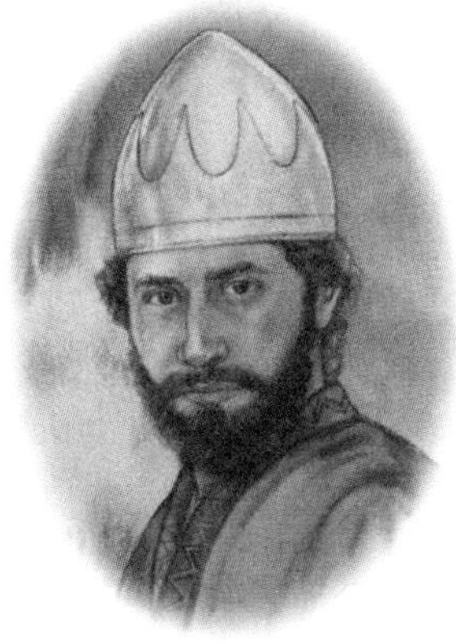

King David wrote many different kinds of psalms, including psalms of worship to God. These worship psalms express David's gratefulness for the goodness of God and for God's protection. They encourage believers and teach them how to worship God properly.

Read the verses in I Chronicles 16. Complete the instructions showing ways you can worship God.

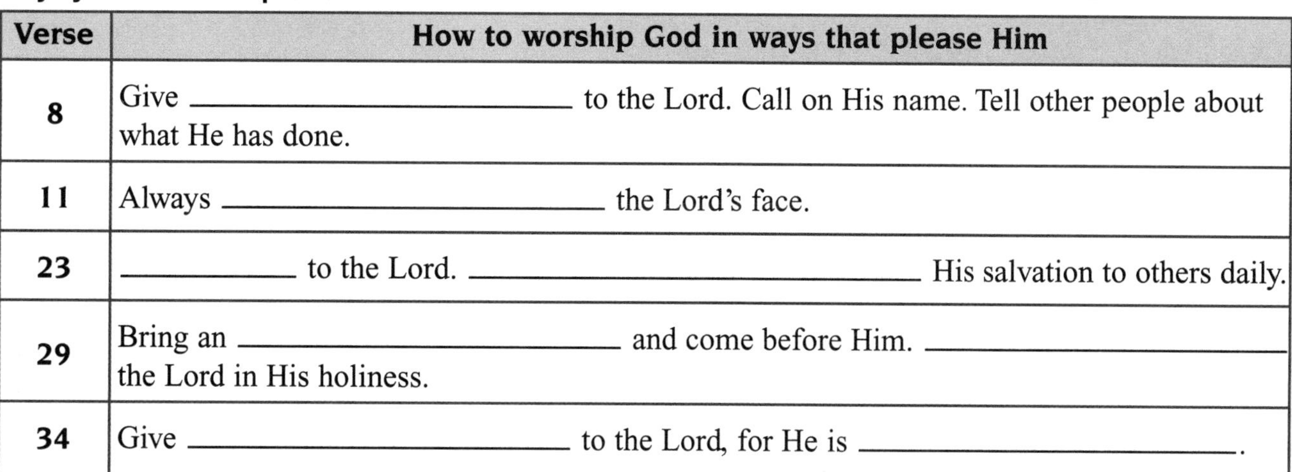

Verse	How to worship God in ways that please Him
8	Give ____________________ to the Lord. Call on His name. Tell other people about what He has done.
11	Always ____________________ the Lord's face.
23	__________ to the Lord. ________________________ His salvation to others daily.
29	Bring an ____________________ and come before Him. ____________________ the Lord in His holiness.
34	Give ____________________ to the Lord, for He is ____________________.

Something to Think About

Worship

Name ______________________

CHRISTIAN Living Skills

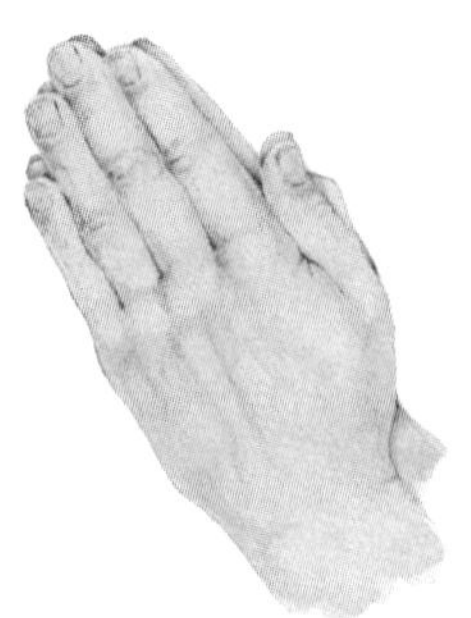

It is important for you to understand that worshiping God is more than **doing** something to show love, honor, and respect for Him. God is concerned about your heart. Christians know that all of their actions of worship (giving an offering, singing, reading Scripture, etc.) are just outward expressions of their inward spirit. God is displeased with the wrong kind of worship. Be careful! If you do things that look like you're worshiping God, but your heart is not in them, you are sinning against God.

Read John 4:23-24. Describe how God wants you to worship Him.

____

____

Read the scenarios and mark a ✔ in the box that describes the kind of worship taking place. If it is false worship, write why it is displeasing to God. If it is true worship, explain why God is pleased.

Scenario	True Worship	False Worship	Why is it displeasing or pleasing to God?
During the singing, Jessica mouthed the words to the hymns, but she was thinking about how she could get her dad's permission to go over to a friend's house after church.			
Stephen was hoping that his Sunday school teacher would call on him to pray out loud before class. He wanted the other kids to know how spiritual he was.			
Mitch's family has been praying for his dad to find a new job. When God provided a job for his dad, Mitch couldn't wait to tell his friends about how God had answered his prayers.			

What About Me?

Worshiping God reminds you that He is your provider. It allows you to express your gratefulness to Him for His goodness to you and it can show others how much you love Him. How do YOU worship God? Is it with a heart of gratefulness? Is your spirit praising God for His faithfulness to you?

Take time at home and think about your attitudes and actions toward worship. Carefully consider the following questions.

Do you focus on praising God when you are singing in church?

Is God pleased with the way you worship Him?

Do you worship God by telling others about His goodness to you?

Do you spend time thanking God for how He provides for you?

The questions to which you answered "no" or "sometimes" show areas you need to change in how you worship God. Ask God to help you worship Him in a way that is pleasing and honoring to Him.

Only Until . . .

Name ____________________

Identify the person that matches each description.

______ 1.	I am the grandmother of Joash.	A. Jehoiada
______ 2.	I became king at the age of seven.	B. Zechariah
______ 3.	I am the priest who anointed the young king.	C. princes of Judah
______ 4.	We are the men who gave the king bad advice.	D. Joash
______ 5.	I am the son of Jehoiada.	E. Athaliah

King Joash followed the godly advice of others in the early years of his reign. Jehoiada loved God and directed Joash according to God's Word. Joash did right as long as Jehoiada was alive, but as soon as Jehoiada's influence ended, Joash went the way of the world.

Many people in churches know how to act like Christians. But when they are removed from godly influences, they follow the worldly ways of the unsaved. For someone to live for God at all times, he must accept Christ as his Savior and desire to obey God's Word whether others around him do or not.

Unscramble the words to find ways a Christian can remain faithful to God.

A Christian should . . .

1. **DARE** ____________ God's Word (Deut. 17:19).
2. **BYOE** ____________ God's Word (Acts 5:29).
3. avoid **FLINUS** ____________ situations (James 4:7).
4. not listen to the **SULENOC** ____________ of ungodly people (Ps. 1:1).

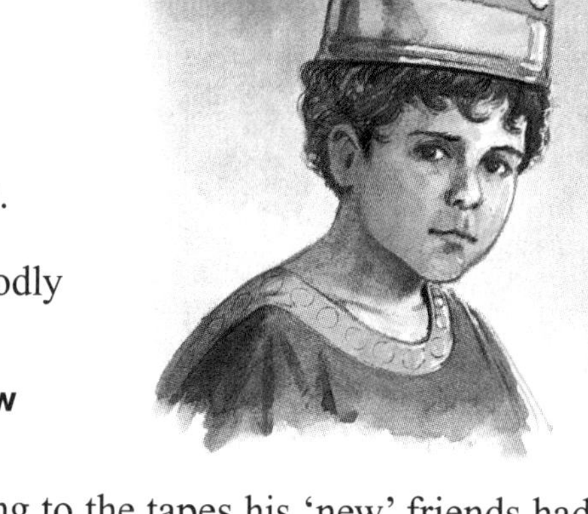

Read the story. Choose a truth from the list above. Write how Adrienne might use it to help Kirk return to following Christ.

Adrienne ran out her front door to meet Kirk. It had been months since Kirk's family had visited. Their parents were old friends, so the families got together several times a year. Kirk always seemed to have a science project brewing. On his last visit, he brought pulleys and heavy string to run 'tests' from the tree in the back yard.

As she neared the car, Adrienne gave a gasp as a head of purple hair appeared. Adrienne soon found that Kirk hadn't brought any science stuff on this trip. He said he had better things to do like listening to the tapes his 'new' friends had given him. Adrienne asked if he would attend the bonfire that evening at her church. She told him that several friends he had met the last visit were looking forward to seeing him again. Without looking, Kirk said he wasn't going to church much any more, so he'd rather not go.

At the bonfire, Adrienne found a quiet time to talk to the youth leader about the changes in Kirk. The leader reminded her of some truths from the Bible that she might share with Kirk.

Truth: ____

Adrienne would tell Kirk that the Bible says ______________________________

Singing with Understanding

"Great Is Thy Faithfulness" (vv. 1-3)

Name ______________________

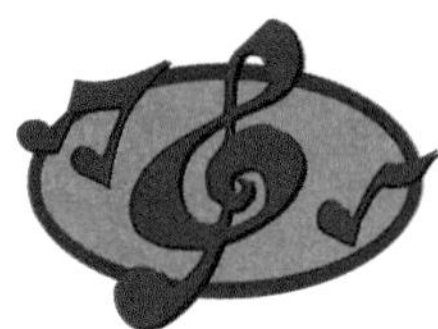

Read verses 1-2 of the hymn on page 315. Read the Scripture passages and compare the words of Scripture to the hymn. Write the phrases from the hymn that remind you of each Bible passage.

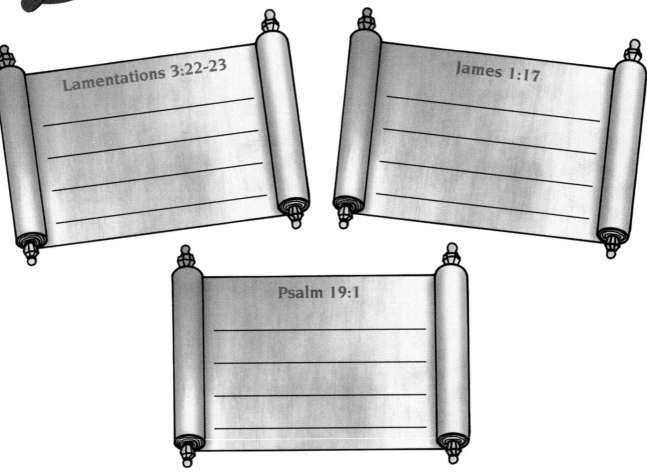

Lamentations 3:22-23

James 1:17

Psalm 19:1

Read verse 3 of the hymn. List blessings from the hymn and then add others you think of on your own.

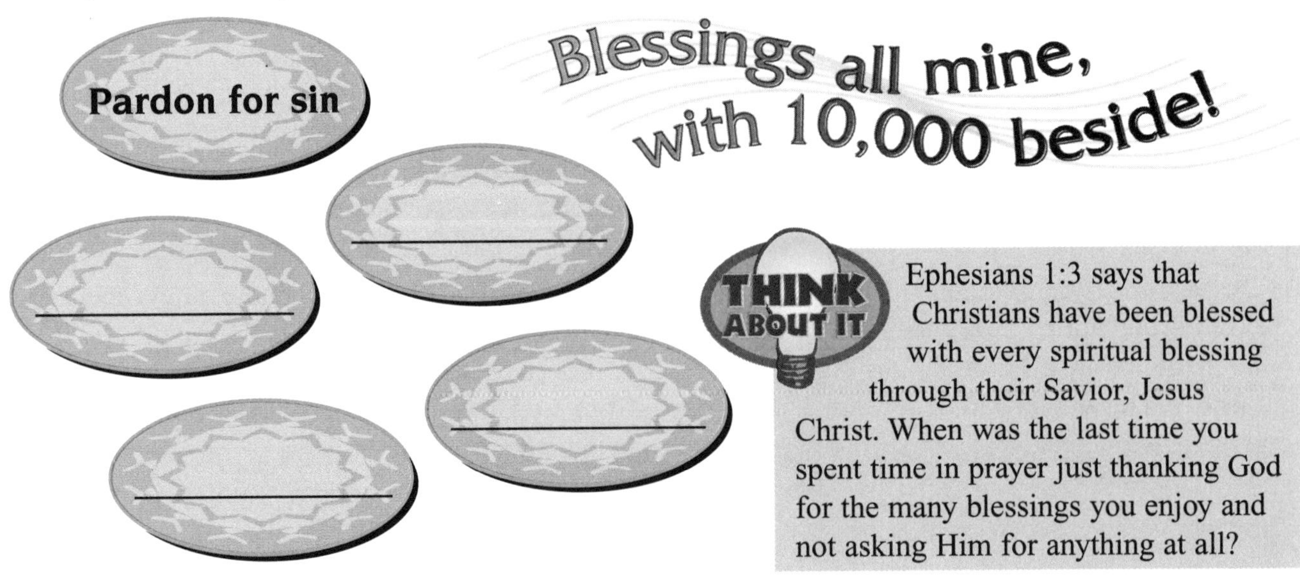

Pardon for sin
Blessings all mine, with 10,000 beside!
THINK ABOUT IT

Ephesians 1:3 says that Christians have been blessed with every spiritual blessing through their Savior, Jesus Christ. When was the last time you spent time in prayer just thanking God for the many blessings you enjoy and not asking Him for anything at all?

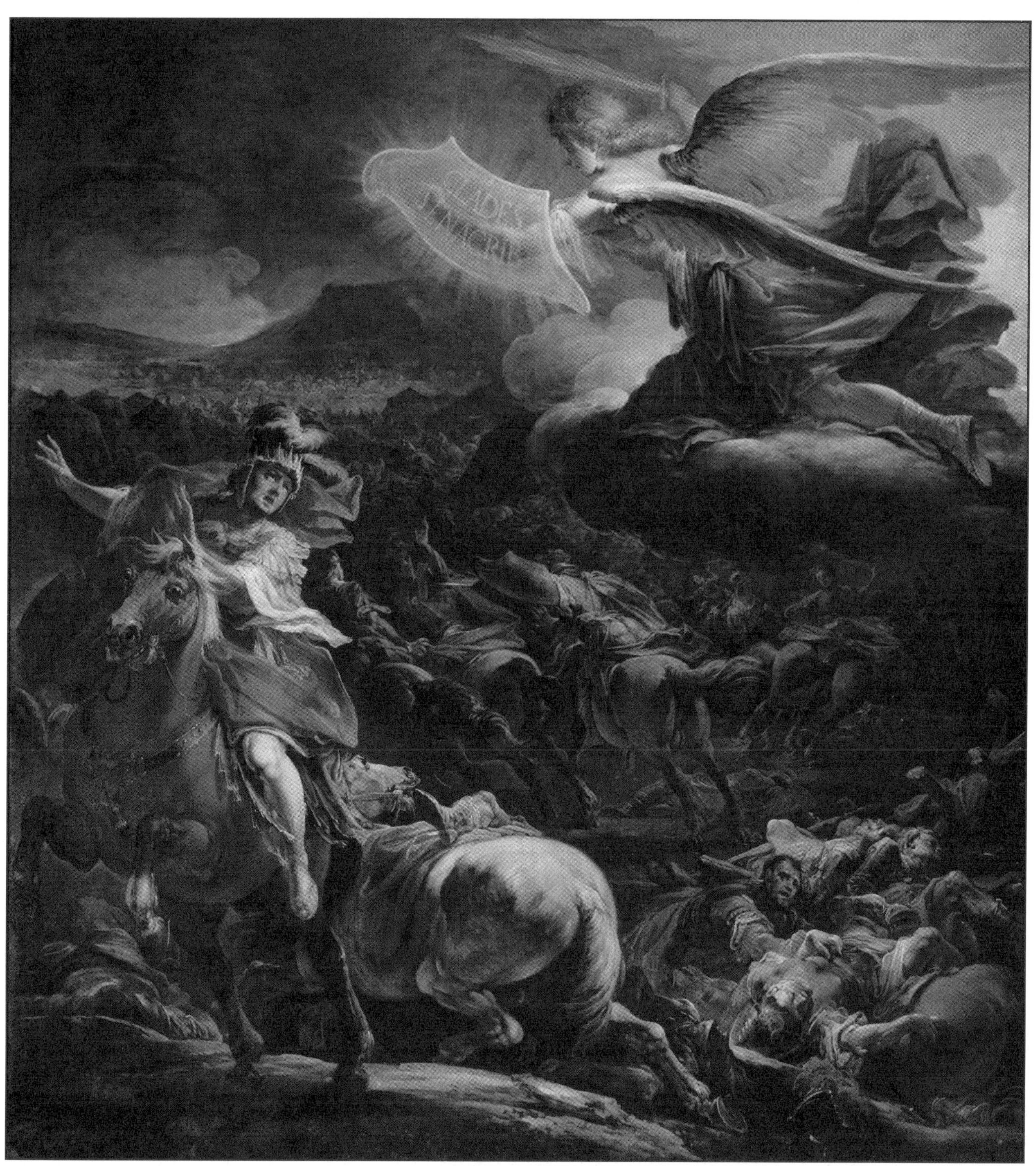

The Destruction of the Army of Sennacherib

Ilario Spolverini

Name ______________________

The Destruction of the Army of Sennacherib

by Ilario Spolverini (1657-1734)

Ilario Spolverini (Ē´lär ē ō Spōl və rē´nē) liked to paint excitement in scenes of violent battles or bandit attacks. In the accounts given in II Chronicles 32:1-22 and Isaiah 36-37, Hezekiah and his people were trapped in Jerusalem without hope of rescue until Hezekiah and Isaiah prayed and depended upon God.

This painting is one of seven paintings on the theme of justice and mercy. Some historians think that these paintings may have been made for a legal foundation or for a group that provided charity to the poor. Paintings that were exhibited in public places often contained themes that were instructional for the employees of those places. Each of the paintings in this set was painted by a different artist; one is dated 1733. Since they were all made to hang together in the same building, scholars think that all the works of the set were painted during the same time period.

The horses in the foreground look terrified. The men do not look confident either. King Sennacherib is in the front left with his crown clearly identifying him. Facing him diagonally across the painting is a fierce angel with a sword of flame. All around are dead and dying men. The grey horse behind the king has fallen and lost its rider. Men flee on horseback in all directions away from the angel's sword. In the left middle ground are the tents that the invaders have been living in. On this bright moonlit night, only the people of Jerusalem in the background are sleeping. The Lord's angel is battling the Assyrian army. On his shield is written "CLADES SENACRIB," Latin words meaning "Disaster to Sennacherib."

When Spolverini painted his horses running away from the dreaded angel, he showed them with their back feet together and their front legs stretched out before them. (In this position, the horses would have to jump like rabbits.) Modern photography has allowed us to see that one back foot and one front foot hit the ground at the same time. Today, artists can represent horses running more realistically than Spolverini could.

Following the Right Leader

II Kings 18-20

Name ______________________

Hezekiah began his reign by eliminating false religions and restoring the worship of God to the land of Judah. As King Hezekiah led in the observance of the Passover, many of the people from Israel returned to Jerusalem and joined with Judah in this important feast of praise and remembrance. When the land was invaded by Assyria and Jerusalem was under siege, Hezekiah looked to God for help. Hezekiah wisely followed the words of Isaiah and left the battle to the Lord.

Fill in the circle next to the correct answer.

1. The people of Jerusalem were urged to surrender to King Sennacherib and to rebel against Hezekiah and his God. The people responded by ______ (II Kings 18:36).
   - ○ agreeing that God was as powerless as the gods of other nations
   - ○ remaining faithful to Hezekiah and to God
   - ○ surrendering Jerusalem as they were taken away captive

2. God answered the prayers of Hezekiah and Isaiah by ______ (II Kings 19:35).
   - ○ killing the Assyrian soldiers during the night
   - ○ providing them with safe passage out of the city as it was attacked
   - ○ giving King Sennacherib access to the city through Hezekiah's tunnel

3. God fulfilled two prophecies made by Isaiah concerning the battle and the enemy. These prophecies were that ______ and that the Assyrian king would die by a sword (II Kings 19:7, 32, 37).
   - ○ Hezekiah would see Jerusalem captured
   - ○ the enemy would be defeated before they could shoot an arrow at the city
   - ○ Sennacherib would stop water from flowing into the city

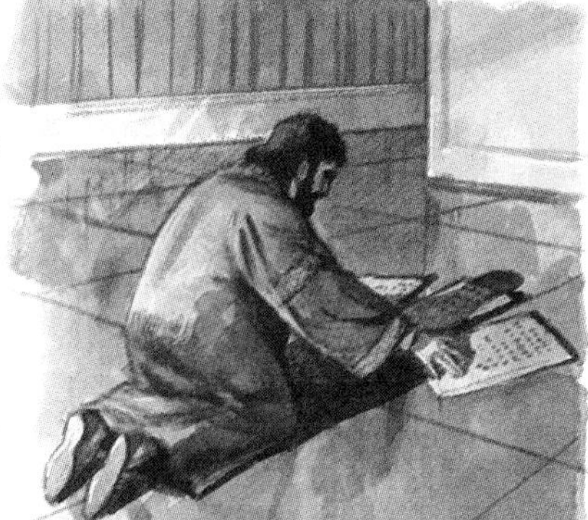

As Hezekiah followed God, the people followed Hezekiah.

Number the events in order. Use II Kings 20:1-11 for help.

- ___ God promised to answer Hezekiah's prayer.
- ___ Hezekiah prayed as he faced death.
- ___ As a sign to Hezekiah, God changed the movement of the earth so that the sun's shadow moved ten degrees backwards.
- ___ Isaiah directed Hezekiah to use figs to recover.
- 1 Isaiah visited the dying King Hezekiah.

For Your ENLIGHTENMENT — **The Dial of Ahaz**

The instrument used by Hezekiah to tell the time of day was a carefully placed staircase upon which the rays of the sun moved up and down. The time was revealed by the placement of shadows on the steps. The miracle that Hezekiah asked for was for the shadow to move back up the steps, therefore lengthening the time of daylight. The stairway is named after Hezekiah's predecessor, King Ahaz, who had it built.

Godly Leaders

Name ____________________

The Bible gives guidelines for leaders to follow. Godly leaders look to God and His Word for help.

Multiply each number by 6.

A	B	D	E	F	H	I	L	M
5	8	3	9	7	11	10	2	6

Multiply each number by 8.

N	O	P	R	S	T	U	V	W	Y
10	11	9	8	2	3	5	12	7	4

Use the code to spell the characteristics a godly leader should have. You may use your Bible for help.

1. A godly leader is ___ ___ ___ ___ ___ (Ps. 27:1).
   16 30 96 54 18

2. A godly leader is a ___ ___ ___ ___ ___ ___ ___ to bring others to salvation (Ps. 51:12-13).
   56 60 24 80 54 16 16

3. A godly leader reads and ___ ___ ___ ___ ___ God's Word (Josh. 1:8).
   88 48 54 32 16

4. A godly leader ___ ___ ___ ___ ___ for God's guidance (Ps. 143:10).
   72 64 30 32 16

5. A godly leader ___ ___ ___ ___ ___ ___ ___ to godly counsel (Ps. 1:1).
   12 60 16 24 54 80 16

6. A godly leader is ___ ___ ___ ___ ___ ___ about accomplishments (Prov. 16:19; 29:23).
   66 40 36 48 12 54

7. A godly leader avoids sin and ___ ___ ___ ___ ___ teaching (Titus 2:11-12).
   42 30 12 16 54

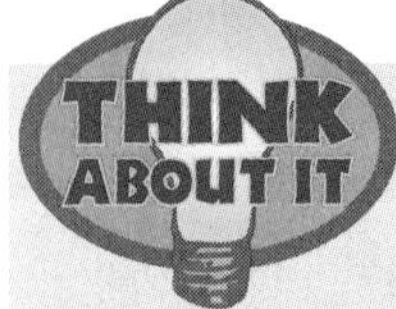
THINK ABOUT IT

Are there any characteristics of a godly leader that are not characteristics every Christian should have? ____________

A leader has more opportunities to influence people. But everyone influences other people. Do you have a godly influence on others?

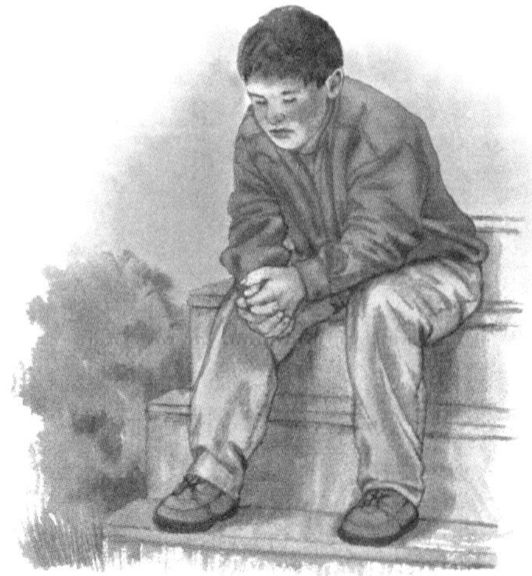

The Bible says you are to pray for those who are over you. Have you prayed for your leaders today?

Prophecies to Kings

Name ______________________________

Christians usually think of prophecies as being about the coming and death of Christ or about the end times. But the Bible contains many other prophecies. God gave the following prophecies concerning three kings of Judah.

Prophecies

Isaiah prophesied to King Hezekiah concerning Sennacherib, the king of Assyria. This prophecy from God contained three parts.

Write the letter of the verse in which the prophecy was fulfilled next to each prophecy.

_____ 1. Sennacherib would return home (II Kings 19:6-7).	A. II Kings 19:37
_____ 2. Sennacherib would die by a sword (II Kings 19:6-7).	B. II Kings 19:35
_____ 3. God would protect Israel (II Kings 19:30-34).	C. II Kings 19:36

When King Jeroboam took leadership of the tribes of Israel which split away from Judah, he created places for false worship to keep people from returning to Jerusalem. God sent a messenger to deliver a prophecy to Jeroboam.

Complete each sentence.

1. The man of God told Jeroboam that ____________________ would destroy the high places and burn their priests (I Kings 13:2).
2. Josiah was the sixteenth king over Judah after the prophecy was made to Jeroboam.

   During Josiah's reign, ______________________________ was found during the temple restoration (II Kings 22:8, 10).
3. After reading the law of God, King Josiah made a ____________________ to follow God and His Word (II Kings 23:3-4).
4. To restore proper worship of God, Josiah led the people in destroying idols, altars, and

   high places of false worship. Josiah also ____________________ the priests and burned their bones in fulfillment of the prophecy made to Jeroboam (II Kings 23:14-15, 20).

King Jehoshaphat began his reign as a godly king. Toward the end of his reign, he began to trust in alliances with other nations rather than God.

Answer the question.

What prophecy was made by Eliezer concerning the alliance between Jehoshaphat and Ahaziah?

(II Chron. 20:37) ____

The Way of the Word

Name ______________________

Use words from Psalm 119:9-12 to complete the sentences.

1. The Christian is to keep his life and his walk with God clean and pure. He can only do this by ______________________ according to God's Word (Ps. 119:9).
2. Some believers may think that they have to think about God and His Word only when they are in church, in Bible class, or having devotions. David tells us that the Christian is to seek God with his ______________ (Ps. 119:10).
3. It is not always possible to carry a Bible everywhere as a defense against sin. But a Christian can still have God's Word with him wherever he goes and whatever he is doing by ______________________ (Ps. 119:11).

Read the story. Use Psalm 40 to answer the questions.

Shannon stared at the test questions, listening to the quiet sound of pencils scratching around her. "I've got to focus," she thought. "I've got to think about geography instead of Mom's lab report." Her mother was going to find out the results of some medical tests today. Shannon had found it hard to concentrate on anything until she knew whether or not her mom had cancer.

Shannon looked up at the clock. Only ten minutes left to finish the test. The verses Pastor Conner had read from Psalm 40 last week came back to her mind. *Often we are so concerned about our problems that we forget to look to God for help with them,* Pastor had said. "Here I am," thought Shannon, "right in the middle of a problem, and I haven't even asked for help yet."

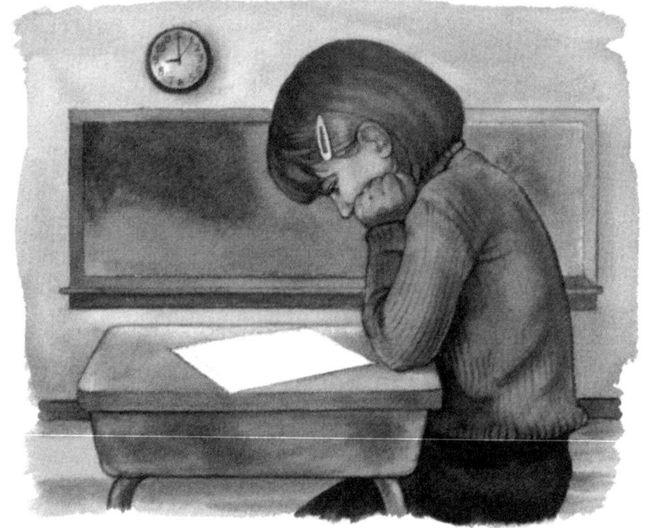

What should Shannon ask God to help her do?

____

____

1. After praying and asking God for help, what are you to do until He answers? (Ps. 40:1) ______________________
2. If your words influence others for Christ, how do you think your trust and obedience might influence them? ______________________
3. God has done and continues to do wonderful things. If the psalmist were able to share them all, how many would there be? (Ps. 40:5) ______________________

What Does God Say About My Work Habits?

Name ______________________

CHRISTIAN Living Skills

God is concerned about the way you fulfill the responsibilities He has entrusted to you. The choices you make today will become the *habits* that will influence the success of your work for the rest of your life. A **habit** is any action that is done so often that you can do it without thinking about it, such as brushing your teeth or tying your shoe.

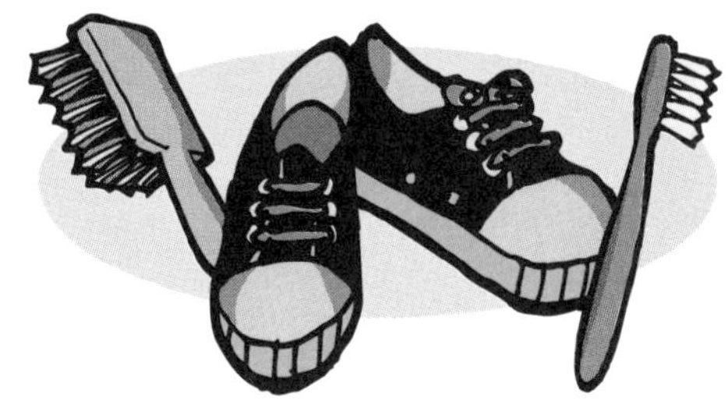

List several habits that have become part of your life.

______________________ ______________________

______________________ ______________________

Read Colossians 3:17 and describe the attitude you should have toward the way you do your work.

____

Read each verse and think about specific ways you can please God in your work. Complete the chart.

Reference	God's Command/Warning About My Work	What I Can Do to Please God in My Work
I Corinthians 14:40		
Proverbs 21:5		
I Thessalonians 4:11-12		

Read II Thessalonians 3:6-15 and answer the questions.

1. What is the cause-effect relationship found in verse 10? ______________________

____

2. How does this cause-effect relationship demonstrate God's justice? ______________________

____

3. According to these verses, why do you think it is important that Christians have good reputations in the way they do their work? ______________________

Something to Think About

My Work Habits

Name ______________________________

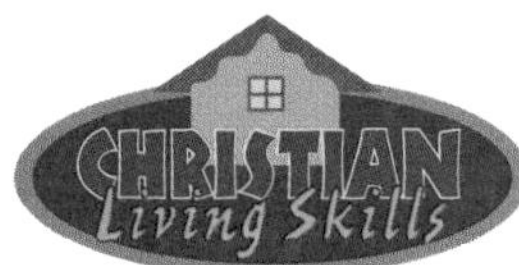
CHRISTIAN
Living Skills

There are many Christlike character qualities that you should be developing into **work habits** as you seek to please God.

Using the clues, complete the puzzle to discover these qualities.

Clues

diligence	**honesty**	**endurance**
prompt	**initiative**	**thorough**
responsible	**trustworthy**	**organization**
creative	**loyal**	**attentive**

Down:

1. The ability to begin and carry out a task
2. Completing the details of a task
5. The ability to face and conquer challenges in a task
7. The ability to work on the task in an orderly manner
10. Having new ideas in approaching a task

Across:

3. Telling the truth about every issue
4. Dependable; reliable; able to accomplish the assigned task
6. Able to be trusted to make the right decision
8. Completing the assigned task on time
9. Giving steadfast allegiance to something or someone
11. Industriousness; hard work
12. Giving careful attention to instructions and details of a task

1 2 3 4 5 6 7 8 9 10 11 12

What About Me?

Take time at home to think about your work habits. Carefully consider the following questions.

1. What three qualities describe your work habits? ______________ ______________ ______________
2. Which quality would your teacher say describes your work habits? ______________
3. Which quality would your teacher say does NOT describe your work habits? ______________
4. What three qualities do you need to develop in your work habits?

   ______________ ______________ ______________

5. Choose one quality to work on. What action can you take to make it become a work habit for you?

   ____

The Kings of Judah

The twelve tribes of Israel were united during the time of Saul, David, and Solomon. Because of Rehoboam's harsh treatment of the people, ten of the tribes split and made Jeroboam king over Israel, the Northern Kingdom. The two remaining tribes under the rule of Rehoboam became known as Judah, the Southern Kingdom. Twenty kings ruled over Judah after Solomon. The records of the lives of these kings are in I Kings, II Kings, and II Chronicles. For some kings, several chapters record the events of their reigns. The reigns of others are described in a few verses. These accounts tell not only the ages of the kings, the lengths of their reigns, and the battles they fought, but also about their character and relationships to God. The records for most of the "good" kings include statements that the kings "did that which was right in the sight of the Lord."

Evil Kings

Good Kings

1. **Rehoboam** He sought the advice of young counselors and was extremely harsh to the people. The kingdom split during his reign.
2. **Abijah** He was defeated by Jeroboam in efforts to reunite the kingdom.
3. **Asa** He removed the idol worship from the land. He trusted God for their victories in battle.
4. **Jehoshaphat** He was one of Judah's wealthiest kings. He feared God and was greatly blessed.
5. **Jehoram** He killed his six brothers to become king. He continued in sin, even after God spoke to him through Elijah.
6. **Ahaziah** He ruled for less than 1 year, then was killed in battle.
7. **(Queen) Athaliah** She was the mother of Ahaziah and the only queen to rule over Judah. To assure her throne, she sought to kill all heirs to the throne.
8. **Joash** He was hidden from Queen Athaliah and his life was spared. He became king at age 7.
9. **Amaziah** He followed God for most of his reign, and then began trusting in himself and suffered serious defeat in battle.
10. **Uzziah** (Azariah) He became king at age 16. He followed God through the influence of the prophet Zechariah. Late in his reign he performed priestly duties in the temple, and God punished him with leprosy.
11. **Jotham** This follower of God brought strength to the land by building the armies and fortifying the cities.
12. **Ahaz** He closed all worship in the temple. Because of his wickedness he was defeated in battle and lost much of the wealth of the kingdom.
13. **Hezekiah** God greatly blessed this king who loved Him. Hezekiah removed idol worship and restored worship in the temple and the observance of the Passover. God gave Hezekiah a sign when granting Hezekiah a longer life.
14. **Manasseh** He became king at age 12. All the good accomplished by Hezekiah was destroyed by Manasseh, who caused the people to sin more than the heathen nations. Manasseh repented and turned to God when taken captive by the Assyrians.
15. **Amon** He followed the wicked influence of his father. After 2 years as king, he was murdered by servants.
16. **Josiah** He became king at age 8. He removed the idol worship, rebuilt the temple, and observed the Passover.
17. **Jehoahaz** He was placed on the throne by the pharaoh of Egypt. The pharaoh removed him from office after only 3 months.
18. **Jehoiakim** The brother of Jehoahaz was also made king by the pharaoh. He was defeated as he led an uprising against Babylon.
19. **Jehoiachin** He became king at age 18 and reigned 3 months. During his reign, Judah was taken captive by the Babylonians and the temple treasures were taken to King Nebuchadnezzar.
20. **Zedekiah** During his reign, the Babylonians destroyed and burned Jerusalem, tortured him, and killed his sons.

The Kingdom Divided

I Kings 12-14

Name ______________________________

The twelve tribes of Israel remained united as one nation through the reigns of Saul, David, and Solomon. God had granted Solomon the wisdom to rule the country. Solomon wisely chose godly men to help advise him. The people knew that they could come to King Solomon and receive wise responses.

After Rehoboam became king, Jeroboam and the people came to him with a request to lighten the yoke placed upon them by Solomon.

Answer the questions.

1. What does the word *yoke* mean in I Kings 12:4? (You may use the glossary.) ________________
2. Who did King Rehoboam first go to for counsel? (I Kings 12:6) ________________
3. What advice did they give? (I Kings 12:7) ________________

   ____
4. Who else did Rehoboam look to for counsel? (I Kings 12:8) ________________
5. The young men advised Rehoboam to increase the yoke of the people and to treat them more harshly. Whom did Rehoboam listen to? (I Kings 13-14) ________________
6. What was the reaction of the people to Rehoboam's announcement? (I Kings 12:19-20)

   ____

For Your ENLIGHTENMENT Only the tribes of Judah and Benjamin remained under the rule of the house of David. This kingdom that remained in the south with Jerusalem as its capital became known as ***Judah.***

Ten tribes of Israel chose to make Jeroboam their king. Jeroboam was not from the line of David and introduced idol worship to keep the people from returning to the temple in Jerusalem. He placed golden calves in Bethel and in Dan for the people to worship. This Northern Kingdom chose Samaria as its capital and became known as ***Israel.***

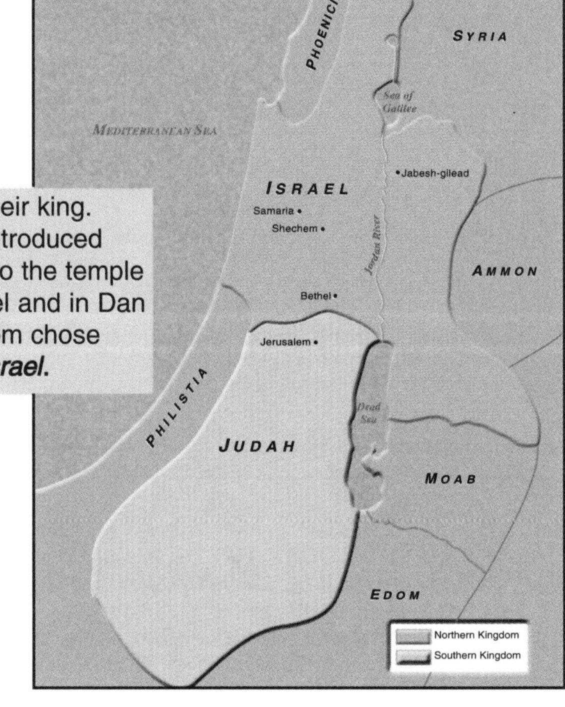
Divided Kingdom—
Israel and Judah
Phoenicia
Dan
Syria
Sea of Galilee
Mediterranean Sea
Jabesh-gilead
Israel
Samaria
Shechem
Jordan River
Ammon
Bethel
Jerusalem
Philistia
Dead Sea
Judah
Moab
Edom
Northern Kingdom
Southern Kingdom

THINK ABOUT IT Whom do you go to for advice—your friends or an adult? Remember Rehoboam the next time you have a problem to solve or a big decision to make. Look to your parents, a teacher, or another adult who will give you advice that follows God's Word.

What Does God Say About Choosing Friends?

Name ______________________________

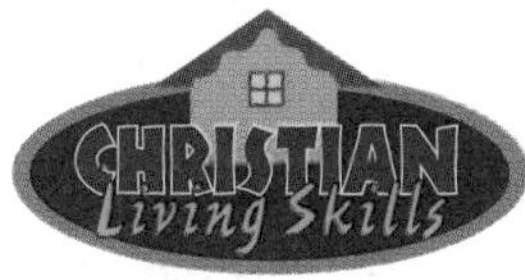
CHRISTIAN
Living Skills

While your friendships are important to you and to God, you must remember that your friends should never be the *most* important thing in your life. **Peer pressure** is the pressure put on you by your friends to love what they love. It can cause you to become like your friends if you allow them to influence your attitudes and actions.

If you have friends that love God, then peer pressure can be a good encouragement to you. However, if you have friends that love the world, you're headed for trouble. You should never love anything or anyone more than you love God. In His Word, God gives you good advice for choosing friends.

Read Proverbs 13:20. Complete the statements.

God is teaching me in this verse that I should ______________________________.

He is warning me not to ______________________________.

Read the verses and complete the statements to find out how to choose good friends.

Proverbs 17:17 — I should choose a friend who will ______________________________.

Proverbs 28:7 — I should choose a friend who does not ______________________________.

Proverbs 16:28 — I should choose a friend who will not ______________________________ or ______________________________ friends.

Psalm 119:63 — I should choose a friend who ____________________ God and who will ______________________________ God's Word.

A good friend is not afraid to be honest with you. The Bible teaches that he will tell you what needs changing in your attitude because he cares about you. A good friend will encourage you to do what is pleasing to God and will be loyal to you in the tough times. Taking the time to find this kind of friend is worth it!

Read the following verses from Proverbs 27 and match them to the correct statement.

A. verse 6 B. verse 9 C. verse 17

_____ 1. A true friend challenges me to make good decisions and develop Christlike character, which will protect my testimony and please God.

_____ 2. A true friend isn't afraid to confront me when I do wrong, even if he knows it will hurt my feelings, because he is concerned that I choose to please God.

_____ 3. A true friend is valuable to me because he gives me good advice that will encourage me to obey God.

Something to Think About

Choosing Good Friends

Name ______________________

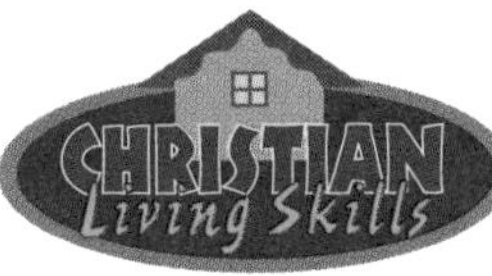
CHRISTIAN
Living Skills

What kind of person do you consider to be a true friend? What kind of character do you think a true friend should have? What are you looking for in a friend? It is important that you know the kind of friend that pleases God so that you won't be deceived by people who may be "friendly," but who don't love God or want to please God in all that they do. Remember, you will become like your friends!

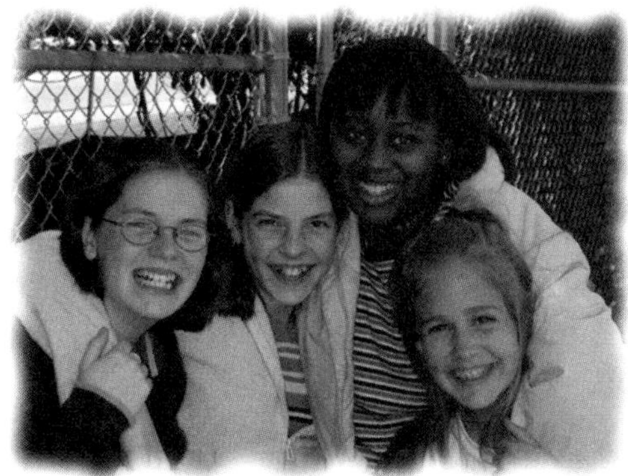

Read each scenario and determine the choices you should make about your friends.

Scenario	What Should You Do?
Stephen is your new neighbor, and your mom has encouraged you to have a good testimony with him. You want to go over to his house on Saturday, but you know that his parents allow him to play computer games your parents do not allow you to play. Stephen tells you not to mention the computer games to your parents. Instead, he suggests that you just tell them you're going to be playing baseball.	
Several girls you know like to hang out at the mall. They are always talking about the newest fads and buying popular magazines to find out what the movie stars are wearing. They talk like they have fun, and they love to sing the latest songs they hear on the radio. They invite you to go to the mall with them.	

What About Me?

Take time at home to think about your friends.

List the top six qualities you look for when choosing your friends.

______________ ______________ ______________

______________ ______________ ______________

- **Go back to your list and circle the qualities that please God.**
- **Study your list and think about the friends you enjoy spending time with most.**
- **Complete the following chart by putting a ✔ in the correct box.**

Questions for Thought	Yes	No
Is God pleased with my choice of friends?		
Do my friends love God and want to please Him?		
Do my friends prove that they care about me by being honest with me when I'm wrong?		
Do my friends honor and obey their parents?		
Do my friends encourage me to honor and obey my parents?		
Are my parents pleased with the kind of friends I have?		

The Way of Joy

Name ______________________

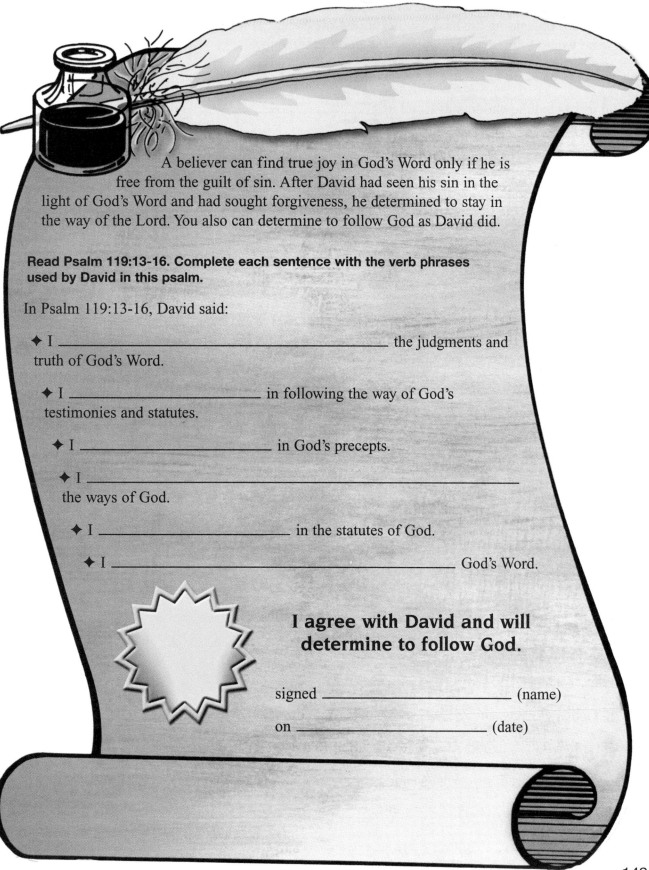

A believer can find true joy in God's Word only if he is free from the guilt of sin. After David had seen his sin in the light of God's Word and had sought forgiveness, he determined to stay in the way of the Lord. You also can determine to follow God as David did.

Read Psalm 119:13-16. Complete each sentence with the verb phrases used by David in this psalm.

In Psalm 119:13-16, David said:

- ✦ I ______________________ the judgments and truth of God's Word.
- ✦ I ______________________ in following the way of God's testimonies and statutes.
- ✦ I ______________________ in God's precepts.
- ✦ I ______________________ the ways of God.
- ✦ I ______________________ in the statutes of God.
- ✦ I ______________________ God's Word.

I agree with David and will determine to follow God.

signed ______________________ (name)

on ______________________ (date)

High Places

Name ______________________

As Israel was preparing to enter the Promised Land, God gave Moses specific instructions for possessing the land. God expected obedience. Disobedience to God's Word would bring the consequences of God's judgment.

eyes
destroy
disobedience
drive out
thorns
tribes

Read Numbers 33:50-56 to complete the instructions given to Moses.

1. God instructed the children of Israel to ______________________ all the inhabitants of the land.
2. They were to ________________ all their images and idols and their high places.
3. They were to take possession of the land and divide it by families according to their __________.
4. God said that the inhabitants of the land would continually annoy them like pricks in their ________________ and ________________ in their sides if not driven out.
5. If their ______________________ continued, God would do to the children of Israel as He wanted done to the inhabitants of the land.

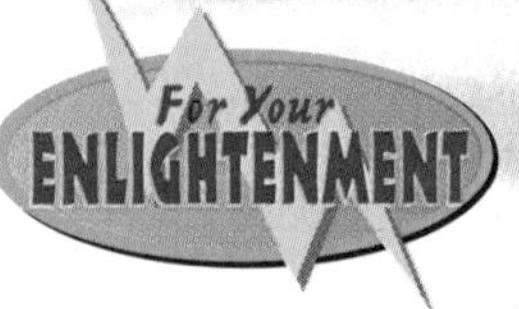
For Your
ENLIGHTENMENT

Some of the kings of Judah permitted high places to remain for use in worship to God. This method of worshiping God was not in His plan for the people.

The Scriptures record that Hezekiah and Josiah removed the high places, but they were rebuilt by wicked kings.

High places were used in many pagan forms of worship. These altars for sacrifices and incense were often on hilltops or raised mounds of earth. Some religions included the sacrificing of children. This practice was followed by two kings of Judah.

Use your knowledge of the kings to answer the questions.

1. Did the children of Israel successfully remove the inhabitants and their religions? ____________
2. How were the enemies like annoying pricks and thorns to the people?

   ____

3. Did God approve when the kings of Judah permitted high places of worship? ____________
4. Where were God's people supposed to go to offer their sacrifices? ______________________
5. God keeps His promises. What should the kings of Judah have known would happen when they continued to disobey God? ______________________

   ____

Alliances

Name ______________________

God's Word says that even though Christians live in the world, they are not to be joined improperly with the things and people of the world. The godly kings usually had peaceful relationships with other nations; but God often used battles to show these godly kings their need to repent of wrongdoing. Some kings chose to join with other nations rather than to trust God to help them in battle. These battles often ended in defeat.

Make an *X* to mark the type of alliance each king of Judah had with another king or nation.

		Alliance that honored God and His desires	Alliance for self that dishonored God
1. The Lord was with King Asa of Judah. Some of the tribes of Israel saw this and joined Judah to worship in Jerusalem.	**II Chron. 15:9-12**		
2. King Asa paid the Syrians to battle Israel.	**II Chron. 16:7**		
3. Nearby countries made peace with King Jehoshaphat when they heard that the Lord fought his battles.	**II Chron. 20:29-30**		
4. King Jotham trusted God for victory over the Ammonites. God gave him victory and the Ammonites paid tribute to Judah.	**II Chron. 27:5-7**		
5. King Ahaz used the treasure of the temple to pay the Assyrians to help in a battle that was a judgment from the Lord.	**II Chron. 28:16-21**		
6. King Josiah ignored God's warning and joined the king of Assyria in fighting against Egypt. Josiah was killed in the battle.	**II Chron. 35:20-24**		

Length of Days

Name ____________________

God promised David that as long as his descendants continued to walk in the truth of God's Word, there would continue to be a descendant of David on the throne. Only God's mercy permitted the evil kings to reign.

Read Psalm 91:14-16 and Proverbs 3:1-3. Answer the questions.

1. What does God promise in both of these passages?

   ____
   ____
   ____
   ____

2. What is man's responsibility to receive these promises?

   ____
   ____
   ____
   ____
   ____

■ = good king ■ = bad king

Kings of Judah

Rehoboam
Abijah
Asa
Jehoshaphat
Jehoram
Ahaziah
Q. Athaliah
Joash
Amaziah
Uzziah
Jotham
Ahaz
Hezekiah
Manasseh
Amon
Josiah
Jehoahaz
Jehoiakim
Jehoiachin
Zedekiah

5 10 15 20 25 30 35 40 45 50 55 60

Years of Reign

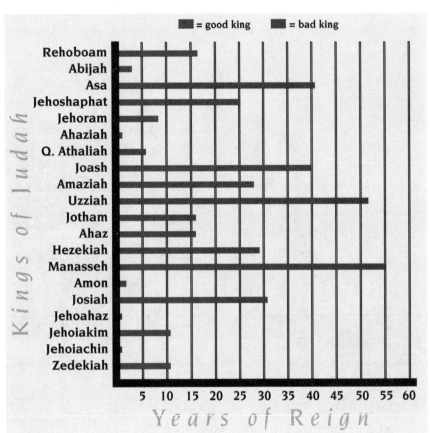

Use the kings graph to answer the questions about the good and evil kings.

1. Which group has more kings? ____________________
2. Which group has more who reigned over 20 years? ____________________
3. Why do you think certain kings had longer reigns? (*Hint:* Remember the verses above.)

   ____
4. Why do you think God might have extended the reign of Manasseh? (II Chron. 33:12-16)

   ____

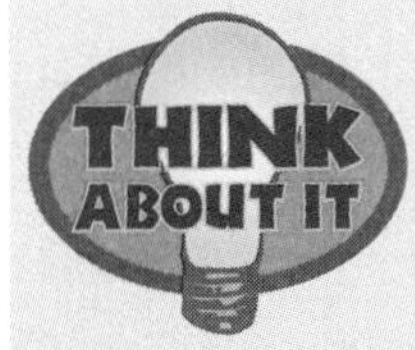
THINK
ABOUT IT

God continued to give kings of Judah opportunities to do right and serve Him. God loves all men and desires that they love Him and choose the salvation He provides. The kings knew the truth of God's Word, but more than half chose to turn from Him. You have heard the truth of God's Word. Do you choose to follow Him?

Get the Bible Reading H.A.B.I.T.

Name ____________________

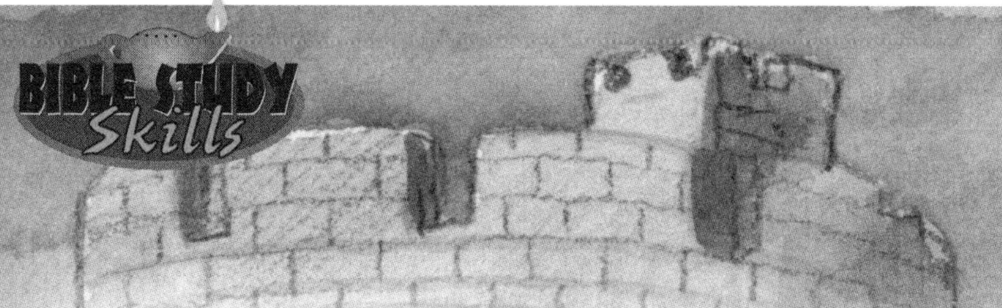
BIBLE STUDY
Skills

Have a special time set aside each day to read your Bible. If possible, make it the same time every day.

Ask God to teach you from His Word. Remember to thank Him for helping you to understand and apply it.

Be still and give your attention to what you are reading.

Investigate the Scripture by asking yourself questions about it.

Take time to look up words and ideas you do not understand.

As you read the Scripture for each day, write the date in the box.

God is able to do much more than Christians can ask or think. **Ephesians 3:20-21**	God promises to meet Christians' needs for His own glory. **Philippians 4:19-20**	God provides for Christians' financial needs as they give to His work. **II Corinthians 9:7-11**	God uses other Christians to supply the needs of His people. **Philippians 4:10-14**	We must not trust in riches but in God who provides them. **I Timothy 6:17-19**
Put on the armor of God to be strong to stand against Satan. **Ephesians 6:10-13**	Protect yourself with truth, righteousness, and a prepared gospel witness. **Ephesians 6:14-15**	Faith is the Christian's shield, salvation his helmet, and God's Word his sword. **Ephesians 6:16-17**	Christians must pray for boldness for themselves and others. **Ephesians 6:18-20**	Christians can stand fast because their comfort and hope are in God. **II Thessalonians 2:15-17**
Christians should warn sinners, encourage the weak, and do good to all. **I Thessalonians 5:14-15**	Love God, not the temporary things of this world. **I John 2:15-17**	Meekness is one of the fruits of the Spirit. **Galatians 5:22-23**	If Christians walk in the Spirit, they will not be proud and envious. **Galatians 5:24-26**	Christians should live in harmony and respond to others with humility. **Romans 12:14-17**
All things work together for Christians' good to make them like Christ. **Romans 8:28-30**	No bad thing can separate Christians from Christ's love. **Romans 8:31-39**	Whoever is born of God does not habitually sin. **I John 3:5-9**	Godly sorrow for sin brings about true repentance. **II Corinthians 7:9-11**	When others are caught in sin, Christians should help to restore them with meekness. **Galatians 6:1-5**

Praying with Purpose

Name ______________________________

God is omniscient and already knows Christians' needs and desires, so why do they pray? Those who pray do so because they have a sincere desire to please God and relate to Him as His child. Sincere prayer quickly teaches us that many purposes are accomplished by prayer.

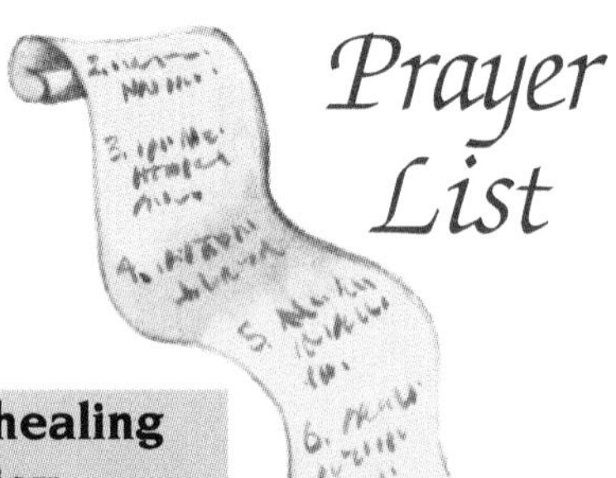
Prayer List

Complete the puzzle by writing a word from the word bank to match each underlined definition.

understanding	**healing**
temptation	**joy**
pleases	**blessings**
thanks	**presence**
praise	

Across

1. Prayer offers God the admiration and exaltation He is worthy to receive (Ps. 67:3).
3. Prayer strengthens the believer against the attraction to do wrong (Matt. 26:41).
7. Prayer brings God's gifts and favor (Matt. 7:11).
8. Prayer helps the believer increase in judgment and discretion (Jer. 33:3).

Down

1. Prayer delights God (Prov. 15:8).
2. Prayer completes the believer's deep and lasting satisfaction (John 16:24).
4. Prayer gives the believer assurance of God's closeness (Ps. 145:18).
5. Prayer gives restoration of health to the spirit of the believer (James 5:15).
6. Prayer helps the believer express the gratitude God deserves (Eph. 5:20).

These are only a few of the purposes for praying.

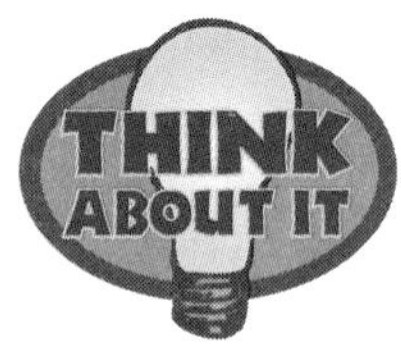
THINK ABOUT IT

Add to the list by writing more purposes here and giving Scripture references for them. You may use a Bible concordance for help.

____

____

REMEMBER!

God does not answer *yes* to every prayer, even if it is prayed for the right purposes. Sometimes He answers *no* or *wait,* but a Christian who prays with a purpose can always be assured that God will hear and give the best answer.

Apart from the Crowd

Daniel 1

Name ______________________

King Nebuchadnezzar conquered Jerusalem in the land of Judah. He stole the treasures from the temple of God and took them to the house of his god. Many people were taken captive and brought to Babylon. Some young men were chosen to be taught in the king's palace.

Answer the questions. You may use your Bible for help.

1. How were the chosen men to prepare themselves before going before the king? (Dan. 1:5)

____

____

2. How long were the young men to prepare before going before the king? (Dan. 1:5) ____________

> God had given His people strict laws about what they could eat and drink. Even though these men were not in their homeland, they wanted to honor God.

3. Did Daniel eat what was given to him? Why or why not? (Dan. 1:8)

____

4. What concern did the chief official have about changing the food of Daniel and his friends? (Dan. 1:10)

____

____

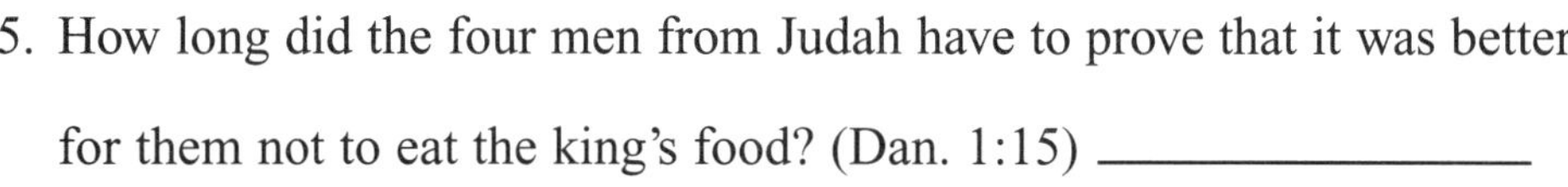

5. How long did the four men from Judah have to prove that it was better for them not to eat the king's food? (Dan. 1:15) ____________

6. In addition to good health, how did God bless these men for their obedience to His Word? (Dan. 1:20)

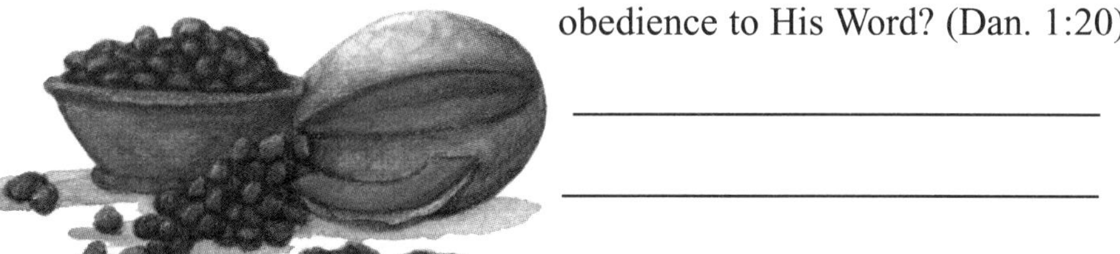

____

____

____

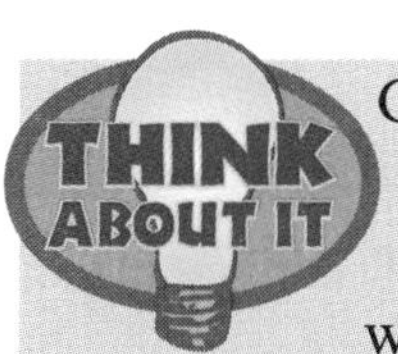
THINK
ABOUT IT

God provided Daniel with the boldness he needed to do right. Before this time came, Daniel had already established a good testimony with the chief official. This good testimony gave Daniel the freedom to make the request that the official change their food. What testimony do you have with those in authority over you?

Draw lines to match the new Chaldean names to the Hebrew names of four of the young men from Judah (Dan. 1:6-7).

7. Belteshazzar	Hananiah
8. Shadrach	Azariah
9. Meshach	Daniel
10. Abednego	Mishael

Continuing to Stand

Daniel 3

Name ______________________________

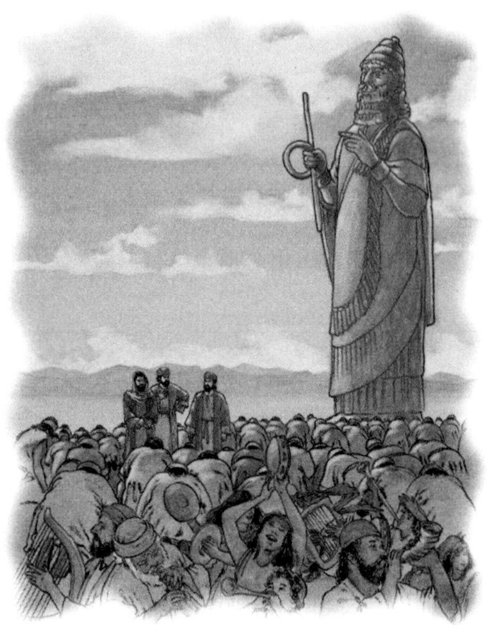

After Daniel interpreted King Nebuchadnezzar's dream, he was made a ruler over the province of Babylon and governor over the wise men of the land. Daniel then advised the king to place Shadrach, Meshach, and Abednego over the affairs of the province of Babylon. Although Shadrach, Meshach, and Abednego were now in positions of authority, they still had to choose to obey God and follow His Word.

The idol Nebuchadnezzar created was threescore or sixty cubits high and six cubits wide. A cubit equals about 1.5 feet. Sixty cubits equals ninety feet.

Draw an outline representing the size of the image on the graph. Each line represents two cubits.

Write *T* if the statement is true and *F* if the statement is false. If the statement is false, correct it.

______ 1. All the people in the land were to bow in worship before the image each time they heard the herald shout.

____

______ 2. Some Chaldeans went to the king and reported that the Jews over the province of Babylon did not bow because they worshiped another God.

____

______ 3. The punishment for not bowing was to be cast into the fiery furnace.

____

______ 4. Nebuchadnezzar was pleased that Shadrach, Meshach, and Abednego chose to follow their God.

____

______ 5. God protected the three in the furnace by sending His Angel to protect them.

____

______ 6. Nebuchadnezzar recognized that only God could deliver men from the fire.

____

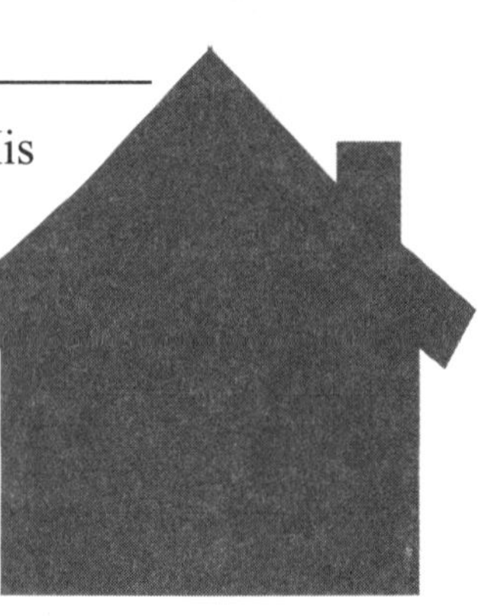

There Is a Season

Ecclesiastes 3:1-3

Name ______________________________

God is all-knowing. He has a plan for His creation. As you read His Word, you will discover His way and purpose.

God's creation is orderly and timely. At the Creation, God set the seasons in motion so they occur regularly each year. Christ often used planting and harvesting as illustrations to teach Christians to spread the gospel to others.

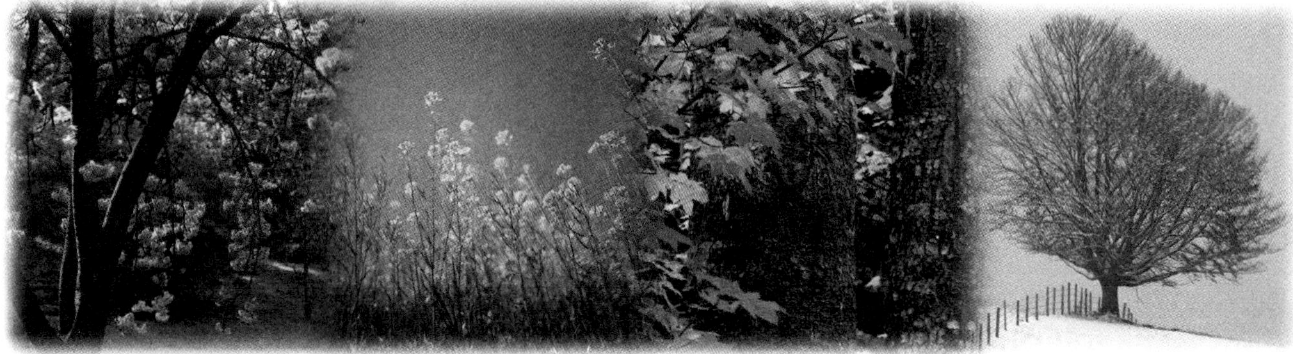

God had a purpose for each event in the Bible to happen when it did.

Write the letter of the correct phrase to complete each sentence.

1. Christ said the blind man had been **born** blind ________, not because of the sin of his parents (John 9:1-3).
2. Christ knew that God had appointed a time for Him to **die** ________ (John 12:27-33).
3. God commanded that every Israelite family **kill** a spotless lamb ________ (Exod. 12:5-7, 13-14).
4. Jesus **heal**ed the son of the nobleman so that ________ (John 4:50-53).
5. God commanded the Israelites to **break down** altars as they entered the promised land ________ (Exod. 34:12-14).
6. Nehemiah told the Jews that they should **build up** the walls of Jerusalem ________ (Neh. 2:17).

A. so that they would not begin to worship other gods

B. to show the works of God

C. for the blood to be used as a sign for the death angel to pass over them

D. so it would no longer be a reproach or testimony against the Jews

E. for all men

F. the nobleman and his family would believe in Christ

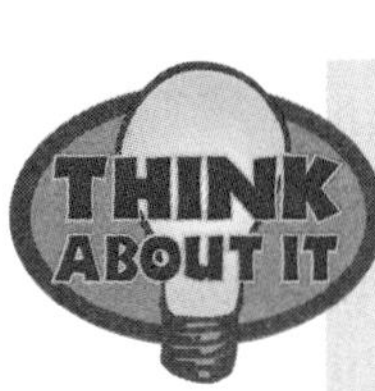
THINK
ABOUT IT

God has a purpose for each event in your life. Do you see everything as coming from Him? What about when things seem to go wrong? Perhaps God is trying to teach you or someone watching you a lesson through the trial. Ask God to help you see His hand working in your life.

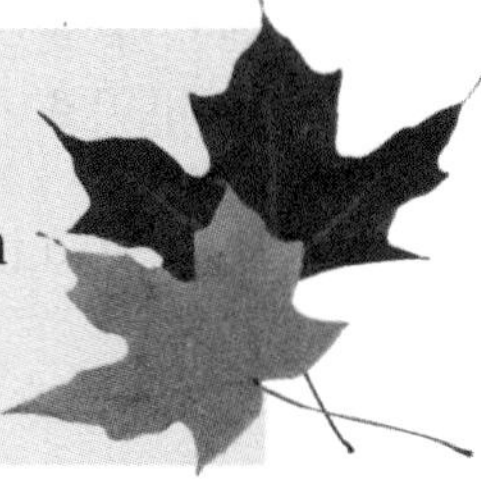

Purged for Purity

Name ______________________________

From Bible times to the present, metals found in the earth have been precious to man. Over the centuries, man has devised various methods to remove metal from rock (ore) and to purify the metal so it can be used. **Metallurgy** is the scientific process of separating metals from their ores and preparing them for use.

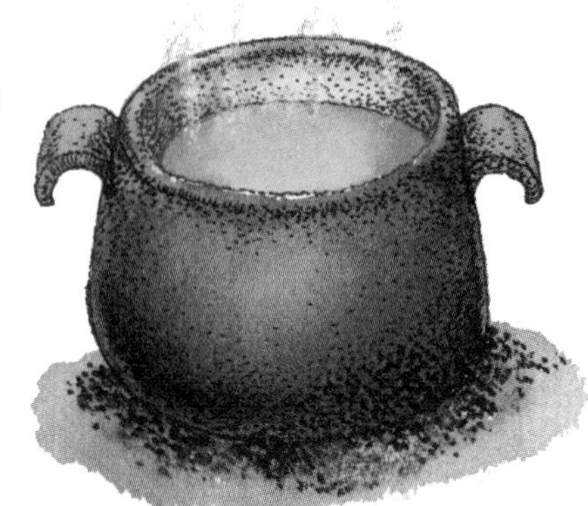

The Scriptures use some of the terms of metallurgy to describe the process God uses to prepare believers for His service. Several different methods are used to extract metal from ore. The processes of **extractive metallurgy** are compared to God's refining process.

Write the reference that correctly matches the step of God's refining process.

Psalm 119:11 | Proverbs 27:9-12, 17 | Jeremiah 33:7-8 | Zechariah 13:9

Extractive Metallurgy	God's Refining Process
Step 1. Mineral Dressing In this cleansing process, the ore is ground and placed in water and chemicals. As bubbles of gases are added to the water and the mixture is stirred, the chemicals cause the minerals to stick to the bubbles. The bubbly froth containing the metal is removed, leaving waste in the water.	In ______________________________, God's Word shows Christians that God let the Jews become captives of other nations so that the Jews would receive forgiveness from their sin. God sends events and people into the lives of Christians so that they might look to God for cleansing and separation from sin.
Step 2. Roasting This step removes impurities from the metal ore. The ore is heated in air, causing the impurities to combine with oxygen and be removed from the metal.	In ______________________________, God's Word shows Christians that memorizing Scripture helps each Christian recognize sin and remove it from his life.
Step 3. Sintering When the temperatures are high enough during the roasting process, particles of metal will combine to form lumps. These lumps make the ore easier to handle in further processes.	In ______________________________, God's Word tells Christians to value their godly friendships. When trials and pressures come, close relationships with other believers help Christians avoid sin and make right choices.
Step 4. Smelting The ore is combined with other minerals and placed in a special furnace. The ore is exposed to high temperatures, removing oxygen from the ore. The impurities form a liquid that floats and is skimmed from the top. The remaining metal is ready for further processing.	In ________________________, God's Word shows Christians that the Israelites were tried with the fire of captivity and refined to become a people that would honor the Lord. In the same way, the heat and pressure of trials should draw Christians closer to God and His Word and further from their sin. Through this process, Christians become ready for the Lord to begin using them and molding them for His service.

What Does God Say About Being Different from the World?

Name ______________________

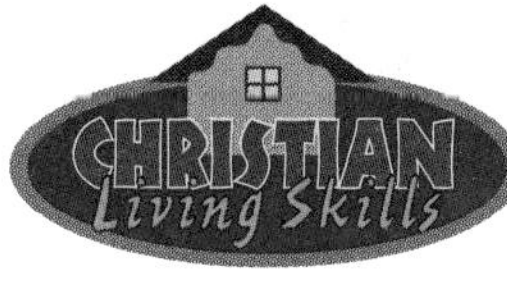
CHRISTIAN
Living Skills

Although Christians get sick, hungry, and tired like everyone else, their souls have been saved by the blood of Jesus Christ. They are destined to spend eternity with God. This should make a difference in the way Christians live while on earth. They know that this world is not their final home. They also know that heaven's glory is beyond anything they can imagine.

Read I Peter 2:9 and answer the questions.

1. What was God's purpose for setting apart Christians as a chosen, royal people that belong to God?

____

2. According to this verse, what is a Christian's motivation for showing God's praise to others?

____

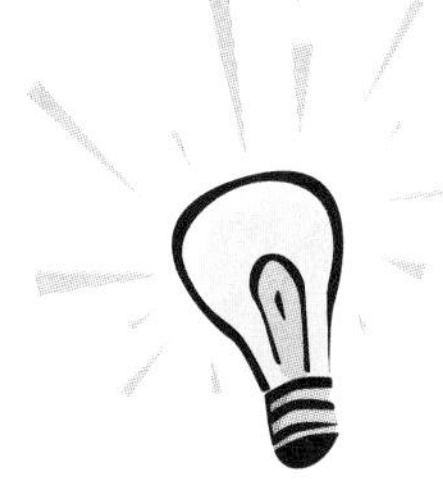

Being a Christian isn't always easy.

When you are called by God to make a difference in this world, you must realize that YOU *must be different too.*

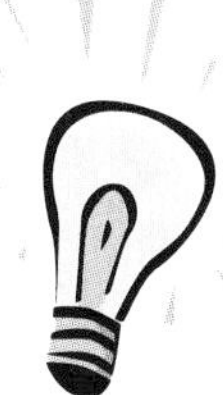

Read Matthew 5:14-16 and describe how each verse challenges you to affect the lives around you.

vs. 14 ______________________

vs. 15 ______________________

vs. 16 ______________________

One of the major differences Christ will make in your life is that you will begin to think like Him. You will love what He loves, and you will hate what He hates. Most of all, you will want to please your heavenly Father just as He does.

Match the verse to the correct statement about what Christians should love and hate. The verses and statements can be used more than once.

_______ 1. They should love God.

_______ 2. They should hate pride.

_______ 3. They should hate perverse talk.

_______ 4. They should hate evil.

_______ 5. They should love what is good.

A. Psalm 97:10

B. Proverbs 8:13

C. Amos 5:15

Something to Think About

Being Different from the World

Name ___________________________

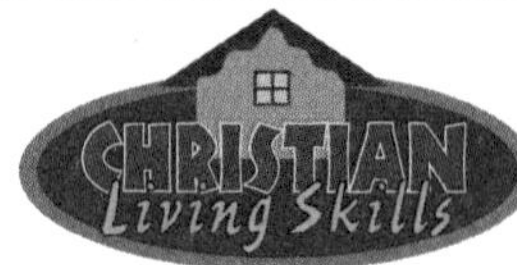
CHRISTIAN
Living Skills

Loving God and hating evil go together. You can't separate them. It's easy to understand that a holy and righteous God hates the evil ways of Satan. All Christians will say that they love God and hate evil. However, the real test of what they love the most is best demonstrated by their actions.

Read the scenarios and decide if the person was demonstrating a love for God or a love for evil. If a love for evil was demonstrated, write what a Christian should have done in that situation. If a love for God was demonstrated, tell how the person demonstrated it.

Scenario	Love for God	Love for Evil	What should have been done? (or) How was God pleased?
Elizabeth wanted the other girls to accept her, but it seemed like they were always gossiping about other people. Elizabeth decided to gossip with them rather than be the one about whom they gossiped.			
Cole found out that his older brother had some magazines containing indecent pictures hiding under his bed in their room. Cole didn't want to make his brother mad, but he knew that God was not pleased. Cole was also concerned about his brother loving evil things. Cole asked his brother to throw the magazines away.			

What About Me?

Loving God and hating evil will set you apart from the world. It may even make you different from others who say they are Christians. Are you willing to do what God says, no matter what? It may require sacrifice, and you may even suffer persecution for doing what is right, but God will richly bless you, and you will please Him.

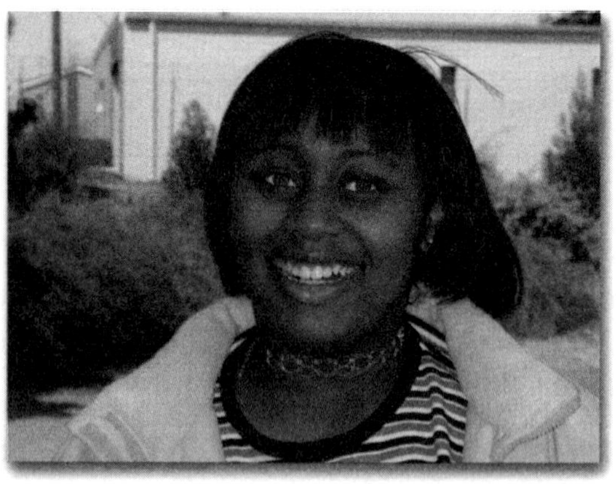

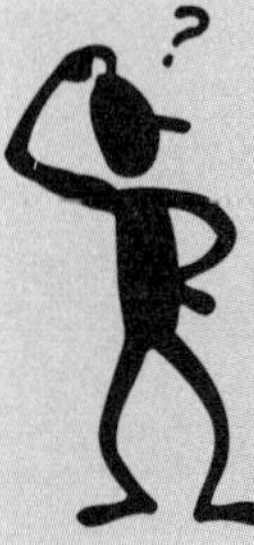
?

Take time at home to think about the following questions.

Would your friends say that you are a light to people around you?

Are you too scared to kindly confront someone for doing wrong?

Are you willing to take whatever persecution might come from doing right?

Do you hate evil the way God hates evil?

Prophet Focus

Ezekiel (ca. 597 B.C.)

Name ____________________

Ezekiel, a priest in Judah, was taken to Babylon during the second captivity. God sent a vision in the form of a whirlwind to Ezekiel. In this vision, God placed Ezekiel as a watchman to the children of Israel. Through these prophecies, Ezekiel was to sound out the alarm of God's coming judgment. To emphasize that Ezekiel was to speak for Him only, God caused Ezekiel's tongue to stick to the roof of his mouth. From then on, Ezekiel could only speak when God gave him the ability and the words to say.

Ezekiel received signs from God to help the people understand what would happen to Jerusalem. Many of these signs were like small dramas for Ezekiel to act out before the people. The first set of signs pictured details of Babylon's siege before and during the destruction of Jerusalem. God desired that the people repent and be saved. Punishment would come to those who did not repent. The people did not think it was right for God to punish sinners. They did not want to hear Ezekiel's messages, so they tried to harm him.

After years of prophesying, Ezekiel found out that Jerusalem had been conquered. Ezekiel's prophecies had come true; now some of the people began to believe his messages from God.

Most of the people living in Israel did not follow God. Even the destruction of Jerusalem did not bring them to repentance. Ezekiel now prophesied God's message revealing that blessings would come to the remnant of people who survived the captivity and remained faithful.

God used a vision of a field of dry bones that grew flesh and returned to life to picture the hope that some people who were dead in their sin would one day return to God and receive life. Later, God instructed Ezekiel to take two sticks and hold them together to become one to demonstrate the promise that the divided kingdoms would be reunited. Ezekiel's final vision from God gave hope that a new temple and a new city would be built some day.

Ezekiel prophesied for about fifty-two years. During this time, he was ridiculed and humiliated as he proclaimed and demonstrated God's truth. Ezekiel remained faithful to God and claimed the promises of eternal life and the kingdom to come.

Answer the questions.

1. Where were the people of Israel when God began speaking through Ezekiel? ____________
2. Did the people believe God's messages? ____________
3. What event caused some of the people to begin to believe that Ezekiel was speaking the truth?

   ____
4. Did this event cause the people to repent of their sins? ____________
5. Why do you think the people did not repent? ____________
6. What should you do when God reveals sin in your life? ____________

   ____

I'm Accountable for Me

Bible Study of Ezekiel 18:14-32

Name ______________________

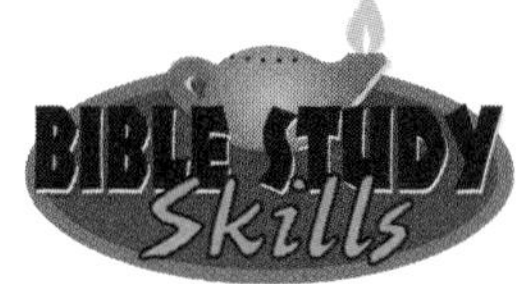
BIBLE STUDY
Skills

When was the last time you heard someone say, "That's not fair"? Sometimes people even say that about God and His punishment of sin. God talks about this in His Word. Is God fair? Does He enjoy punishing sin? The people of Judah were asking these questions as they were held captive in Babylon. God gave Ezekiel His answers to share with the people.

Read Ezekiel 18:14-32 and answer the questions.

Ezekiel 18:14-19

1. If a son has a wicked father, what choices does the son have concerning his own life? (v. 14)

   ____

   ____

2. What blessing will come to the son that follows God? (v. 17*b*) ______________________

   ____

3. What will happen to the sinful father? (v. 18) ______________________
4. Should the son bear the punishment of the father's sin? (v. 19) __________

Ezekiel 18:20-22

5. What clear statement is made about a soul that sins? (v. 20) ______________________
6. Is it fair for God to say that a righteous person bears the results of his own righteousness and a wicked person bears the results of his own wickedness? (v. 20) __________
7. What hope does a wicked person have for eternal life? (v. 21) ______________________

   ______________________ What is this verse talking about? ______________________

8. Does God remember the sins of believers once they ask forgiveness? (v. 22) ______

Ezekiel 18:23-25

9. In your own words, what are the people saying in verse 25? ______________________

   ____

10. Have you ever thought it was unfair for God to send unbelievers to hell? __________

    Do your thoughts and feelings change the truth of God's Word? __________

Ezekiel 18:26-32

11. God once again shows the people that He is fair. But what do the people say in verse 29?

    ____

12. What does God want His people to do? (v. 30) ______________________
13. As they repent, what will God make new? (v. 31) ______________________
14. When sinful people die, what is God's response? (v. 32) ______________________

Pride Abased

Daniel 4

Name ______________________

Nebuchadnezzar, the powerful king who overthrew the mighty Assyrians and who destroyed Jerusalem, had to face a situation he could not control. Many years had passed since his first dream and its interpretation by Daniel. Nebuchadnezzar experienced a new dream that made him afraid. He called on his wise men to help him, but they could not interpret the dream. Daniel was called, and through God's power he explained the meaning of the dream: If Nebuchadnezzar puffed himself up in pride because of his great kingdom, then God would take away his kingdom. This powerful king would become like a beast in the field and realize that God rules over all the earth.

Answer the questions.

1. If Daniel had successfully interpreted Nebuchadnezzar's first dream, why do you think the king waited before calling Daniel this time? ______________________

____

2. Nebuchadnezzar was fearful about his dream. He was seeking peace. What characteristic about Daniel did the king notice as he requested an explanation of his dream (Dan. 4:5, 9)?

____

____

3. Why do you think Daniel was not worried about the unknown? ______________________

____

____

4. Think about situations when you are fearful. Are you fearful because you don't have control? What should you do when you find yourself in a fearful situation?

____

Number the events in the life of King Nebuchadnezzar in order. Read Daniel 4:27-37 for help.

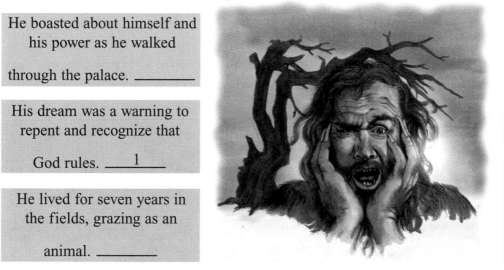

He boasted about himself and his power as he walked through the palace. ________

His dream was a warning to repent and recognize that God rules. ___1___

He lived for seven years in the fields, grazing as an animal. ________

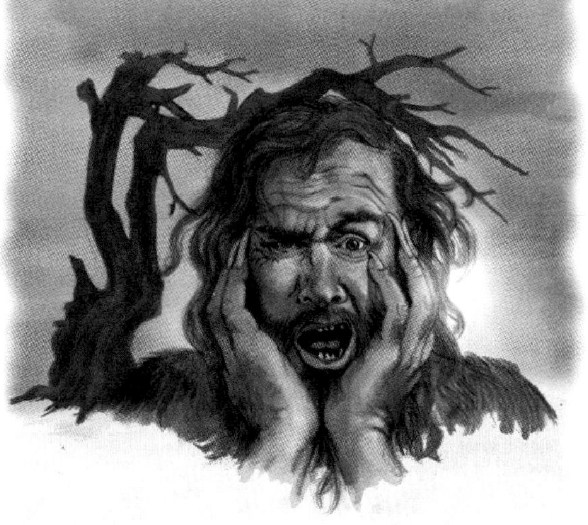

As his understanding returned, he praised God and recognized that God is in control. ________

A voice from heaven told him that his kingdom was taken from him. ________

Message for the King

Daniel 5

Name ____________________

Answer the questions. Refer to Daniel 5 in your Bible for help.

1. What vessels did King Belshazzar use to drink wine at the banquet?

2. Whom did the men praise as they drank?

3. How did God deliver His message to King Belshazzar?

4. What was the king's reaction to the writing?

5. Who remembered that Daniel had the power of God to interpret?

6. Daniel reminded Belshazzar of another king that God had humbled. Which king was he speaking about?

7. Who did the message say would take away the kingdom?

8. When did the attack take place?

What Does God Say About Being Fearful?

Name ______________________

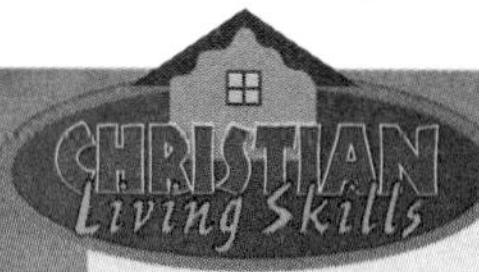
CHRISTIAN
Living Skills

What makes you fearful? Deep water? Heights? Low grades? New people? Being alone? **Fear** is that feeling of being afraid or scared of something. It is an emotion with the power to control you—but only if you let it!

Read II Timothy 1:7 and answer the questions.

1. What kind of spirit has God given Christians?

   ____

2. What does NOT come from God according to this verse? ______________________

3. Where do you think the feeling of being scared or afraid comes from?

   ____

You may have heard of people who have phobias. This word is from the Greek word *phobos,* which means "fear." A **phobia** is a fear that is so strong that it controls your actions. Allowing your fear to control you comes when you focus on yourself or your circumstances. God has given Christians reminders about allowing their thoughts and actions to be controlled not by fear, but by Him.

Read each verse. Write in your own words God's instructions to you about being fearful.

Proverbs 3:25 ______________________

____

Psalm 23:4 ______________________

____

Isaiah 51:7*b* ______________________

____

Instead of being fearful, God wants you to learn to trust Him. He loves you and will always do what is best for you. Every time you find yourself tempted to be afraid, ask God to help you to trust in Him and His protection.

Use the glossary to write the definitions for the noun and verb forms of *trust.* Answer the question.

Noun: ______________________

____

Verb: ______________________

Question: In your own words, describe what it means to trust in God.

____

Something to Think About

Being Fearful

Name ______________________

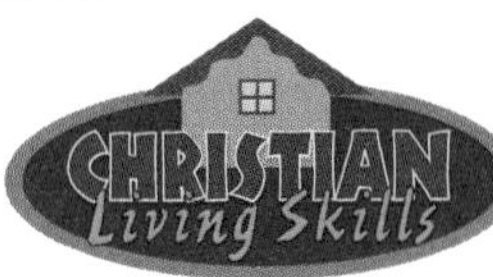
CHRISTIAN
Living Skills

When you become fearful about something, you worry about it. You spend time thinking about something you can't control. God is in control of what happens in your life, and He wants you to trust Him. He gives Christians the ability to make wise decisions with the help of His Holy Spirit. He expects them to make responsible decisions about where they go and what they do. He also expects you to believe Him when He says that He will take care of you.

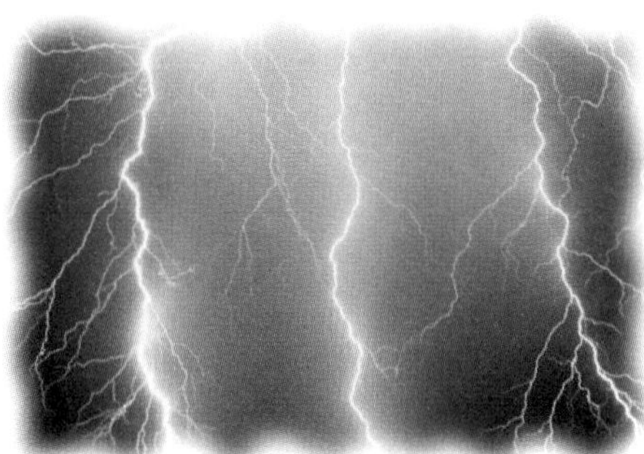

Match the verse to the correct statement about what you should do when you are fearful.

_____ 1. I Peter 5:7

_____ 2. Proverbs 3:7

_____ 3. Psalm 56:3-4

A. I should stop being afraid because I trust in God.

B. I should not trust myself. I will fear the Lord and get away from evil things.

C. I should tell Jesus all about my cares and anxiety because He cares.

The Right Kind of Fear

It may surprise you to find out that God tells you that there is a good kind of fear that you *should* have. Sometimes people are confused about the different ways God uses the word *fear* in the Bible. One kind of **fear** means being so afraid of something that someone can't do what God wants him to do. This kind of fear is a sin because the person is not trusting God to take care of him.

The other kind of **fear** means to have so much respect and reverence for God that one does everything he can to obey Him no matter what. Fearing God is more than being impressed by His power. You must realize that He has the power to judge YOU for your sins. Having this kind of good fear will help you overcome the temptation to sin because you understand the seriousness of its consequences. The more you get to know God and His character, the more you will understand how much He hates sin.

What About Me?

Take time at home to think about what things make you fearful and whether you fear God. How do YOU deal with the wrong kind of fear? Do YOU have the right kind of fear? Follow the directions.

1. List several things about which you are fearful.

   ____________ ____________ ____________

2. Write one way you can please God in how you handle your fear.

   ____

3. Write about an area in which you need to learn to trust God and how you're going to change to please Him.

   ____

4. List three ways you can show that you *fear* God.

   ____________ ____________ ____________

Darius, Daniel, and the Den

Daniel 6

Name ______________________________

Daniel's testimony before God was seen by the king and other officers and leaders. King Darius loved the good character he saw in Daniel and placed him over all the officers and leaders. These men hated Daniel and tried to use his testimony to bring him harm.

Write the character trait next to each description.

concerned	**deceitful**	**encouraging**	**faithful**
grieved	**humble**	**jealous**	**obedient**

	the attitude of the other leaders toward Daniel after he was placed over them
	the way in which the other leaders caused the king to create the new law restricting prayer

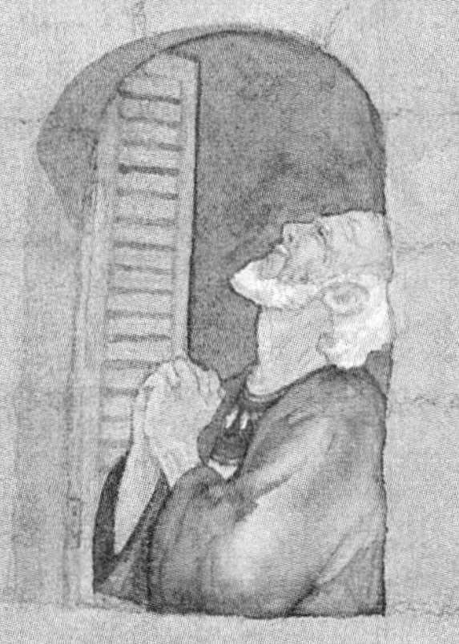

	how King Darius felt when he found that Daniel's regular prayers to God caused Daniel to break the new law
	the king's words to Daniel, reminding him that God could deliver him
	shown by the king's thoughts for Daniel throughout the night

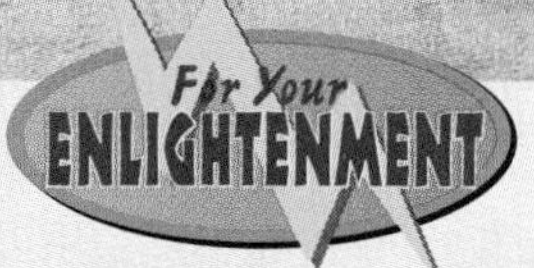
For Your
ENLIGHTENMENT

A Persian or Median king was the supreme ruler and authority of the land. It would have been seen as a sign of weakness for a king to change his mind. As a result, laws established under the Medes and Persians were unable to be amended or changed. A new law had to be made in order to reverse an old one.

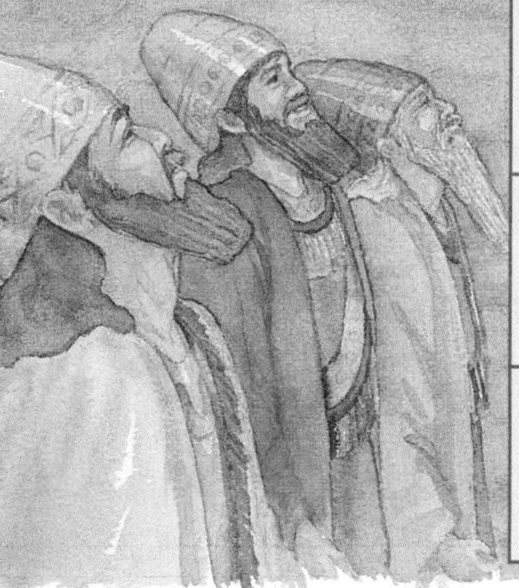

	Daniel continued to pray and followed God's Word rather than man's law.
	Daniel went willingly without complaint when taken to the lions' den.
	Daniel gave the praise to God for delivering him from the lions.

The system of law and government for the Medes and Persians was highly organized. The Medes and Persians often left existing leaders in their positions of authority as lands were conquered. This may be why Daniel remained in authority when the Medes and Persians took control of Babylon.

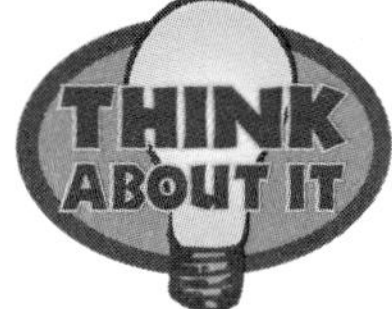
THINK
ABOUT IT

What character traits do you think describe you? Which ones should you work on?

Singing with Understanding

"Standing on the Promises" (vv. 1-2)

Name ____________________

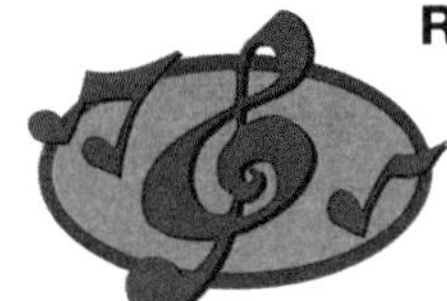

Read verses 1-2 of the hymn on page 316 and answer the questions.

1. What do you think it means to stand on the **promises** of God?

____

____

____

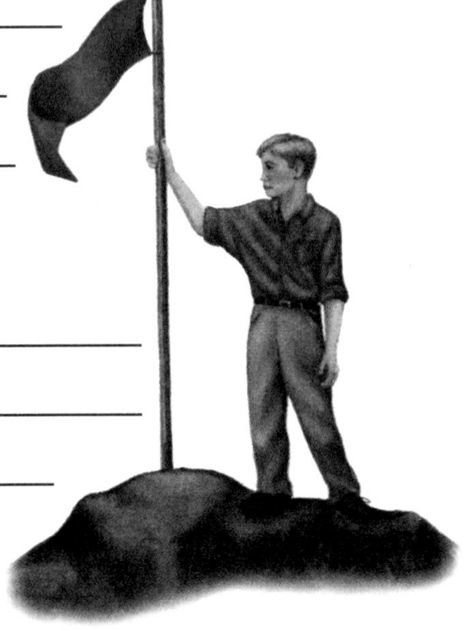

2. What are some **promises** from God's Word that have helped you in times of doubt or fear?

____

____

____

____

Read the following verses and complete the sentences.

3. **Acts 16:31**—God **promises** to save those who ______________ on Jesus Christ.

4. **John 6:37**—God **promises** that anyone who ______________ to Him will never be rejected.

5. **Hebrews 13:5**—God **promises** never to ______________ us.

6. **Jeremiah 31:34**—God **promises** to ______________ our sin and ______________ it no more.

7. **Romans 8:38-39**—God **promises** that nothing can ______________ us from His love.

8. **James 1:5**—God **promises** to give ______________ to those who ask Him.

9. **Psalm 91:15**—God **promises** to ______________ us when we call upon Him and to be with us in times of trouble.

Beauty and Character

Esther 1–2:20

Name ______________________

When you are making an important choice, do you ever look at the life of a person in authority to see how he has made similar choices? The women in the kingdom of King Ahasuerus looked to Queen Vashti as a model for behavior.

Answer the questions. You may use your Bible for help.

1. How would Vashti's disobedience to the king affect the women of the land? (Esther 1:17)

   ____

2. As part of her punishment, Vashti would no longer come before the king. What other punishment was given her according to the law of the Medes and Persians? (Esther 1:19)

   ____

3. What kind of new queen did the king look for? (Esther 2:2) ______________________

4. Mordecai had been brought to the land when Jehoiachin, a king of Judah, was captured by which Babylonian king? (Esther 2:6) ______________________

5. Esther had been orphaned. Although Mordecai was a cousin to Esther, how did Mordecai treat her? (Esther 2:7) ______________________

6. Each woman had to go through a time of purification before the king would consider her to be his next queen. How long did the purification process take for Esther? (Esther 2:12)

   ____

7. Why do you think Mordecai wanted Esther to keep her Jewish heritage a secret from the king? (Esther 2:10, 20) ______________________

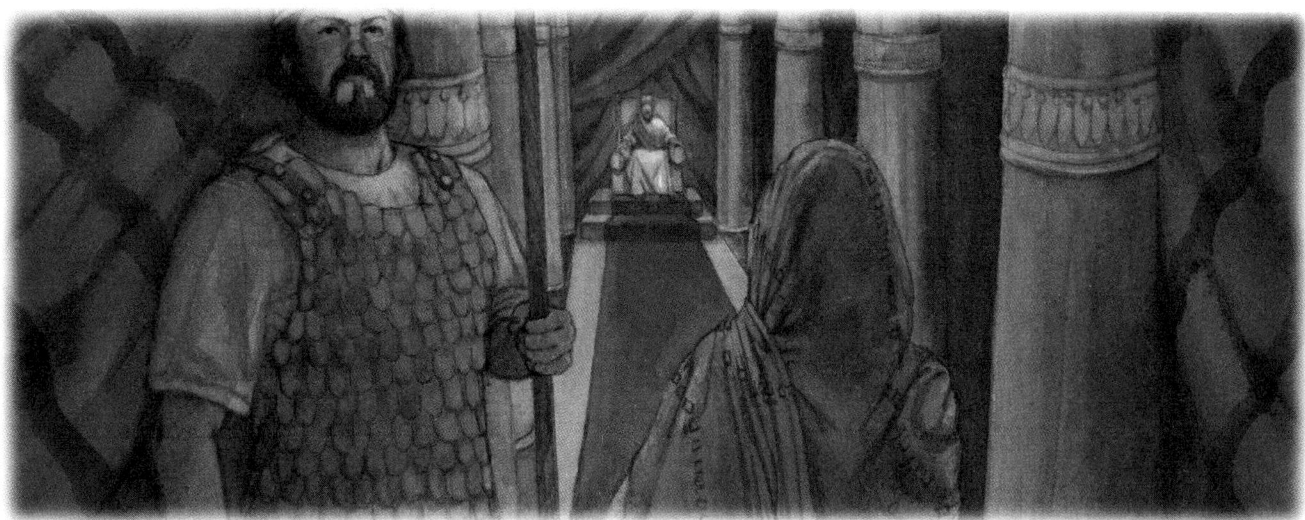

The Appropriate Time

Ecclesiastes 3:4-9

Name ______________________

Has your parent or teacher ever told you that something you did was inappropriate behavior? You were probably acting incorrectly for the place you were in. There is an appropriate time and place for everything.

In each pair, mark an *X* on the activity that is appropriate.

1. _____ a child crying when he falls
   _____ a child crying to get something in a store
2. _____ laughing at a friend's funny picture drawn during church
   _____ laughing at an actor during a funny skit
3. _____ getting gifts for a birthday
   _____ getting a second helping before others have had any
4. _____ tearing out a hem to lengthen pants
   _____ tearing a friend's paper to make others laugh
5. _____ keeping quiet when you see someone do wrong
   _____ keeping quiet to not hurt someone's feelings
6. _____ talking about someone you don't like
   _____ talking to the teacher about a problem

What about other things you do? Do you do "good" things at the wrong times? For example, it is good to help your brother fold his clothes, but if you were told to practice the piano at that time, is it right to be folding laundry?

Read James 4:17 and answer the questions.

7. What does God call it when you don't do what you know is right? ______________________
8. What is one thing that you know to do but your parent has to regularly remind you about?
   ____
9. When you fail to do this particular thing, what does God call it? ______________________
10. What can you do to keep from sinning? ______________________
    ____
    ____

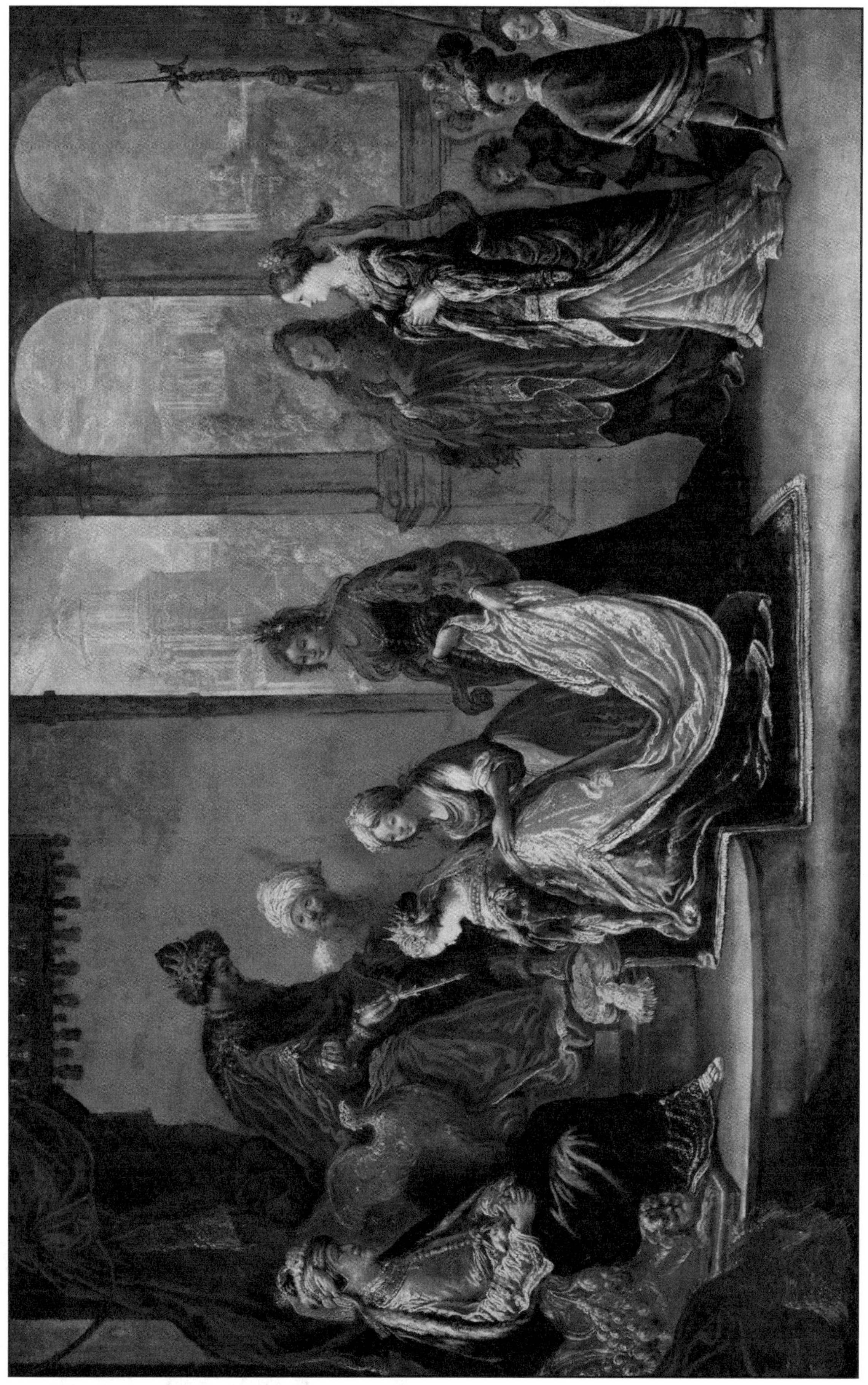

Esther Before Ahasuerus
Claude Vignon

Bob Jones University Museum & Gallery, Inc.

Name ______________________

Esther Before Ahasuerus

by Claude Vignon (1593-1670)

Claude Vignon (Klōd Vēn yōn´) had great advantages since his father was a personal servant of Henry IV, king of France. When Vignon was twenty-six, he left home and went to Rome where he met students of famous masters. For a while, Vignon painted in the style of Rome, dark paintings with deep shadows, strong highlights, and very realistic scenes. He made two trips to Spain to visit artists there but returned to Paris in 1624 to become a court painter to Louis XIII.

Back in France, Vignon changed from the dark style of Rome to paint more colorful, decorative paintings. He liked elegant clothes and shimmery fabrics and became very skillful at painting little blobs of paint to resemble lace and jewels. Vignon also had a knack for inventing imaginary architecture. In this painting, the rows of arches behind the ladies-in-waiting were just drawn on the canvas and left unpainted. The artist painted the garden and oriental architecture inside the arches.

The subject of Esther and Ahasuerus was perfect for Vignon's new style of painting. Esther lived in Persia; though Vignon had never been there, he read the story and allowed his imagination to work. He invented luxurious clothing, curious foreign-looking hats, and architecture to make his painting look exotic and rich. He invented an elegant throne with eagles on the arms for King Ahasuerus. The account depicted here is told in Esther 4:7–5:2. The satisfied-looking man seated next to the king may be Haman, the king's closest officer. Vignon shows the king's sympathy toward Esther as Ahasuerus bends down to extend his scepter and stroke her hair. Though Esther boldly approaches the king, she keeps her eyes downcast but does not appear fearful. The person on the other side of the king who looks a little surprised may be Mordecai, Esther's cousin.

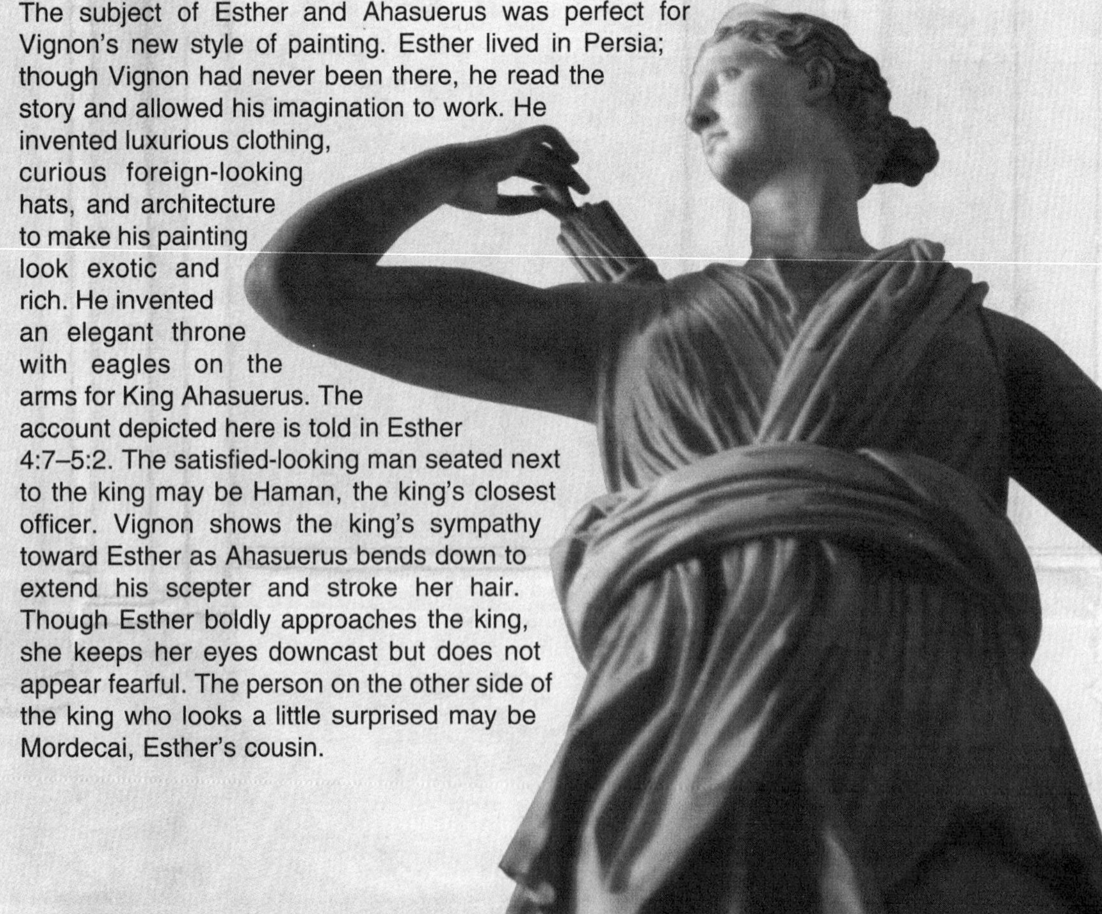

Name ______________________

Who Am I?

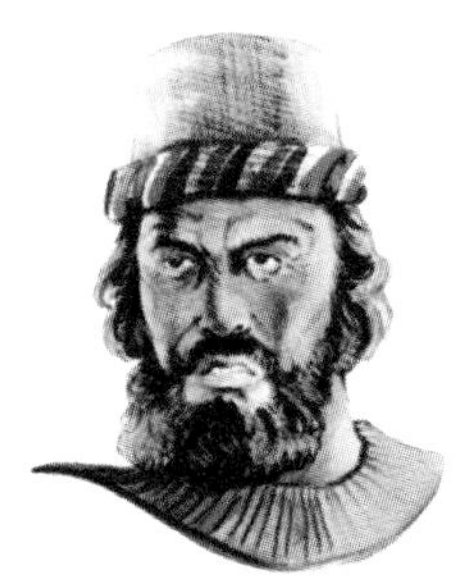
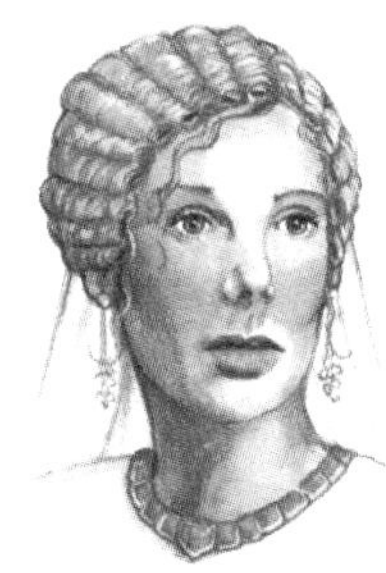
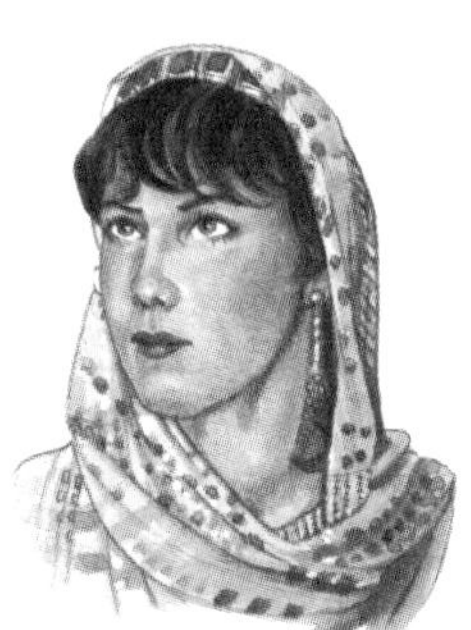
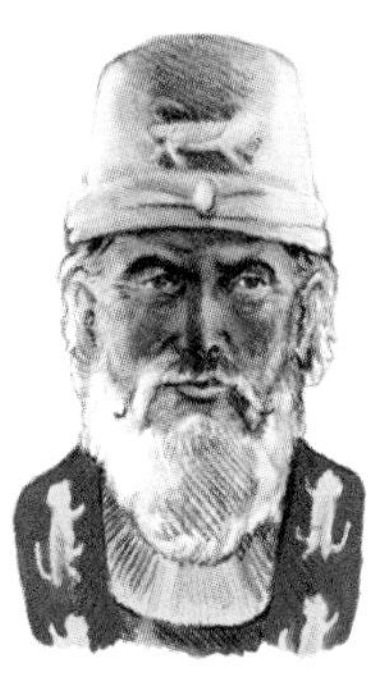
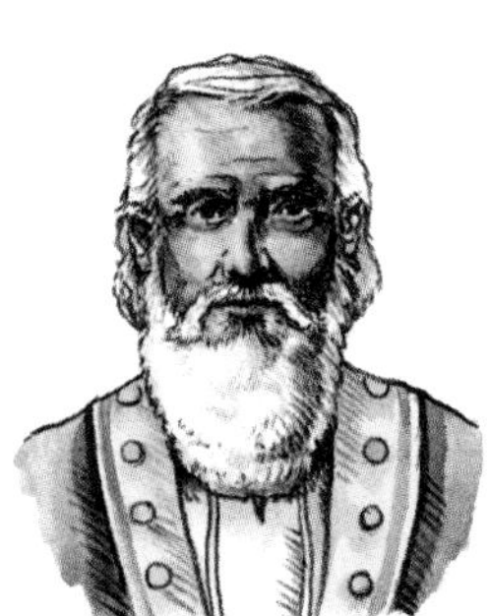

Write the letter of the correct person next to each statement.

A. Haman **B. Vashti** **C. Esther** **D. Ahasuerus** **E. Mordecai**

_____ 1. I am the king that rules all the land from India to Ethiopia.

_____ 2. I am a Jewish young lady who became the queen.

_____ 3. Because the king placed me over all the princes, everyone is to bow to me in reverence.

_____ 4. As a Jew, I cannot bow to anyone other than God.

_____ 5. I was removed from being queen because I disobeyed the king.

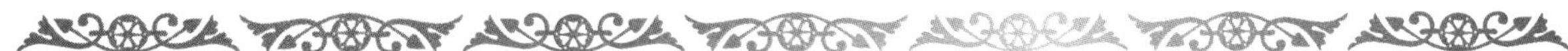

Number the events in order.

_____ Esther asked the king to release the Jews from the sentence of death.

_____ Mordecai told Esther to go before the king and intercede for her people.

_____ The king had Haman hung on the gallows Haman had prepared for Mordecai's execution.

_____ Esther went to the king, even though she had not been invited.

__1__ Because of his hatred for Mordecai, Haman led the king to believe that the Jews were causing trouble and breaking the king's laws.

_____ Esther invited the king and Haman to two special banquets.

_____ When Mordecai heard that the king passed a law to destroy all the Jews, he came to the king's gate clothed as a mourner in sackcloth and ashes.

Word Study

Name ______________________________

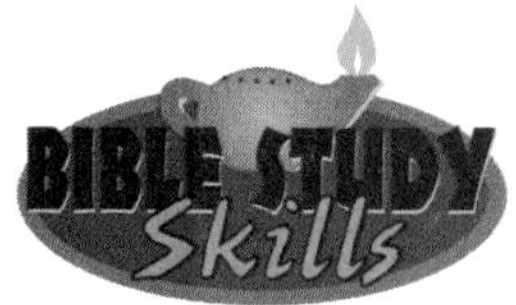
BIBLE STUDY
Skills

Studying the Scripture and other sources to find out what God says about a particular word is called a **word study.**

To study the word *provide,* start by reviewing the resources available to you.

PROVIDENCE (Lat. *providentia,* "foreseeing"). In theology, this word refers to God's preparation for the management of His universe and His continual care and control over it.

Step 1: Look in **dictionaries** for the meaning of the word. A Bible dictionary will provide connections to Scripture and give possible biblical application. If your chosen word is not found, try other forms of the word. *Provide* is not in the Bible dictionary.

1. What form of *provide* is in the Bible dictionary? ______________________

PROVIDE, Gen.22:8, God will *p* himself a lamb
30:30, when shall I *p* for mine own house
Ps.78:20, can he *p* flesh
Mt.10:9, *p* neither gold nor silver
Lk.12:20, whose shall those things be thou hast *p*
33, *p* bags that grow not old
Rom.12:17; 2 Cor.8:21, *p* things honest
1 Tim.5:8, if any *p* not for his own
Heb.11:40, having *p* better thing for us
PROVISION, Gen.42:25; 45:21, *p* for the way
Josh.9:14, the men took of their *p*
Neh.13:15, in the day in which they sold *p*
Ps.132:15, I will abundantly bless her *p*
Lk.9:12, into villages to buy *p*

Step 2: Look in a **concordance.** Is the word found in your Bible? If so, it will be in a concordance. Look up the references and read the verses. Find out how God uses the word.

2. Which reference is probably the account of God's providing a sacrifice when Abraham went to offer Isaac? ______________________

3. What two verses are in the concordance for "*p* things honest?"

____

Step 3: Look at **cross-references.** Are there letters or numbers on words in the verses alerting you to look at the reference column? Are words from the verse defined? Is there a cross-reference leading you to other verses to read?

12 Romans

(4) The Christian and those outside of God's family

17 Recompense to no man [x]evil
for evil. [y]Provide things honest in
the sight of all men.
18 If it be possible, as much as
lieth in you, live peaceably with
all men.
19 Dearly beloved, avenge not
yourselves but, *rather,* give place
unto wrath; for it is [z]written,
[aa]Vengeance *is* mine; I will repay,
saith the Lord.
20 Therefore, [bb]if thine enemy
hunger, feed him; if he thirst,
give him drink; for in so doing
thou shalt heap coals of fire on
his head.

instant. 1 Th.5:17
u Heb.13:16; 1 Pet.4:9
v v. 20; Lk. 6:28; cp. Mt.5:44
w Lit. *them that are lowly*
x 1 Pet.3:9
y Lit. *take thought for things honorable*
z *Inspiration*: v. 19; Rom. 14:11. (Ex.4:15; 2 Tim. 3:16)

II Corinthians 8

21 [b]Providing for honest things,
not only in the sight of the Lord
but also in the sight of men.
22 And we have sent with them
our brother, whom we have often
proved diligent in many things,
but now much more diligent,
upon the great confidence which
I have in you.
23 Whether *any do inquire* of
[c]Titus, *he is* my partner and
[d]|fellow worker| concerning you;
or our brethren *be inquired of,*
they are the [e]messengers of the
[f]churches, *and* the glory of Christ.
24 Wherefore, show ye to them,
and before the [f]churches, the
proof of your [g]love, and of our
[h]boasting on your behalf.

b Cp. Prov. 3:4; 1 Pet.2:12
c v. 16; 2 Cor.7:13–14
d KJV *fellow-helper*
e Cp. Phil. 2:25
f *Churches* (local): vv. 23,24; 2 Cor.11:8. (Acts 8:3; Phil. 1:1, *note*)
g *Law* (of Christ): v. 24; 2 Cor. 10:5. (Jn.13:34; 2

4. Are the two verses talking about something God will provide or about Christians? ______________

5. Which verse has cross-references to other verses about providing? ______________________

Step 4: Record your findings in a notebook. Keeping a record will remind you of answers you have found in God's Word. Your notebook will be a good source to help you find answers from God.

What Does God Say About My Appearance?

Name ______________________________

CHRISTIAN Living Skills

Does your outward appearance matter?

When you meet someone, your first impression of that person comes from what he looks like. You form an opinion about that person by clothes, hairstyle, expressions, and what is said. You look at the outward appearance. God does not look on the outward appearance to find out about a person because He can see into the heart (I Sam. 16:7). People cannot see into the heart of a person, but they can often get a good idea of what a person is like by his outward appearance. *What you look like on the outside is a picture of your heart.*

Read the verses. Match the reference to the phrase that describes the importance of a person's outward appearance.

_____ 1. David cleaned up and changed his clothes before entering the house of the Lord.

_____ 2. Priests were required to wear special garments to properly perform their duties.

_____ 3. The difference between a man and a woman should be easily recognized by their appearance.

_____ 4. Esther knew that to enter the king's presence and gain his approval, she must be properly attired.

_____ 5. An immoral woman can be recognized by the kind of clothes she wears.

A. Deuteronomy 22:5

B. Leviticus 16:4

C. II Samuel 12:20

D. Proverbs 7:10

E. Esther 5:1-2

What does the Bible mean when it says Christians should not love the world?

When God refers to the **world** in this way, He is not talking about His creation. Here the world refers to all the plans, ideas, theories, fads, music, fashions, and entertainment that do not reflect God's holiness. In this sense, the world is Satan's working to turn people's hearts against God.

The Bible warns Christians to avoid falling into Satan's trap of following the trends of the world. The appearance of a Christian should be different from the appearance of an unsaved person. Much like a uniform identifies which team a player is on, your appearance tells others whose team you are on—God's or the world's.

Read the verses. Complete the sentences about what God says your attitude should be toward the world.

I John 2:15-17 I must not __________ the world. If I love the world, the love of the ______________ is not in me. Everything that is in the ________________ is not from God, and it will ______________ away. If I do the ________________ of God, I will live ________________.

Romans 12:2 I should not be ________________ to this world, but should be ________________ by renewing my __________ so that I can know what God's __________ is for me.

Name ____________________

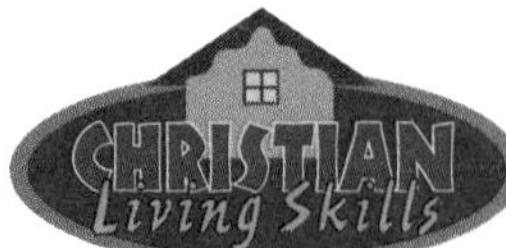
CHRISTIAN
Living Skills

God's Word has much to say about the outward appearance of Christians. Below are a few answers to questions you might have about how to make right choices about your appearance.

What about fads?

A fad is a fashion statement that is popular for a limited time with a limited group of people. When a person participates in a fad, he becomes identified with the group or culture that is promoting that fad. *A Christian should not identify with the world and should avoid participating in the world's fads.* (I Cor. 7:31)

What about modesty?

One dictionary defines **modesty** as "an avoidance of extremes in dress and action." For a Christian, this means that he must carefully avoid any action or style of clothing that identifies him with the world or draws attention to a particular part of his body. *The Bible teaches that both boys and girls are to be modest.* God also gives a specific command to girls to dress in clothes that adequately cover their bodies so that they do not distract from their public testimony of Christlikeness. (I Tim. 2:9-10)

What about the clothes I wear?

The clothes you put on your body are important because they make a public statement about what you believe about God. Do you choose clothing that is moderate or extreme? modest or sensual? too tight or too baggy? too short or too long? too sloppy or too sheer? These extremes draw attention to your body and away from Jesus Christ and tell others that you don't care what opinion they get from you about the Savior.

What about body piercing or tattooing?

Historically, tattooing and body piercing have always been a mark of identification with a certain social class, tribe, or religion. Leviticus 19:28 says that God's people are not to make any marks or tattoos on their bodies. Tattoos and body piercing have an association in today's culture as well. *They identify you with the world, which is rebelling against God. Since a Christian's body is the temple of the Holy Spirit, he has the responsibility of taking care of it.*

What About Me?

Making right decisions about your appearance is actually very simple. Just ask yourself, "Does this identify me with the world or with my Savior?" Your appearance should be a picture of the love and respect you have for your Creator.

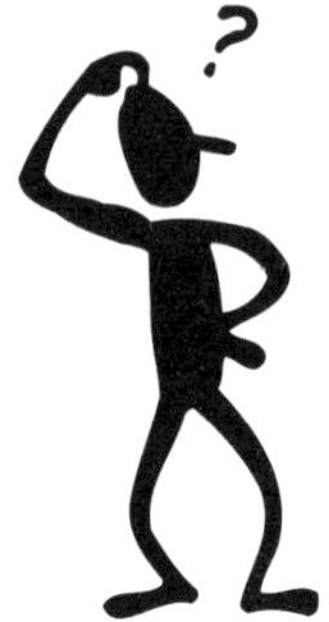

Take time at home to think about the following questions.

Does my clothing picture the love and respect I have for God?
What message does my hairstyle give to others?
Do I enjoy participating in the latest fad or fashion of the world?
When people look at me, what are they most likely to notice first?
Am I more concerned about pleasing God or "fitting in" with my friends?
Have I damaged my body for the sake of fads or fashions?
Is God pleased with my appearance?

It Shall Be Forever

Ecclesiastes 3:14

Name ______________________

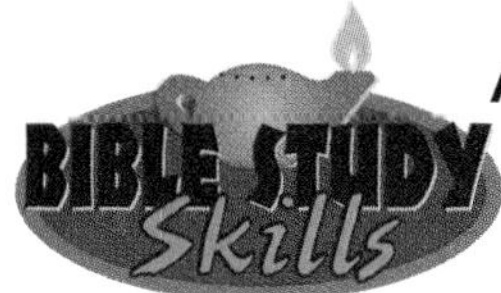
BIBLE STUDY
Skills

Answer the questions.

1. How long will God's works last? ______________________

2. Write three things about God that you know do not change. ______________________

______________________ ______________________

God is eternal and does not change. Key words from this statement that might be found in a concordance are *eternal* and *change*.

Use the entries to answer the questions.

3. What are most of the *eternal* entries about? ______________________

4. Which reference calls God eternal? ______________________

5. Across the page is another entry with a meaning similar to *eternal.* What is the word? ______________________

6. What other verses talk about God as *everlasting?* ______________________

ESTRANGED, *see also* DESECRATED
Job 19:13; Ps.78:30; Ezek.14:5
ETERNAL, Dt.33:27, the *e* God is thy refuge
Isa.60:15, will make thee an *e* excellency
Mt.19:16; Mk.10:17; Lk.10:25; 18:18, what shall I do that I may have *e* life
25:46, righteous into life *e*
Mk.3:29, is in danger of *e* damnation
10:30, receive in age to come *e* life
Jn.3:15, believeth in him have *e* life
4:36, gathereth fruit unto life *e*
5:39, scriptures, in them *e* life
6:54, drinketh my blood hath *e* life
68, thou hast words of *e* life
10:28, give sheep *e* life
12:25, hateth life, shall keep it to life *e*
17:2, give *e* life to as many
3, this is life *e*, that they might know thee
Acts 13:48, many as were ordained to *e* life
Rom.2:7, who seek for glory, *e* life
5:21, grace reign to *e* life
6:23, gift of God is *e* life
2 Cor.4:17, an *e* weight of glory
18, things not seen are *e*
5:1, house *e* in the heavens
Eph.3:11, according to *e* purpose
1 Tim.6:12,19, lay hold on *e* life
Ti.1:2; 3:7, in hope of *e* life
Heb.5:9, author of *e* salvation
6:2, doctrine of *e* judgment
9:15, promise of *e* inheritance
1 Pet.5:10, called to *e* glory by Christ
1 Jn.1:2, *e* life, which was with the Father
2:25, this is the promise, even *e* life
3:15, no murderer hath *e* life
5:11, record, that God hath given to us *e* life
13, know that ye have *e* life
20, this is true God, and *e* life
Jude 7, vengeance of *e* fire
1 Th.4:17, so shall we *e* be with the Lord
5:15, *e* follow that which is good
2 Tim.3:7, *e* learning
Heb.7:25, he *e* liveth to make
EVERLASTING, Ex.40:15; Num.25:13, an *e* priesthood
Ps.90:2, from *e* to *e* thou art God
139:24, lead me in way *e*
Prov.8:23, I was set up from *e*
10:25, righteous is an *e* foundation
Isa.9:6, called the *E* Father
26:4, in the Lord is *e* strength
33:14, with *e* burnings
35:10; 51:11; 61:7, *e* joy
45:17, with *e* salvation
54:8, with *e* kindness
55:13, for an *e* sign
56:5; 63:12, an *e* name
60:19,20, an *e* light
Jer.31:3, with an *e* love
Hab.3:6, the *e* mountains
Mt.18:8; 25:41, into *e* fire
19:29, inherit *e* life
25:46, into *e* punishment
Lk.16:9, into *e* habitations
18:30, in age to come *e* life
Jn.3:16,36, believeth shall have *e* life
4:14, water springing up into *e* life
5:24, heareth my word hath *e* life
6:27, food which endureth to *e* life
40, seeth Son may have *e* life
12:50, his commandment is life *e*
Acts 13:46, unworthy of *e* life
Rom.6:22, free from sin, the end *e* life
Gal.6:8, of Spirit reap life *e*
2 Th.1:9, punished with *e* destruction
2:16, given us *e* consolation
Jude 6, reserved in *e* chains
Rev.14:6, having the *e* gospel

CHANGE (*n.*), Job 14:14, till my *c* come
Prov.24:21, meddle not with them given to *c*
CHANGE (*v.*), Ps.15:4, sweareth and *c* not
102:26, as vesture shalt thou *c* them
Mal.3:6, I the Lord *c* not
Rom.1:23, *c* glory of uncorruptible God
1 Cor.15:51, we shall all be *c*
2 Cor.3:18, *c* from glory to glory

7. What two references say *change not?*

____

8. Ecclesiastes 3:14 gives a cross-reference to the Psalm 19:9 note. What is the definition of *fear of the Lord* in the footnote? ______________________

Ecclesiastes 3:14

14 I know that, whatsoever God doeth, it shall be forever; [p]nothing can be put to it, nor any thing taken from it; and God doeth *it*, that *men* should [q]fear before him.

p Jas.1:17
q See Ps.19:9, *note*

Psalm 19:9

8 The statutes of the LORD *are* right, rejoicing the heart; the commandment of the LORD *is* pure, enlightening the eyes.
9 The [2]fear of the LORD *is* clean, enduring forever; the [e]|ordinances| of the LORD *are* true *and* righteous altogether.

[1](19:7) Whereas the law of the Lord is summarized in the Ten Commandments, it comprises all God's revealed truth—in David's day, the Pentateuch; today the whole Bible.
[2](19:9) "The fear of the LORD" is an O.T. expression meaning *reverential trust,* including the hatred of evil.

THINK ABOUT IT

Have you trusted the eternal, unchanging God for salvation? Are you developing a hatred of evil?

Prayer and Prophecy

Daniel 9

Name ______________________

The coming of Christ was still hundreds of years away, but God gave Daniel a message of assurance concerning the coming Messiah.

To interpret the prophecy of Daniel 9, it is generally accepted that 1 week equals 7 years, so 7 weeks would equal 49 years.

Answer the questions. You may use your Bible for help.

1. Daniel had been studying the prophecies about the captivity in Babylon in the writings of which prophet? (Dan. 9:2) ______________
2. The prophecies reminded Daniel of the reason God let His people be defeated and taken captive. Why were the people now in Babylon? (Dan. 9:5) ______________
3. What did Daniel do when he put on sackcloth and ashes? (Dan. 9:3-5) ______________
4. What hope did Gabriel's message from God bring to Daniel? (Dan. 9:21-22, 25) ______________

Write *T* if the statement is true and *F* if the statement is false.

_____ 5. Only some men are guilty of disobedience and rebellion.

_____ 6. God shows mercy on those who confess and turn from their sin.

_____ 7. God promises salvation even to the sinners who will not repent.

_____ 8. Daniel looked ahead to the promised Messiah that would forgive sin and provide salvation.

_____ 9. Daniel put on sackcloth and ashes to humble himself before God.

_____ 10. The 7 weeks in Daniel 9 equals 49 years.

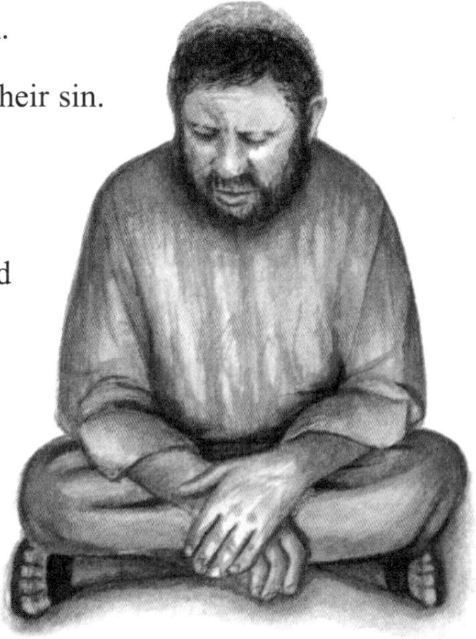

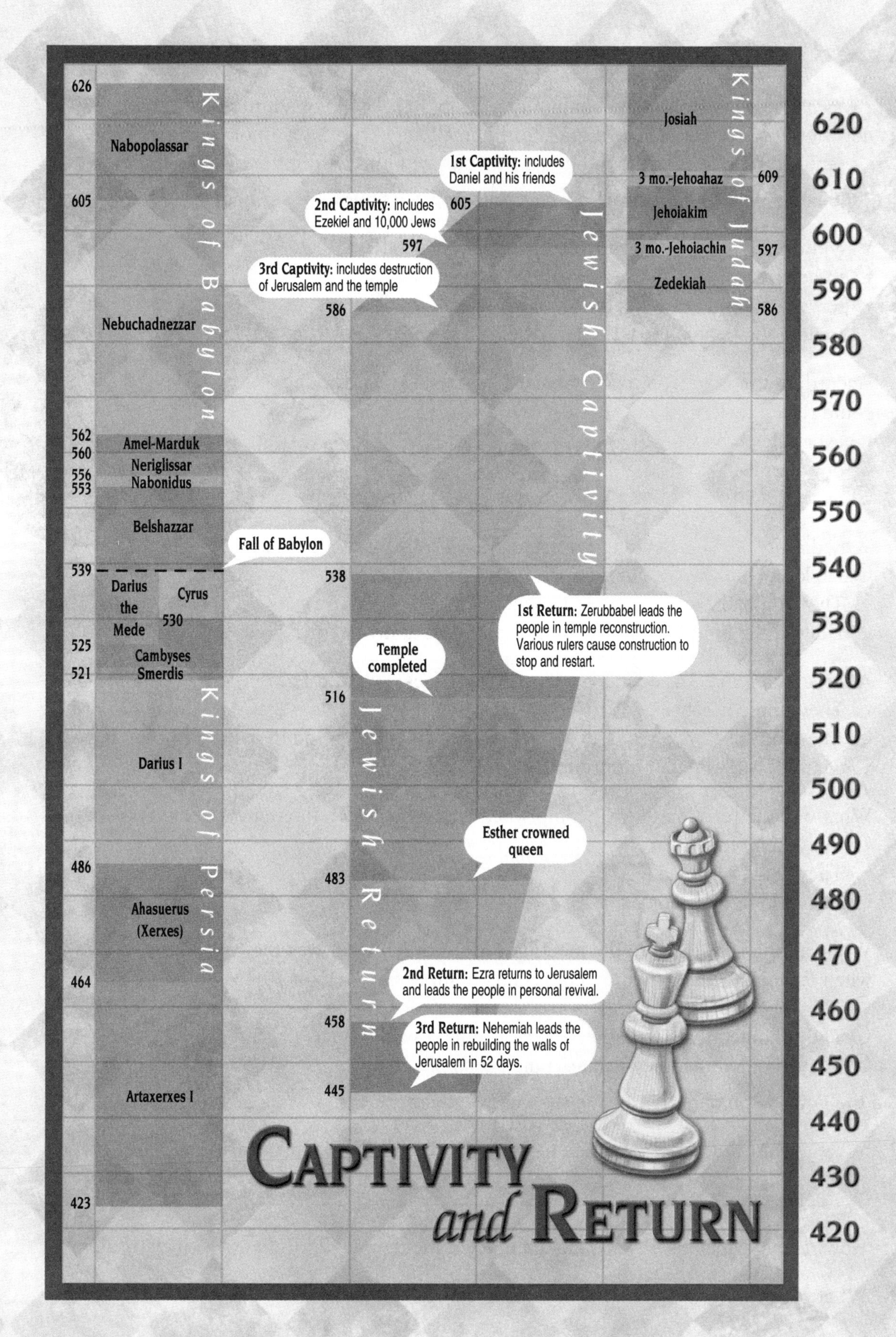
Captivity and Return
Kings of Babylon
Kings of Persia
Kings of Judah
Jewish Captivity
Jewish Return
626
Nabopolassar
605
Nebuchadnezzar
562
Amel-Marduk
560
Neriglissar
556
Nabonidus
553
Belshazzar
539
Fall of Babylon
Darius the Mede
Cyrus
530
525
Cambyses
521
Smerdis
Darius I
486
Ahasuerus (Xerxes)
464
Artaxerxes I
423
1st Captivity: includes Daniel and his friends
605
2nd Captivity: includes Ezekiel and 10,000 Jews
597
3rd Captivity: includes destruction of Jerusalem and the temple
586
538
1st Return: Zerubbabel leads the people in temple reconstruction. Various rulers cause construction to stop and restart.
Temple completed
516
Esther crowned queen
483
2nd Return: Ezra returns to Jerusalem and leads the people in personal revival.
458
3rd Return: Nehemiah leads the people in rebuilding the walls of Jerusalem in 52 days.
445
Josiah
3 mo.-Jehoahaz
609
Jehoiakim
3 mo.-Jehoiachin
597
Zedekiah
586
620
610
600
590
580
570
560
550
540
530
520
510
500
490
480
470
460
450
440
430
420

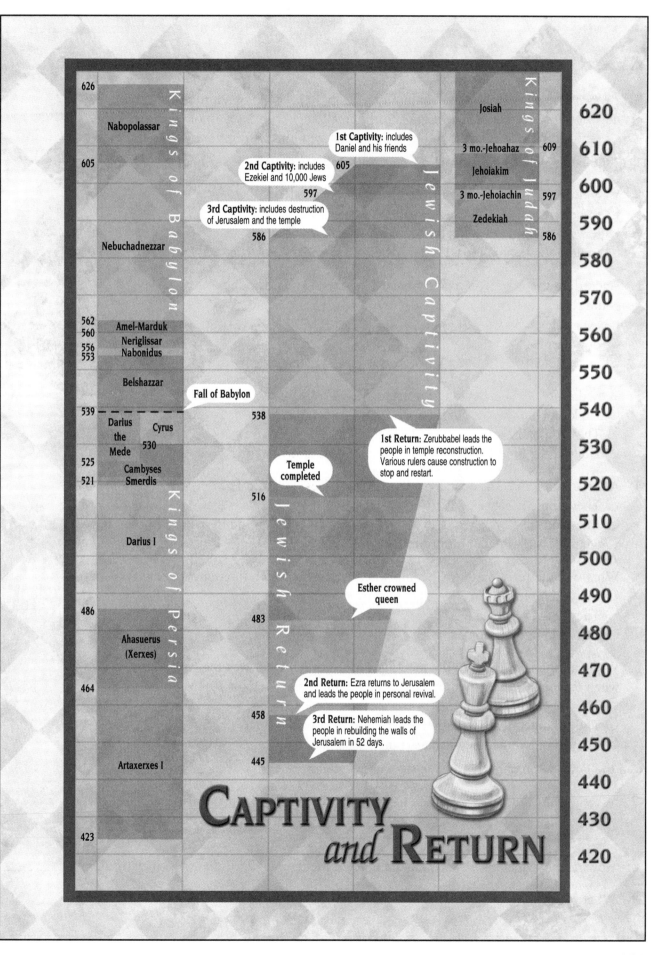

To Teach the People

Ezra 7-10

Name ______________________

Ezra was a priest in the Jewish community of Babylon. The king admired him and knew his devotion to God. Because of Ezra's testimony, King Artaxerxes I not only granted Ezra's request to go to Jerusalem, but also encouraged him with gifts for the temple.

Fill in the circle next to the correct answer. You may use your Bible for help.

1. Why did Ezra want to return to Jerusalem? (Ezra 7:10)
   - ○ to help rebuild his house
   - ○ to help rebuild the walls of Jerusalem
   - ○ to help the people learn the law of God

2. According to the letter King Artaxerxes sent with Ezra, which Jews could return to Jerusalem? (Ezra 7:13)
   - ○ every Jew who wanted to go
   - ○ only Ezra
   - ○ every Jew living in Babylon who was commanded to leave the city

3. Why didn't Ezra ask the king for protection for the journey? (Ezra 8:21-23)
   - ○ He knew the way would be safe.
   - ○ The king had already offered to send men.
   - ○ He told the king that God's power could defeat any enemy.

4. After arriving in Jerusalem and offering sacrifices, why did Ezra mourn? (Ezra 9:1-3)
   - ○ The temple had been destroyed again.
   - ○ Many of the Jews already in Judah had sinned against God by taking foreign wives.
   - ○ Many Jews wanted to return to Babylon.

5. What was the reaction of the people when confronted with their sin? (Ezra 9:4, 10:9)
   - ○ They trembled.
   - ○ They fled to Babylon.
   - ○ They hid in their homes.

6. When all the men came to the meeting in Jerusalem, what was their response when Ezra challenged them to confess their sin to God? (Ezra 10:12)
   - ○ They began to stone Ezra.
   - ○ They shouted that they agreed with Ezra and would do as he said.
   - ○ They shouted that they wanted other gods.

Use the timeline on page 179 to answer the questions.

7. What event occurred a few years before the Jews began to leave Babylon?

   ____

8. How many years after Zerubbabel completed the temple did Ezra arrive in Jerusalem? __________

9. What other event in Jewish history occurred during this time?

   ____

Bearing the Burden

Nehemiah 1-6

Name ______________________

Use the timeline on page 179 to answer the questions.

1. How long after Ezra went to Jerusalem did Nehemiah go? ______________________
2. Who was the king over Persia at the time of Nehemiah? ______________________
3. Why did Nehemiah leave Babylon? ______________________ ______________________
4. How long had it been since the walls of Jerusalem were destroyed? ______________________
5. How long did Nehemiah's project take to complete? ______________________

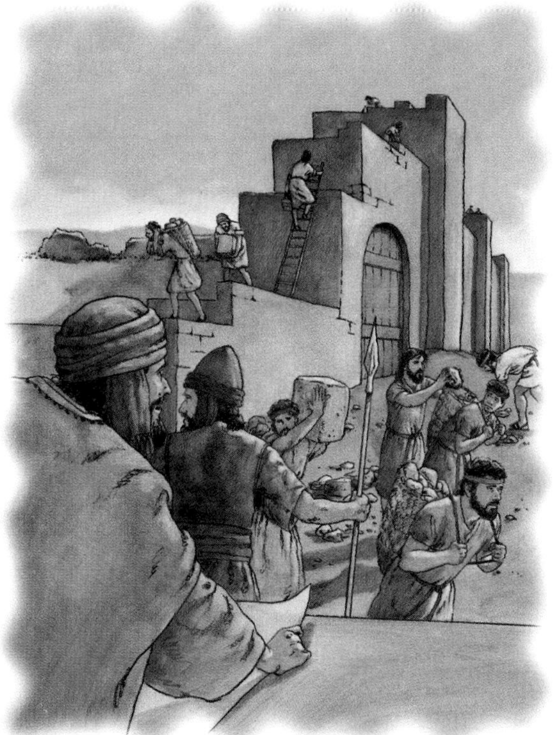

Write the letter of the correct word or phrase to complete each sentence.

_____ 6. Nehemiah was the _____ for the king.

_____ 7. Nehemiah's countenance was sad because he had heard that _____.

_____ 8. Nehemiah _____ before making his request of the king to go to Jerusalem to rebuild the walls.

_____ 9. Nehemiah encouraged the Jews by telling them _____.

_____ 10. Sanballat and Tobiah, leaders of neighboring lands, tried to _____.

_____ 11. As a result of the threats of Sanballat and Tobiah, the _____; some would stand guard while the others continued to work.

_____ 12. Even though men were standing guard, the workers _____ while they worked.

_____ 13. To stay ready in case of an enemy attack, the workers _____.

A. how God had directed and blessed in bringing him to Jerusalem
B. also carried or wore weapons
C. workers were divided
D. prayed for wisdom
E. cupbearer
F. slept in their clothes
G. hinder the work on the walls
H. the walls of Jerusalem had never been rebuilt, leaving the city unprotected

Singing with Understanding

"Standing on the Promises" (vv. 3-4)

Name ______________________

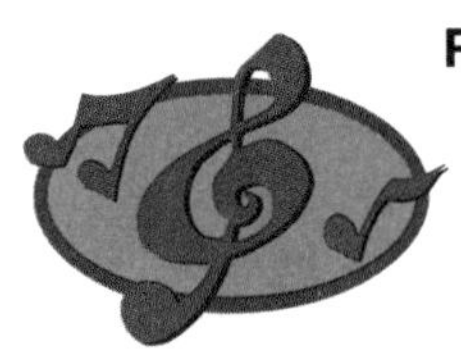

Read verses 3 and 4 of the hymn on page 316.

1. What is the *Spirit's sword,* according to Ephesians 6:17?

____

2. Who helps us understand the truth of God's Word, according to John 16:13?

____

The primary way that God speaks to Christians is through His Word. It is only by the Spirit's guidance that you can understand how the promises in God's Word apply to you as an individual. The Spirit also teaches Christians how to claim those promises to help them overcome temptation and rest in the Savior who loves them.

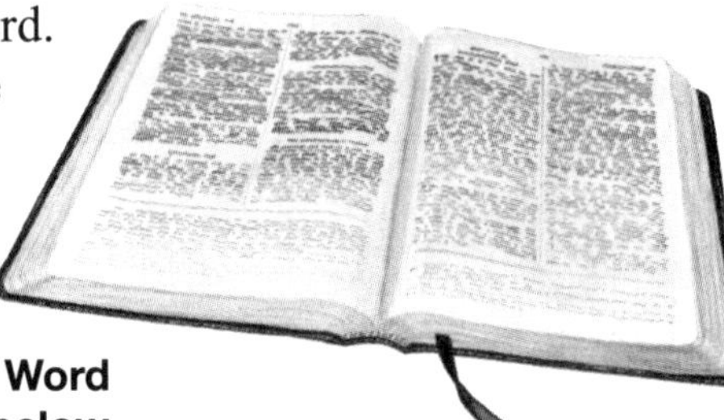

Using a concordance or your memory, write a promise from God's Word that you can "stand on" when faced with each of the temptations below.

"Do you really think you could ever be saved? Look at what a sinner you are!"

Promise:

____

____

____

"God has forgotten about you and your needs."

Promise:

____

____

____

"Do you really think God can help you? Maybe you'd be better off taking matters into your own hands."

Promise:

____

____

____

What Does God Say About My Time?

Time Management

Name ______________________

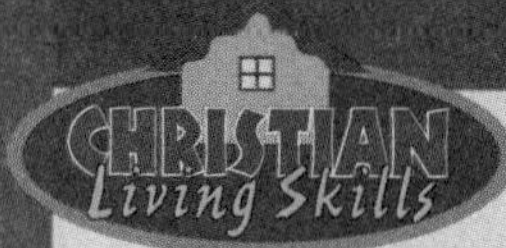

CHRISTIAN
Living Skills

Time is a gift from God. Your entire life will be measured by pieces of time—seconds, minutes, hours, days, and years. God is the Creator and the sustainer of time. Before He created time, He decided on an exact point in time for you to be born, to live, and to die.

Read Psalm 31:15 and complete the sentence explaining what this verse means.

This verse means that ______________________

God has appointed a time for everything that happens on earth. He has put **you** at this particular time in history for a purpose. He has given you the family you have for a reason. You are your age by God's design. There is a perfect time for every event that occurs in your life.

Read Ecclesiastes 3:1-8. List some of the words that describe events for which God has given us time.

__________ __________ __________

__________ __________ __________

Read Ecclesiastes 3:11*a* and answer the question.

When did God make everything beautiful? ______________________

God has much to say about the way you use the time He has entrusted to you. He wants you to remember that your days are limited and precious and should be used wisely.

Read the verses and match them to the correct statements. The verses match to more than one statement.

_____ Your life is like a vapor or a mist that won't last long.

_____ Be wise about how you live your life.

_____ Understand what the Lord's will is for how you spend your time.

_____ Ask God to help you value the number of days you have to live.

_____ You do not know what will happen tomorrow.

_____ Apply your heart to gaining wisdom.

A. Psalm 90:12

B. Ephesians 5:15-17

C. James 4:14

Something to Think About

Time Management

Name ______________________

CHRISTIAN *Living Skills*

You are responsible for what you do with God's gift of time. The way you direct or control the use of your time is called **time management.** God has given you the freedom to choose how you spend your time, but you cannot choose the consequences. Remember that you will give an account to God for the way you use the time He has given you.

What About Me?

Study the principles. Take time at home to complete the chart evaluating your time management habits.

TIME Management Principles

Target Priorities

Priorities are activities that are most important to us and that take up our time. They should include your responsibilities to God, your parents, your teachers, and your church.

Write down some of YOUR God-given responsibilities that YOU must make a priority.

God: ______________________ Parents: ______________________

Teachers: ______________________ Church: ______________________

Identify Distractions

Distractions are things that hinder you from accomplishing God's will in the right time. Avoid becoming distracted as you work! Distractions could include good things (friends, sports, books) or bad things (wrong music, worldly TV programs, laziness).

Make a list of things that distract YOU from using your time wisely.

______________________ ______________________ ______________________

Master Organization

Organization is putting everything around you in its proper place so that you can easily get your work done. You should carefully inspect every area in which you work and do what you need to do to get yourself organized! (Sort piles, throw trash away, file papers, etc.)

Make a list of all the places where YOU work and live.
Circle the ones that you need to organize.

______________________ ______________________ ______________________

Evade Procrastination

Procrastination is putting off your responsibilities until a later time. If you'll be honest with yourself, you'll realize that it is laziness in managing the time God has given to you.

Make a list of the responsibilities in which YOU are tempted to procrastinate.

______________________ ______________________ ______________________

Get the Bible Reading H.A.B.I.T.

Name ______________________________

BIBLE STUDY Skills

Have a special time set aside each day to read your Bible. If possible, make it the same time every day.

Ask God to teach you from His Word. Remember to thank Him for helping you to understand and apply it.

Be still and give your attention to what you are reading.

Investigate the Scripture by asking yourself questions about it.

Take time to look up words and ideas you do not understand.

As you read the Scripture for each day, write the date in the box.

Christ revealed salvation to all men and taught them how to live. **Titus 2:11-12**	Christians should be watching for the second appearing of Christ. **Titus 2:13-14**	Salvation is through belief on the Lord Jesus Christ. **Acts 16:30-31**	The Scriptures make it clear that Jesus is the Christ. **Acts 18:24-28**	God intends salvation for Gentiles as well as for Jews. **Ephesians 2:11-13**
In His earthly life, Jesus openly displayed that He was God. **I John 1:1-3**	Christ's life on earth teaches Christians how to be godly. **I Timothy 3:15-16**	Jesus is the image of God, and through Him Christians learn of God. **II Corinthians 4:3-6**	Jesus Christ is eternally the same. **Hebrews 13:7-8**	Whoever does not believe Jesus Christ came in the flesh is not of God. **II John 7-9**
God's power is the same great power that raised Christ from the dead. **Ephesians 1:15-20**	Christ has power over all other powers and over the church. **Ephesians 1:21-23**	In His death, Christ triumphed over all rulers. **Colossians 2:13-15**	Christ will reign until He has conquered all His enemies. **I Corinthians 15:21-26**	Jesus gives Christians victory over death and the grave. **I Corinthians 15:54-57**
Christ's death and resurrection were planned by God. **Acts 2:22-24**	David prophesied that Christ would rise from the dead. **Acts 2:25-31**	God has raised Jesus and exalted Him to sit at His right hand. **Acts 2:32-33**	God has made Jesus, whom man crucified, both Lord and Christ. **Acts 2:34-36**	We must repent and be baptized in the name of Jesus Christ. **Acts 2:37-39**

Bible Study Methods

Topical

Name ______________________

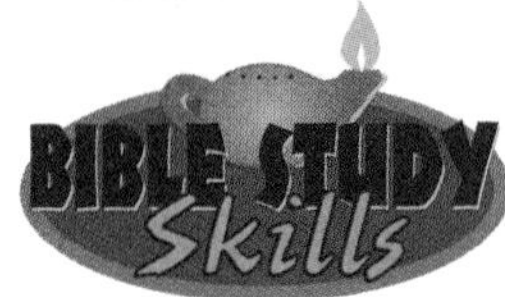

BIBLE STUDY
Skills

A *topical* Bible study examines a single topic as it is found in the Scriptures. It differs from *synthetic* Bible study by examining a specific subject rather than a broad theme. Think of topical study as looking at one room instead of an entire house plan. Concordances, topical Bibles, cross-references, and Bible dictionaries are useful for topical Bible study.

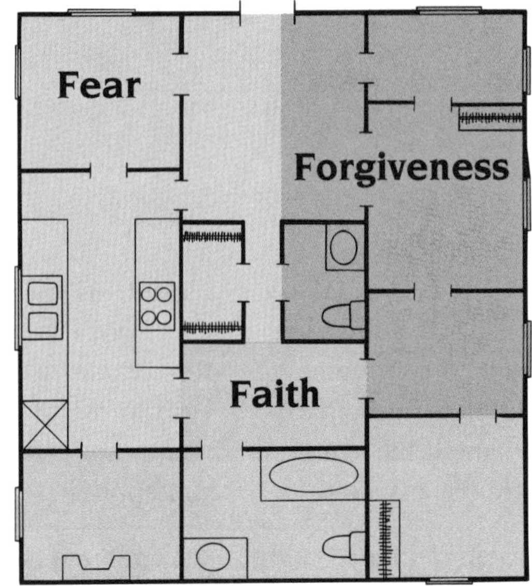

Fear
Forgiveness
Faith

Choose one of the topics above and complete the study guide. Give Scripture references to support your answers.

List some Old Testament Scriptures that refer to the topic.

______________________ ______________________ ______________________

List some New Testament Scriptures that tell about the topic.

______________________ ______________________ ______________________

Name some Bible characters who learned about the topic.

______________________ ______________________ ______________________

Briefly tell what Jesus Christ said about the topic.

____

____

What else would you like to learn about the topic?

____

____

Clear Messages

Luke 1:26-56 *and* 2:21-39

Name ______________________________

Match the truth about Christ next to the person who said it.

_____ 1. Gabriel

_____ 2. Elisabeth

_____ 3. Mary

_____ 4. Simeon

_____ 5. Anna

A. He said that Christ would provide salvation for the Gentiles and for Israel (Luke 2:28-32).

B. He said the baby was the Son of God and would one day sit on the throne of David in an everlasting kingdom (Luke 1:26-35).

C. She shared the good news that those seeking redemption through the promised Messiah should look to this baby (Luke 2:36-38).

D. She said God would fulfill His promises as He had for Israel and Abraham (Luke 1:46-55).

E. The Holy Spirit helped this person know that Mary's baby was the Lord (Luke 1:41-45).

The Bible is sometimes called God's Word. In the first chapter of John, Christ is also called the Word. Christ *manifested,* or clearly demonstrated, God's message of salvation to all people.

Read John 1:1-14. Mark an *X* next to the six truths about Christ proclaimed in this passage.

_____ 6. Christ was from the beginning, before creation.

_____ 7. Christ came to heal the sick.

_____ 8. Christ is God.

_____ 9. Christ created all things.

_____ 10. Christ raised people from the dead.

_____ 11. Christ is the light of salvation to men.

_____ 12. Christ calmed the sea.

_____ 13. Christ is the Son of God made flesh.

_____ 14. Christ is full of grace and truth.

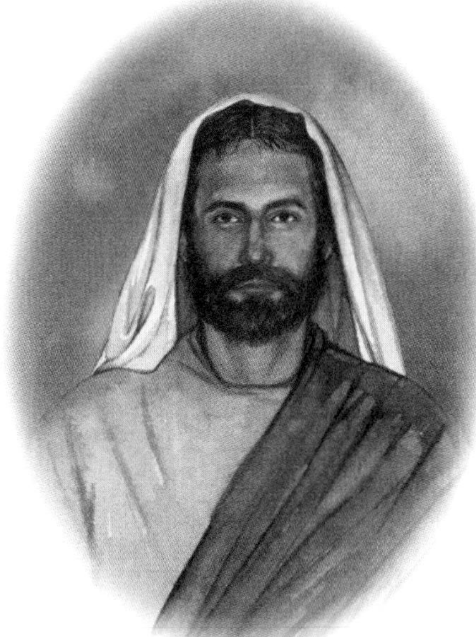

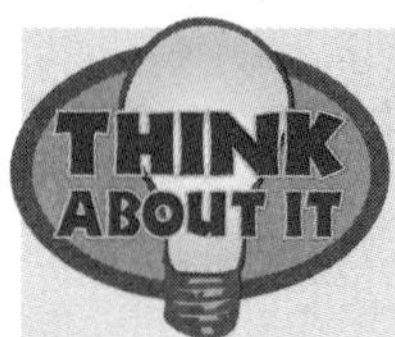
THINK
ABOUT IT

God provided a clear message of who Christ is and why He came to earth. Have you accepted the salvation found in this truth from God? If you have, do you know someone that needs to hear God's message of salvation? Take time to talk with that person about Christ.

Obedient to the Father

Luke 2:40-52; 4:16-30

Name ______________________

God chose Mary and Joseph to be the earthly parents of Jesus. They demonstrated their obedience to God as they went to Jerusalem each year for the Passover feast. God sent Christ to earth to do His will. As He grew, Jesus demonstrated His obedience to His Father before those around Him.

Fill in the circle next to the answer that correctly completes each sentence.

Luke 2:40-52

1. Jesus was ______ years old at this time.
   ○ twelve ○ thirty
2. Mary and Joseph searched for ______ days before finding Jesus in Jerusalem.
   ○ thirty ○ three
3. The knowledge and understanding of Jesus amazed the ______ at the temple.
   ○ scholars ○ widows
4. Jesus had expected Mary and Joseph to know that He would be doing the business of ______ in His Father's house.
   ○ His Father ○ a carpenter

Luke 4:16-30

5. At the synagogue in Nazareth, Jesus read from the book of ______.
   ○ Isaiah ○ Deuteronomy
6. After reading, Jesus said that He was the fulfillment of this ______.
   ○ time ○ Scripture
7. By the way Jesus spoke, the people wondered how He could be ______ son.
   ○ Joseph's ○ God's
8. Through examples of Elijah and Elisha, Jesus reminded the people that a ______ is not accepted in his own country.
   ○ priest ○ prophet
9. The people became ______ at what Jesus said.
   ○ overjoyed ○ angry
10. The people led Jesus out of the city to ______ a high hill.
    ○ hear Him preach from ○ cast Him off

What Does God Say About Being a Friend?

Name ______________________

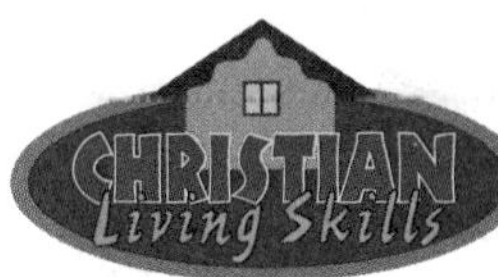
CHRISTIAN
Living Skills

If you want to have good friends, you must BE a good friend. The kind of friend you are is a result of the choices you make. The choices you make show the kind of character you have. Your **character** is what you think and who you are.

Read the verses for clues to complete the puzzle and discover qualities that describe a good friend. (*Note:* Words will be written across, down, up, and backwards.)

faithful	**godly**	**courageous**	**compassionate**	**considerate**
patient	**honest**	**kind**	**unselfish**	**forgiving**

Across

3. **Zechariah 7:9**—shows sympathy for someone else
4. **Ephesians 4:32*b***—grants pardon to someone without holding a grudge
6. **I Timothy 4:8*b***—lives a holy life that pleases God

Down

1. **Titus 3:2**—is gentle and considers the needs of others
2. **Joshua 1:6**—is fearless in the face of difficulties

Up

5. **Ephesians 4:25**—tells the truth in all situations
7. **Ephesians 4:32*a***—does good things for others; is thoughtful
10. **I Thessalonians 5:14*b***—waits cheerfully on others

Backwards

8. **John 15:13**—puts the needs of others before self
9. **I Timothy 6:12*a***—stands up for and lives by what he believes

1 2 3 4 5 6 7 8 9 10

God wants you to be a good friend. You will have a great effect on your friends, and your friends will also greatly affect you. Being a good friend will not come easily. You must work on developing your character by making choices that please God. God always blesses obedience!

Read Psalm 1 and follow the instructions.

1. List the three kinds of people with whom you should avoid being friends (v. 1).

   ______________________ ______________________ ______________________

2. In what should you enjoy spending time? (v. 2) in the ______________ of the ______________.
3. What is the outcome of the wicked? (vv. 4-6) ______________________
4. As you make right choices to become a good friend, who will watch over you? ______________

Something to Think About

Being a Friend

Name ______________________

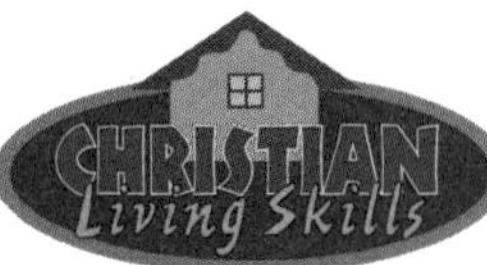
CHRISTIAN
Living Skills

Being a good friend is a responsibility you should take seriously. Friendship requires you to make some decisions between pleasing God and pleasing your friends. Sometimes your friends may not like it when you decide to do what is right. This is when you will find out who your true friends really are. True friends are those who want you to please God.

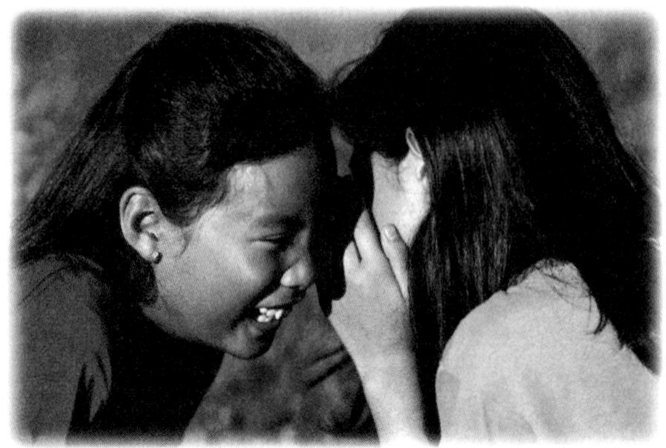

Read the scenarios and determine what action you should take to demonstrate true friendship.

Scenario	What should you do if you want to be a true friend?
You and your friend Kaitlyn went to Brittany's birthday party. While you were watching Brittany open her presents, Kaitlyn whispered a few comments to you, making fun of Brittany's house and the clothes she was wearing.	
You saw your friend Hudson find five dollars on the ground at recess. Hudson decided not to turn it in to the teacher. When your teacher asked whether anybody found the five dollars that another student lost at recess, Hudson didn't say anything.	
Caleb's mom has been in the hospital for the past month, and she doesn't seem to be getting better. You have noticed that Caleb seems very sad and discouraged.	

What About Me?

Take time at home to think about the kind of friend you are.
List four things your friends would say describing the kind of friend you are to them.

______________________ ______________________

______________________ ______________________

Think about the list you have made. Complete the chart.

Questions to Think About	Yes	No
Do I encourage my friends to love and obey God?		
Do I care enough about my friends to be honest with them when they are doing wrong?		
Do I encourage my friends to honor and obey their parents?		
Can my friends count on me to do the right thing?		
Do I look for ways to encourage my friends?		
Do I ever use my friends to get what I want?		
Am I being the kind of friend to others that I want them to be to me?		

The Word from God

History of the Bible

Name ____________________

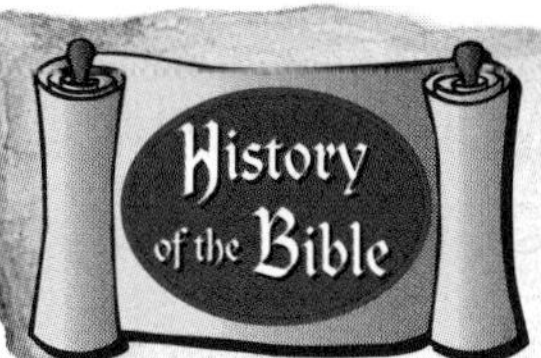
History of the Bible

For hundreds of years God's Word was spoken directly to men, then passed on by word of mouth. But for His written Word, God used holy men, devoted to Him, to record the Scriptures that we call the Bible. Now, thousands of years after the first books were written, we have the complete Word of God, which leads us to salvation through Christ and guides us in our relationships with God and other men.

Because **papyrus sheets** were strips of plant stems pressed together, they did not have the durability of today's paper. For this reason, the sheets would tear or fall apart if sewn into a book form. Gluing sheets of papyrus into scrolls was the best way to make "books" from this fragile material.

In II Peter 1:21, God tells us that He used holy men to record the Scriptures as the Holy Spirit directed them. The **original** writings, called **autographs,** are the only *inerrant* copies *inspired* by God. These copies no longer exist since they were written on *papyrus,* the common writing surface of those days.

Papyrus was not very durable, and temperature changes and moisture would cause it to rot in less than 100 years. Papyrus writings that exist today were preserved because of a dry desert climate.

Define each word using the glossary.

1. inerrant ____________________
2. inspiration ____________________

Write the word which best completes each sentence, using the information about the history of the Bible.

1. Today the Scriptures from God are called the ______.
2. The writing material on which the original Word of God was written was ______.
3. It has been thousands of years since the first ______ of the Bible were written.
4. Because God's Word was inspired, the ______ writings were inerrant.
5. The original writings are called ______ because they were written by the original authors.
6. Because God breathed the Scriptures as holy men recorded them, we know that the Bible is ______.

Write the letters from the shaded boxes to complete the sentence.

Since the first copies of the Scriptures were written on papyrus, they eventually became known as the Bible from the Greek word ___ ___ ___ ___ ___ ___, which means "papyrus" or "book."

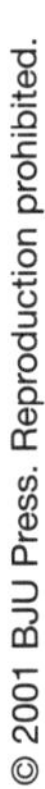

Preserving the Word

History of the Bible

Name ____________________

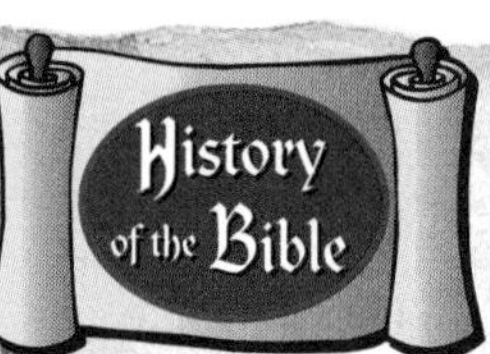
History
of the Bible

The earliest books of the Bible were written around 1500 B.C. The apostle John wrote the last book, Revelation, around A.D. 100. The Old Testament was written in Hebrew and Aramaic, and the New Testament was written in Greek. **Scribes** worked diligently to make more copies of the Word of God. These hand-written **manuscripts** are the basis for the English Bibles we have today.

As these manuscripts were collected, a standard was set to determine whether they were the Word of God. Many writings exist which were written at the same time as the books of the Bible. Some writings might seem very close to Scripture, but are not included in the **canon** because they do not meet all the standards.

As writing processes developed, the use of **parchment** and **vellum** replaced papyrus. At first the parchment was made into scrolls, but scrolls had several drawbacks. They were bulky to move around, and the writing was limited to one side. Eventually it was found that parchment pages could be stacked and sewn together to form a type of book called a **codex.** Often a stiff material such as wood was used to cover a codex. Both sides of the codex pages could be used, which helped make the copies lighter and easier to carry.

Hebrew scribes took great care to preserve the accuracy of the Scriptures as they made copies. Between A.D. 300 and 500, the scribes, known as Masoretes, developed elaborate procedures for standardizing the copies they made. They measured the lines in each column, counted the characters (letters) on each line, and measured the spaces between characters and words. These precautions and others helped preserve the accuracy of the Word of God.

The **scribes** were Jewish scholars. These men were priests who preserved, copied, and interpreted the law of God.

A **canon** was originally a reed or rod used as a measuring stick. When applied to Scripture, the term *canon* means the books included in the Bible. These writings had to measure up and meet standards set to determine whether they were truly inspired by God.

The **Apocrypha** is a group of books included in some Bibles. Although some people consider them Scripture, they are not included in the canon.

Parchment is a material made from the skins of calves or goats and is used for writing or painting. A finer form of parchment is called **vellum**.

Write the letter of the word next to the correct definition.

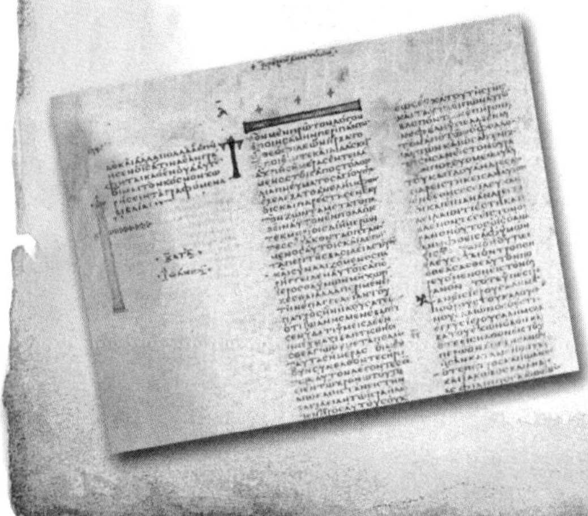

_____ 1. hand-written copies of the Bible

_____ 2. an early type of book which replaced scrolls

_____ 3. the books recognized as the inspired Word of God

_____ 4. men who copied the Scriptures

_____ 5. a material made from animal skins which replaced papyrus

A. codex
B. scribes
C. parchment
D. manuscripts
E. canon

Clearly God

John 8:1-31

Name ______________________

People who seek forgiveness should look to God and His Word. No man has the ability to forgive sin—only God can forgive. The scribes and the Pharisees tried to find fault in Jesus' actions and in His teaching. They refused to believe that He could forgive sin.

Fill in the circle for the phrase that correctly completes each sentence.

1. In the Old Testament, Samuel was commanded to anoint a king to follow Saul. God directed him to the family of Jesse. Samuel wanted to anoint the son who looked the best, but God told Samuel that _____ (I Sam. 16:7).
   - ○ Saul was tall and strong, but made a poor king
   - ○ man looks at the appearance, but the Lord looks at the heart
   - ○ he needed to go to another family

2. Once while Jesus was teaching, a paralyzed man was lowered through the roof by his friends. Jesus told the man his sins were forgiven. The Pharisees said that _____ (Luke 5:20-24).
   - ○ only God can forgive sins
   - ○ the man's faith healed him
   - ○ the man was not really paralyzed

3. Later in His earthly ministry, Jesus said that the scribes' and Pharisees' actions were done only so that they would appear righteous before men. Christ described the scribes and Pharisees as beautiful on the outside, but _____ (Matt. 23:27-28).
   - ○ full of pride
   - ○ full of a wealth of Bible knowledge
   - ○ full of dead bones and uncleanness

4. The scribes and Pharisees tried to give Christ a problem too difficult to answer correctly when they brought a sinful woman to Him. Christ _____ (John 8:10-11).
   - ○ quoted the law of Moses and had the woman stoned
   - ○ rebuked the scribes and Pharisees for attempting to trick Him
   - ○ saw the woman's need of salvation and forgave her sin

5. The Pharisees accused Jesus of lying about who He was since no one could testify that what Jesus said was true. Christ _____ (John 8:13, 18).
   - ○ said that God the Father testifies that Jesus is God
   - ○ had no reply to their accusation
   - ○ performed a miracle to prove that He is God

THINK ABOUT IT

The scribes and Pharisees knew the Scriptures and should have been the first to recognize that Jesus was the promised Messiah. But they had made practicing religion a way of life, full of laws to be obeyed to earn salvation. To the people, the scribes and Pharisees looked like they loved and obeyed God. But God, able to look on the hearts of these men, said that they lacked spiritual life.

Consider your spiritual condition. Are you _____

- ○ like the Pharisees—obedient and spiritual on the outside, but spiritually dead on the inside?
- ○ like the followers of Christ, and can you say "I have found the Savior and He is alive in me"?
- ○ like others who were seeking the Savior—interested, but not yet trusting Him?

Humble as a Servant

Philippians 2:7-8

Name ______________________

Christ was a Servant dedicated to God. He accepted doing God's will on earth. Just as Jesus had power to calm the wind and the waves, He could have avoided the humiliation and trials He endured on earth. Like a true servant seeking to fulfill the wishes of his master, Christ submitted to and obeyed His Father.

For Your ENLIGHTENMENT In Israel, servants were usually owned by the wealthy. Some servants were foreigners, while others were poor Jews. If a man owed a debt to another man, he made himself a servant until the debt was paid.

Jewish law contained rules concerning servants:
- They were not to be mistreated.
- They were entitled to observe the Sabbath and other holidays.

The Jews treated their servants much better than other cultures did. Servants were almost like family members. Most servants were given the same privileges in society as their masters, except that they could not own property.

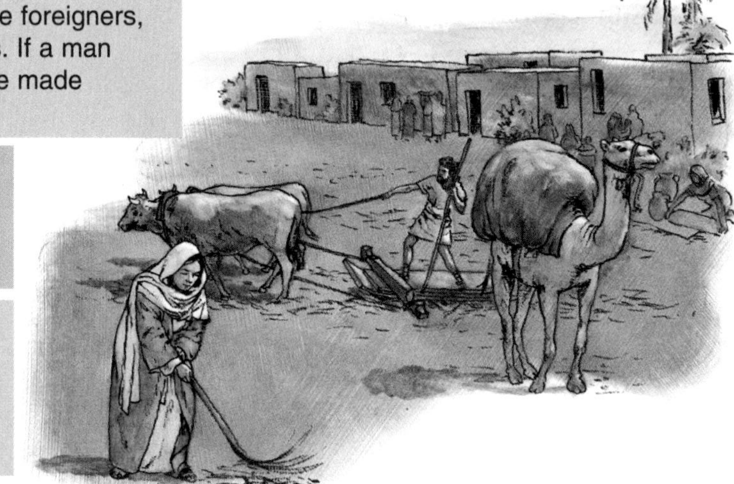

Read Philippians 2:7-8 and answer the questions.

1. What two characteristics did Christ demonstrate? ______________________
2. What benefit did Christ's obedience bring to mankind? ______________________

In the Bible, Christ is not the only person identified as a servant. In some cases, God calls a person His servant to show the relationship of that person to Him. Sometimes the writers of Scripture identified others as servants of God. There are also Scriptures in which the writer declared himself to be a servant of God as he introduced himself to others. For example, Paul often introduced himself as a servant of God, and he also identified individuals as servants when he wrote Scripture.

For each passage, write the name of the person who is called a servant, then mark who identified him as a servant.

	Name of the servant		Identified as a servant by		
			God	the writer of the book	himself
1.		Numbers 14:20-24			
2.		I Samuel 3:10			
3.		Job 1:8			
4.		Romans 16:1-2			
5.		James 1:1-3			

Deity Revealed

John 8:31–9:41

Name ______________________

Braille is a system of raised dots that can be read by touch. Sixty-three different characters can be formed using the basic Braille cell, which is three dots high and two dots wide.
The first ten letters of the alphabet are formed using combinations of the top four dots of the cell.

A B C D E F G H I J

The next ten letters are formed by adding the lower left-hand dot.

K L M N O P Q R S T

The last five letters (except *w*) and some small words are formed by adding the lower right-hand dot.

U V X Y Z and for of the with

Nine other speech sounds and the letter *w* are made by omitting the lower left-hand dot.

ch gh sh th wh ed er ou ow W

Use Braille to spell the words that complete each sentence.

1. Sinners are enslaved to sin, but they can find freedom from sin by knowing

   ____ ____ ____ ____ ____. (John 8:32)

2. The Jews said that Abraham was their father; then they said that God was their

   Father, but Jesus said the ____ ____ ____ ____ ____ was their father. (John 8:44)

3. The blind man was born blind to show the ____ ____ ____ ____ ____ of God. (John 9:3)

4. The Pharisees' ____ ____ ____ ____ ____ prevented them from accepting the testimony of the healed man.

Answer the questions.

5. What evidence did Jesus say showed that His accusers were not children of God? (John 8:44-47)

   ____

   ____

6. Jesus called Himself "I AM." How did the Jews react? (John 8:58-59)

   ____

   Why? ____

7. Jesus compared those without salvation to blind men. What did the Pharisees, who were spiritually blind, need? (John 9:5) ______________________________

Singing with Understanding

"Our Great Savior" (vv. 1-3)

Name ______________________________

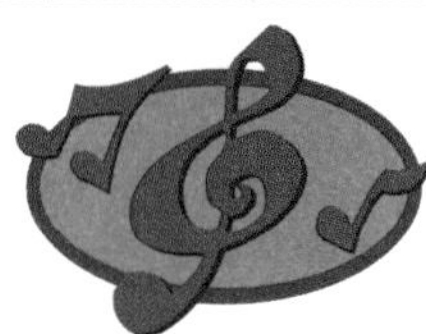

Read verses 1-3 of the hymn on page 317 and answer the questions.

1. To whom did Jesus show that He was a friend? ____________________
2. What did Jesus provide in times of weakness, temptations, trials, and failure?

   ____

3. What did Jesus provide for those with sorrow and broken hearts?

   ____________________ and ____________________

Other friends may fail you, but Jesus loves you with an everlasting love. Have you felt His comfort during a time of sorrow or His strength during a time of temptation?

Comfort

Write about a time of sorrow in which Jesus comforted you.

____
____
____
____
____
____
____
____
____
____

Victory

Write about a time of temptation in which Jesus gave you victory.

____
____
____
____
____
____
____
____
____
____

Translating the Word

History of the Bible

Name ______________________

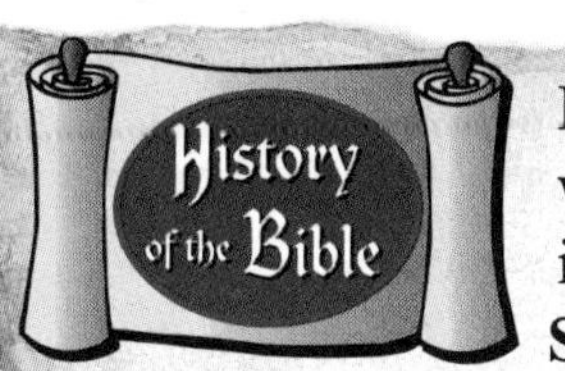
History of the Bible

Before the time of Christ, Old Testament Scriptures were translated into other languages. The most important translation made from 250-100 B.C. was the **Septuagint.** The Septuagint was a translation of the Hebrew Old Testament into Greek. Christ and the disciples quoted from the Septuagint.

Although everyone had a spoken language, not all people had a written language. As languages developed and alphabets formed, the Bible could be translated more. In most nations, schooling was limited to the religious and political leaders. These leaders made the decisions whether or not to translate the Scriptures and make them available for reading. The common people had to rely on the religious leaders to interpret and deliver the Word of God to them.

No language can directly translate word for word. Often it is necessary for translators to choose the best way to *render* a word in their own language for the idea God is expressing. Much care and effort was given by the translators to ensure that the Word of God remained accurate. Some written languages were new and still developing, so changes in wording were made on new copies.

By the early A.D. 400s the leading nations of the world—Egypt, Syria, and Rome—had the complete Bible in their own languages. The Roman translation of the Bible in Latin, called the **Vulgate,** was the version used throughout Europe for centuries. As the nations of Europe developed and the Roman Empire fell, the Roman Church still influenced the government. Rulers used the people's dependence on the religious leaders to interpret the Latin Scriptures as a way to maintain control over the people.

For the translators to **render** God's Word in their own languages means that they put the Bible's ideas and thoughts into words they could understand.

As the Roman Empire spread, Latin became the common language rather than Greek. The word *vulgate* means "common." The overwhelming acceptance of Jerome's Latin Vulgate prevented future vulgates from being written.

Write *S* next to the phrases describing the Septuagint and *V* next to the phrases describing the Vulgate.

______ 1. the translation written before the time of Christ

______ 2. the translation written in Latin

______ 3. the translation written after the time of Christ

______ 4. the translation written in Greek

______ 5. the translation used by Christ and the disciples

______ 6. the translation used by the Roman Church

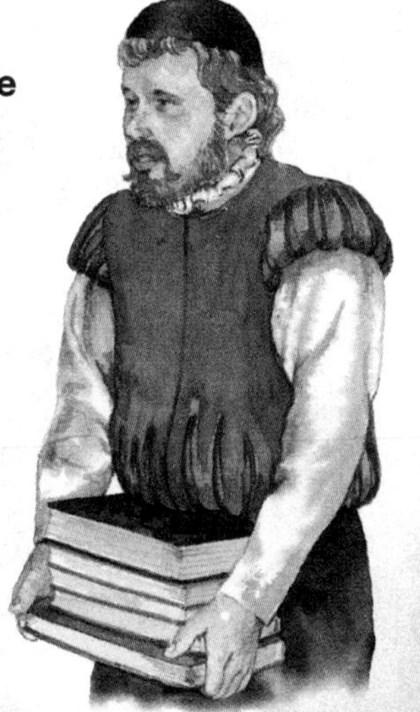

History of the English Bible

Name ______________________

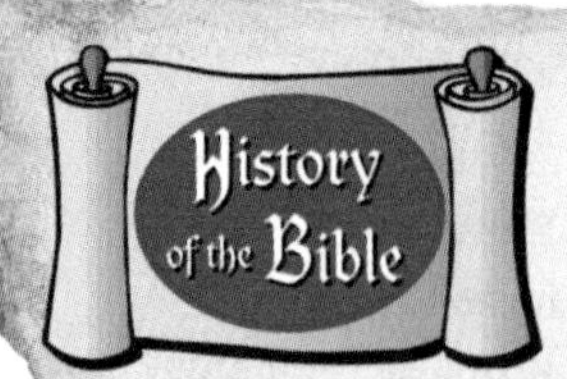
History
of the Bible

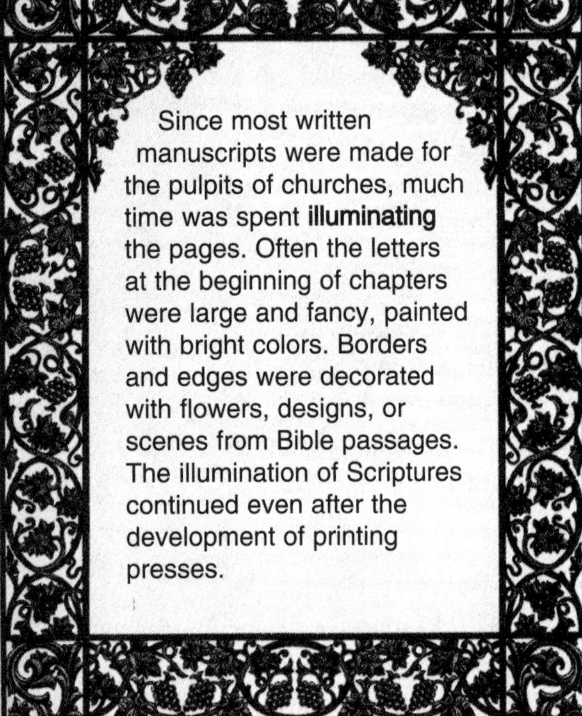

Since most written manuscripts were made for the pulpits of churches, much time was spent **illuminating** the pages. Often the letters at the beginning of chapters were large and fancy, painted with bright colors. Borders and edges were decorated with flowers, designs, or scenes from Bible passages. The illumination of Scriptures continued even after the development of printing presses.

ST. JOHN 3:16

him should not perish, but have eternal life. John 3:36
16 For God so loved the world,
that he gave his only begotten Son,
that whosoever believeth in him
should not perish, but have everlasting life. Rom. 5:8
17 For God sent not his Son into

King James Version

nall life.
16 ¶ *For God so loued þ world, that
he gaue his only begotten Sonne: that
whosoeuer beleeueth in him, should
not perish, but haue euerlasting life.
17 * For God sent not his Sonne in-

King James Facsimile

lo: filius hominis qui est in celo. Et si-
cut moyses exaltavit serpentem in de-
serto · ita exaltari oportet filiū hominis:
ut omnis qui credit in ipso nō pereat:
sed habeat vitam eternā. Sic enī deus
dilexit mundū ut filiū suū unigenitū
daret: ut omnis qui credit in eū non
pereat: sed habeat vitam eternā. Non
enim misit deus filiū suū in mundū

Gutenberg translation

15 That whosoeuer beleeueth in him, should
not perish but haue eternall life.
16 ✠ ⁵For God so loued the world, that hee
hath giuen his only begotten Sonne, that whosoeuer beleeueth in him, should not perish, but haue
euerlasting life.
17 ∵ ⁶For God sent not his Sonne into the

Geneva

ge Leben haben.
16 Also hat GOtt die Welt geliebet,
daß er seinen eingebohrnen Sohn gab,
auf daß alle, die an ihn glauben, nicht ver-
lohren werden, sondern das ewige Leben
haben. 1. Joh. 4, 9.
17 Dann GOtt hat seinen Sohn nicht

German translation

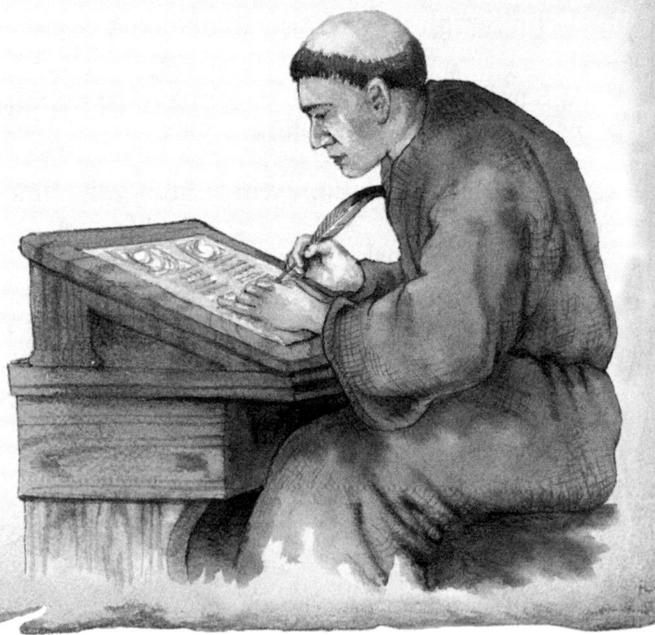

What Does God Say About Kindness?

Name ____________________

CHRISTIAN Living Skills

You are surrounded by people every day whether you are at home, in the car, in the classroom, on the athletic field, or at church. How you treat these people is a direct result of the condition of your heart.

Read I John 4:8-11 and answer the questions.

1. How did God show His love for you? ____________________
2. Since God showed you His love, what should you do? ____________________
3. If you do not love others, what is true? ____________________

Kindness is demonstrating your thankfulness to God by showing love and compassion to those around you. This includes your friends, your teachers, and even your family members. God's Word teaches you that kindness is a result of Christlike love and is a quality that describes a true Christian.

Read each verse and complete the statement using principles about kindness.

Romans 12:10
I should demonstrate true ____________________ to others by ____________________ them above myself.

Galatians 6:10
Every time I have the ____________________, I should do ____________________ to others, especially those who are Christians.

Proverbs 11:17
If I want to do something good for myself, I should show ____________________ to others.

Ephesians 4:32
I should be kind and ____________________ to others. I should ____________________ them just like God has forgiven me for Jesus' sake.

Proverbs 3:27
I should never withhold ____________________ from others, especially when it is within my ability to do something.

Something to Think About

Treating Others with Kindness

Name ______________________

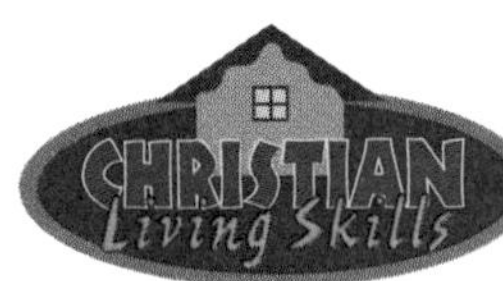
CHRISTIAN
Living Skills

Showing genuine kindness to others means making your attitude, your words, and your actions all reveal the same thing—Christlike love. One of the most challenging places to show kindness is in your own home. Satan tempts you to be selfish and unkind to your family members.

Read the scenarios and write one way that each person could demonstrate kindness.

Scenario	How can kindness be demonstrated?
Jessica's little sister Amy asked her for help in reviewing the spelling words for tomorrow's test. Jessica knows that Amy is trying to make a perfect score on the test. However, Jessica's favorite TV program is about to start.	
Phil's dad has been working late hours to be able to pay off some bills, and he usually gets home after Phil is in bed. The kitchen trashcan is full, but Phil's dad is usually the one who takes out the garbage.	
Angela's mom received a call from a friend who asked her to go up to the hospital to visit an elderly lady. After she left, Angela noticed that the laundry was dry but had not been folded and put away. The dinner dishes weren't finished either. Angela wanted to spend time playing a computer game.	
Ben's older brother Tom has been teasing him again because Ben does not make very good grades in science. Yesterday, when Tom got his science test back, *he* did not make a passing grade.	

What About Me?

Recognizing that unkind words and actions are really just proof of a prideful heart can be painful. However, if you confess your pride and unkindness to God, He will forgive you and help you to make permanent changes in the way you treat others.

Read II Peter 1:5-8. Describe the character of a believer using the qualities listed in these verses.

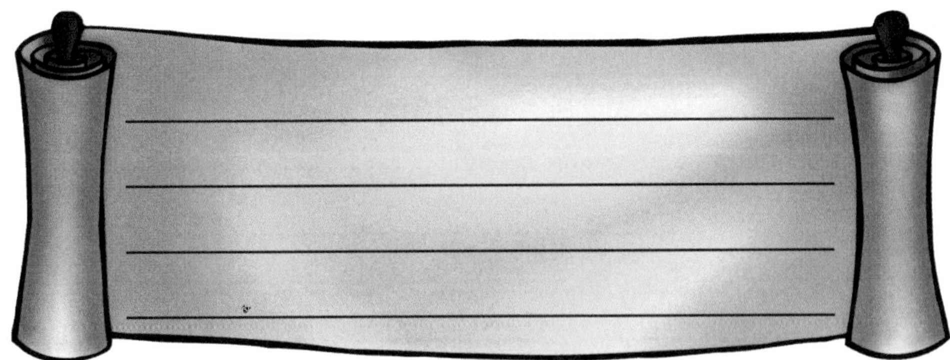

Take time at home to think about the following questions.

Would your parents say that you consistently demonstrate kindness to them?
What two things can you do to show kindness to a family member today?

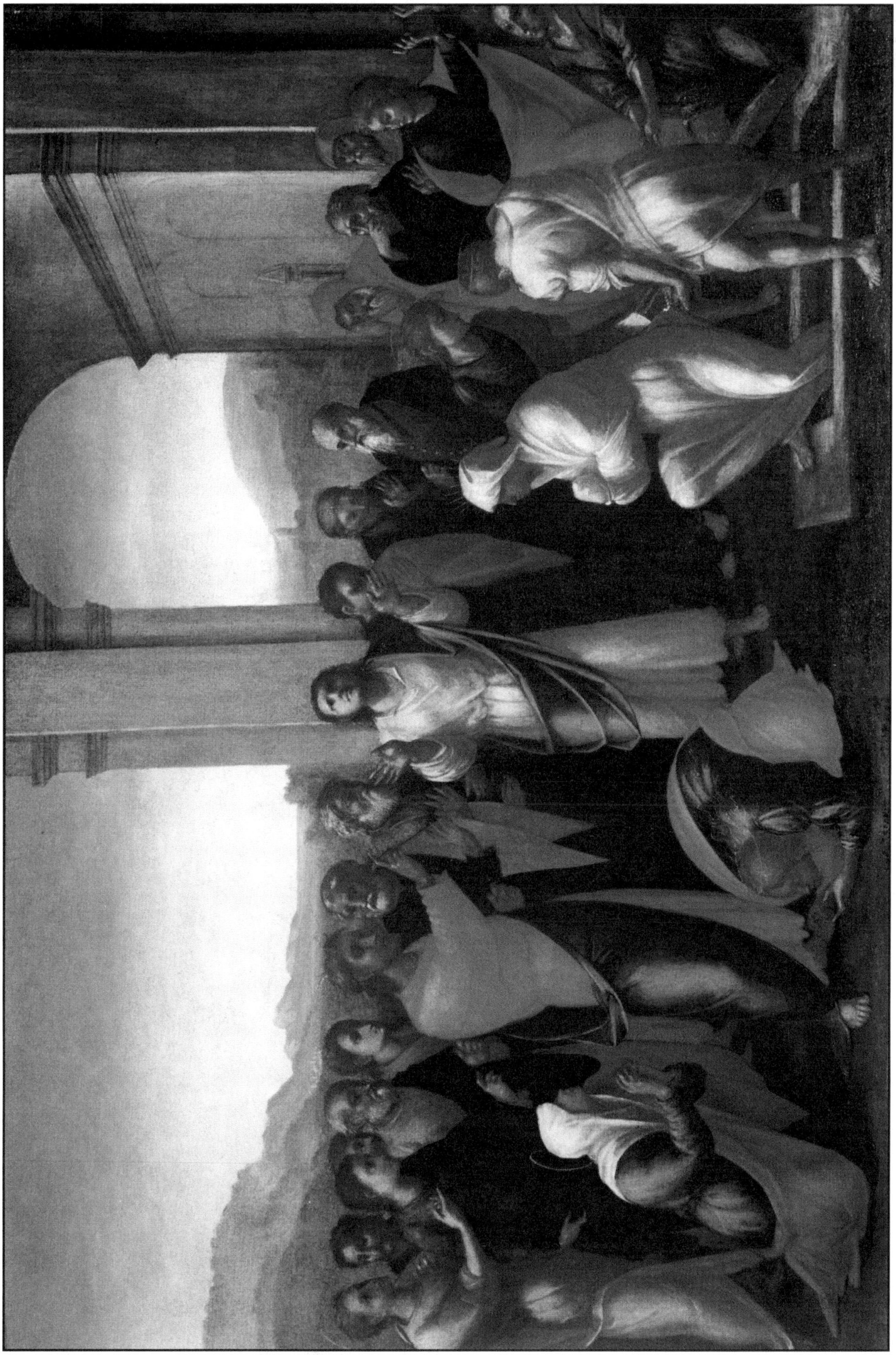

Raising of Lazarus

Francesco Granacci

Bob Jones University Museum & Gallery, Inc.

Name ______________________

Raising of Lazarus

by Francesco Granacci (1469-1543)

As a young man, Francesco Granacci (Frän chĕs´kō Grän ä´chē) was an apprentice to the painter Domenico Ghirlandaio, as was another boy, Michelangelo. Francesco was older than Michelangelo, but the boys became good friends and remained friends even after they were no longer working together. Granacci was also familiar with the work of Raphael and Leonardo da Vinci, who were working in Florence at the same time he was. Some of Granacci's paintings show the influence of these artists on him.

After years of training, Granacci was recognized as a master himself and opened his own studio to make his living as a painter. During the Renaissance, artists made most of their artworks for churches, so most paintings had biblical themes. Christ's raising of Lazarus from the dead is a fairly rare theme in art. This painting, *Raising of Lazarus*, was not entirely painted by Francesco Granacci; apprentices from his studio probably contributed to the work.

Note that the scene reflects Granacci's time, not New Testament times. The artist has marked the center of the painting by a large pillar that forms one end of an arch in the background. The person at the center of the composition has eleven people on each side of him. The key figures of Christ and Lazarus are placed almost equally on each side of the center of the painting. Other characters in the scene include Mary, Martha, and many of Jesus' disciples. Of course, Mary is bowed low, anointing the feet of Jesus. The disciples have halos painted above their heads.

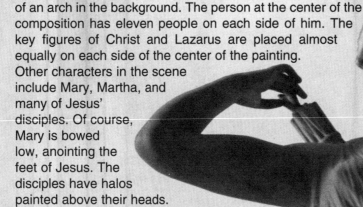

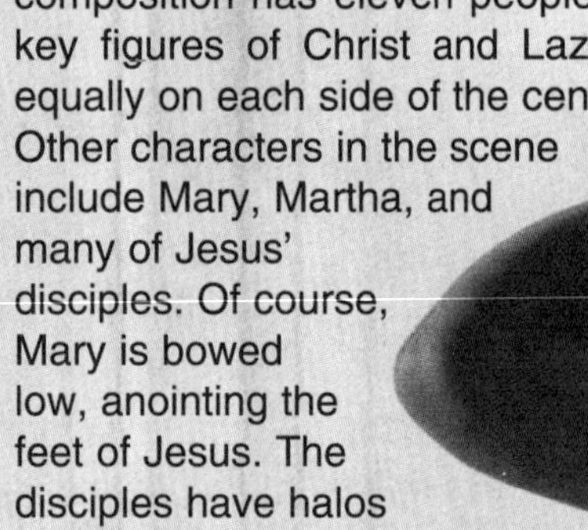

The details of this event are found in John 11:38-44. The two men on the right are lifting the heavy stone that was on the tomb. The people behind them do not look very happy about opening the tomb. One man holds his nose at the stench of the decaying body, which has been in the tomb for three days. The person in the exact center of the painting has his eyes lifted up toward heaven, for he has obviously seen a miracle.

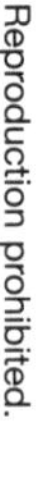

Above Every Name

Philippians 2:9-10

Name ______________________

Christ came to earth as the humble Servant of His Father to die for the sins of men and provide them salvation. Even though Christ became a man, He remained God. As a man, Christ knows our needs by experience; and as God, Christ provides for our needs. The many names or titles for Christ illustrate His ability to meet each need specifically.

Jesus was the name given by God to the human Christ. In Matthew 1:21, the angel said He was named Jesus because He would save people from sin. In Acts 4:8-12, Peter identified Jesus as the only name able to provide salvation.

Use Philippians 2:9-10 to answer the questions.

1. In what position has God placed the name of Jesus? ______________________
2. What is the response of every living thing to the knowledge that Jesus Christ is the Lord?

   ____
3. What attitude does bowing demonstrate? ______________________

   ____

Christ has other names that illustrate salvation.

Draw a line to match the name of Christ to the correct statement and reference.

4. Christ provides light in this world of darkness (John 8:12).	Lamb of God
5. Christ shed His blood as the sacrifice for the sin of man (Isa. 53:4-7).	Redeemer
6. Christ was sent by God for this purpose (I John 4:14).	Light of the World
7. Christ's death purchased salvation, which frees man from sin (Gal. 3:13-14).	Savior

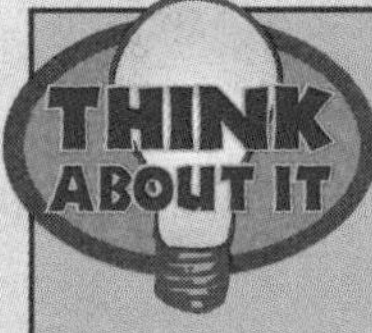
THINK ABOUT IT

Christ became man and offered Himself as a sacrifice for your sin. He did this seeking nothing in return from man except faith, praise, and honor. Have you demonstrated faith in Christ and shown Him praise and honor today?

Power for a Purpose

Miracles of Jesus

Name ____________________

Christ showed the power of God in the miracles He performed on earth. While many people accepted that Jesus was the Messiah and believed on Him, the religious leaders did not accept Christ's miracles or that He was God.

Christ came to the earth to do the will of His Father. There was a purpose in everything Jesus did while here.

Write the letter of the phrase that correctly completes each sentence.

1. Jesus said that the works He did were to ______ (John 5:36).
2. Jesus said that the Jews should look at His miracles to ______ (John 10:37-38).
3. After the crowd saw Jesus heal a paralyzed man, they ______ (Matt. 9:8).
4. When the Pharisees accused Jesus of blasphemy, He healed the paralyzed man so they would ______ (Luke 5:24).
5. Jesus cast out demons and healed the sick to ______ (Matt. 8:16-17).

A. fulfill prophecy
B. show men that God the Father sent Him
C. gave praise and glory to God
D. know that He is God
E. know that He has power to forgive sins

The miracles of Jesus demonstrated His power over His creation.

Write the area of power that Jesus demonstrated as He performed each miracle.

health death nature spirits

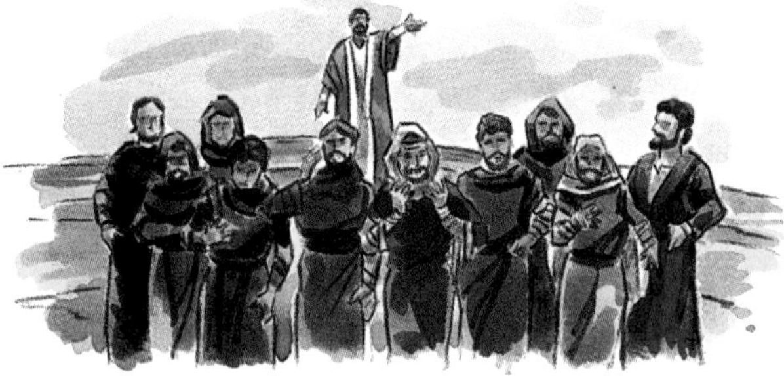

When He healed the ten lepers in Luke 17:11-14, Jesus demonstrated power over ____________________.

Matthew 8:28-34 records that Jesus sent demons from two men into a herd of pigs. This demonstrated Jesus' power over ____________________.

When Jesus died and rose again, He demonstrated power over ____________________.

In Mark 4:35-41, the disciples awakened Jesus because they had sailed into a storm. When Jesus calmed the storm, He demonstrated power over ____________________.

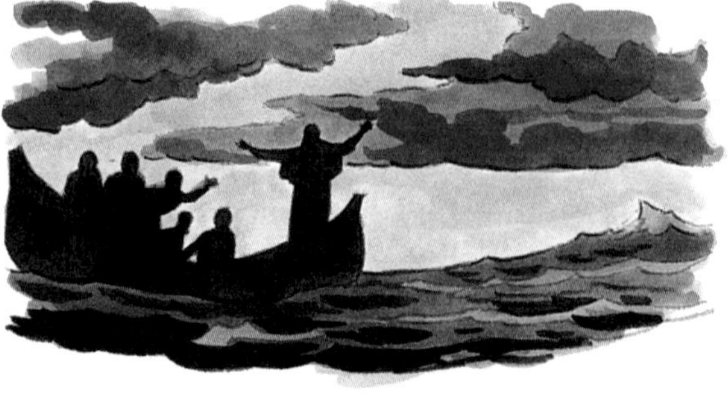

What Does God Say About Being Thankful?

Name ______________________

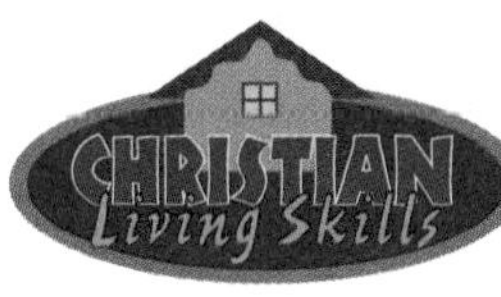
CHRISTIAN
Living Skills

God has done good things for you. If you are a Christian, your heart wants to praise God for His many blessings. Giving thanks to God is a natural and right response for a Christian and comes from realizing that God provides for him.

Write a sentence explaining what it means to be thankful.

____

____

A good thing to do when you are tempted to complain about your circumstances is to list reasons you should be thankful. Counting blessings is important! It keeps you from discouragement and reminds you of God's love.

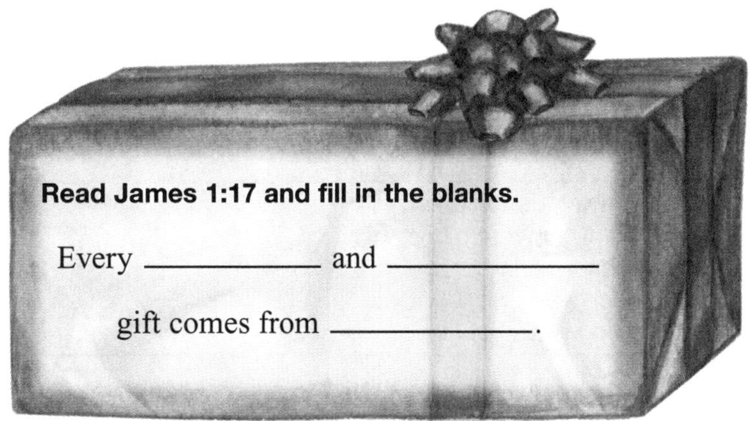
Read James 1:17 and fill in the blanks.
Every __________ and __________
gift comes from __________.

Read the verses and complete the crossword puzzle of *good gifts* from God for which you can be thankful.

Across:

1. I am thankful that God hears and answers my ______ (Ps. 66:19-20).
2. I am thankful for ______ that teaches me how to please God (II Tim. 3:16-17).
3. I am thankful for faithful ______ (Prov. 17:17).
5. I will rejoice that God has provided ______ for mankind (Ps. 98:2-3).
7. I am thankful that I can go to ______ to worship God (Ps. 122:1).
8. I am thankful for the ______ that God provides (I Tim. 6:8).

Down:

1. I am thankful for the ______ God has given me (Deut. 5:16).
4. I should give thanks to the Lord because He is ______ (Ps. 106:1).
6. I will give thanks to God who gives me the ______ through Jesus (I Cor. 15:57).

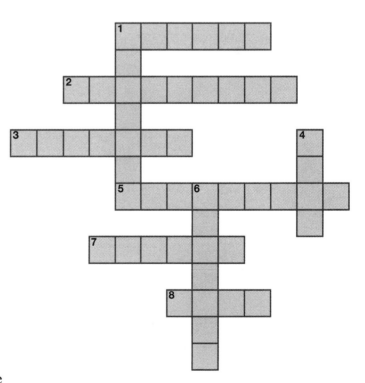
1
2
3
4
5
6
7
8

Something to Think About

Being Thankful

Name ______________________

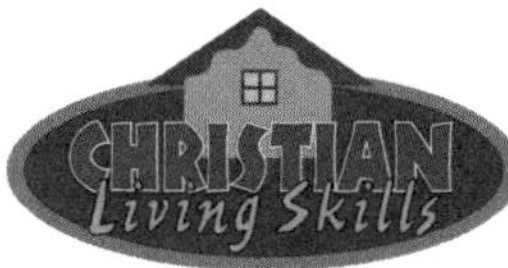
CHRISTIAN
Living Skills

The real test of thankfulness comes when things are NOT going your way. What do you do when you get a low grade on a test? What about when you aren't allowed to go someplace with your friends? What's the attitude in your heart when your dad loses his job or when your little sister spills paint on your assignment? God reminds His children that He is just as concerned about their attitudes in the tough times as He is in the good times.

Read I Thessalonians 5:18 and fill in the blanks.

I should give ______________ in all ______________________________ because this is God's ______________ for me in Christ Jesus.

Read each scenario and write one thing each person can be thankful for in that situation.

Scenario	For what can you be thankful?
You've been praying that you would get a specific thing for your birthday. Your birthday comes and goes, and several people give you gifts, but you don't get what you were hoping for.	
You just found out that you made the team. Your best friend also made the team.	
You tried out for the lead part in the church program. You practiced hard to do well at the tryouts. When the parts were announced, you got a part in the program, but another boy got the part you wanted.	

It is important to have a thankful heart for what God and others have done for you. It is just as important to express your thankfulness to them.

What About Me?

Take time at home to think about your attitude.
List two ways you can express your thankfulness to God.

1. ______________________________
2. ______________________________

List two ways you can express your thankfulness to others for what they have done for you.

1. ______________________________
2. ______________________________

Write the names of two people for whom you are thankful and complete the chart.

Name	What I am going to do to express my thankfulness to them:

The Word for the People

History of the Bible

Name ______________________

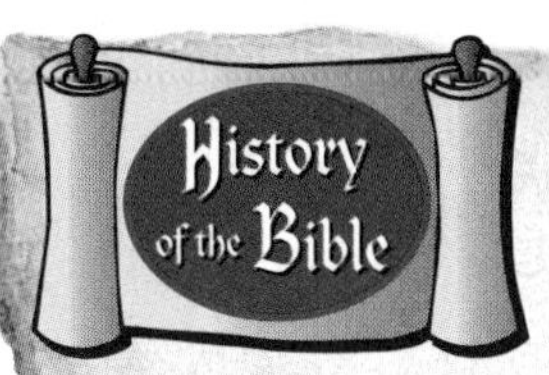
History of the Bible

Peter Waldo and several men translated parts of the Latin Vulgate into French in the 1170s. He and his followers used this translation to preach in France until persecution stopped them.

One important English translation was led by John Wycliffe. While at Oxford University in England, Wycliffe read the Latin Scriptures. He saw that many of the teachings of the Roman Church were contrary to the truth found in the Bible. He knew that the common people needed access to the Bible rather than depending on the teaching of church leaders. Still using the parchment and codex forms for his manuscripts, Wycliffe, with the help of other men, translated the Vulgate into English. Published in 1382, Wycliffe's translation infuriated the church and government leaders. By 1408, it had become illegal to translate the Bible into English without special permission. It was over a hundred years before this permission was granted.

In 1455, the invention of moveable type by Johannes Gutenberg made the reproduction of books by printing presses much faster than copying handwritten manuscripts. The Gutenberg Bible, a copy of the Latin Vulgate, was the first book Gutenberg produced on his press. Thirty years after Gutenberg's death, most European countries had printing presses. As scholars continued to read the Latin Vulgate, the eyes of many were opened to the truth of Scripture. They saw the need for every man throughout Europe to read the Bible for himself. The printing press was instrumental in providing better access to Scripture.

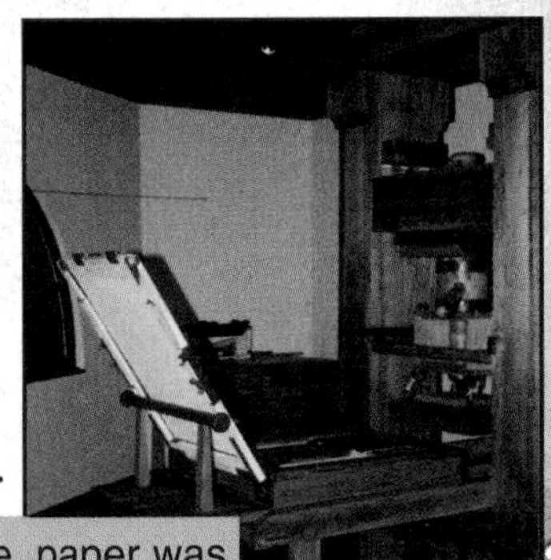

Gutenberg printed 200 Latin Bibles on paper and 30 on vellum. At this time, paper was made from rags. For this reason, the white pages of these early Bibles still look white today. Paper was not made of wood and plant fibers until around 1800. The acidic content of plants causes many types of paper to turn yellow and brown with age.

Mark an *X* in the correct column.

	Waldo	Wycliffe
1. translated from the Latin Vulgate		
2. translated into French		
3. translated into English		
4. translation was a hand-written manuscript		
5. preached from his translation		
6. translation caused the government to ban translations into English		

Complete the sentences.

1. Although not a translator, ______________________ made moveable type for the printing press which helped provide Bibles in the languages of the people.

2. The first book printed on the Gutenberg press was ______________________.

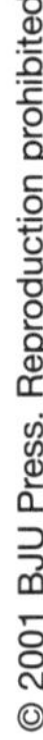

The Word Brings Reformation

History of the Bible

Name ______________________

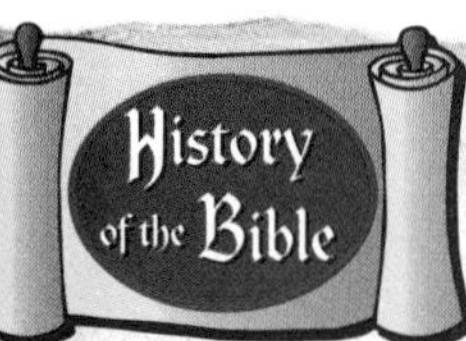
History of the Bible

One of the first Bible translators to use the printing press was the Dutch scholar Erasmus. Using the best manuscripts he could find, Erasmus compiled a Greek/Latin New Testament in 1516. Each page of this New Testament contained one column of Latin and one column of Greek. This New Testament would be a main source for many future European translations.

Like John Wycliffe, Martin Luther also saw the errors of the Roman Church. After confronting the church with its error, Martin Luther composed many writings dealing with the truth of the Bible and error in the teachings and practices of the Roman Church in Germany. Martin Luther used Erasmus's New Testament as he translated the Bible into German. Luther's German New Testament was printed in 1522, and his complete Bible was published in 1534.

Since translations other than Latin had been illegal in England since 1408, it wasn't until 1525 that a new English translation appeared. William Tyndale, an Oxford scholar like Wycliffe, also saw the need for an English Bible to be available to the common people. Tyndale did not have the freedom to work in England without persecution. He went to Martin Luther in Germany as he began his translation work. Although they did not agree on the interpretations of specific passages, Luther and Tyndale did agree that the Bible is the only authority. Instead of translating from Latin into English as Wycliffe had done, Tyndale translated from Erasmus's Greek New Testament. Tyndale's Bibles were printed in Germany, and then smuggled into England for the people to read.

Many of Tyndale's English New Testaments were burned by church leaders throughout England. Reformers possessing Tyndale New Testaments were often arrested and **martyred** by being beheaded or burned at the stake. Although he was not in England, Tyndale was also watched by spies of the church. He was finally arrested and burned at the stake after being betrayed by a friend.

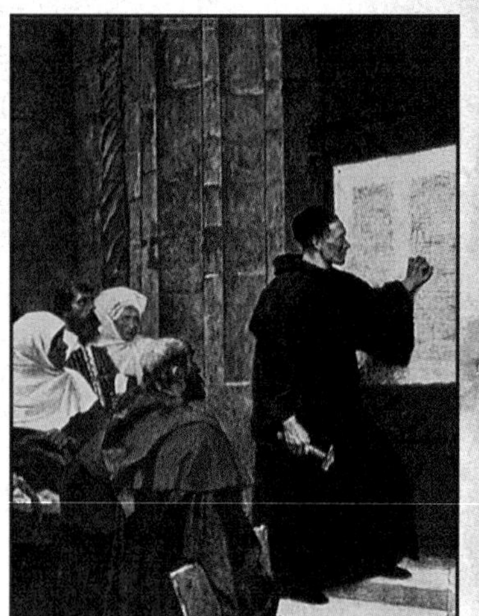

Answer the questions.

1. In what two languages was Erasmus's New Testament? ______________________
2. Both Martin Luther and William Tyndale translated and published their works in Germany. Which man worked on an English translation? ______________________
3. Which man was martyred for his work? ______________________
4. What work did both Luther and Tyndale translate from? ______________________
5. Did Luther and Tyndale agree on all their interpretations of Scripture? ______________________
6. What did Martin Luther and William Tyndale agree on? ______________________

Singing with Understanding

"Our Great Savior" (vv. 4-5)

Name ______________________

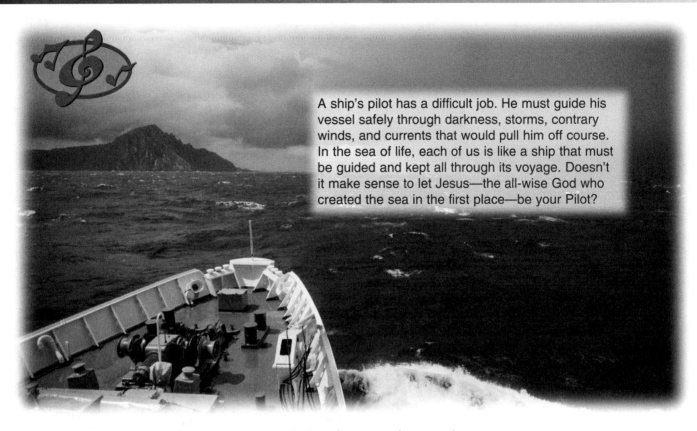
A ship's pilot has a difficult job. He must guide his vessel safely through darkness, storms, contrary winds, and currents that would pull him off course. In the sea of life, each of us is like a ship that must be guided and kept all through its voyage. Doesn't it make sense to let Jesus—the all-wise God who created the sea in the first place—be your Pilot?

Read verses 4 and 5 of the hymn on page 317 and answer the questions.

1. What kinds of things in a person's life might be considered "tempests"?

____

____

2. What does the hymn say Christians should do when stormy nights overtake them?

____

3. What does a person have to do to have Jesus as his Friend, Strength, Help, Guide, Keeper, and Pilot? ______________________________

____

4. What does God freely grant to Christians when they receive Him? ______________

5. For how long will Christ be with believers? ______________________

Jesus has promised to save, help, keep, and love Christians to the end! Spend a few moments thanking Him for being such a great Savior and wonderful Friend.

Taking the Word to Others

Name ______________________________

In the New Testament, missionaries such as Paul traveled to many places and shared the gospel of Christ. Often Paul would remain in a city for months or even years until a church was started and was strong enough for him to move on. As he ministered to the people, Paul made his living by making and mending tents.

The governments of some countries do not permit missionaries to pastor or start churches. However, these countries often allow foreigners to come as teachers, doctors, or other types of workers. Christians go to these countries and work at these jobs while they witness for Christ and disciple new believers. This type of missionary is called a *tentmaker* after the example of Paul.

Read the information and answer the questions.

1. Are all missionaries pastors? ______________
2. Does every country allow missionaries to come and start churches openly? ______________
3. What is a tentmaker? ______________________________

____

Research and find the answers as directed. (Hint: You may ask your pastor, read missionary letters or prayer cards, write to a mission board, or read a biography about a missionary.)

4. Many missionaries start schools to train nationals to be pastors to their own people.
   Write the name of a missionary who works with a Bible school.

   ____

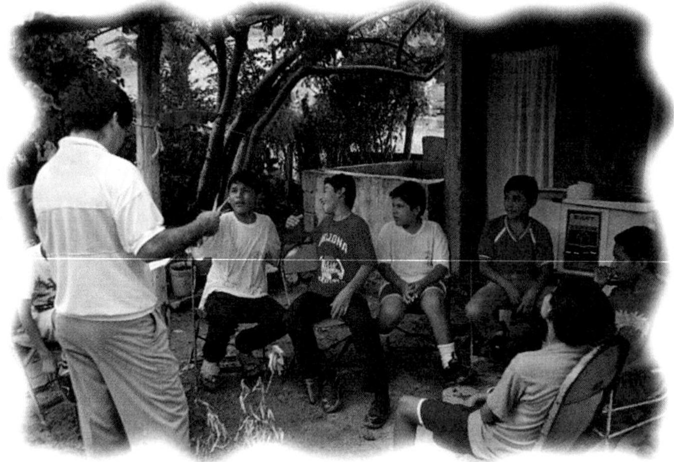

5. Some missionaries work in clinics or help with medical needs as a way to bring people to hear the gospel.
   Write the name of a missionary who uses medicine to share the gospel.

   ____

6. Missionaries might work other jobs as a way to minister to people on the field.
   Write the name of a missionary who works a regular job while ministering to others.

   ____

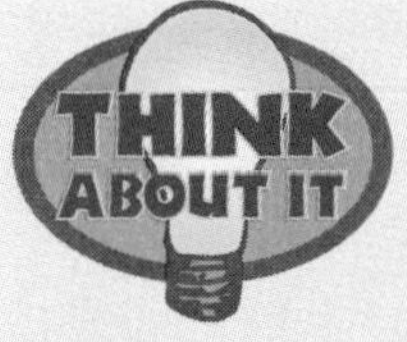
THINK
ABOUT IT

God can use people of all skills and abilities to share His Word with others. What job would you like to have when you finish school?

____

How could God use you in that job to share the gospel?

____

His Glory Seen

Matthew 17:1-9; Mark 9:1-10

Name ______________________

For more than two years, the disciples had watched Jesus forgive sin, perform miracles, and teach God's truth. The disciples were beginning to understand more about Jesus. Jesus continued to patiently teach the disciples about His purpose on earth. Their knowledge that Jesus was sent by God was becoming the realization that Jesus *is* God. Then one day, Jesus showed three of them something they would never forget.

Fill in the circle next to the correct answer. You may use your Bible for help.

1. Jesus took ______ up to a mountain (Mark 9:2).
   - ○ all of his disciples
   - ○ Peter, James, and John
   - ○ Matthew, Mark, and Luke
2. In awe, the disciples saw the clothing and appearance of Jesus ______ (Matt. 17:2).
   - ○ become shining bright
   - ○ become a brilliant blue
   - ○ become like that of a priest
3. While Jesus stood talking with Moses and Elijah, Peter said he wanted to remember the occasion by ______ (Mark 9:5).
   - ○ singing a hymn
   - ○ building tabernacles
   - ○ offering a sacrifice
4. God spoke from a ______ as He blessed Jesus (Matt. 17:5).
   - ○ dove
   - ○ whirlwind
   - ○ cloud
5. At the sound of God's voice, the disciples ______ (Matt. 17:6).
   - ○ sang a hymn
   - ○ fell on their faces
   - ○ looked up to see God
6. God's blessing included a command for the disciples to ______ (Mark 9:7).
   - ○ listen to Jesus
   - ○ bow in worship
   - ○ build tabernacles
7. Jesus told the disciples to tell no man what they saw until ______ (Mark 9:9).
   - ○ three days had passed
   - ○ He was arrested
   - ○ He had risen from the dead

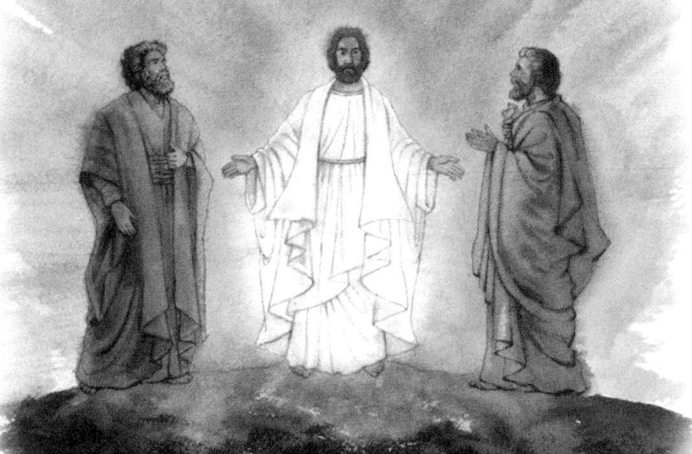

THINK ABOUT IT

Some say that since Christ is not physically on earth today, He does not continue to perform miracles. But each soul that is saved and each life that is changed are miracles demonstrating God's power over sin. Do you take time to thank God for providing His Word and the way of salvation? Like the disciples, do you walk with Christ daily and seek to learn about Him?

Every Tongue Confess

Philippians 2:11-12

Name ______________________

Read Philippians 2:11-12 and fill in the circle next to the correct answer.

1. In Philippians 2:11, *every tongue* means ______.
   - ○ flaps under the laces of shoes
   - ○ languages
   - ○ all people
2. In Philippians 2:11, *confess* means ______.
   - ○ to admit doing wrong
   - ○ to acknowledge belief in
   - ○ to make known sin
3. Every person will proclaim that Jesus Christ is ______.
   - ○ the Savior
   - ○ the Messiah
   - ○ Lord
4. Belief in Christ gives God ______.
   - ○ glory
   - ○ pride
   - ○ a throne in heaven
5. A Christian should do good works in order to ______.
   - ○ receive salvation from God
   - ○ obey God and glorify Him
   - ○ become a church member

Salvation is only through faith in Christ. Christians who believe that Jesus is the Savior and have made Him the Lord of their lives will demonstrate their salvation to others through what they do and say. Their works will give evidence of their belief.

Knowing of Cynthia's love for flowers, Cynthia's mother gave her the care of the flowerbed at the corner of the house. Cynthia often spent time in her garden. That fall she prepared the soil by removing the weeds and stones. Once the ground was prepared, she planted the flower bulbs she had carefully selected from the store. During the winter and spring months, she prayed for snow and gentle rains to water her bulbs. As the weather grew warm she thanked the Lord for the bright sun that would help them grow. Soon Cynthia saw the plants appear and grow taller and stronger. As the blossoms began to open, Cynthia's anticipation of their colors and fragrances also grew. What Cynthia hadn't anticipated was her younger brother, Rusty, and his best friend, Scott. The boys were in the yard every day the weather permitted. Rusty knew all about Cynthia's flowers from her daily reports on their growth. But when a foul ball sent a baseball close to the house, all thoughts of the flowers vanished as Rusty raced to catch the ball. With the ball safe in his glove, Rusty looked down at the broken stems under his feet. Immediately he thought of Cynthia and what her reaction would be to her ruined flowers. He called to Scott and the two solemnly entered the house to find Cynthia.

Choose one or more truths about God that you would try to demonstrate if you were Cynthia. Write how your choice applies to this situation between Cynthia and Rusty.

- ○ God is just and requires punishment for sin.
- ○ God forgives the sin of those who repent.
- ○ God controls all things and nothing happens that He doesn't know about.

____

What Does God Say About Authority?

Name ______________________________

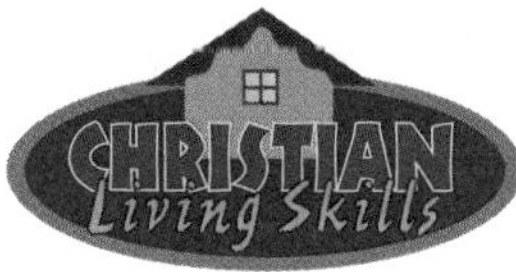
CHRISTIAN
Living Skills

Everyone lives under the authority of someone else. A child lives under the authority of his parents. A student is under the authority of his teacher. An employee is under the authority of his employer. Even the President of the United States is under the authority of the Constitution. Every person, family, and government leader is under God's authority.

God is the highest authority and is over every other authority.

Read I Chronicles 29:10-11 and answer the questions.

1. List three of the five attributes for which King David praised God (verse 11).

   ______________________ ______________________ ______________________

2. Over what does King David say God is exalted? ______________________________

What power does an authority have over you?

Someone who is in authority over you has God-given responsibilities. The Bible says that God holds your authorities accountable for how they fulfill their responsibilities.

Read II Samuel 23:3 and Proverbs 29:12. Describe how someone in authority is to govern those for whom he is responsible.

____

____

What is your attitude toward the authority that God has placed in your life?

The Bible teaches that God's blessings are on those who obey and respect the authorities God has placed in their lives. **Obedience** is doing what you're told to do. Showing **respect** is demonstrating honor by avoiding attitudes and words that discredit or insult.

Read Romans 13:1-2. Write in your own words the four principles that teach you about attitudes toward authorities.

Verse 1*a*
Verse 2*a*
Verse 1*b*
Verse 2*b*

Something to Think About

Authority

Name ______________________________

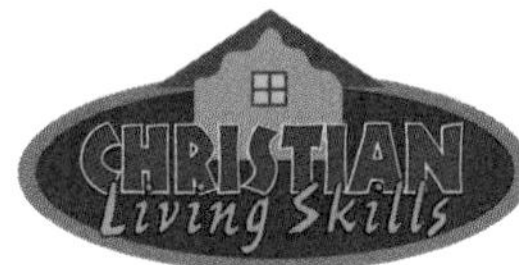
CHRISTIAN
Living Skills

Who are my authorities?

An authority can be described as someone who has the power to enforce rules, demand obedience, and administer punishment for disobedience. God has placed authorities in your life to help you. The Bible teaches that the only time you should fear your authorities is when you disobey them (Rom. 13:3-5). You will be under authority for your entire life. The sooner you learn to honor and obey authority, the sooner you will find joy and contentment.

Read each scenario. Complete the chart.

Scenario	Fill in the correct circle.	If needed, explain what the person should have done to respectfully obey.
Devin dribbled the basketball down the court. Suddenly, a player on the other team tripped him and knocked the ball out of bounds. The referee gave the ball to the other team and didn't call a foul on the player who tripped Devin. Devin yelled, "That's not fair!" as he returned to position.	○ obeyed with respect ○ obeyed with disrespect ○ disobeyed	
There is a new law in Brad's state requiring everyone to wear a seatbelt while in a moving vehicle. Although Brad and his family were not accustomed to wearing them, they made an effort to obey the law by reminding each other.	○ obeyed with respect ○ obeyed with disrespect ○ disobeyed	
Tina's room was a mess. When Tina was watching TV, her mom turned the TV off and sent Tina to clean her room. Tina went to clean her room and slammed the door, grumbling and complaining.	○ obeyed with respect ○ obeyed with disrespect ○ disobeyed	
The sixth grade teacher was sick. Karley and some of her classmates tricked the substitute into letting them have an extra recess.	○ obeyed with respect ○ obeyed with disrespect ○ disobeyed	
Justin's new Sunday school teacher had an unusual way of speaking. While she taught, Justin listened quietly, but he snickered behind her back and talked to his friends about how strange her voice sounded.	○ obeyed with respect ○ obeyed with disrespect ○ disobeyed	

What About Me?

Take time at home to answer the following questions about your reactions and attitudes toward the authorities that God has placed in your life.

Do I demonstrate respect for and obedience to my parents?
Do my friends know that I love God by the way I show respect for my authority?
Would my friends say that I demonstrate respect for and obedience to my teachers?
Have I experienced the joy that comes from showing true respect for my authority?

The Word We Read

History of the Bible

Name ______________________________

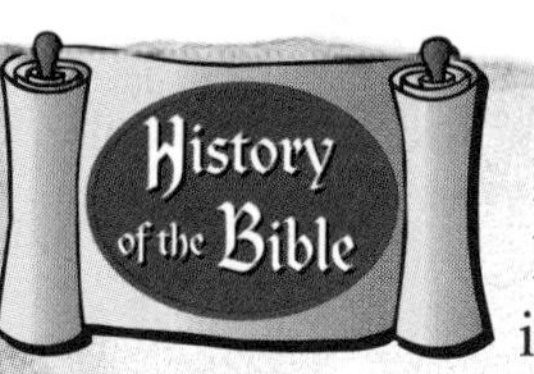

History of the Bible

During the Reformation, Myles Coverdale with the help of John Rogers translated the Old Testament into English to add to Tyndale's New Testament. This complete translation, known as the **Coverdale Bible,** was printed in 1535. Under the pen name of Thomas Matthew, Rogers published the **Matthew Bible** in 1537. The first English Bible translation authorized by the Church of England was called the **Great Bible.** This Bible, named for its extreme size, was published by Coverdale in 1539 at the request of King Henry VIII, who was head of the Church of England.

The **Geneva Bible,** completed in 1560, was the first Bible to divide the chapters into verses. This Bible also included extensive notes in the margins to help explain each chapter. For the next one hundred years, this would be the English Bible of choice.

During the reign of King James I, the Anglican church leaders desired a Bible for the people, but without the notes of the Geneva Bible which often condemned Anglican teachings and practices. Fifty-four scholars gathered to evaluate existing translations and conduct research. By 1611, the first edition of the **King James Version** was printed. Throughout the history of the Bible, no other Bible has been printed more than the King James Version.

Because the English language has continued to develop and the meaning of words has changed, other English versions of the Bible have been published during the last one hundred years. Many modern translations and versions exist today. Some express verses in a conversational style. Others group verses into paragraphs or use quotation marks to provide clarity to the reader. The intent of many of these versions is to provide the Word of God in the everyday language of the people.

The Geneva Bible is the translation quoted by **William Shakespeare** in his famous plays.

New versions must be read with discernment. Many versions try to deny the deity of Christ or the virgin birth, or they try to reduce the importance of salvation through faith in Christ alone. Look to parents and spiritual leaders for guidance if you are looking to read from a different version. (Remember: Accuracy is more important than readability.)

Write *T* if the statement is true and *F* if the statement is false.

______ 1. The first English version authorized by the Church of England was the Great Bible.

______ 2. The first Bible to divide chapters into verses was the Geneva Bible.

______ 3. The Great Bible was named for its great importance.

______ 4. Myles Coverdale published only one version of the Bible.

______ 5. The notes in the Geneva Bible condemned the wrong Anglican practices.

______ 6. The first edition of the King James Version was printed in 1611.

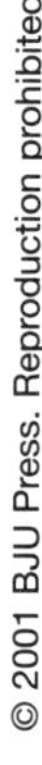

Name ______________________

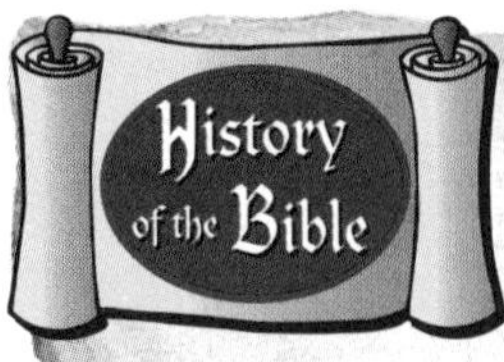
History
of the Bible

All of the main languages of the world now have translations of the Bible, but there are still many areas of the world where the people do not have a Bible in their own language. Some people still do not even have a written form of their spoken language. Some missionaries prepare themselves to help meet these needs before they go to the mission field.

These missionaries often take *linguistics* courses to help them learn how to develop alphabets, record spoken words, and translate verses. But having the Bible in print is only part of the job. The people must also be taught to read and write their own language. Many years and even lifetimes are spent by missionaries to provide the Word of God in the language of the people.

Today the Bible is not only in the form of a printed and bound book. The Bible has been printed in Braille and recorded on tapes and compact discs. Computer programs provide several versions of the Bible at once, as well as concordances and other resources to help Bible study. Some electronic Bibles are small enough to be carried in a pocket. In this age of technological advances, the Bible has once again been put into the language of the people.

Many missionaries go to language school to study a foreign language. Studying **linguistics** is not the same. The study of linguistics concentrates on learning the principles behind sounds and structures of how words go together to form languages.

Mark the types of Bibles found in your home and answer the questions.

- ☐ Reference Bible
- ☐ Electronic pocket-sized Bible
- ☐ Braille Bible
- ☐ Pocket Bible
- ☐ Audio Bible
- ☐ Study Bible
- ☐ Bible on computer
- ☐ Bible in another language
- ☐ Large decorative family Bible

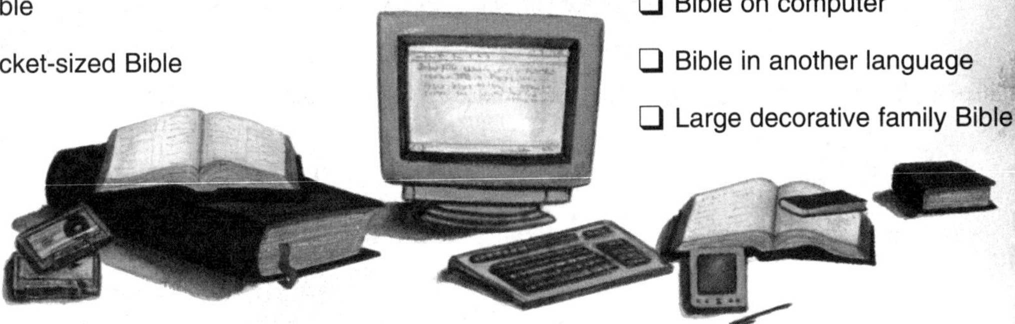

1. With the Bible so readily available, it seems everyone should be a Bible scholar. Why don't more people know the truth found in God's Word?

____

2. What should you do with the Bible you have? ______________________

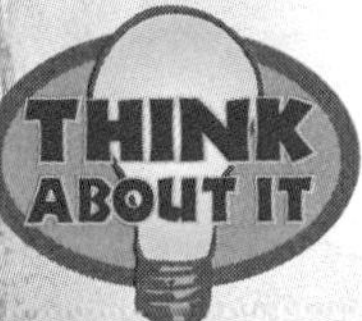
THINK
ABOUT IT

Suppose you were given the responsibility to translate a portion of Scripture for someone to read. What passage or account would you choose?

The reference or account I would translate first is ______________________.

This passage is important to translate first because

____.

Get the Bible Reading H.A.B.I.T.

Name ____________________

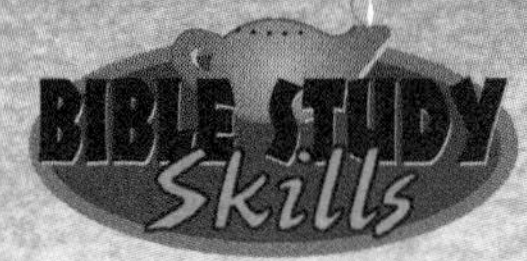

Have a special time set aside each day to read your Bible. If possible, make it the same time every day.

Ask God to teach you from His Word. Remember to thank Him for helping you to understand and apply it.

Be still and give your attention to what you are reading.

Investigate the Scripture by asking yourself questions about it.

Take time to look up words and ideas you do not understand.

As you read the Scripture for each day, write the date in the box.

Christ loved us and died for us when we were sinners. **Romans 5:6-8**	Christ's death made peace between man and God. **Ephesians 2:14-17**	Because of Jesus, believers have access to God and a place in His family. **Ephesians 2:18-20**	Now that Christ has died for Christians, they should live for Him. **II Corinthians 5:14-17**	Through Christ, God saved Christians and showed them His kindness and love. **Titus 3:3-7**
If Christ had not been raised, the preaching and faith of Christians would be in vain. **I Corinthians 15:12-15**	If Christ had not been raised, believers would not be forgiven of sin. **I Corinthians 15:16-18**	Because Christ is risen from the dead, believers have hope in Him. **I Corinthians 15:19-20**	Jesus is the only name through which we can be saved. **Acts 4:12**	Christians can know that God has given them eternal life through His Son. **I John 5:11-13**

A Pattern for Prayer

Name ______________________

Many Christians come to their prayer time as they would come to a business meeting. They bring a list of complaints and requests, and they try to conclude their business with God as quickly as possible and get on to something else. Others can think of little to say, so they spend their prayer time daydreaming or repeating words they have memorized. You can avoid this by using a simple guide for your prayer time.

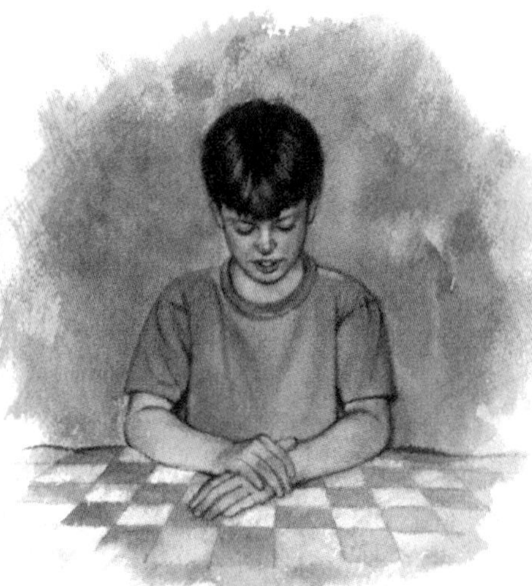

Adoration
Confession
Thanksgiving
Supplication

Read the psalm and list some of the creations of God that give Him the praise He deserves.

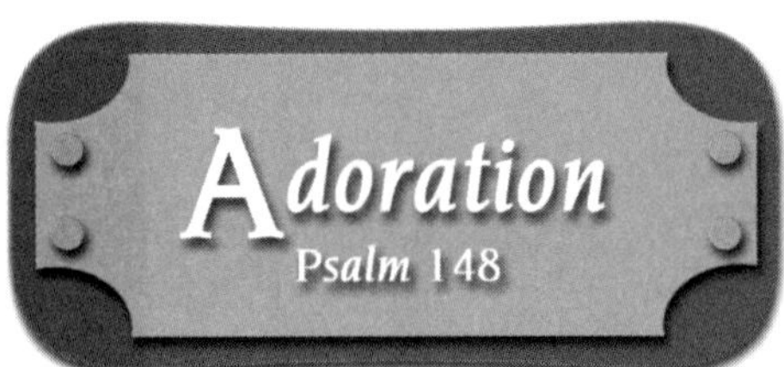
Adoration
Psalm 148

______________ ______________
______________ ______________
______________ ______________
______________ ______________

Praise and adore God as His other creatures praise Him.

Read each verse and answer the questions.

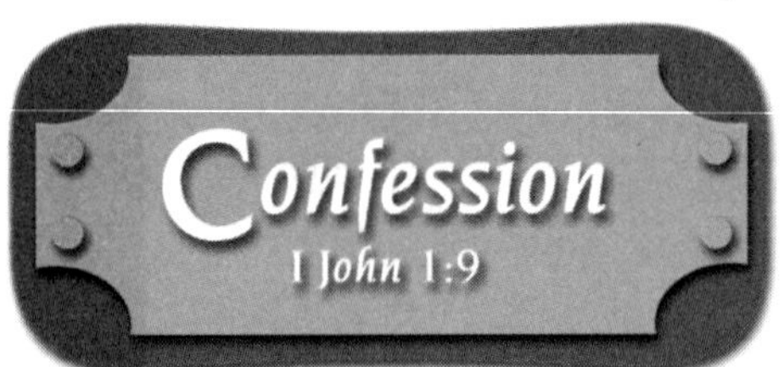
Confession
I John 1:9

Sin hinders fellowship with God. What is necessary to restore this fellowship? ______________

Confess your sins to God, asking for His forgiveness and cleansing.

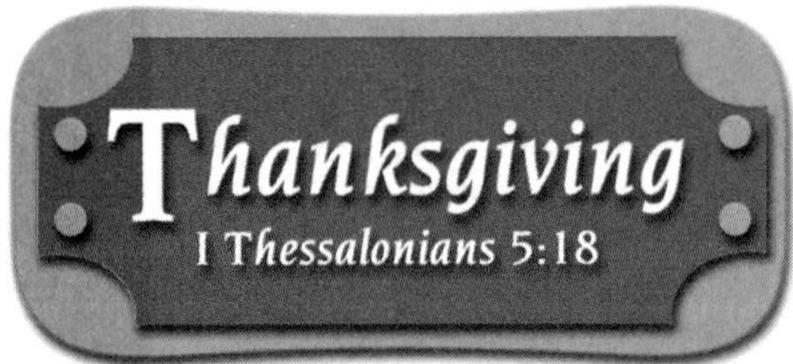
Thanksgiving
I Thessalonians 5:18

In what circumstances should you give thanks?

____

Thank God for all the things in your life.

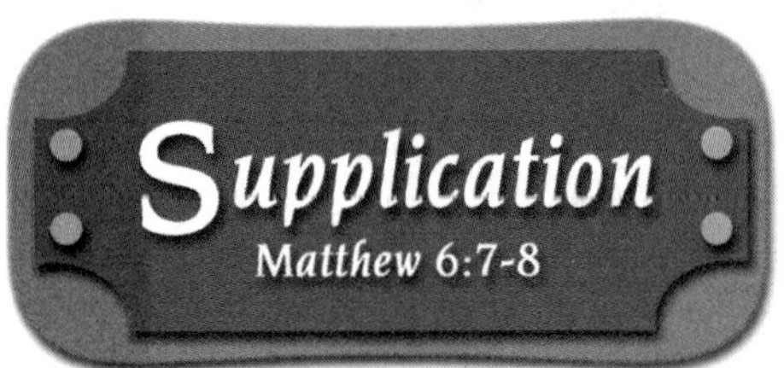
Supplication
Matthew 6:7-8

When you ask for things in prayer, will God give you everything you ask? Why? ______________

____

Ask God to give you and others what is needed.

What is the greatest gift God ever gave?

____

Using Cross-References

Name ______________________________

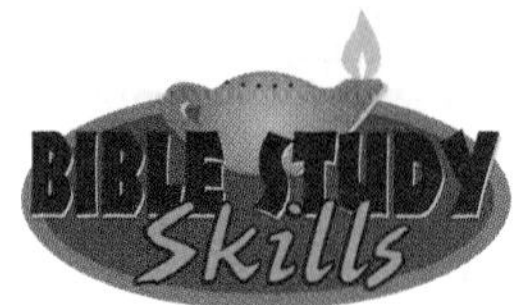

BIBLE STUDY
Skills

Cross-references are helpful in finding out more about a certain word, topic, account, or idea. Learn to make use of these Bible study tools.

Use the cross-references to learn more about the days that preceded the Crucifixion of Christ.

Look at the cross-references indicated by the letter *c*. Write the numbers of the three verses in **Matthew 21** where the idea of inspiration can be found.

____

Matthew 21:9 records the shouts of the people praising Jesus as He entered Jerusalem. They quoted a part of what verse in the Psalms?

____

Look at the cross-references for the word *prophet* in **Matthew 21:11**. Write the reference where a note about *prophet* may be found.

____

Read the verses cross-referenced by the letter *e* in **Matthew 21:13**. Which verse says God has seen how His house has become a "den of robbers"?

____

Chapter subtitles help the reader quickly find sections of Scripture. Which other Gospels contain the account of *Jesus' authority challenged?*

____

21:8 MATTHEW 21:29

colt, and put on them their
clothes, and they set *him* thereon.
8 And a very great multitude
spread their [a]garments in the way;
others cut down branches from
the trees, and [b]|spread| *them* in
the way.
9 And the multitudes that went
before, and that followed, cried,
saying, Hosanna to the Son of
David! [c]Blessed *is* he that cometh
in the name of the Lord! Hosanna
in the highest!
10 And when he was come into
Jerusalem, all the city was moved,
saying, Who is this?
11 And the multitude said, This
is Jesus, the [d]prophet of Nazareth
of Galilee.

Jesus drives traders from Temple
(Mk.11:15–18; Lk.19:45–47;
cp. Jn.2:13–16)

12 ¶ And Jesus went into the
temple of God, and cast out all
them that sold and bought in the
temple, and overthrew the tables
of the money-changers, and the
seats of them that sold doves,
13 And said unto them, It is
[c]written, [e]My house shall be called
the house of prayer, but ye have
made it a den of thieves.
14 And the [f]blind and the lame
came to him in the temple, and
he healed them.
15 And when the chief priests
and scribes saw the wonderful
things that he did, and the children crying in the temple, and
saying, Hosanna to the [g]Son of
David! they were [h]|very| dis-
pleased,
16 And said unto him, Hearest
thou what these say? And Jesus
saith unto them, Yea; have ye
never [c]read, [i]Out of the mouth of
babes and sucklings thou hast
perfected praise?
17 And he left them, and [j]went
out of the city into [1]Bethany; and
he lodged there.

The barren fig tree
(Mk.11:12–14, 20–26)

18 ¶ Now in the morning, as he
returned into the city, he [k]|was
hungry|.
19 And when he saw a [l]fig tree
along the way, he came to it, and
found nothing on it but leaves
only, and said unto it, Let no fruit
grow on thee henceforward forever. And presently the fig tree
[m]withered away.
20 And when the disciples saw
it, they marveled, saying, How
soon is the fig tree withered away!
21 Jesus answered and said unto
them, Verily I say unto you, If ye
have [n]faith, and doubt not, ye
shall not only do this *which is*
done to the fig tree, but also, if ye
shall say unto this mountain, Be
thou removed, and be thou cast
into the sea, it shall be done.
22 And [o]all things, whatever
ye shall ask in prayer, believing,
ye shall receive.

Jesus' authority challenged
(Mk.11:27–33; Lk.20:1–8)

23 ¶ And when he was come into
the temple, the chief priests and
the elders of the people came unto
him as he was teaching, and said,
By what authority doest thou
these things? And who gave thee
this authority?
24 And Jesus answered and said
unto them, I also will ask you one
thing, which, if ye tell me, I like-
wise, will tell you by what
authority I do these things.
25 The [p]baptism of [q]John, from
where was it? From heaven, or of
men? And they [r]reasoned with
themselves, saying, If we shall
say, From heaven; he will say unto
us, Why did ye not then believe
him?
26 But if we shall say, From men;
we [s]fear the people; for all hold
John as a [t]prophet.
27 And they answered Jesus,
and said, We cannot tell. And he
said unto them, [u]Neither tell I you
by what authority I do these
things.

Parable of the two sons

28 ¶ But what think ye? [v]A *cer-*
tain man had two sons; and he
came to the first, and said, Son,
go work today in my [w]vineyard.
29 He answered and said, I will

a Cp. 2 Ki. 9:13
b KJV *strawed*
c *Inspiration:* vv. 9,13,16; Mt.21:42. (Ex.4:15; 2 Tim.3:16); Ps. 118:26
d Dt.18:15,18; Mt.2:23; 16:14; Lk.4:16–29; Jn.6:14; 7:40; 9:17; Acts 3:22–23; see Lk. 24:19, *note*
e Isa.56:7; Jer.7:11
f Cp. Lk. 14:21; Acts 3:1–10
g Mt.1:1; Jn.7:42; cp. Jer. 23:5–6
h KJV *sore*
i Ps.8:2; cp. 1 Cor.1:26–29
j Mk.11:11
k KJV *hungered.* Mk.11:12–14; cp. Jn. 4:6
l Lit. *a solitary fig tree.* Lk.13:6–9
m *Miracles* (N.T.): vv. 18–22; Mk. 1:26. (Mt.8:3; Acts 28:8)
n Mt.17:20; Lk. 17:6; 1 Cor. 13:2; Jas.1:6
o Mt.7:7–11; Mk. 11:24; Lk.11:9; Jn.15:7; 1 Jn.3:22; 5:14–15
p Jn.1:29–34; see Acts 8:12, *note*
q Jn.1:15–28
r Cp. Lk. 5:21
s v. 46; Mt.14:5; Lk.20:6; cp. Prov. 29:25; Mk.6:25
t Mt.14:5
u Cp. v. 32; Mt.3:3
v *Parables* (N.T.): vv. 28–32; Mt. 21:33. (Mt.5:13; Lk. 21:29)
w v. 33; Mt.20:1; cp. Isa. 5:7; Mt. 28:19; Jn.15:1–5

1(21:17) Bethany, two miles east of Jerusalem and the home of Lazarus, was a frequent stopping place for Christ (Lk.10:38–42; cp. Mk.11:1–11; Lk.19:29–35; Jn.12:1–8). With no other place was the human Christ so tenderly associated. Here also was manifested His divine power in the resurrection of Lazarus (Jn.11:41–44).

1028

Read the footnote about Bethany in **Matthew 21:17**. What miracle did Jesus perform there?

____

The Lord's Supper

Matthew 26:17-30

Name ______________________

The disciples had entered Jerusalem triumphantly and joyfully as their beloved Master was praised and worshiped by the people. Later, as they sat around the table with Him preparing to partake of the traditional Passover, He shocked them with the news that one of them would betray Him. Their hearts became sorrowful. As they reflected on what would happen to their Master, Jesus provided them with a way to remember Him. He assigned new meanings to the bread and drink of the Passover. In doing this, Jesus provided a reminder not only to the disciples, but also to present-day Christians of His willing sacrifice for our sins. This reminder has become an **ordinance** of the New Testament church.

Answer the questions.

1. What did Jesus say the bread represented? (Matt. 26:26) ______________________
2. What did Jesus say the liquid in the cup represented? (Matt. 26:27-28) ______________________
3. For what purpose did Jesus shed His blood? (Matt. 26:28) ______________________

   ____
4. Paul gives Christians instructions about participating in the Lord's Supper in I Corinthians 11:23-29. Why do Christians continue to participate in this ordinance? (I Cor. 11:25)

   ____
5. Why would it be inappropriate for non-Christians to observe the Lord's Supper?

   ____

   ____

Using the information found in the Catechism about God's ordinances on page 381, answer the questions.

6. What is an ordinance?

   ____

   ____

   ____

7. The Lord's Supper is an ordinance that helps Christians remember Christ's **death** on the cross. What is another ordinance observed by Christians that is a picture of Christ's **resurrection**? ______________________

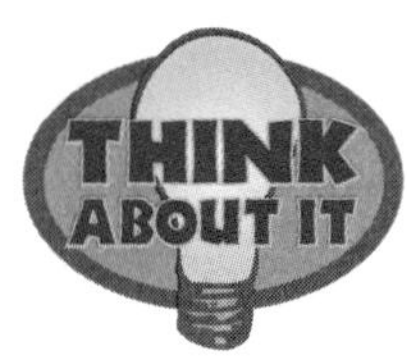
THINK
ABOUT IT

Have you participated in these ordinances? If so, what do they mean to you?

Falsely Accused

Matthew 26:30-75; John 18:12-24; Mark 14:53-65 Name ____________________

After Judas betrayed Jesus in the garden of Gethsemane, Jesus was taken to the Jewish religious leaders. The events that followed were illegal according to both Jewish and Roman law. The Pharisees and chief priests violated their responsibility to be just and truthful leaders in an effort to get rid of Jesus.

Match the requirements of the laws with what actually happened when Jesus was tried, accused, and condemned to die.

Requirements for condemning someone to death at the time of Christ	What actually happened to Jesus was . . .
_____ 1. A trial must be conducted openly in the daytime (Matt. 26:31; 27:1).	A. Jesus was asked to defend Himself, and He was not given the opportunity to have anyone else speak in His defense.
_____ 2. The accusations of the witnesses against the accused person must agree (Mark 14:56).	B. Jesus was tried during the night, and condemned by the Jewish leaders at daybreak.
_____ 3. The witnesses against the accused person must tell the truth (Matt. 26:59-61).	C. Jesus did not break the law, but was accused because religious leaders were envious of His authority and popularity with the people.
_____ 4. A person may be brought to trial only for breaking the law (Matt. 27:18; Mark 15:10).	D. Many people falsely accused Jesus, but none of the witnesses agreed with each other.
_____ 5. The accused person must be given the opportunity to allow other people to speak in his defense (Matt. 26:62-68).	E. Jesus was found innocent again and again but was still condemned to die.
_____ 6. The accused person can be put to death only if found guilty (John 18:38; 19:4, 6; Luke 23:13-15).	F. The religious leaders couldn't find any witnesses against Jesus. Finally two people came forward and lied about something Jesus had said.

Answer the questions.

1. How did Jesus respond when He was falsely accused? (Matt. 26:60-63)

   ____

2. By saying that Caiaphas would someday see Him in the clouds at the right hand of God, Jesus was clearly claiming to be God. What did Caiaphas call this statement? (Matt. 26:63-65) ____________________

3. Read the definition for *blasphemy* in the glossary. Write the part of the definition that describes how Caiaphas thought Jesus blasphemed.

   ____

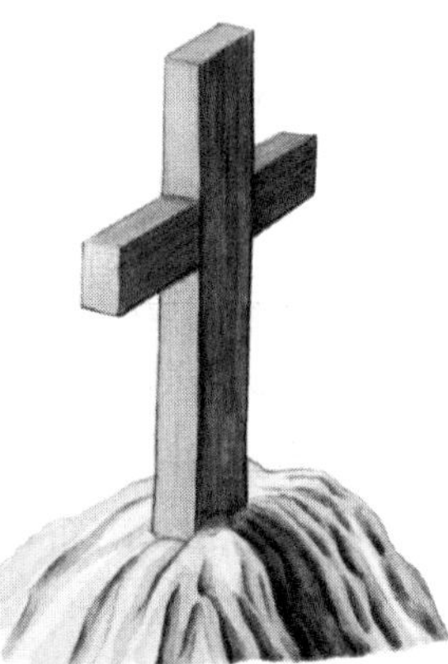

Overcoming Failure

Matthew 26:31-35, 69-75

Name ______________________

Peter believed in Jesus. He had traveled with Jesus around the country, watched His miracles, and listened to His teachings. Peter knew Jesus was the Son of God, and he had come to love Jesus as his Master. He loved Jesus so much that he even promised to die for Him if necessary. But when the real test of Peter's devotion came, he failed miserably. What happened? How could someone who was so eager to prove his loyalty to Jesus turn around and deny Him that same day? Peter failed because he was afraid to suffer for Christ.

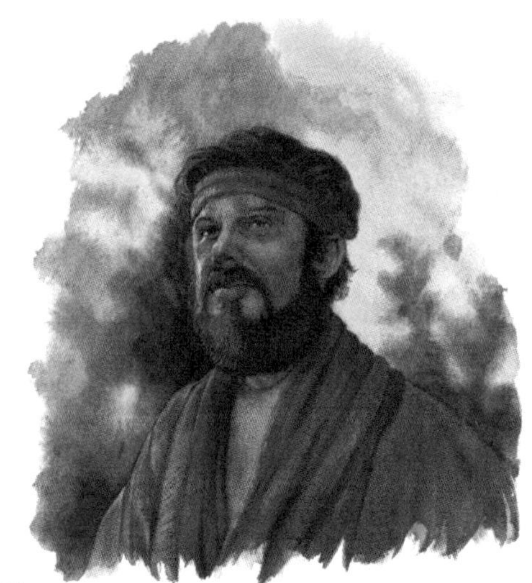

Think about Peter's actions and answer the questions.

1. What did Peter say he would never do? ______________________
2. Do you think Peter meant to keep this promise? __________ Did he? __________

   What *did* he do? ____
3. List two things a Christian might do that would be a denial of Christ.
   - ◆ ____
   - ◆ ____

Although Peter failed, God was not finished with him. Peter's grief over his failure led to his repentance and his restored fellowship with Jesus after the Resurrection. Peter became a strong testimony of God's forgiveness to the early church. Peter's response to his failure is a good example for today's Christians.

Read each verse and write in your own words what you should do when you fail God.

1. **Psalm 32:5** ____
2. **Psalm 143:10** ____

WARNING!
When you fail, you can't just try to do better next time. Remember that victory over failure must start with confession!

Read Proverbs 28:13 and fill in the blanks.

Anyone who tries to ______________________ his sin will not prosper.

Only those who ______________________ and ______________________ their sins will find ______________________.

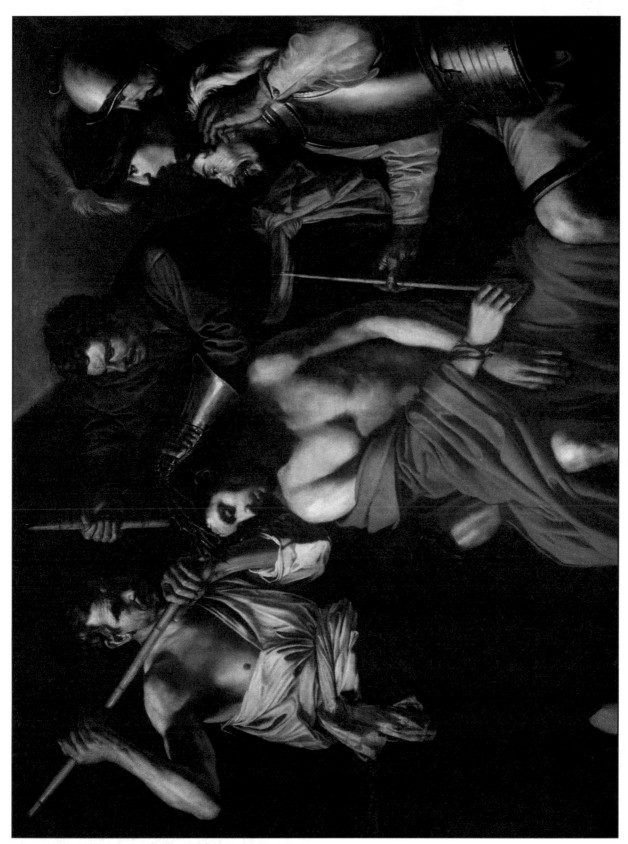

The Mocking of Christ
A Northern Follower of Caravaggio

Bob Jones University Museum & Gallery, Inc.

Name ______________________

The Mocking of Christ

by a Northern Follower of Caravaggio

Unlike the other artists studied, the name of this artist is unknown. Because of his style of painting, we do know that he probably studied in Rome during the early seventeenth century with a teacher named Manfredi, who used the modern style of a man named Caravaggio.

Caravaggio had invented a new way to depict a dramatic scene. He placed his characters in dark places with a little light coming through a window or from a candle. He also persuaded his friends to pose as characters for his pictures. He even dressed them in costumes to make the effect more realistic. Many painters dressed their characters in modern seventeenth-century clothing. Notice that the soldiers look more like those of the seventeenth century rather than Roman soldiers of Bible times. Painters often showed Jesus and His disciples in robes of nomadic Arabs.

The story depicted here is told in Matthew 27:27-30. Many details are shown—Christ wearing a robe and a crown of thorns, a soldier extending a piece of bamboo as a royal scepter, and another soldier kneeling in front of Christ, laughing as several men are beating Christ on the head. Notice that one man in the picture seems to be shocked or surprised. Why do you think the man placing the thorned crown on Jesus' head is wearing a glove? What kind of people do you think these men are? The Bible does not tell us much about the men who tortured Jesus except that they were soldiers. It simply lists what they did and said. The artist had to think about the story and what kind of people he wanted to put into his picture. He used what he knew about human nature to build a dramatic scene.

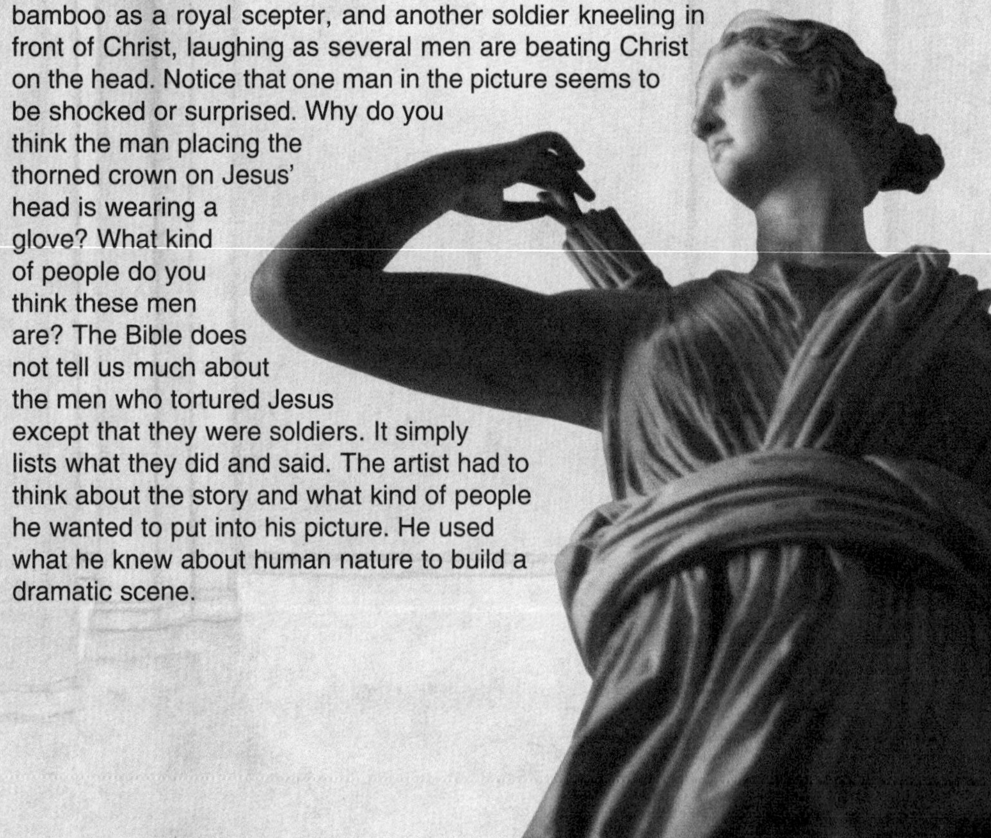

Name Above All Names

Matthew 27:1-54; Luke 23:1-25

Name ______________________

Jesus Christ is known by many names. Each name given to Him describes His authority, His character, or His actions. All of these names point to the deity of Christ and are names which are above every other name.

Complete the puzzle. You may use your Bible for help.

Across

2. ______ asked Jesus if He really was the King of the Jews (Matt. 27:2,11).
5. The soldiers called Jesus the ______ ______ ______ ______ when they mocked Him (Matt. 27:29).
7. At Christ's death, the ______ realized Jesus was the Son of God (Matt. 27:54).

Down

1. The chief priests, scribes, and elders called Jesus the ______ ______ ______ when they were mocking Him (Matt. 27:41-42).
3. Those who mocked Jesus said He called Himself the ______ ______ ______ (Matt. 27:43).
4. The crowd wanted ______ to be crucified (Matt. 27:22).
6. Jesus called Himself the Son of ______ (Matt. 26:64).

Write the names of Jesus found in the verses *in the order that they appear*.
If the name is a title that describes His position of authority, draw a crown in the square (crown).
If the name describes His character, draw a heart (♥).
If the name describes His actions, draw a hand (hand).
Some names have more than one description symbol. Draw all the symbols that apply for each name.

Isaiah 9:6

W______________________

M______________________

E______________________

P______________________

Revelation 19:16

K______________________

L______________________

John 10:11

S______________________

Luke 2:11

S______________________

C______________________

Sinless Suffering

I Peter 2:21-23

Name ______________________

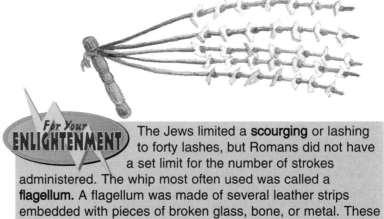

Jesus set a high standard for Christians to follow. Christians can expect to suffer for their faith. It may be verbal insults or threats. It may be physical abuse, imprisonment, or even death. They should not be surprised when it happens. The world hates Jesus Christ, so if you are a Christian, you can expect the world to hate you as well. When faced with suffering, you will also be faced with the decision of how to respond to it. God's Word gives the answers by focusing on Jesus' response to suffering.

For Your ENLIGHTENMENT The Jews limited a **scourging** or lashing to forty lashes, but Romans did not have a set limit for the number of strokes administered. The whip most often used was called a **flagellum.** A flagellum was made of several leather strips embedded with pieces of broken glass, bone, or metal. These sharp pieces would grab and cut into the skin as the leather made contact. Often a scourging would cause death.

Read I Peter 2:21-23 and answer the questions.

1. According to verse 21, what is one reason Christ suffered?

____

2. List two ways that Jesus suffered.

____

3. How did Jesus respond when the people insulted and abused Him?

____

4. How should a Christian respond when someone criticizes or insults him because of his faith in Jesus?

____

You might have heard about Christians in other countries who are suffering painful persecution for their faith in Christ. While not all Christians may suffer like these people, they will have many opportunities to stand firm and unashamed for their Savior.

Read each scenario and write responses that follow the example of Christ.

Scenario	A response that follows Christ's example would be...
Dean plays baseball at the park with some of the boys from his neighborhood. One day, Tom brought cigarettes to the park to try out with the boys. Dean knew that God would not be pleased, so he told them he was going home. The other boys called him a "sissy" and made fun of him.	
Eileen tried to tell her cousin, Maycee, about Jesus. Maycee didn't want to listen and changed the subject every time Eileen brought it up. Eileen heard Maycee tell her friends that Eileen was weird. Eileen wanted to help Maycee, but her feelings were hurt.	

What Does God Say About Being Angry?

Name ______________________________

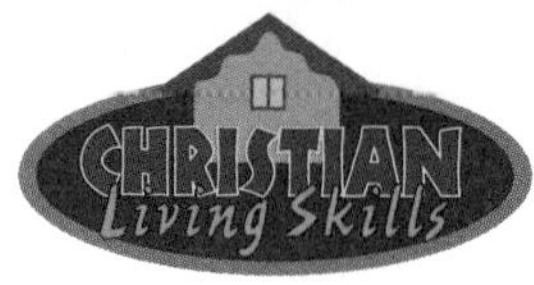
CHRISTIAN
Living Skills

Have you ever been mad at somebody?

Anger is a powerful emotion. It is a strong feeling of displeasure when something does not go your way. Anger is a choice. No one can force you to become angry. Someone may do something that tempts you to get mad, but the choice to become angry is *yours*. Some people react with harsh words, others with silence, and still others with violence. Sinful anger leads to negative consequences.

Read the verses and complete the chart to find out the negative consequences of sinful anger in the lives of these men.

Person	What reason is given for the anger?	What did his anger lead him to do?	What were the negative consequences of his sinful anger?
Cain Genesis 4:3-15	Cain was angry because God did not accept his offering. (Gen. 4:5)	(Gen. 4:8)	God cursed Cain. The land would not produce food for him, and he became a wanderer. (Gen. 4:11-12)
Asa II Chronicles 16:1-10	Asa was angry because the seer said that God was displeased with Asa's actions. (II Chron. 16:7-10)	Asa put Hanani, the seer, in prison and oppressed some of the people. (II Chron. 16:10)	(II Chron. 16:9,12)

Not all anger is sinful. The Bible says that God is angry with sin (Ps. 7:11). Anger that is a result of seeing an injustice or wrong thing being done is known as **righteous anger.** Christians should imitate Christ in being angry about sin and its destruction in the lives of people. However, the Bible also says that God is merciful and patient and that He is willing to forgive their sins immediately when they confess them to Him.

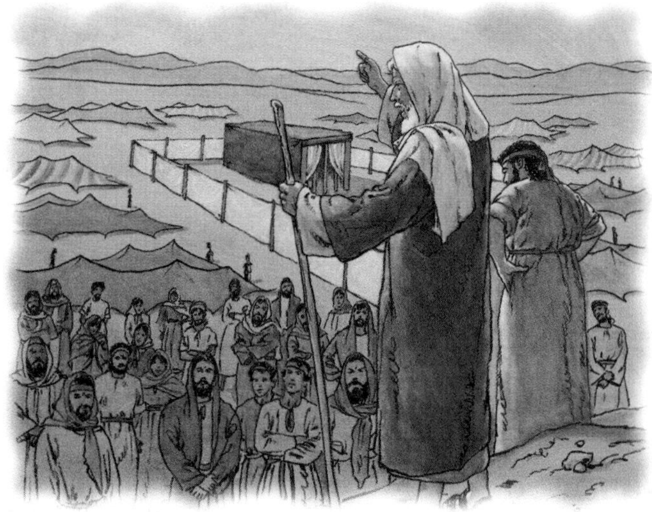

Read the verses and complete the chart.

	Who felt righteous anger?	Why did he feel righteous anger?
Exodus 32:17-20		
John 2:13-16		

Something to Think About

Being Angry

Name ______________________

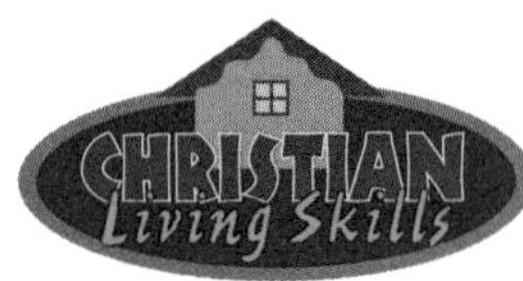
CHRISTIAN
Living Skills

Christians must learn to control their emotions when something does not go their way. Anger that controls you and drives you to react with a lack of self-control is sin and is a direct result of pride in your heart. God's Word warns Christians about the dangers of sinful anger.

Read the verse and match the references to the correct warning about people who allow themselves to react in sinful anger.

_____ 1. A person who gets angry easily does foolish things. A. Proverbs 29:22

_____ 2. An angry person causes problems and commits many sins. B. Proverbs 14:17

Read the verses. Complete the statements of advice to a friend who wants to find out how to avoid sinful anger.

Ephesians 4:31

You must get rid of

____________________.

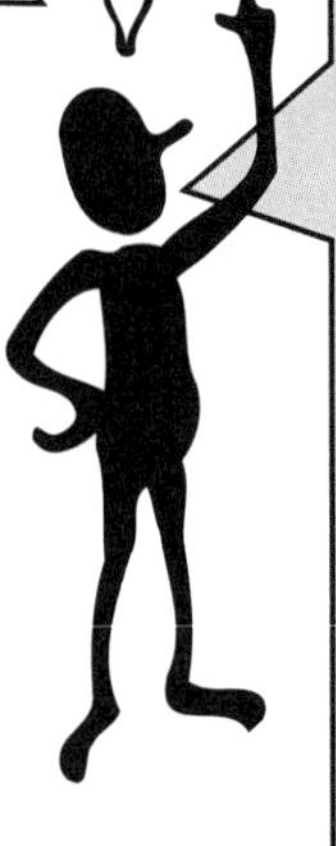

James 1:19-20

Three things to remember when you are tempted to become angry are to

1) Be ______________ to listen,

2) Be ______________ to speak,

3) Be slow to ______________

You should remember this because anger does not ______________

____

____

Proverbs 22:24-25

You should never be friends with

____

because you might ______________

____

____

What About Me?

Take time at home to think about your reaction when faced with the choice to become angry. Ask God for help in overcoming sinful anger.

What situations cause me to become angry?

How do I react when I am frustrated or irritated?

Do I need to confess the sin of anger to God?

Do I need to apologize to someone for my wrong behavior when I was angry?

Do I get angry when I see sin around me?

Is God pleased with my attitude toward sin?

Lost Sheep

I Peter 2:24-25

Name ______________________

We deserve to die for our sins. We can do nothing to gain salvation. Jesus Christ willingly took our sins upon Himself and died on the cross. Because Jesus died for your sin, the price has been paid. Now you are faced with the choice of either receiving Him or rejecting Him. *What will you do?*

Read I Peter 2:24-25 and answer the questions.

1. What does it mean that Jesus bore your sins in His body? ______________________

   ____

2. According to verse 24, why did Jesus die? ______________________
3. To what animal are we compared? ______________________

Sheep are not very smart. They are totally dependent on their shepherd to lead them to good pasture, to find clean water, and to protect them from storms and wild animals. Sheep can't even get up on their own if they turn themselves over on their backs. Interestingly, the Bible often refers to people as *sheep* in need of a loving and merciful Shepherd.

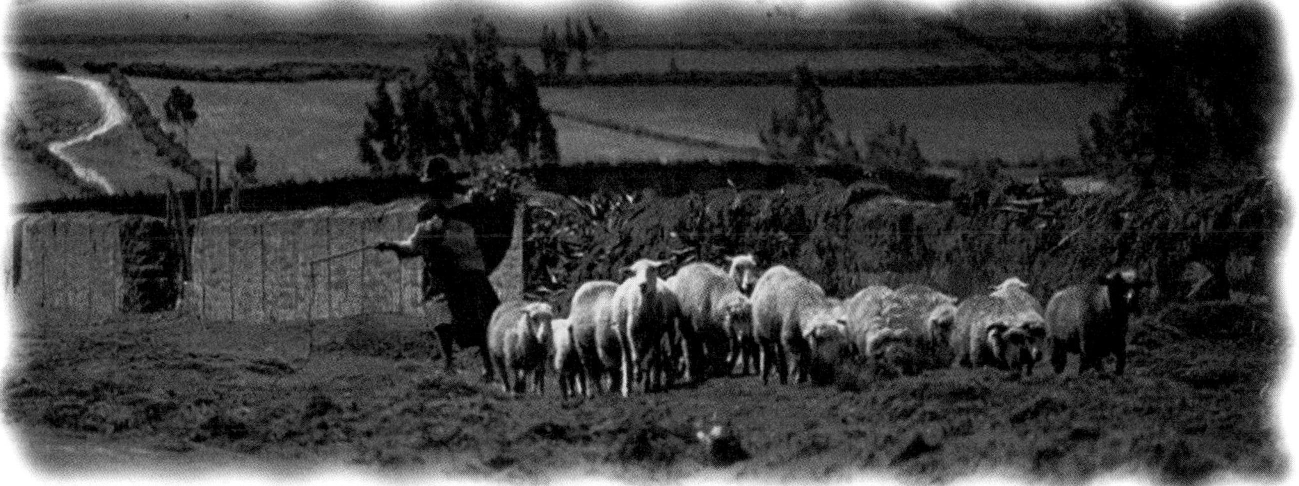

Think about how sheep need a shepherd. Think about how people need a Shepherd. Complete the comparisons. In the last row, write your own comparison between people and sheep.

Sheep		People
Sheep need a shepherd to protect them from wild animals.	⟷	*People need protection from ____.*
Sheep need ____.	⟷	People need a Shepherd to provide food and shelter for them.
Sheep need a shepherd to find and save them when they get lost from the flock.	⟷	*People need to be saved from ____.*
Sheep need ____.	⟷	*People need ____.*

Miraculous Resurrection

Matthew 27:55–28:20

Name ______________________

Match the correct person to each action.

______ 1. Joseph of Arimathea	A.	paid the guards money to lie about Jesus' resurrection
______ 2. Mary Magdalene	B.	met with Jesus on the mountain in Galilee
______ 3. an angel	C.	met the women on their way into Galilee
______ 4. Pilate	D.	buried Jesus in his tomb
______ 5. the disciples	E.	gave permission for the tomb to be sealed
______ 6. the guards	F.	went to Jesus' grave to look at the tomb
______ 7. Jesus	G.	spread the rumor that the disciples had stolen Jesus' body
______ 8. chief priests & Pharisees	H.	sat on the stone that was rolled away from the tomb

Describe what the following people might have been thinking when Jesus died.

1. **the disciples:** ______________________________

2. **the chief priests and Pharisees:** ______________________________

Describe what the same people might have been thinking when Jesus arose.

1. **the disciples:**

____

____

____

2. **the chief priests and Pharisees:**

____

____

____

Describe what the death and Resurrection of Jesus mean to you.

THINK ABOUT IT

For me the death and Resurrection of Jesus mean . . .

____

____

____

Fulfilled Prophecy

Bible Study

Name ____________________

Read the verses to discover the prophecies about the arrest, crucifixion, and resurrection of Jesus. Complete the chart.

Old Testament Reference	Prophecy	New Testament Fulfillment
Zechariah 11:12	Jesus would be betrayed for thirty pieces of silver.	**Matthew 26:15**
Zechariah 11:13	Money would be returned and used to purchase a potter's field.	**Matthew 27:5-7**
Psalm 27:12		**Matthew 26:59-61**
Isaiah 53:7		**Matthew 26:62-63**
Isaiah 50:6		**Matthew 26:67, 27:30**

Old Testament Reference	Prophecy	New Testament Fulfillment
Psalm 22:18	Jesus' enemies would cast lots and divide His clothing among themselves.	**Matthew 27:35**
Isaiah 53:12	Jesus would be numbered with transgressors (the thieves) in his death, and He would bear the sin of many.	**Matthew 27:38**
Psalm 69:21		**Matthew 27:34, 48**
Psalm 22:1		**Matthew 27:46**
Psalm 34:20		**John 19:33-36**

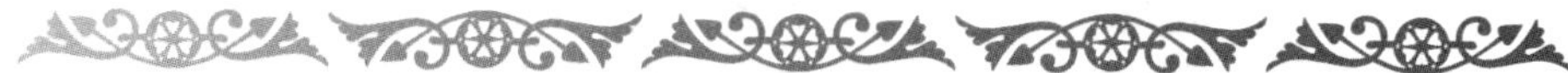

Old Testament Reference	Prophecy	New Testament Fulfillment
Psalm 16:10		**Matthew 28:5-7**

Singing with Understanding

"Christ the Lord Is Risen Today: (vv. 1-4)

Name ____________________

Read the words of the hymn on page 318. Use the clues given to complete the puzzle. All of the words are taken from the hymn.

1. Christ needed to die only once to ____________________ all. (v. 3)
2. Men and angels proclaim the news that Christ the ____________________ is risen. (v. 1)
3. Christians can sing praise because Christ ____________________ again. (v. 3)
4. ____________________ had no power to forbid Christ's resurrection from the grave. (v. 2)
5. When Christ comes for Christians, they will be made ____________________ Him. (v. 4)
6. Christians can raise their ____________________ high because Christ is risen. (v. 1)
7. Christ is our glorious ____________________. (v. 3)
8. Christ's death and resurrection opened the way to ____________________. (v. 2)

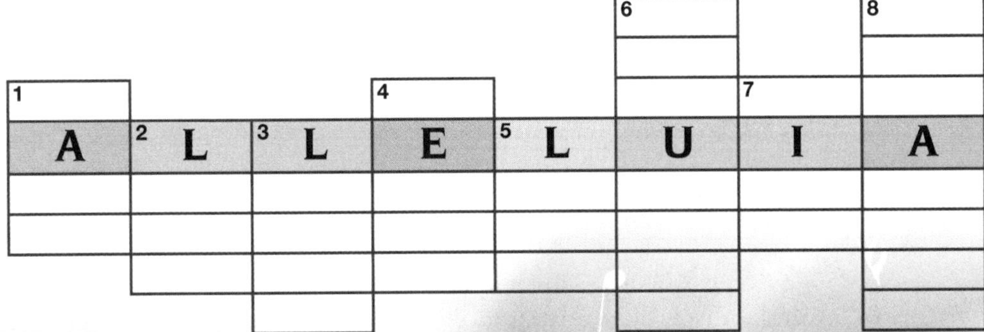

1 A
2 L
3 L
4 E
5 L
6 U
7 I
8 A

For Your ENLIGHTENMENT

Alleluia is a Hebrew word meaning "praise the Lord." It is translated roughly the same way in any language. Because *allelula* occurs so often in our hymns and songs, we often sing it without really thinking about what it means. As you sing "Christ the Lord Is Risen Today" this Easter, think of the great victory the Savior has won for you. He has made it possible for you to join Him in heaven one day and stay there with Him for all eternity! Isn't that thought enough to help you sing *alleluia* and really mean it?

Alleluia

Christ, Our Redeemer

Name ______________________________

God's Word reminds Christians of the wonderful gift of redemption through Jesus Christ. His death on the cross provides salvation from sin and eternal fellowship with God. Such a gift is priceless!

Follow the directions below to make a prism prompter to learn about redemption through Christ.

1. **Cut out the square on the heavy dark lines.**
2. **Turn the square over so it is print-side down.**
3. **Fold the square diagonally. Open it and fold it on the other diagonal. Open it again.**
4. **Fold each corner so the point touches the center. Turn it over and again fold each corner so the point touches the center. Crease.**
5. **Fold the square in half vertically. Crease. Open it and fold it in half horizontally. Crease.**
6. **Slide your thumbs and your first fingers into the tabs to open the prism prompter.**
7. **Ask a partner to choose a picture. Open and close the prism prompter as you alternate between each side spelling the word on the picture.**
8. **Ask your partner to choose a letter inside the prism prompter. Open the tab and read the verse.**

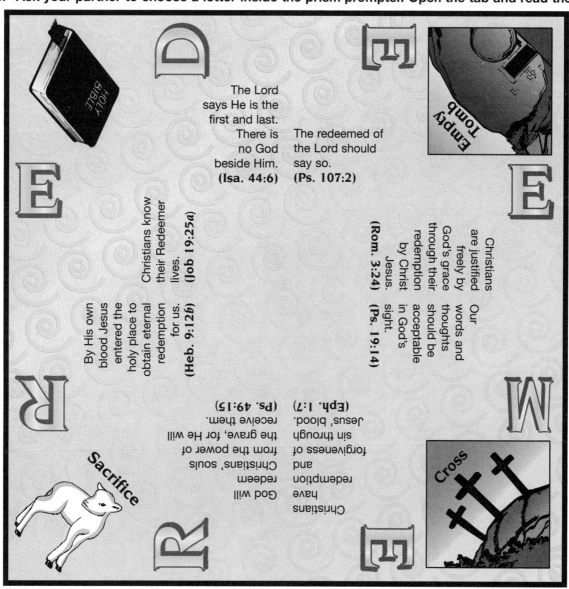

HOLY BIBLE
D
E
Empty Tomb
The Lord says He is the first and last. There is no God beside Him. (Isa. 44:6)
The redeemed of the Lord should say so. (Ps. 107:2)
E
E
Christians know their Redeemer lives. (Job 19:25a)
By His own blood Jesus entered the holy place to obtain eternal redemption for us. (Heb. 9:12b)
Christians are justified freely by God's grace through their redemption by Christ Jesus. (Rom. 3:24)
Our words and thoughts should be acceptable in God's sight. (Ps. 19:14)
R
M
God will redeem Christians' souls from the power of the grave, for He will receive them. (Ps. 49:15)
Christians have redemption and forgiveness of sin through Jesus' blood. (Eph. 1:7)
Sacrifice
Cross
R
E

What Does God Say About My Abilities?

Name ______________________________

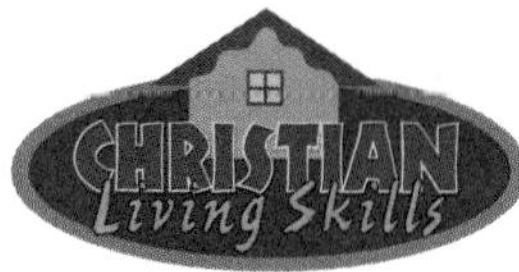
CHRISTIAN
Living Skills

You are miraculously designed.

God created you with a unique personality and set of abilities. As you look around and notice the talents of others, you may feel like you somehow missed out. It might seem like everyone else is smarter, more athletic, or more musical than you are. Don't be deceived! Don't waste your time comparing yourself to someone else. God knew you before you were born, and He has given you every talent you need to serve Him.

Read Psalm 139:13-16. Use these verses to complete the statements to describe to someone how much God knows about and cares for him.

Verse 13 God created you and knew who you were when you were still in ______________________

Verse 14 We are each ________________ and ________________________ made by God.

Verse 14 We know that God does ______________________________________ works.

Verse 16 Everything about you was written in God's ________________ before you were born.

You are responsible for how you use your God-given abilities.

A Christian should want to bring glory to God in the way he uses his talents. As you make choices about the activities in which you want to be involved, remember to make time to develop skills that will be useful in God's service in the future.

Read the verses and match them to the correct statements about your God-given abilities.

______ 1. **I Peter 4:10**

______ 2. **Colossians 3:23-24**

______ 3. **Ephesians 4:12**

A. I should use my gifts to glorify God.
B. I should use my gifts to build up the body of Christ.
C. I should make every effort to use my gifts to minister to others.

Beware of pride!

Satan would love to distract you from glorifying God by focusing your attention on your abilities. There are two extremes that might describe you.

1.) You might think that you are very talented and enjoy letting others see your special ability. This shows a prideful heart!
2.) You might know that you have a certain talent, but you're too embarrassed to use it in public because of what others might say, or too scared to try because you might fail. This attitude shows that you are more concerned about what others think about you than what God tells you to do. This also shows a prideful heart! Don't be deceived! Be grateful for the abilities that God has given to you and do your best to please Him by taking every opportunity to use them because you love Him.

Read the verses and complete the statements.

Matthew 6:1 A Christian's purpose for using his abilities should not be to

be ____________ by other people.

Hebrews 13:6 The Lord is

our ________________.
Therefore, we don't need to be afraid of what man can do to us.

Something to Think About

My Abilities

Name ______________________

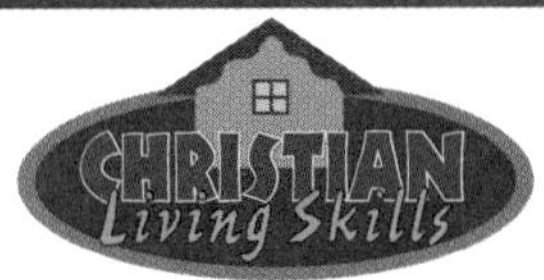
CHRISTIAN
Living Skills

What is your definition of "success?"

Fame? Popularity? Prosperity? Straight As? The world believes that success is getting something you want, no matter what it is. The world tells us that we should dream about what we want, set high goals, work hard, and proudly enjoy the satisfaction that comes from achieving our goals. You probably noticed as you read the last sentence how selfish the world's focus is. True success does not come from getting what you want. True **success** is finding out what God created you to do and focusing all your energy on becoming who God wants you to be.

Read the following list of abilities and circle the ones you believe God has given to you (even if it's a talent you're not very good at yet). Write in the blanks other talents you have that are not listed.

Playing ball	Singing	Playing a musical instrument	Running fast	______
Making friends	Fixing things	Getting good grades in writing	Gymnastics	______
Being a leader	Acting	Speaking in front of others	Being responsible	______
Swimming	Drawing	Getting good grades in math	Making things	______
Painting	Cooking	Speaking a foreign language	Being organized	______

Choose two of your talents and write how they can be used for God's glory.

Talent/Ability	One way this ability could be used to glorify God is...

What About Me?

What is your motive? Why do you want to do your best? What drives you to achieve? Sadly, many Christians have gotten caught up in the pursuit of selfish ambitions that will never make them happy. They may be working hard to do their best, but their motives are wrong. While Christians should make every effort to work hard and do their best, their motives are different from the world. *A Christian should desire to honor God by faithfully using his gifts to bring glory to God, not to himself.*

Take time at home to think about and answer the following questions.

What is my motive for doing my best?	○ I want to impress other people with my abilities. ○ I want to glorify God with my abilities. ○ I want to feel good about myself.
What am I doing with the gifts God has given to me?	○ I try to get out of using them as much as possible. ○ I concentrate on only one skill that I like the most. ○ I look for opportunities to practice and improve all my skills.
What is my attitude toward the abilities God has given to me?	○ My abilities don't seem to be as good as someone else's are. ○ I wish that God had given me different abilities than the ones I have. ○ I am learning to be thankful for the unique abilities God has given me.

Get the Bible Reading H.A.B.I.T.

Name ______________________________

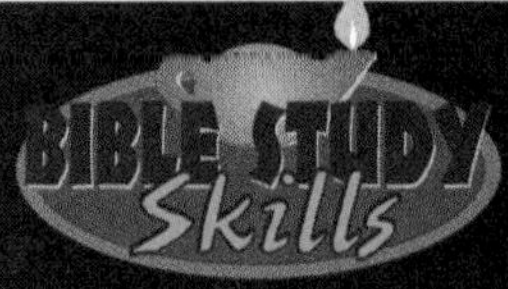
BIBLE STUDY
Skills

Have a special time set aside each day to read your Bible. If possible, make it the same time every day.

Ask God to teach you from His Word. Remember to thank Him for helping you to understand and apply it.

Be still and give your attention to what you are reading.

Investigate the Scripture by asking yourself questions about it.

Take time to look up words and ideas you do not understand.

As you read the Scripture for each day, write the date in the box.

God ordained preaching as a means to bring souls to Christ. **I Corinthians 1:17-21**	God has made Christians ambassadors to tell the world to be reconciled to God. **II Corinthians 5:18-21**	The gospel Christians should preach is to confess Christ and believe. **Romans 10:8-10**	Whoever calls on the name of the Lord shall be saved. **Romans 10:11-13**	People will not be reached for Christ without preachers of the gospel. **Romans 10:14-17**
Godly Christians may be called upon to suffer persecution. **II Timothy 3:10-12**	Jesus never forsakes Christians when they suffer for Him. **II Corinthians 4:8-9**	When Christians suffer, they identify with Christ and manifest His life. **II Corinthians 4:10-11**	Suffering should not turn Christians from testifying of the gospel. **Acts 20:22-24**	Christians should conduct themselves in a manner worthy of the gospel. **Philippians 1:27-30**
The gospel is the power of God; Christians should never be ashamed of it. **Romans 1:14-16**	Christians are obligated to preach the gospel. **I Corinthians 9:14-16**	Christians should speak the gospel not to please men, but God. **I Thessalonians 2:1-4**	Christians should give the gospel gently, from a heart of love. **I Thessalonians 2:5-8**	Christians should keep their lives pure and blameless to be effective witnesses. **Philippians 2:14-16**
Jesus intended that the gospel go to the Gentiles as well as the Jews. **Romans 15:8-12**	Souls truly won to Christ should show evidence of the Spirit's work. **Romans 15:13-14**	Any soulwinning that Christians accomplish is a manifestation of Christ's power, not their own. **Romans 15:15-19**	The gospel should be preached in places where Christ has never been named. **Romans 15:20-21**	Christians should pray fervently for missionaries. **Romans 15:30-32**

Prayer Promises

Name ______________________

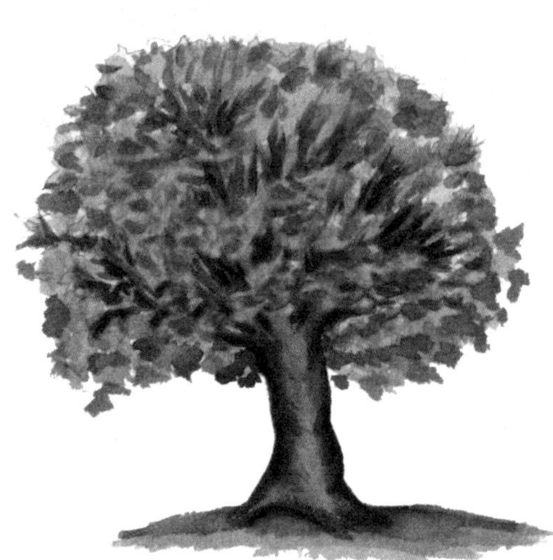

The disciples marveled when they saw a fig tree wither at the words of Jesus (Matt. 21:18-20). They were probably even more startled when He told them that they could move mountains with prayer. However, Jesus told them there was a condition that had to be met before their prayers were granted. The prayer had to be *in faith*, with no doubting. Looking at God's promises stated in His Word will help Christians to pray in faith. The conditions that go with these promises can be met with the help of the Holy Spirit.

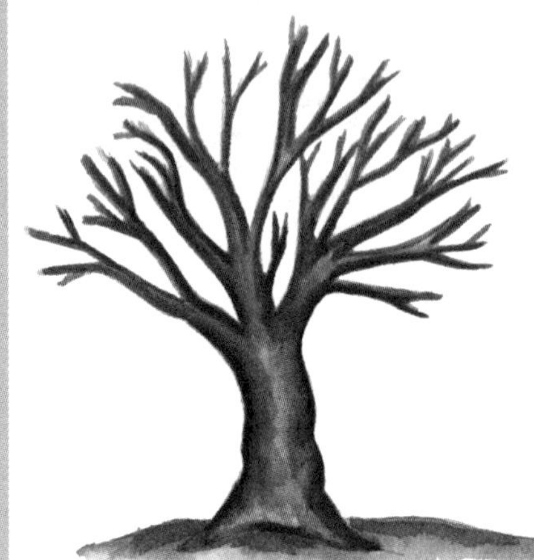

Read each Scripture. Complete the chart by writing the condition or promise.

	Condition (If you...)	Promise (Then...)
Isaiah 40:31	wait on God and place your hope and trust in Him,	
Jeremiah 33:3		God will answer and tell you great and mighty things.
Matthew 6:14	forgive others,	
John 14:14		God will answer your prayer.

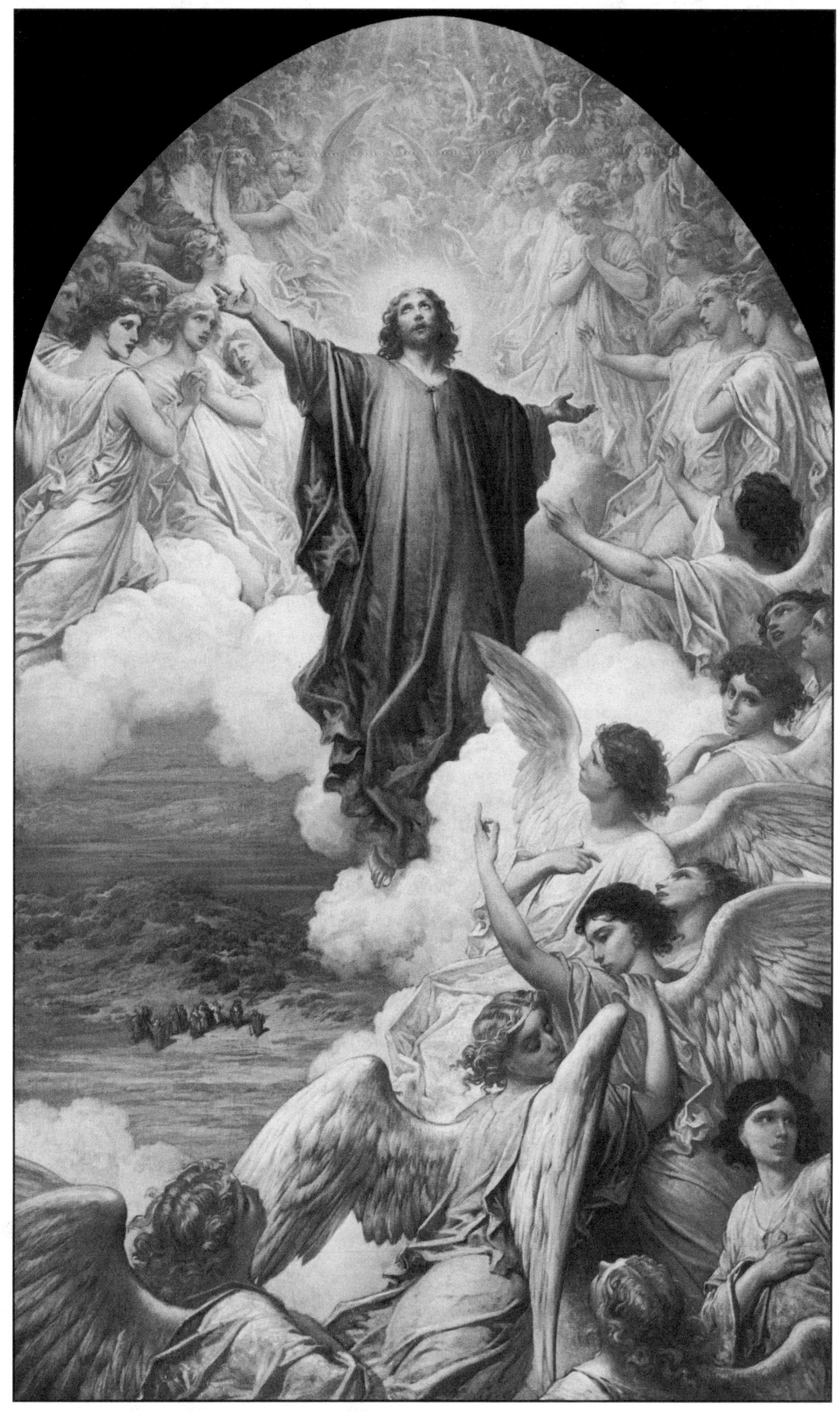

The Ascension

Gustave Doré

Bob Jones University Museum & Gallery, Inc.

Name ______________________

The Ascension

by Gustave Doré (1832-1883)

In contrast to some artists, Gustave Doré (Gŏŏ stäv′ Dô rā′) did not go to school to study painting. He was a very talented child who wanted to become a great painter. His hero was an artist whom he wanted to imitate. While Doré was still a teenager, he got a job illustrating a magazine. Early success attracted him, and he never went to art school. Doré never became a great oil painter, but he did become a great illustrator.

In addition to his illustrations, Doré began painting large oil paintings on religious subjects. In France, despite royal commissions for religious paintings, his paintings were never very popular. But in 1870, Doré opened a gallery in London to show his religious pictures. The people in London loved them. They called Doré the Painter-Preacher. Doré illustrated a Bible which was published as the Doré Bible.

This painting was one of those that Doré exhibited in London. The scene in this painting is the ascension of Jesus into heaven (Acts 1:9). In his painting, Doré places us among the angels welcoming Jesus back to heaven. The angels form a large curve surrounding Jesus. Notice the position that Jesus is in—like that of a cross, but more triumphant.

Doré was a Romantic painter, meaning an artist who paints emotional subjects in a touching way. Look at the faces of the angels. What emotions do they seem to have?

One of the interesting details in this painting is the view you have of the ground. What do you think is happening? Who do you think these people are? Doré was one of the first artists who painted a view of the earth from high above it. Before people could fly in airplanes, they didn't know what the earth looked like from above. But in the nineteenth century, people began flying in hot air balloons. One of Doré's friends took him ballooning. As was his custom, Doré took a sketchbook with him; evidently he drew the ground as seen from the balloon, and those sketches formed the basis of this part of the painting.

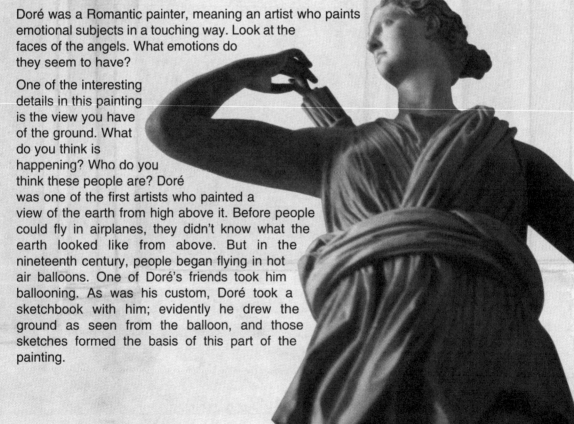

Last Words

Acts 1

Name ______________________

After the Resurrection, Jesus appeared to the apostles many times before ascending into heaven. On the day of His ascension, Jesus gave His apostles a promise and a command before He returned to heaven.

Write the letter of the correct definition next to each word.

______ 1. apostles

______ 2. resurrection

______ 3. ascension

______ 4. disciples

A. Christ's going upward into heaven
B. the name used for the men who had been closest to Christ
C. the name used for followers of Christ
D. act of coming to life again

Answer the questions.

1. What was the promise Christ gave His apostles before He ascended? (Acts 1:8)

____

2. What was the command Christ gave the apostles before He ascended? (Acts 1:8)

____

After Christ's ascension, the remaining eleven apostles chose another man to join them so that the group would once again have twelve.

Circle the names of the twelve apostles in the Book of Acts.

Peter Judas Simon Silas Andrew

Bartholomew Barsabas Matthias James Justus

Barnabas John James Philip Thomas

Joseph Matthew

For Your ENLIGHTENMENT In Bible times, the **casting of lots** was sometimes used to determine God's will. It is not exactly known what casting lots involved. Some believe that small marked pebbles were tossed during the selection process. Men are reminded in Proverbs 16:33 that although lots might be used, God controls all things.

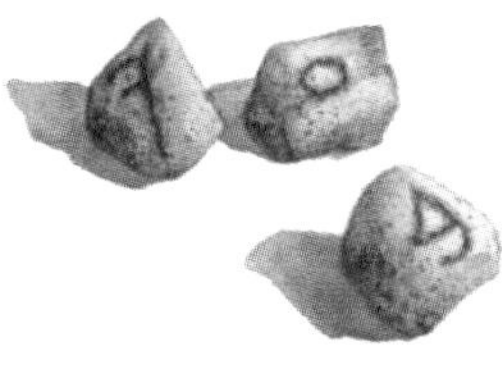

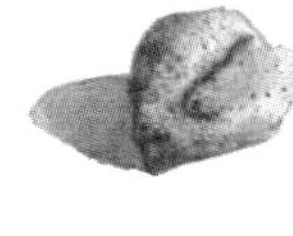

Using a Bible Commentary

Name ______________________

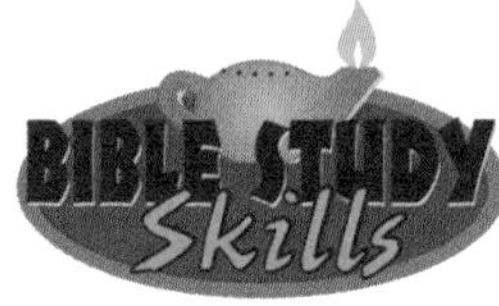
BIBLE STUDY
Skills

Commentaries are written by Bible scholars to help readers understand Scripture. Often commentators give background or information about the setting and define words as they explain or make comments on verses. Some commentators use quotation marks around verses as they paraphrase the words for better understanding.

Use information from the commentary to answer the questions.

Acts 2
1 And when the day of Pentecost was fully come, they were all with one accord in one place.
2 And suddenly there came a sound from heaven as of a rushing mighty wind, and it filled all the house where they were sitting.

Acts 2 Exposition

I. Pentecost: the Coming of the Spirit. vv. 1-13.

There were three great yearly festivals that brought crowds of pilgrims and worshipers to Jerusalem: Passover, Pentecost, and Tabernacles. Pentecost was celebrated 50 days after the Passover (Lev. 23:15-17). It was also known as the feast of the firstfruits because the first-ripe harvest was then brought to the temple. Thus, it was the day when the Lord began His spiritual harvest of souls (John 4:35). "And when the day of Pentecost had fully come, they were all together in one place" (v. 1). [See note on 2:1.] This certainly included the 120 already mentioned, as well as others from Galilee who had come for the festival. On this special occasion the Lord sent His Holy Spirit upon the church (John 16:7). There were two outward signs of His coming: one of sound and one of sight. "Suddenly there came a sound from heaven as of a rushing mighty zephyr, and it filled the whole house where they were sitting" (v. 2). This is a deliberate contrast between words for power and a word that denotes the gentlest breath of air that could be detected (Trench, *Synonyms*, pp. 275-78). A zephyr is a light breath of air that could be detected on the cheek, but it is not strong enough to cause leaves to move. This contrast is a beautiful image of the working of the Spirit of God. He is the infinite Spirit of almighty power, but He works with compassionate kindness, never crushing people into line, but like a dove, gently wooing men to the love of God. The *as* makes clear that there was no wind, just the sound.

1. What three festivals brought people to Jerusalem?

____

____

____

2. Who does the commentator define as *they* in verse 1?

____

____

____

____

3. What were the two types of signs that the Lord sent with the coming of the Holy Spirit?

____

4. According to the verses at the top of the commentary page, what was the sound the people heard?

____

5. What word does the commentator use for wind as he translates the verse? ______________________

6. How is this word defined? ______________________

____

7. Do you think the people felt the wind or only heard the noise from it?

____

Sharing Salvation

Acts 2

Name ______________________________

The day of Pentecost was a time of festival in Jerusalem. Many Jews from the surrounding countries came to the city to celebrate and worship. God chose this special day to send the Holy Spirit to believers.

Through the power of the Holy Spirit, believers were able to share the gospel in the native languages of the unsaved visitors. God used Peter to preach and declare that whoever called on the name of the Lord would be saved. Just as on the day of Pentecost, God uses Christians like Peter to share the truth of the gospel with unbelievers.

Answer the questions.

1. The people heard the sound of a rushing wind when the Holy Spirit came.

   What was seen above the heads of the believers? (Acts 2:3) ______________________________

2. Does the Bible say whether anyone could feel the heat or get burned by the fire? ______________

3. What brought others to the believers? (Acts 2:5-6) ______________________________

4. The people were surprised when they came to the believers. What did they

   hear that surprised them? (Acts 2:6-12) ______________________________

   ____

5. What prophet did Peter refer to as he preached? (Acts 2:16) ______________________________

6. After the people heard Peter's sermon, what did they do? (Acts 2:37-41)

   ____

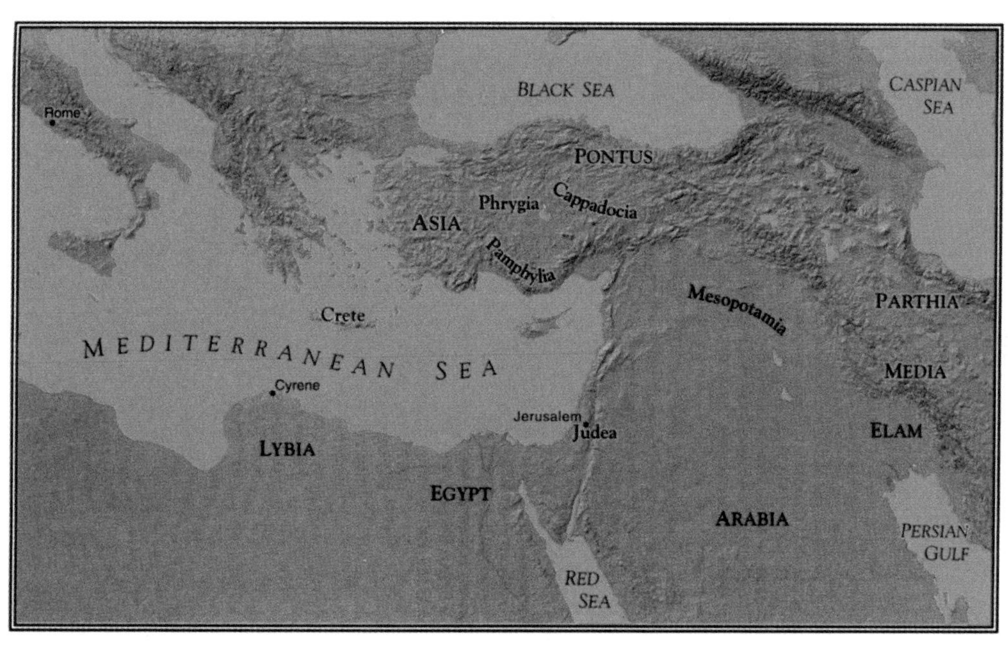

BLACK SEA
CASPIAN SEA
Rome
PONTUS
Phrygia
Cappadocia
ASIA
Pamphylia
Mesopotamia
PARTHIA
Crete
MEDITERRANEAN SEA
MEDIA
Cyrene
Jerusalem
Judea
ELAM
LYBIA
EGYPT
ARABIA
PERSIAN GULF
RED SEA

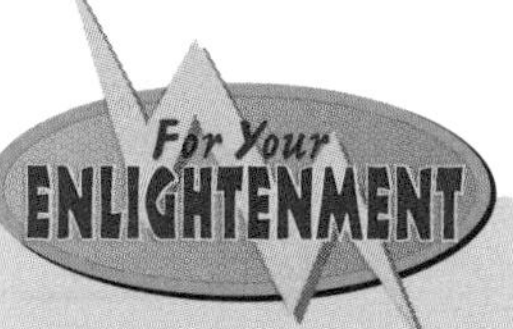

For Your
ENLIGHTENMENT

As Galileans, Peter and the other believers would not have known the fifteen or more foreign languages represented by the people who came. Those who listened expressed their astonishment and recognized this ability as from God (Acts 2:7-12).

Ambassadors for Christ

Acts 3:1–4:30

Name ______________________

The Jews set aside three times each day to pray in the temple (9:00 A.M., 12:00 noon, 3:00 P.M.). Peter and John were going obediently to the temple to pray when they met a lame beggar. The followers of Christ took every opportunity to point others to their Savior.

Answer the questions.

1. What did Peter and John give to the man begging for money? (Acts 3:6)

____

2. After accusing the crowd of not accepting Christ and killing Him, what did Peter tell them they needed to do? (Acts 3:14-15, 19) ______________________

3. Even though the religious leaders could not say anything against the healing of the lame man, they did not want anyone to preach about Jesus. How did Peter and John respond to this restriction? (Acts 4:16-20) ______________________

____

An **ambassador** is someone who is chosen to represent a person, organization, or nation. The United States has ambassadors to most other nations of the world. These ambassadors are appointed to represent the president and the country to the nations in which they serve. Many other nations have ambassadors which represent their governments in America.

While ambassadors are in other countries, they display the flag of their country at the embassy building in which they work.

The biblical use of *ambassador* includes the idea of a messenger delivering a message. Peter and John were ambassadors for Christ. They represented Christ with the message of salvation as they witnessed to those around them.

Draw the flag design for each reference next to the correct description of an ambassador for Christ.

1. Acts 1:8	☐	is blameless and pure; shining as a light in the world
2. Acts 20:24	☐	is not ashamed; is bold and courageous
3. Philippians 1:20	☐	shows love for the lost by sharing the gospel
4. Philippians 1:27	☐	is selfless; thinks Christ, not self
5. Philippians 2:15	☐	has power from the Holy Spirit
6. I Thessalonians 2:8	☐	stands together with other believers

What Does God Say About My Self-Esteem?

Name ______________________

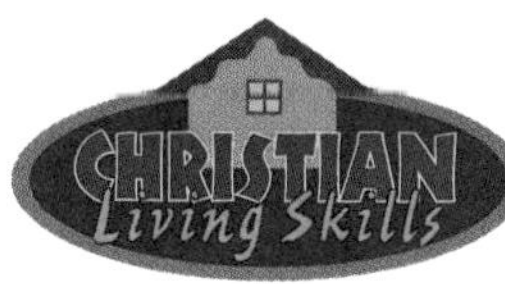
CHRISTIAN
Living Skills

Do you love yourself?

According to the Bible, you do. You'll do whatever you think is best to take good care of yourself. The world calls this love you have for yourself **self-esteem.** In fact, you love yourself so much that Jesus sets up your self-love as a standard for loving others. He tells you that in order for you to fulfill His second great commandment, you should love your neighbor as much as you already love yourself (Matt. 22:39).

Read Ephesians 5:29 and summarize it in your own words.

____

____

Face reality!

God created you with a special purpose in mind. He loved you so much that He sent His Son, Jesus, to die on the cross for your sins. However, the reality is that you are a sinner and can never do anything to save yourself. Your value as a person does not come from you, your talents, or your personality. It comes from the fact that God is merciful and loves you. Everything you have is a gift from God for which you can take no credit. Don't be deceived by the world into becoming prideful about yourself.

Remember that you are nothing without Christ.

What kind of attitude should you have toward yourself? To find out what God says in Romans 12:3, carefully follow the directions. Write the words on the lines as you move; then read the message.

1. From Start, go down 1 space ____________
2. Go right 2 spaces and down 2 ____________
3. Go up 2 spaces and left 1 ____________
4. Go down 2 spaces ____________
5. Go left 1 space and up 1 ____________
6. Go right 2 spaces ____________
7. Go left 1 space and up 2 ____________
8. Go down 3 spaces and left 1 ____________
9. Go up 1 space and right 1 ____________
10. Go up 2 spaces and right 1 ____________

Start	highly	should
Do	think	you
yourself	you	more
than	of	not

Something to Think About

My Self-Esteem

Name ______________________

Christian Living Skills

How do you view yourself?	
The world says...	**The Word of God says...**
focus on feeling good about yourself.	focus on becoming like Christ.
make pleasing yourself your first priority.	make pleasing Christ your first priority.
look for ways to do things for *you*.	look for ways to serve others.
you are a basically good, self-sufficient person.	you are a sinner in need of God's saving grace.
happiness comes from getting what you want.	happiness comes from obedience to God.

Study the differences between what the world says and what God's Word says about how you should view yourself. Read the verses and use the chart to answer the questions.

1. **Philippians 2:3** - What should be my attitude in the way I treat others?

   ____

2. **Galatians 6:3** - When am I deceiving myself?

   ____

3. According to the world, what brings you happiness? ______________________
4. **Romans 3:23** - In what ways does a Christian disagree with the world's view that people are basically good? ______________________

   ____

5. List two ways you can make Christ your first priority.

   1. ______________________ 2. ______________________

What About Me?

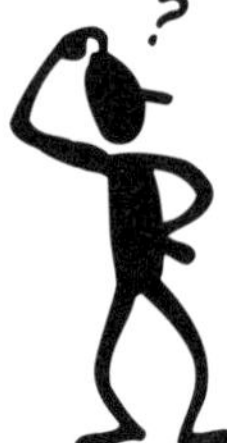

The World vs. The Word

When you have confidence in yourself, the world says you have good self-esteem. It contradicts the view of yourself that the Word of God teaches. Your value as a person comes from God, not you. Don't focus on yourself or on trying to make yourself happy. Instead, focus on becoming more like Christ.

Take time at home to think about the following questions.
Be honest in your evaluation of yourself.

Does my attitude toward others demonstrate a prideful, selfish heart?
Do I look for ways to get what I want, or do I focus on pleasing God?
Do I think more highly of myself than I should?
Do I realize that all I have comes from God and do I give Him the credit for it?

Strength to Suffer

Acts 4:23–5:42

Name ______________________

The Jewish leaders did not approve of the apostles' preaching. They were concerned about the growing number of people following the apostles. Each time an arrest was made, the apostles spoke boldly about Jesus as the Savior. Their preaching to the Jewish council at their trials brought conviction to the hearts of the leaders. This conviction angered the leaders and caused them to want to put the apostles to death. God repeatedly protected and strengthened the apostles and the newly formed church as they continued to share the gospel with others.

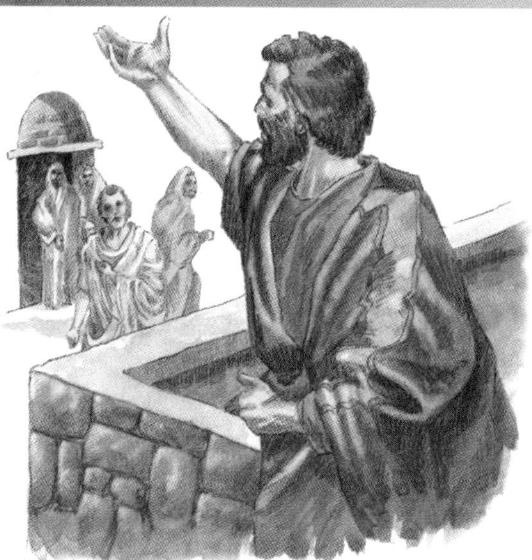

Number the events in order. The first one in each set has been done for you.

_____ 1. The apostles continued to heal the sick and preach about Christ against the wishes of the Jewish leaders.

_____ 2. The angel of the Lord released them from prison.

__1__ 3. Ananias and Sapphira died because they lied about the amount they gave to the church.

_____ 4. The disciples were arrested and placed in prison.

_____ 1. After considering the words of Gamaliel, the council had the apostles beaten, then released.

__1__ 2. The council sent officers to bring the apostles from the temple to their trial.

_____ 3. Peter and the apostles told the council about Christ, and the council wanted to kill them.

_____ 4. Gamaliel told the council that if the preaching of the apostles was of God, there was nothing they could do to stop it.

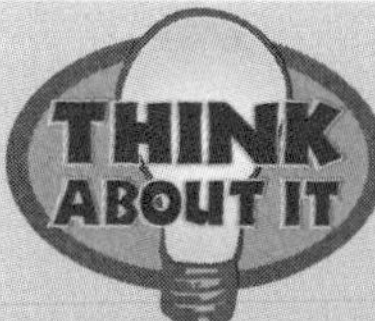
THINK
ABOUT IT

The apostles rejoiced when they suffered for Christ. They considered it an honor to be worthy to suffer. They obeyed the command to preach and believed the promise of Christ that He would be with them and supply them with the power necessary to obey. Christ made the same promise to all believers.

Write two commands God has given you to obey.

1. ____

2. ____

Ask God to provide the strength you need to be bold and obey.

Things Eternal

Colossians 3:1-2, 8-14

Name ____________________

Peter and the early Christians were often persecuted for preaching the gospel and telling others about Christ. They faced their trials on earth by looking to their future home in heaven. Their attitudes toward things and circumstances on earth changed as they grew closer to God.

Today's Christians may not have the same trials and difficulties as those experienced by the early Christians, but they still fight the temptation to focus on the things of the world around them. Remember God's Word as you make decisions throughout the day.

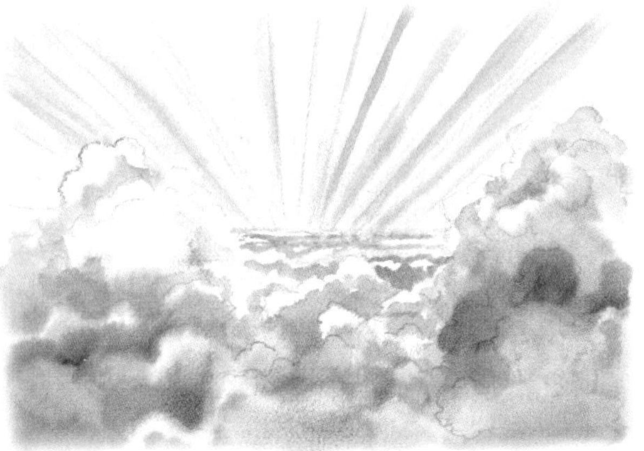

Write the correct word to complete each sentence.

1. Christians should remove sinful practices from their lives and ____________ themselves in the knowledge of God (Col. 3:10).

2. Christians should replace their sinfulness with things of God such as ____________________

    ____

    ____ (Col. 3:12-14).

3. Of the things Christians should add to their lives, the most important one is

    ____________________, which brings a bond of unity between believers (Col. 3:14).

Circle the choice that shows whether the person was thinking on eternal things or things of this earth.

eternal	earthly	1. Kyle spends time daily with God reading His Word and praying.
eternal	earthly	2. Jessica clutches the coins in her pocket as the missionary offering box passes her in Sunday school. She assures herself that plenty will be given by the other students and she can save hers for herself.
eternal	earthly	3. Sarah gives one of her necklaces to a girl in her class that doesn't own any jewelry.
eternal	earthly	4. Jared wants to punch the boy who just insulted him, but Jared stops and asks God to help him be kind instead.
eternal	earthly	5. Kitasha plans a shopping trip with her mom so she will not feel obligated to help her class from church serve supper at the rescue mission.

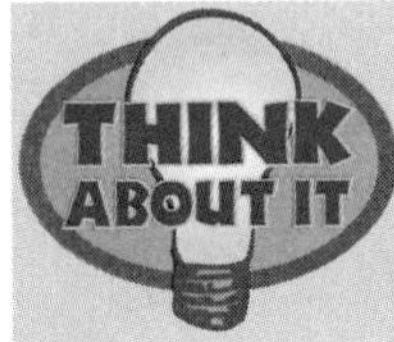
THINK
ABOUT IT

Think about the choices you have already made today. Have you asked God to help you with your decisions? God is always willing and ready to help guide believers. Take a moment to ask God for help and wisdom as you go through today.

Strength to Die

Acts 6-7

Name ______________________

As the early church grew, the apostles needed help meeting the needs of the believers while still preaching the Word. The group of disciples chose seven men to help the apostles. One of the men chosen was Stephen.

Fill in the circle beside the correct word or phrase to complete each sentence.

1. Stephen was chosen because he was full of _____ (Acts 6:5).
   ○ grace and truth ○ faith and the Holy Spirit ○ wisdom and godly knowledge
2. As the Word of God spread and the number of disciples grew, many _____ also trusted Christ (Acts 6:7).
   ○ priests ○ Pharisees ○ Sadducees
3. Men from the synagogue knew that Stephen spoke with wisdom and the Spirit, but they convinced false witnesses to say that Stephen had said _____ God and Moses (Acts 6:9-11).
   ○ truth about ○ he was equal with ○ blasphemies against
4. When Stephen faced the council, his face looked like the face of _____ (Acts 6:15).
   ○ an angel ○ a demon-possessed man ○ John the Baptist
5. The high priest asked Stephen if the accusations against him were true. Stephen answered with a sermon, explaining the history of the Jews and how they repeatedly turned away from God. Stephen then accused the religious leaders of being like their forefathers and _____ the Holy Spirit (Acts 7:51).
   ○ following ○ resisting ○ blaspheming
6. As the religious leaders attacked him, Stephen looked _____ and saw Christ at the right hand of God (Acts 7:55).
   ○ toward heaven ○ at the crowd ○ at the altar
7. The men laid their coats at the feet of _____ while they stoned Stephen (Acts 7:58).
   ○ the Pharisees ○ Stephen ○ Saul
8. Before Stephen died, he prayed that the Lord would _____ (Acts 7:59-60).
   ○ condemn them ○ not hold this sin against them ○ save him from death

Write one thing about Stephen's trial or punishment and his responses that shows Stephen was trusting God.

____

____

____

Not Ashamed

Romans 10:9-13

Name ______________________

Some religious leaders believed on Christ, but were not willing to confess the Lord for fear of being turned away from the synagogue. They were more concerned about what others thought rather than what God thought of them (John 12:42-43). Others, such as Stephen, willingly shared the truth of the gospel with all who would hear. Stephen was willing to die rather than deny that Jesus is Lord.

Read Romans 10:9-13 and answer the questions.

1. What must be confessed? ______________________
2. What about Jesus must be believed? ______________________
3. What is the result of confession and belief in Jesus as the resurrected Lord? ______________________
4. Does the Lord think differently about Jews or Greeks? ______________________
5. Do you think the Lord looks at any of the races differently today? ______________________
6. The Lord is rich with abundant blessings. Who does He bless? ______________________
7. Who is saved? ______________________

Although people often look at the many physical differences between others, the Lord looks only at one difference—their spiritual conditions. God's focus is not on what people look like, how much money they have, or what kind of grades they make. The Lord sees each person as a soul either having or needing salvation. The Lord looks for those seeking salvation and His blessings. He gladly receives all who believe in Him and call on His name.

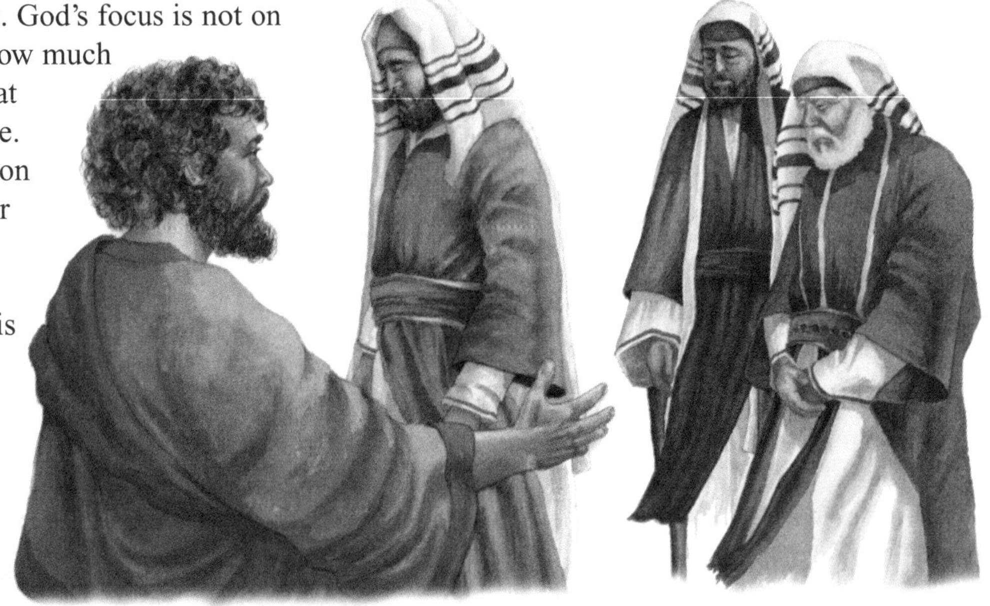

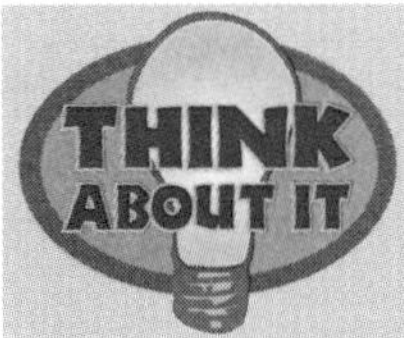
THINK
ABOUT IT

What does God see when He looks at your heart? Does He see a heart that loves Him and has accepted Jesus as Savior? Or, does He see a soul that has heard His message of salvation and has not yet chosen to yield to Him?

What Does God Say About Temptation?

Name ______________________

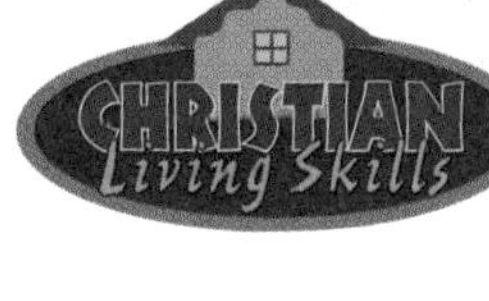

CHRISTIAN
Living Skills

A **temptation** is anything that has the power to attract you to do something wrong. Every person faces temptations to do wrong. Many choose to give in to these temptations. Christians don't have to give in. They have the power of the Holy Spirit to resist. *Remember:* Satan is clever and he can deceive you by making sin look very good. After all, he wants you to fall for it. He would like to destroy you and your Christian testimony.

Read James 4:7 and answer the questions.

1. What are you to do when the devil tempts you to do wrong? ______________________
2. What will happen if you resist the devil? ______________________

While temptations are real and powerful, God will give you the victory over them. His Word provides the keys to victorious Christian living.

Read the verses and match them to the correct statement about temptations.

_____ 1. God knows how to deliver me from temptations.

_____ 2. God will bless me if I endure temptations and trials.

_____ 3. I must watch out for temptations.

_____ 4. Because Jesus was tempted, He is able to help me fight temptation.

A. James 1:12
B. Matthew 26:41
C. Hebrews 2:18
D. II Peter 2:9

The Bible also teaches that your own sinful heart is deceitful and is capable of tempting you to sin against God.

Read James 1:13-16 and complete the statements.

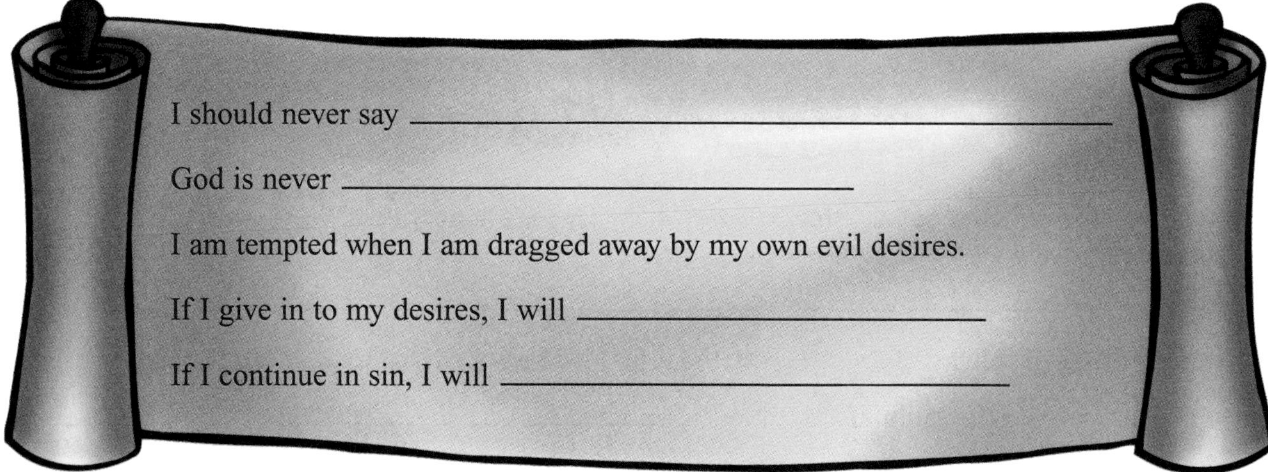

I should never say ______________________
God is never ______________________
I am tempted when I am dragged away by my own evil desires.
If I give in to my desires, I will ______________________
If I continue in sin, I will ______________________

Name ______________________

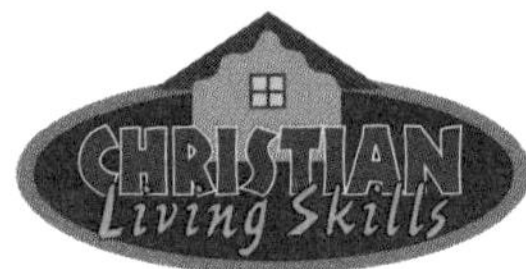
CHRISTIAN
Living Skills

You should be ready for battle when you begin to fight temptation!

It can be an exhausting fight! God has promised Christians the victory over temptation if they will choose to please Him rather than themselves.

Read I Corinthians 10:13 and complete the statements to give advice to someone who needs encouragement to fight temptation.

1. You are not the only one ______________________
2. God is ______________________
3. God will never let you be tempted more ______________________
4. Every time you are tempted, God will provide a ______________________
5. He will help you to be able to ______________________

Use the Word of God to fight your battle!

Ephesians 6:17 calls the Word of God your sword. Any soldier who is getting ready to win a battle must learn to use his weapon effectively. This is also true for you. If you want to win, memorize the Word of God and have this sword of truth ready to use against the attacks of temptations. You have been given everything you need to fight temptation, and there is no excuse for you to lose.

Read the scenarios and verses. Then write the correct reference on the sword to fight that temptation.

When Meshell's mom asked her if she had completed her work, Meshell was tempted to say that she had because she really wanted to spend the night with Kristin.

Psalm 101:3
Proverbs 16:18
Ephesians 4:25

Rachel was curious about the new teen program on TV because she had heard kids at school talking about it. She knew that the characters on the show didn't dress modestly and that they talked about witchcraft.

Joey does better than his brother and sister in math, and he is sure that they must be jealous. He is tempted to look down on them because they don't do as well on their school work.

What About Me?

Take time at home to write out an effective plan of victory for the next time you are attacked by a personal temptation.

TEMPTATION: ______________________

Scripture verse I will use to attack it: (Write the reference.) ______________________

How I will avoid this temptation in the future: ______________________

____

Prophet Focus

Habakkuk (9 B.C.)

Name ______________________

Habakkuk was troubled that, although Judah had become wicked, they seemed to prosper. He thought Judah deserved punishment rather than prosperity. If Habakkuk could see the wickedness of the people, surely God could. The Lord calmly answered Habakkuk's frustration by telling him that He knew Judah was sinning against Him. It was His plan to bring them back to Him by using the mighty Babylonians (Chaldeans) to take Judah captive.

Even though Habakkuk praised God's holiness, he questioned why God would use a nation more wicked than Judah as He judged them for their sin. God assured Habakkuk that wickedness would be punished in His time. Habakkuk was to write God's message for others to see, then wait patiently and watch the Lord work.

The Lord declared five woes or sorrows to the Babylonians and those who sin against Him and His principles.

1. *Woe to him who becomes wealthy and powerful from goods that are not his.*
2. *Woe to him who trusts the splendor and protection of buildings.*
3. *Woe to him who builds a town on the bloodshed of others.*
4. *Woe to him who is friendly to others only to take advantage of them.*
5. *Woe to him who trusts in idols instead of the Lord in His holy temple.*

After receiving answers from the Lord, Habakkuk confirmed his trust in God and His wisdom with a prayer-like psalm. Habakkuk proclaimed that he would rejoice in the Lord and trust Him for strength.

Answer the questions.

1. What two things did Habakkuk think God was not handling properly concerning Judah?

____

____

2. What was God's plan for punishing the sin of Judah? ______________________

____

3. When did God plan to punish the wickedness?

____

4. How did Habakkuk react to God's answers?

____

5. Although the "woes" were directed toward the Babylonians (Chaldeans), do you think Judah was guilty of any of these sins? If so, write the numbers of the ones you think Judah had committed.

____

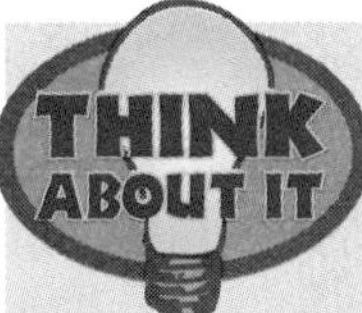
THINK
ABOUT IT

Do you ever feel that God is not handling a situation the way you want? What two things can you remember about God's answers to Habakkuk that can help you when you feel this way?

____

____

Name ____________________

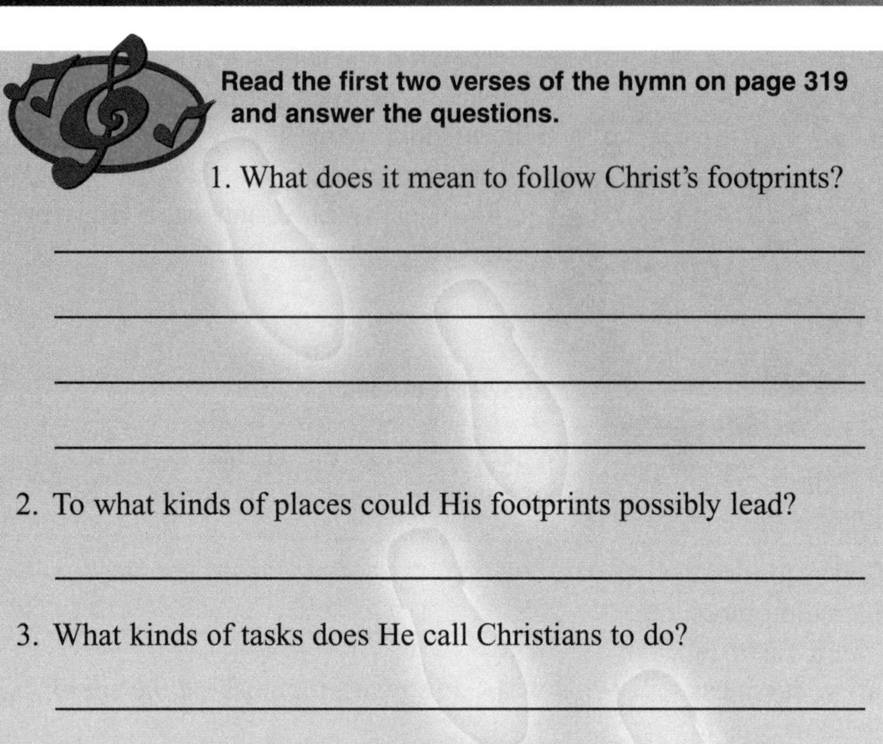

Read the first two verses of the hymn on page 319 and answer the questions.

1. What does it mean to follow Christ's footprints?

____

____

____

____

2. To what kinds of places could His footprints possibly lead?

____

3. What kinds of tasks does He call Christians to do?

____

____

____

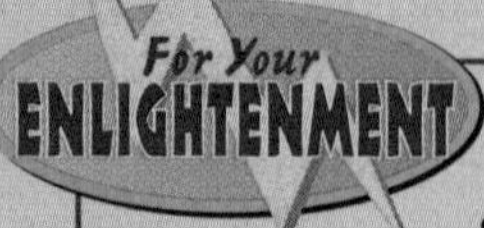
For Your
ENLIGHTENMENT

The name Siloam means "sent." Siloam was the location of the pool where Christ sent the blind man to wash the clay from his eyes. When the man washed the clay away, he could see. In the hymn "Footprints of Jesus," the hymn writer uses the name Siloam to represent the places where we can find weak, faithless people, blinded by their own sin.

Footprints of Jesus
that make the pathway glow

Answer the question using one of the verses in your answer.

4. Why does the hymn writer say that following the example of Jesus will make our pathway glow?

- **Psalm 16:11**
- **Psalm 119:35**
- **Psalm 119:105**
- **Proverbs 4:18**
- **Proverbs 12:28**
- **Proverbs 16:17**

____

____

____

____

____

To Samaria

Acts 8:1-40

Name ______________________

Write the correct word to complete each sentence. You may use your Bible for help.

1. ____________________ scattered believers from Jerusalem into Judea and Samaria (Acts 8:1).
2. Philip went to ____________________ to preach about Christ (Acts 8:5).
3. As Philip spoke and performed miracles, many people believed on Christ and were ____________________ (Acts 8:12).
4. Peter and John came from ____________________ when they heard of the many souls that were saved in Samaria (Acts 8:14).
5. Simon, a man baptized with the believers, offered the apostles ____________________ to purchase the power to give others the Holy Spirit (Acts 8:18-19).
6. Peter told Simon to ____________________ of his wickedness (Acts 8:22).

Find each answer from above in the puzzle below.

H	I	P	S	T	O
R	Y	E	B	E	B
L	S	R	I	J	A
E	A	S	V	E	P
R	M	E	E	R	T
E	A	C	R	U	I
P	R	U	S	S	Z
E	I	T	M	A	E
N	A	I	O	L	D
T	S	O	N	E	P
R	E	N	E	M	A
D	S	T	Y	O	P

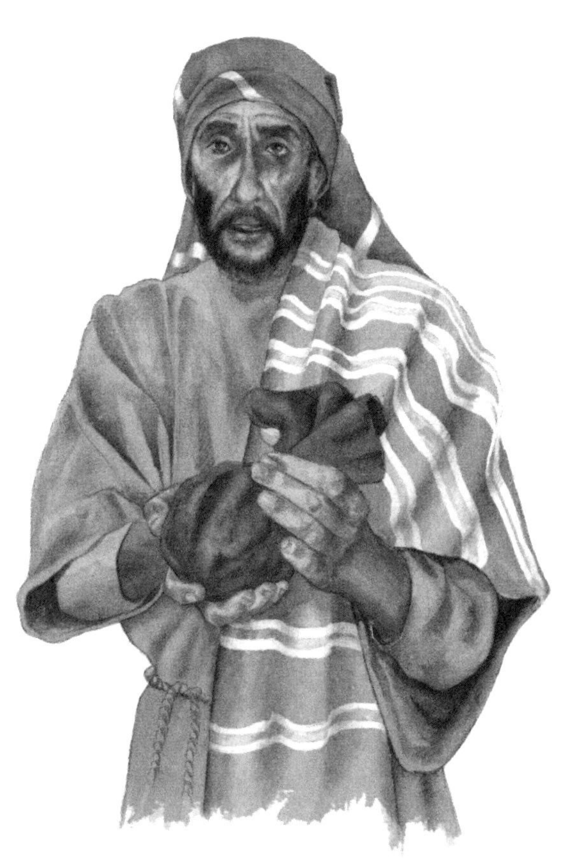

Reading from left to right, write the remaining letters in order to complete the sentence.

Throughout ___ ___ ___ ___ ___ ___ ___, persecution of

___ ___ ___ ___ ___ ___ ___ ___ ___ has helped ___ ___ ___ ___ ___ ___

the gospel rather than ___ ___ ___ ___ it!

From Samaria

Name ______________________________

Persecution in Jerusalem caused Philip to go to Samaria. In Samaria, Philip preached the gospel. Once the body of believers was established, Peter and John returned to Jerusalem, but God had other plans for Philip.

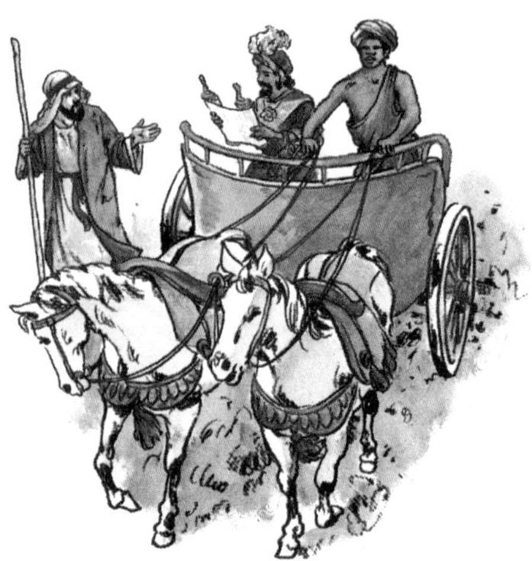

Read Acts 8:25-40 and answer the questions.

1. How did Philip know where to go?

   ____

2. Who had God prepared for Philip to meet? ____________

3. What was the man reading? ____________

4. What was Philip able to teach him through this passage?

   ____

   ____

5. What did the Ethiopian know he must do as soon as he believed on Christ? ____________

6. Those traveling with the Ethiopian must have witnessed his bold testimony as he humbled himself in baptism. Do you think he would have been bold to tell others of Christ when he returned to Ethiopia? ____________

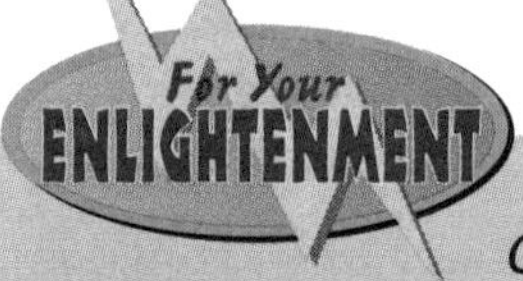
For Your
ENLIGHTENMENT

Queen Candace was an Ethiopian title for the position rather than the specific name of the queen. The title of Pharaoh was used the same way in Egypt.

At this time, personal copies of Scripture were hand copied and very expensive. The Ethiopian probably had some wealth because of his position in the royal court, which made it possible to own a copy.

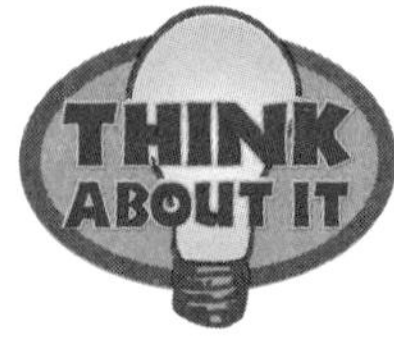
THINK
ABOUT IT

You never know the influence your testimony might have on others—future missionaries and pastors may be around you. Are you a help or a hindrance to their spiritual growth? Are you like Philip and willing to go out of your way to share the gospel?

Have you ever heard someone say that he has read the Bible, but not understood it? Maybe you have said this yourself about certain verses. This is the same thing the Ethiopian told Philip. But Philip was able to clearly explain the Scriptures. How could Philip do this?

Read I Corinthians 2:13-16 and answer the question.

Unbelievers are not able to understand spiritual things. What does a person need to understand the things of God? (I Cor. 2:14) ______________________________

The Holy Spirit lives in every Christian. Pray that God will increase your understanding of spiritual things as you read and study God's Word.

How Shall They Hear?

Romans 10:14-15

Name ____________________

Sometimes when someone looks in an encyclopedia for the answer to a question, other questions come to his mind that need to be answered. As questions continue to arise and are answered, a broader understanding of the subject is formed.

Teachers often use a similar method to help students arrive at correct answers. If the teacher asks a question that cannot be answered by the students, then the teacher may reword the question slightly to include information the students do know. By asking a series of questions, the teacher hopes the students will come to answer the original question.

In Romans 10:13, God uses Paul to state the fact that all who call on the name of the Lord will be saved. This statement is followed by a series of questions to help Christians arrive at God's desired conclusion.

Complete each sentence.

A **preacher** is one who proclaims and teaches God's truth. Today we think of a preacher as a pastor of a church. But any Christian who shares the gospel is a preacher.

1. God says that for people to call on His name, they must ____________________.
2. For people to believe, they must have ____________________ about Christ and salvation.
3. For people to hear about the Savior, they must have a ____________________.
4. For preachers to tell others of Christ, they must be ______________ to the people that need to hear.

Answer the questions.

1. What message do you think God was teaching the believers at Rome? ____________________

____

2. Does this same message apply to Christians today? __________
3. Romans 10:15 says, "as it is written," which means that the following words are from a previous passage of Scripture. Read Isaiah 52:7. According to Isaiah, what things does a preacher do?

____

____

4. Why do you think God says the feet of a preacher are beautiful? ____________________

____

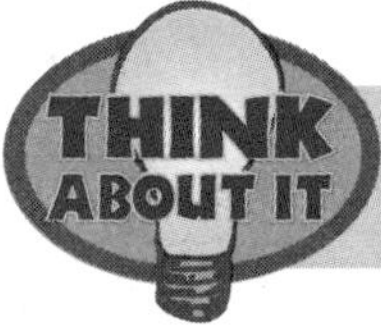
THINK
ABOUT IT

Have you been obedient to preach the gospel of Christ? If so, how have you shared the gospel recently?

Prepared to Give and Receive

Acts 10

Name ____________________

Complete the outline for Acts 10.
Next to each Roman numeral, write the correct heading.
Next to each letter write the correct supporting sentence for each heading.

Peter preached about salvation through Christ.
The Lord prepared Peter to preach to the Gentiles.
Cornelius prayed regularly and gave offerings.
Peter obeyed God and went to Cornelius.
Cornelius was seeking the Lord.
God taught Peter to take the gospel to people whom the Jews considered unclean.

I. ____________________

A. ____________________

B. An angel told Cornelius to send for Peter.

II. ____________________

A. God gave Peter a vision and commanded him to eat the unclean animals, which went against Jewish tradition.

B. ____________________

____

III. ____________________

A. ____________________

B. Cornelius and those who heard Peter accepted Christ and were baptized.

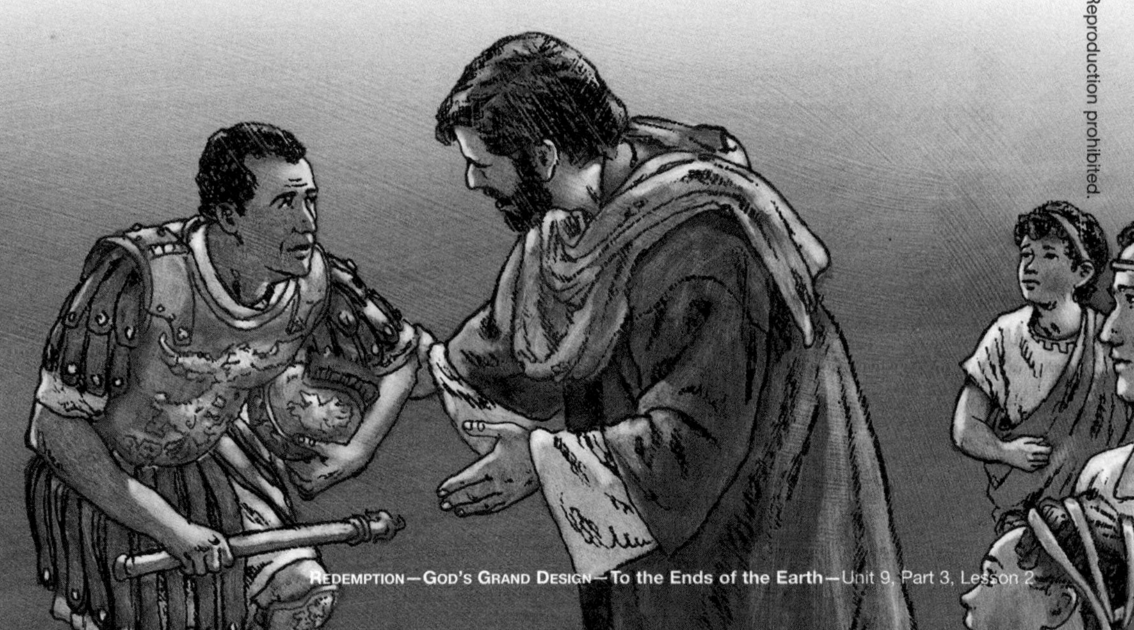

What Does God Say About Witnessing?

Name ______________________________

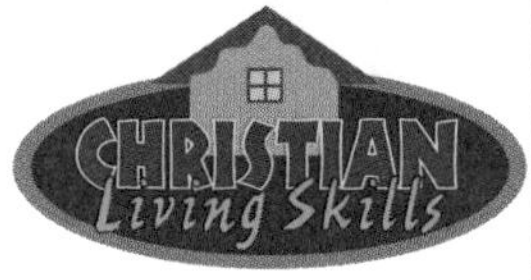
CHRISTIAN
Living Skills

Christians have thrilling news to tell others!

If you won a million dollars, you would want to tell everyone about it. You would be so excited that you probably wouldn't be able to sleep! If you are a Christian, you have even better news—you have personally experienced God's amazing forgiveness of sin. A Christian knows that God has saved him from the consequences of his sin and that he will spend eternity with God in heaven. This is exciting, life-changing news! Christians can't help but want to tell others about how they can be saved from sin too.

Read Matthew 28:19-20 and write God's four commands to Christians in your own words. Also include Jesus' promise to Christians.

____

____

____

Every Christian has a God-given responsibility to tell others about the saving power of Jesus Christ. Doing this is being a **witness** to others about Jesus.

Using the glossary, write the definitions for both the noun and verb forms of *witness.*

Noun: ____

Verb: ____

Christians have suffered persecution for centuries for sharing the good news of salvation. No one wants to hear that he is a sinner and on his way to hell. No one likes to admit that he is wrong. However, a Christian must respectfully and lovingly speak the truth to others, even if he is mocked and made fun of for sharing about Christ.

Read the verses. Write the reference in the puzzle piece with the correct statement about witnessing to others.

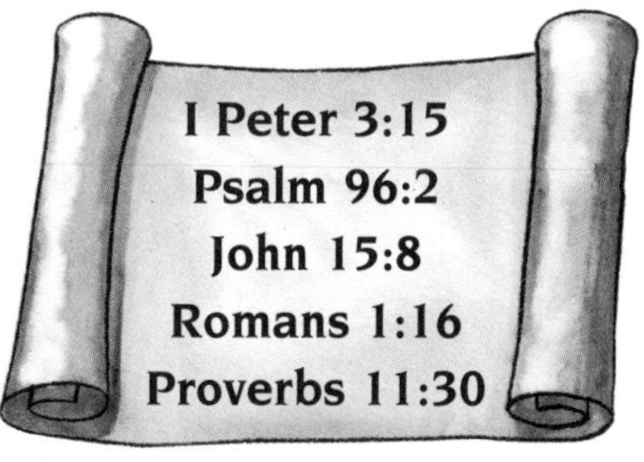
I Peter 3:15
Psalm 96:2
John 15:8
Romans 1:16
Proverbs 11:30

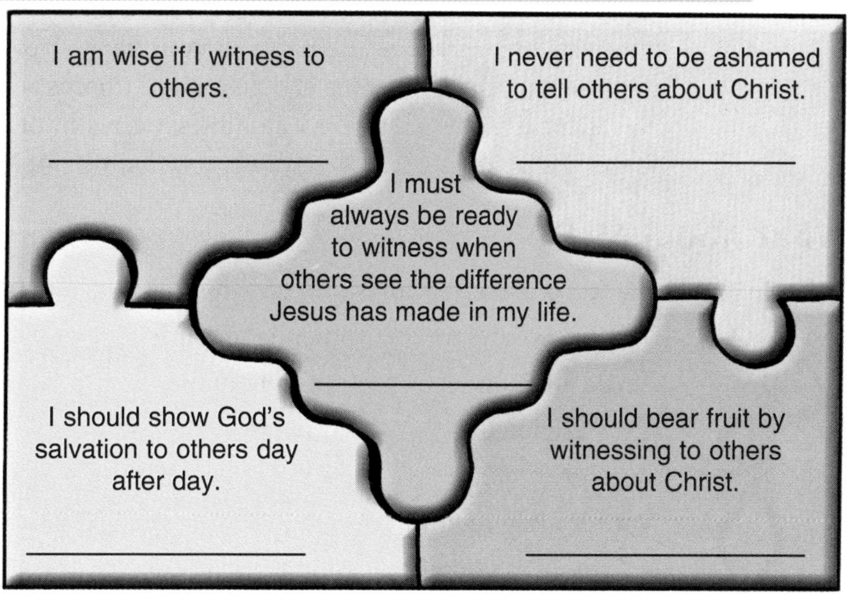
I am wise if I witness to others.
I never need to be ashamed to tell others about Christ.
I must always be ready to witness when others see the difference Jesus has made in my life.
I should show God's salvation to others day after day.
I should bear fruit by witnessing to others about Christ.

Something to Think About

Witnessing

Name ____________________________

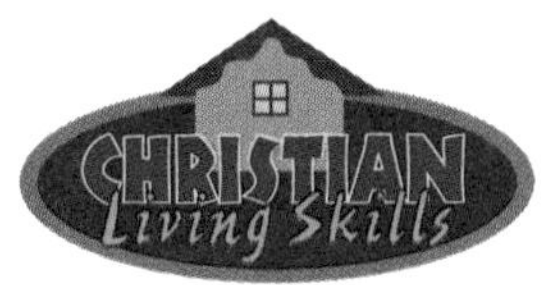
CHRISTIAN
Living Skills

Have you ever witnessed to someone? If you are a Christian, it is your responsibility to tell other people what Jesus has done for you. Can *you* give a good answer to someone if he asks you why you are sure you are going to heaven when you die? What if he asks you who Jesus is? What will you say? Are you ready to witness?

Read the verses and complete the statements which help you witness to someone about Jesus Christ.

Romans 3:23	Everyone has ________________ and fallen short of God's glory.
Romans 6:23	Because we have sinned, we deserve __________. However, God has provided the gift of ________________ through Jesus Christ our Lord.
John 20:31	Jesus is the Christ, the Son of God. If we believe in Jesus, we will have ________.
Ephesians 2:8-9	You are saved by ________. Salvation is a gift from God. Good works cannot save you, or people would ________ about being good enough to earn their own salvation.
Romans 10:9	If you confess with your mouth the Lord Jesus and __________ in your heart that God has raised Him from the dead, you will be __________.

What kind of witness are you?

The most straightforward way to witness to others about Christ is to *tell* them about Him. However, always remember that the way you dress, the expression on your face, the things you do, and your attitude are also witnesses to others about what is in your heart. Never forget the importance of giving other people a good impression of your Savior. Never forget that others are watching your testimony every day. Never forget that there are people around you that do not know Christ.

What About Me?

Take time at home to consider the following questions and evaluate your current witness to others.

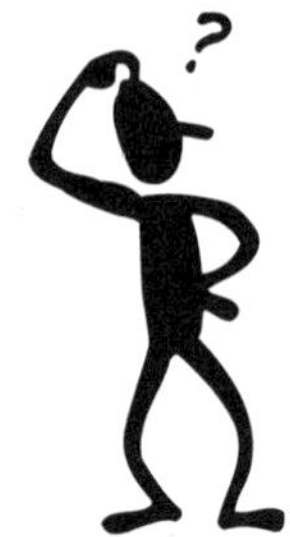

Do I know how to lead someone to Christ?
Have I memorized Scripture to help me lead someone to Christ?
Am I ashamed to be a bold witness for Christ?
Does my attitude give a good impression to others about Jesus Christ?
Am I willing to suffer persecution for telling others about Christ?
Is God pleased with my actions to win others to Christ?

Being a Witness

Making and Using a Tract

Name ______________________

The apostles had witnessed Christ's miracles and teaching while He was on earth. As they spread the message of salvation, they could tell others what they had seen and heard.

Answer the questions.

1. How can believers see Christ work today?

____

____

2. How can believers know what to say about Christ and salvation?

____

____

One way to tell others of Christ is to give a **testimony.** A testimony may include retelling how a believer accepted Christ as Savior. Some testimonies include examples of answered prayer or ways Christ is currently working in the life of the Christian.

Directions for making tract are on page 262.

4

I Corinthians 15:3-4 says
Christ died for our sins,
was buried, and rose again.

5

Ephesians 2:8-9 says
Salvation is a gift from God.
No one is saved by doing good.

6

Romans 10:9 says
Trust Jesus to be your Savior.

7

Romans 10:10 says
A believer tells others
of salvation.

Salvation Tract

Name ______________________

A **tract** is useful when sharing Christ with others. This tract is prepared with suggested verses to help show someone how to find salvation through Christ.

Keep the tract handy to use as you witness and share your testimony. Pray for opportunities to use your tract.

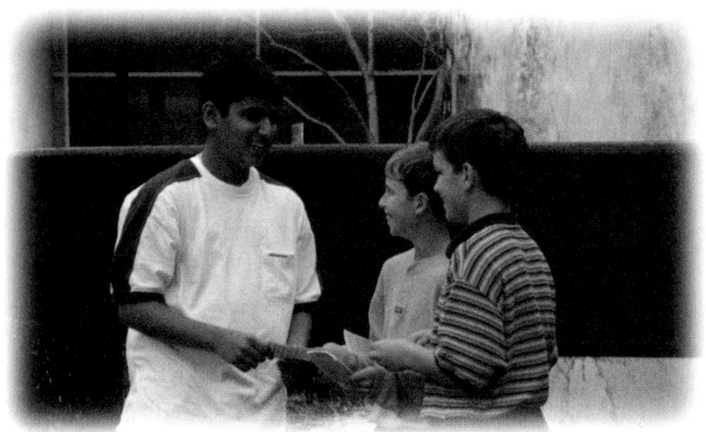

To prepare the tract for use, cut along the bold line around the outside of the tract.

Lay tract with pages 4-7 showing. Fold pages 4 and 7 toward center so edges touch. Crease on dotted lines.

Fold pages 2 and 3 to the inside; crease on dotted line.

Personalize the tract by writing on page 8 the phone number of your church.

Practice using the tract with one or two others in your class or family.

3

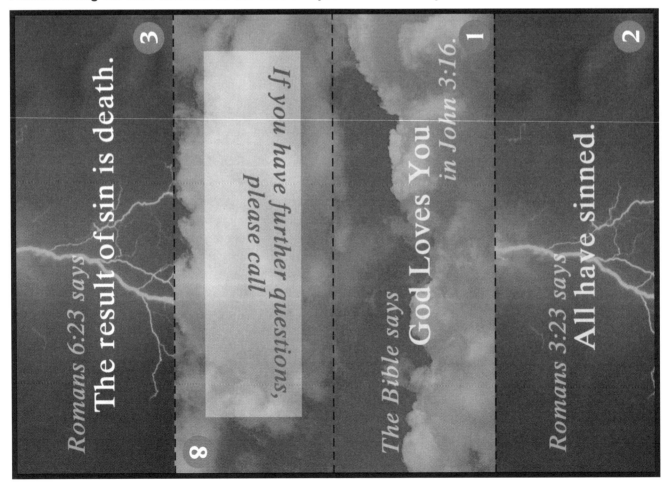

Romans 6:23 says
The result of sin is death.

8

If you have further questions, please call

1

The Bible says
God Loves You
in John 3:16.

2

Romans 3:23 says
All have sinned.

Persecutor to Missionary

Acts 9, 13-14

Name ____________________

Answer the questions.

1. How does Acts 9:1 describe Saul before his conversion? ____________________

2. How does Acts 9:20 describe Saul after his conversion?

Complete the puzzle.

Across

3. The believers in ___ were ministering to the Lord and worshiping when God told them that He was calling Barnabas and Saul to do a work for Him (Acts 13:1-2).
5. As they entered each city, Barnabas and Saul, now called Paul, went to the ___ to speak of Christ to the Jews (Acts 13:5, 14; 14:1).
6. When Paul spoke to the Jews, he showed them that the prophecies given by God were fulfilled in ___ (Acts 13:32-33, 38-39).
8. ___ worked with Barnabas and Saul while they were in Cyprus. He went to Jerusalem rather than continuing with Barnabas and Saul as they sailed to Pamphylia (Acts 13:5, 13).
9. In Lystra the people thought Paul and Barnabas were ___ after they healed a lame man (Acts 14:11).

Down

1. After Paul rebuked a ___ prophet and the prophet was made blind, a government official believed on Christ (Acts 13:6-12).
2. When the apostles would not believe that Saul had become a Christian, ___ took Saul to the apostles and told them of his conversion and preaching of Christ (Acts 9:27).
4. After they returned to Antioch, Paul and Barnabas gathered the ___ together and gave a report of what God had done (Acts 14:27).
6. Because many people followed the preaching of Paul and Barnabas, the ___ and other leaders often stirred the people against them until they left their cities (Acts 13:50; 14:2).
7. Some Jews led the people to turn against Paul and they ___ him. The believers helped Paul until he left for Derbe with Barnabas (Acts 14:19-20).
9. Paul quoted the Old Testament when he told the Jews that God wanted His Word to be a light to the ___ (Acts 13:46-47).

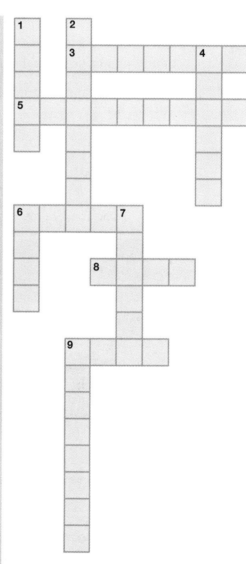

1
2
3
4
5
6
7
8
9

THINK ABOUT IT Before Paul and Barnabas were called by God, they and the Antioch believers were being obedient to what they knew God desired all Christians to do. They were faithful and obedient where they were and God sent them to faithfully and obediently share the gospel with others. Are you faithful and obedient to do what you know the Bible says for you to do? What have you done to obey God today?

Paul, the Missionary Example

Acts 13-14

Name ____________________

Most missionary programs today follow the example set by Paul on his first missionary journey.

Write the letter of the reference of Paul's example in Acts next to the correct sentence about modern missions.

A. Acts 13:1
B. Acts 14:27
C. Acts 13:2
D. Acts 13:4
E. Acts 13:3

_____ 1. God calls missionaries to His service.

_____ 2. Most missionaries have a home church that sends them to the field.

_____ 3. Before missionaries leave for their fields, pastors and spiritual leaders may commission or dedicate them for service.

_____ 4. Missionaries follow the direction of the Holy Spirit as they choose a place of service.

_____ 5. When they return home, missionaries visit their sending churches and report on God's working in their ministry.

From Paul, Christians can learn three main aspects of the ministry of a missionary.

1. By *blazing a trail*, a missionary prepares the way for other missionaries and pastors to follow. Like all Christians, a missionary should not needlessly offend others as the gospel is presented. His desire should be to leave people open for future witnessing opportunities.
2. As missionaries *broadcast the gospel,* they tell all who will listen of Christ and the salvation found in Him. Missionaries use a variety of methods to gain opportunities to talk with people about salvation. A believer may share salvation through tract distribution, visitation, singing, or playing music and giving puppet shows in a park.
3. After a missionary leads someone to accept salvation through Christ, he begins the ministry of *building the believer.* Missionaries help new believers study their Bibles and learn more about Christ while the new Christian starts sharing the gospel with others. Since missionaries are also believers, those at home can help build them by praying for them, writing to them, helping with their physical needs, or actually going to help them with special projects.

Answer the question.

6. What does God command all Christians to do in Mark 16:15?

____

This command makes all Christians missionaries.

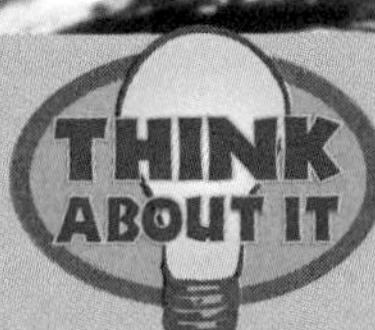
THINK ABOUT IT

Are you obeying this command of God?

What work of a missionary have you done in your neighborhood?

____

How have you helped a pastor or missionary do his work for the Lord?

____

Encouraging Believers

Acts 15:36–18:22

Name ______________________

Answer the questions.

1. Who traveled with Paul on his second missionary journey? (Acts 15:40) ______________
2. Why did the apostles and elders in Jerusalem send decisions with Paul to the elders of the new churches? (Acts 16:4-5) ______________
3. Did God always permit Paul to go to the places he wanted? (Acts 16:6-7) ______________

   How did Paul know where to go? ______________
4. What did God use to tell Paul to go to the region of Macedonia? (Acts 16:9-10)

   ____

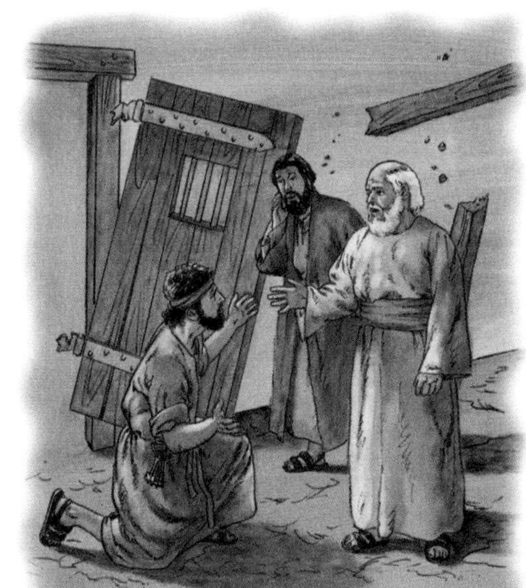

5. Before Paul cast an evil spirit from a girl, the spirit recognized Paul and Silas as servants of God showing the way of salvation. How do you think the evil spirit knew who they were? (Acts 16:17)

   ____
6. When Paul and Silas were in prison, what did they do that might have helped the jailer know they knew the way of salvation? (Acts 16:25)

   ____
7. What promise did God give Paul while he was in Corinth? (Acts 18:9-10) ______________

   ____

How are you to know what to do each day? ______________

How do you know what the Holy Spirit is saying? ______________

____

Remember, in the Old Testament, how Joseph recognized that God used the difficulties in his life for good? How did God use the difficulty between Paul and Barnabas for good (Acts 15:39-40)?

____

____

Often when Paul preached, he told the people about a familiar aspect of their religion and how it lacked truth from God. Paul showed them how Christ is the answer to their needs. What can you learn from this as you share the gospel with others?

____

____

Name ______________________

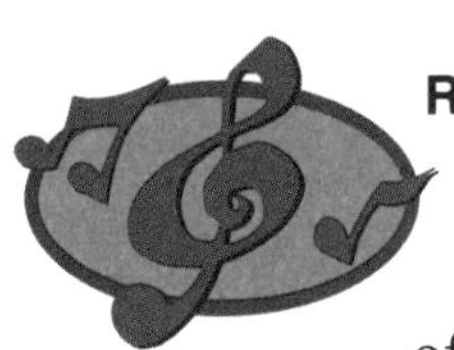

Read verses 3 and 4 of the hymn on page 319 and answer the questions.

1. Where does the journey end for the Christian who follows the steps of the Lord Jesus? ______________________

2. Read Colossians 3:23-24. What is promised to those who faithfully serve Christ?

____

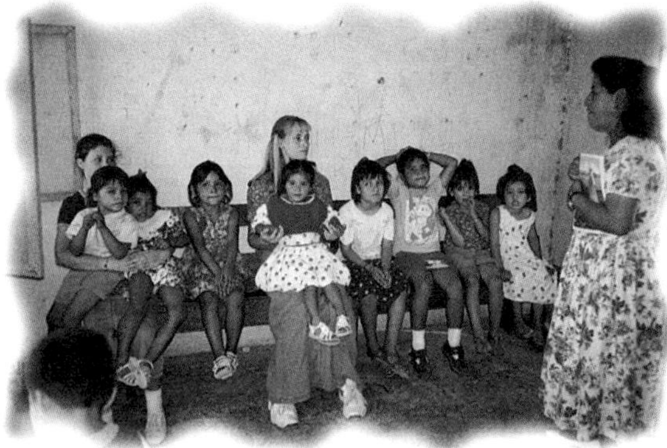

The temple holy

The Lord calls some people to serve Him in a full-time ministry such as pastoring a church, traveling as an evangelist, teaching in a Christian school, working as a missionary nurse or a Bible translator. Perhaps the Lord will call you into such a ministry someday. What could you be doing right now to prepare yourself?

____

____

____

Homes of the poor and lowly

Perhaps you live in an area where there are needy people without Christ. What could you do to help people in need?

Write two of your own ideas.

- I could offer to help them with yard jobs.
- My family and I could donate to the Thanksgiving food basket collection at church.
- I could take them a plate of homemade cookies.
- ______________________
- ______________________

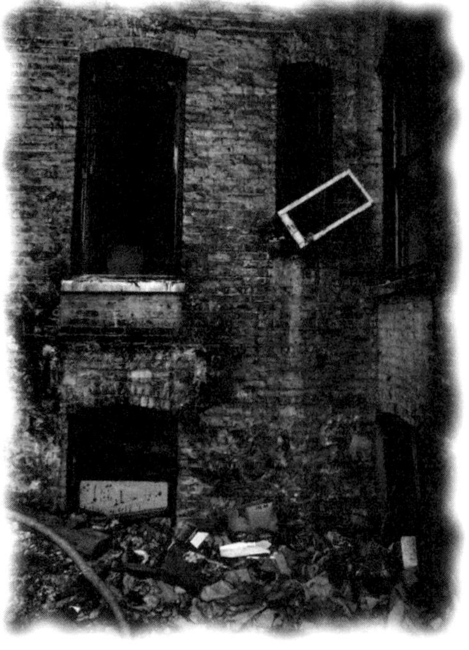

Are you really willing to follow the footprints of Jesus wherever they go?

I Am With You

Matthew 28:19-20

Name ______________________

After His death and resurrection, Jesus appeared to the eleven disciples (apostles) before returning to heaven. Jesus reminded them that He had been given all the power and authority in heaven and in earth. He then gave them a command.

Read Matthew 28:19-20 and answer the questions.

1. Where were the apostles to go? (Matt. 28:19) ______________________
2. What two things were the apostles to do as they went? ______________________
____
3. What were the apostles to teach the new disciples? (Matt. 28:20) ______________________
____
4. As Jesus finished the command, what promise did He give the apostles? ______________________
____
5. How did the apostles know Jesus would keep His promise? ______________________
____
____

Christians are reminded of God's command to witness, but when someone does accept the Lord, what are Christians to do next? Jesus told the apostles to teach the new believers. You may wonder, *How can I teach someone?* Since every situation is different, there is not a specific set of steps to follow. Here are some suggestions you may choose to use.

Write one of your own ideas for each.

If the new believer is someone in your neighborhood, or someone you see frequently,
- have a Christian parent or adult talk with him.
- take him to Sunday school or church with you.
- ask your pastor to visit him.
- ______________________

If the new believer is someone you may never see again,
- give him a tract with the address and phone number of a church printed on it.
- ______________________

For any new believer,
- encourage him to find a Bible and start by reading the Gospel of John.
- encourage him to begin attending a Bible-believing church.
- ______________________

Take time to discuss with your parents and other Christian adults what you should do, so you are ready when the time comes. Be careful about giving your own address and phone number to strangers. Giving the name and address of your church is safer.

Traveling Once More

Acts 18:22–21:19

Name ____________________

Answer the questions.

1. From which city did each of Paul's missionary journeys start? (Acts 18:22-23) ____________
2. Even though Paul did not give the name of anyone starting the trip with him, who does he mention being with him as he left Macedonia for Asia? (Acts 19:22) ____________
3. What goddess did many of the Ephesians worship before they became Christians? (Acts 19:22-27) ____________ How did the conversion of the Christians affect business in the city? ____________
4. What accident and miracle took place as Paul preached one night in Troas? (Acts 20:7-12) ____________
5. What two challenges did Paul give the Ephesian elders when they met together in Miletus? (Acts 20:28-31) ____________
6. Paul was warned that he would suffer harm if he returned to Jerusalem. What was Paul's response to these warnings? (Acts 21:13) ____________

Use the maps of Paul's second and third missionary journeys on pages 344 and 345 to complete each sentence.

1. Paul headed ____________ as he left Antioch at the start of his second and third journeys.
2. Paul traveled by ____________ for most of the first half of each trip.
3. Paul's return trips were both by ____________.
4. During the return trip of his third missionary journey, Paul was probably on a cargo ship since Acts records their stopping daily at ports along the coast and major islands. What advantage to the spreading of the gospel might this boat ride have had over the boat trip of Paul's second missionary journey? ____________

N
W E
S

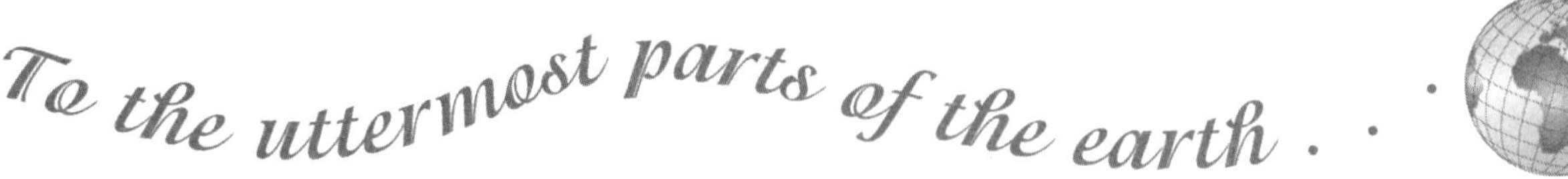
To the uttermost parts of the earth . . .

What Does God Say About Money?

Name ______________________________

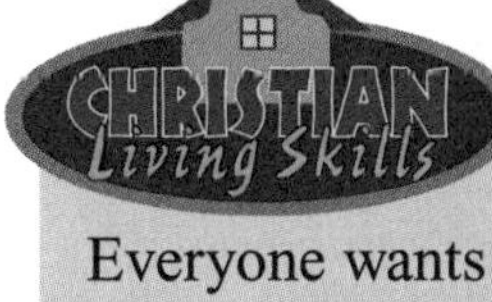
CHRISTIAN
Living Skills

$ The pursuit of money is a dangerous quest in our world. $

Everyone wants it. Everyone wants to spend it. Money is obviously a necessity for survival in our culture. What does God say about money? What should a Christian who wants to please God do with it? God's Word gives advice for the proper attitude you should have toward money.

Read I Timothy 6:10 and fill in the blanks.

The ____________ of money is the ____________ of all kinds of evil.

Many people who have coveted money have __________ themselves with many ______________.

$ Money is a resource given to you by God to accomplish His will. $

You are responsible to be a faithful steward of the money God has given to you. You might hear someone argue that the money he earns belongs to him, not to God. After all, he worked for it, didn't he? Such an attitude reveals the selfish, greedy outlook of that person. Who provided the job for him? Who gave him a healthy body so that he could work? God is our ultimate provider and our trust should be in Him, not in money.

Read Luke 14:28-30 and answer the questions.

1. Why is it important to plan ahead? ____

____

2. What will be the response of people who find out that you didn't plan ahead?

____

$ The key to wise financial planning is budgeting. $

A **budget** is a simple written plan of how the money you earn will be spent.
Wise spending demands wise planning. As you budget your money, it is necessary that you establish priorities. In other words, you must think biblically about the way you spend your cash.

Read the verses and match them to the correct statement about money.

_____	1. Proverbs 15:27	A. I am robbing God if I do not give a tithe to Him.
_____	2. II Corinthians 9:7	B. Greedy people cause problems for their families.
_____	3. Proverbs 28:19	C. Hard work leads to God's provision.
_____	4. Proverbs 23:4	D. I should give generously with a cheerful heart.
_____	5. Malachi 3:8-10	E. Getting rich should not be my purpose for working.

$ Every Christian should express his gratefulness for God's provision. $

The first priority of a Christian should be to show gratefulness for God's provision by giving back to God a part of what God has given to him. This offering given with a cheerful and thankful heart is called the **tithe.** The Bible says that the tithe is 10 percent of all that you earn. God asks Christians to give this money back to Him as a reminder to them that **He** is the One who gave it to them.

Something to Think About

My Money

Name ______________________

Background Information

CHRISTIAN *Living Skills*

Jenna's parents have decided to teach her how to budget money. They know that Jenna wants to go to youth camp at the end of the summer with her church and that she will also want to buy new clothes for the next school year. To teach her the value of money and budgeting, they have decided to give Jenna $8.00 each week for the ten weeks before camp. They have also given Jenna permission to dog-sit for the Clarks, a family in their church, twice each week for one hour each time. The Clarks will be paying Jenna $4.00 each hour to groom and walk their dog.

Jenna's family has been witnessing to their next door neighbor, an elderly widow named Mrs. Yoneida. Mrs. Yoneida has asked Jenna to do some gardening work twice each week for her. Jenna's parents have given her permission and encouraged her to demonstrate responsibility and be a good testimony to their neighbor. Mrs. Yoneida has told Jenna that she will pay her $15 each week for her work.

Jenna wants to figure out how much money she will be earning this summer and how much she must save each week to pay for camp and her clothes for next year. Summer camp costs $155. Jenna's mom suggested that she plan on saving $100 for her new clothes. Jenna is thankful for the opportunities God is giving her to earn money, and she wants to give God her tithe each week. She is also wondering whether she will have any money to spend on other things.

Using the background information, follow the instructions and answer the questions on page 270. Fill in the blanks on page 271 to help Jenna create a successful summer budget. (You can use a separate sheet of paper to do the math.)

Instructions:

1. **Using the background information, fill in Jenna's Weekly Income, Weekly Expenditures, Total Weekly Expenditures and her Total Savings Goal.**
2. **Calculate the amount Jenna needs to save each of the ten weeks for camp and for clothes and write the amount. *(Total Savings Goal ÷ 10 weeks = Weekly Savings Plan)***
3. **Add the sum of the Weekly Expenditures and Weekly Savings Plan to find out how much of each week's money is designated for a specific purpose. Write it in the Weekly Total of Designated Money blank.**
4. **Subtract the Weekly Total of Designated Money from the Total Weekly Income to find out how much money Jenna has left to spend each week. This is her Weekly Total of Undesignated Money.**

Questions:

1. Jenna's parents have told her that she is free to spend her Undesignated Money as she wishes. If Jenna buys a milkshake for $1.29 after she does yard work one day each week, how much money will she have spent on milkshakes by the end of the summer? $ __________
2. When Jenna was moving some flower pots in Mrs. Yoneida's yard, she accidently broke one. The flower pot costs $7.00 to replace. If Jenna uses her Undesignated Money to pay for it, how many weeks will it take her to pay it off? ______________
3. Jenna's grandparents surprised Jenna and sent her $50 for her birthday in July. Decide the amount you think Jenna should put into each category. (Some money should go into each category.)

Tithe:	Clothes Savings:	Camp Savings:	Undesignated:
$ __________	$ __________	$ __________	__________

Name ____________________

CHRISTIAN Living Skills

Use this budget to answer the questions from the previous page.

Jenna's Ten-Week Summer Budget

Weekly Income:

From Parents: $ ________

From Mrs. Yoneida: $ ________

From the Clarks: $ ________

Total (add): $ ________

Weekly Expenditures:

Tithe: $ ________
(10% of total weekly income multiply by 0.1)

Total Savings Goal:

Camp: $ ________

Clothes: $ ________

Total (add): $ ________

Divide by the number of weeks she has to save. (Divide by 10)

Weekly Savings Plan:

For Camp: $ ________

For Clothes: $ ________

Total (add): $ ________

Weekly Total of Designated Money: $ ________ (includes weekly expenditures and weekly savings plan money)

Weekly Total of Undesignated Money: $ ________ (difference of weekly income and total amount of designated money)

What About Me?

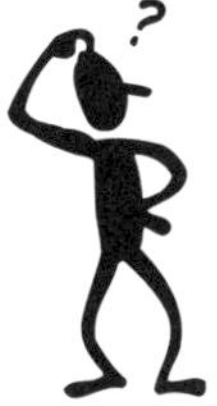

Don't forget that you are accountable to God for the choices you make in spending the money God has given to you. The ability to be generous to others is a direct result of wise planning and budgeting. Be faithful and use self-control when facing decisions about how to use God's money.

Take time at home to answer the questions.

1. Would God say that you are wise in the way you spend your money? YES NO SOMETIMES
2. Do you faithfully tithe the money God allows you to have? YES NO SOMETIMES
3. Do you make selfish choices when spending your money? YES NO SOMETIMES
4. Are you generous, looking for ways to meet others' needs? YES NO SOMETIMES
5. Are you able to save money for a specific purpose rather than just spend it on little things? YES NO SOMETIMES

The questions that you answered NO *or* SOMETIMES *to are the areas in which you need to make changes to please God! Plan today to obey God in the use of the money that He has given you.*

Name ______________________________

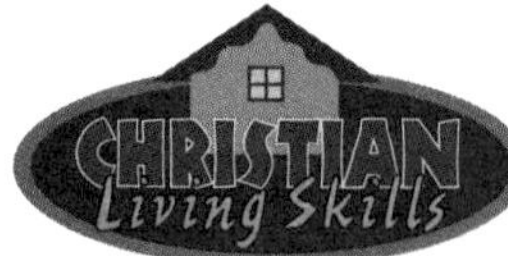
CHRISTIAN
Living Skills

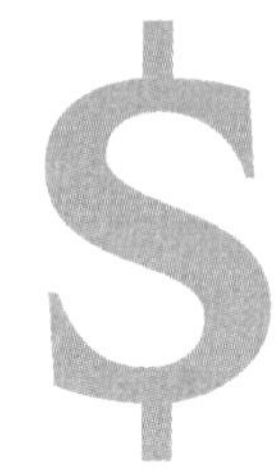

Every time you make a financial decision, ask yourself the following questions:

1. **Have I expressed my gratefulness to God by giving my tithe to Him before I spend anything?**
2. **Will God be pleased about how I am using the money He has entrusted to me?**
3. **Is the choice I'm about to make a selfish choice?**

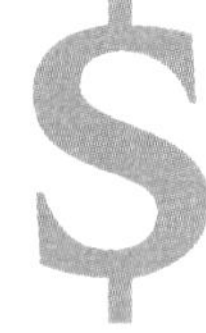

It is never too soon for you to develop good budgeting habits. Remember, you are responsible for how you spend the money God has given to you. Make every effort to make wise decisions! God will bless you for obedience to Him!

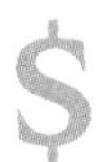

Use the following budget form to evaluate your personal spending habits and formulate a plan to please God by becoming a wise steward of God's money. You may want to refer to Jenna's budget for help.

My Personal Budget

Weekly Income:		**Weekly Expenditures:**	
__________:	______	Tithe:	______
__________:	______	__________:	______
__________:	______	__________:	______
Total (add):	______	*Total*:	______

Total Savings Goal:

__________: ______

__________: ______

Divide by the number of weeks you have to save.

Weekly Savings Plan:

__________: ______

__________: ______

Weekly Total of Designated Money: ______ (includes weekly expenditures and weekly savings plan amounts)

Weekly Total of Undesignated Money: ______ (difference of weekly income and total amount of designated money)

Get the Bible Reading H.A.B.I.T.

Name ______________________

BIBLE STUDY Skills

Have a special time set aside each day to read your Bible. If possible, make it the same time every day.

Ask God to teach you from His Word. Remember to thank Him for helping you to understand and apply it.

Be still and give your attention to what you are reading.

Investigate the Scripture by asking yourself questions about it.

Take time to look up words and ideas you do not understand.

As you read the Scripture for each day, write the date in the box.

At the Rapture, Christ will bring with Him those who died in Christ. **I Thessalonians 4:13-15**	When Christ descends, Christians who are alive will be caught up to meet Him. **I Thessalonians 4:16-18**	God's judgment will come on the earth when no one is expecting it. **I Thessalonians 5:1-3**	Christians should not be taken by surprise. They should be watching for Christ's return. **I Thessalonians 5:4-6**	Christians should be comforted with God's promise to save them from His wrath. **I Thessalonians 5:7-11**
The Lord is coming someday to judge the ungodly. **Jude 14-16**	These people will be mockers, lustful, and without the Spirit. **Jude 17-19**	Christians should continue praying and watching for Christ's coming. **Jude 20-21**	Christians should have compassion on the lost and seek to win them to Christ. **Jude 22-23**	God is able to keep Christians from falling; He is worthy of glory now and forever. **Jude 24-25**
The Lord is faithful; He will help Christians to love Him as they should. **II Thessalonians 3:3-5**	Christians must withdraw themselves from any Christian who is unruly. **II Thessalonians 3:6-9**	Christians should treat an unruly Christian as a brother, not as an enemy. **II Thessalonians 3:14-15**	Christians should keep away from those who promote false doctrine. **Romans 16:17-18**	Christians should be steadfast, always abounding in the work of the Lord. **I Corinthians 15:58**
Christians must be serious, self-controlled, prayerful, and loving since the end is near. **I Peter 4:7-8**	Christians should be joyful when trials come. **I Peter 4:12-13**	Christians should glorify God if He allows them to suffer for being a Christian. **I Peter 4:14-16**	Christians should commit their souls to the keeping of their faithful Creator. **I Peter 4:17-19**	The Lord chastens Christians because they are His children and He loves them. **Hebrews 12:5-7**

Name ______________________

BIBLE STUDY Skills No other Bible study method will be effective unless the **devotional method** is used with it. This very personal method points the Christian to scriptural truth as it is applied to him. By the teaching of the Holy Spirit, a believer is able to claim God's promises, pray according to God's will, avoid error in his thoughts, words, and actions, and do what is right and good. The Holy Spirit will help the believer make application to different parts of his life as he studies the same Scripture again and again. The goal of this kind of Bible study is the completing and the perfecting of the believer's likeness to Jesus Christ.

Choose one of these Scriptures and apply it to the areas of your life that are shown on the bulletin board.

Follow God's Directions Exactly	Joshua 6:1-3, 12-16, 20
Don't Be Lazy, Be Diligent	Proverbs 12:14, 24, 27
Don't Just Say that You Love Others, Show It	I John 3:11-18

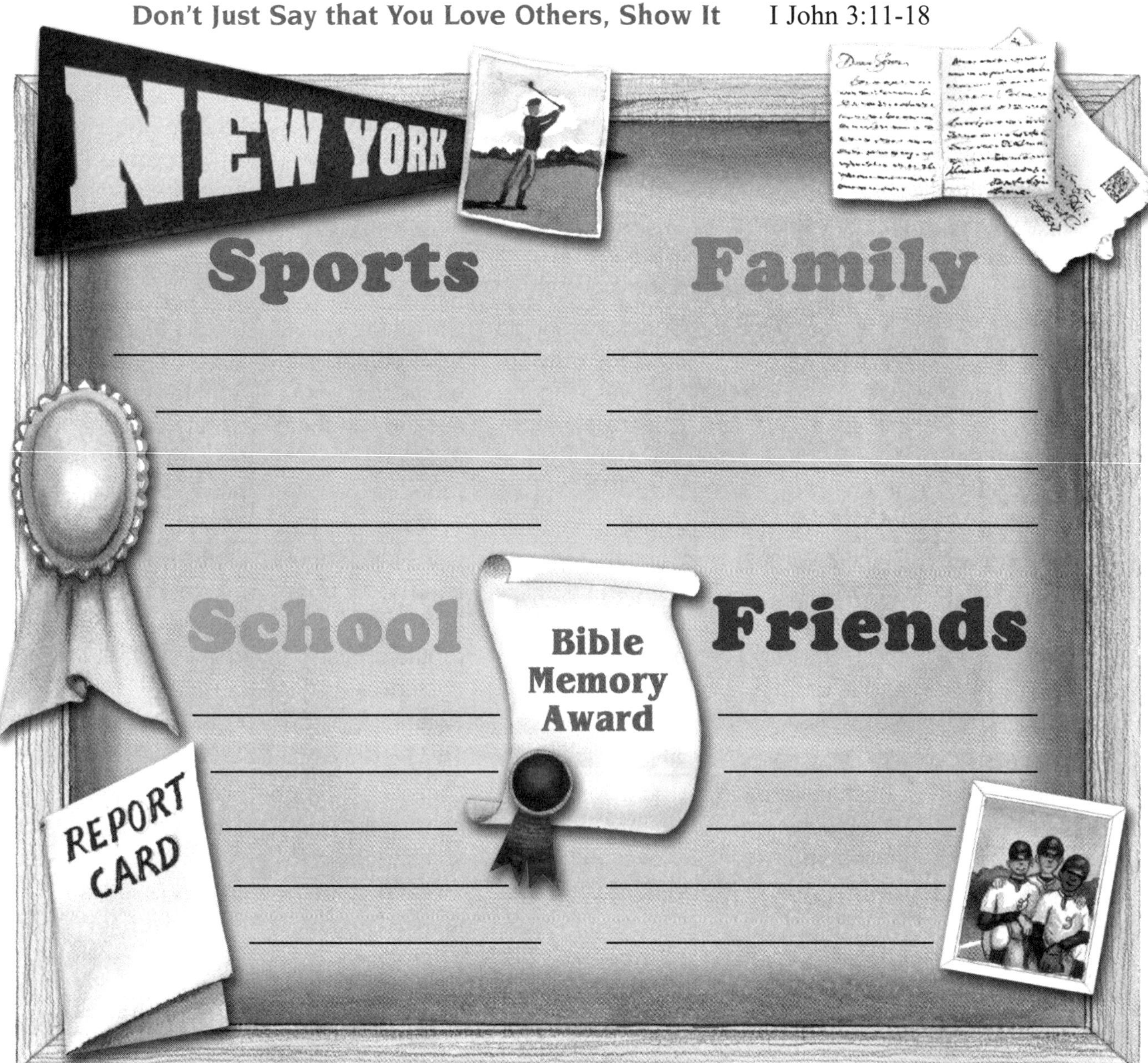
NEW YORK
Sports
Family
School
Bible Memory Award
Friends
REPORT CARD

John's Vision of Christ

Revelation 1:10-20

Name ____________________

The appearance of Christ in heaven was very different from John's memory of Jesus in His human form on earth. Even though John knew that Jesus was the Son of God, seeing Him in His glory must have been an amazing sight to behold!

Read Revelation 1:10-20. Complete the similes that describe the features of Christ.

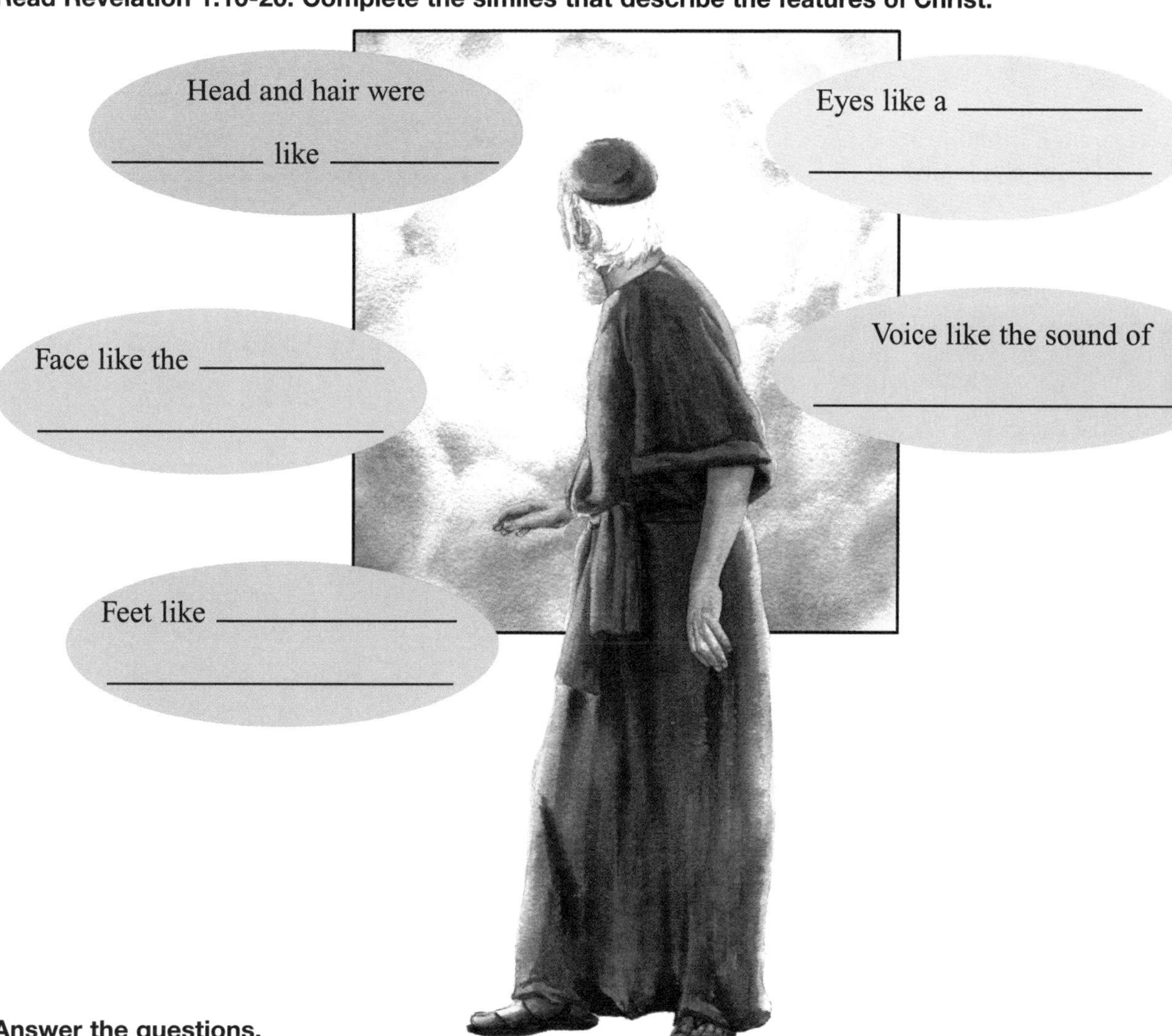

Head and hair were
__________ like __________
Eyes like a __________
____
Face like the __________
____
Voice like the sound of
____
Feet like __________
____

Answer the questions.

1. Christ appeared to John in this glorious form to give him important messages to write down for all believers. One part of this message was a warning about future judgment on the earth. What object coming out of Christ's mouth in the vision illustrates judgment? ____________________

2. Why do you think John fell down when he saw Christ in his vision?

____

____

Blessings Multiplied

Revelation 1:3

Name ______________________

Some people avoid reading and studying the Book of Revelation because they think it is hard to understand. While this may be true, God gives His children a special blessing to encourage them to study His Word. When you come across an event or symbol you don't understand, realize that God can be trusted, and that what He prophesies will come to pass.

Solve the multiplication code to discover how to receive God's special blessing.

Christians will receive God's special blessing if they...

1. ____ ____ ____ ____ the prophecy.
   64 40 12 8

2. ____ ____ ____ ____ ____ ____ to the words of the prophecy.
   125 72 60 20 40 27

3. ____ ____ ____ ____ to heart what the prophecy says.
   20 12 48 40

A = 3 x 2 x 2 ____

D = 2 x 2 x 2 ____

E = 5 x 4 x 2 ____

I = 4 x 3 x 6 ____

K = 8 x 2 x 3 ____

L = 5 x 5 x 5 ____

N = 3 x 3 x 3 ____

R = 4 x 4 x 4 ____

S = 4 x 5 x 3 ____

T = 2 x 5 x 2 ____

Answer the questions.

1. What is prophecy? (Use the glossary.)

____

2. Why is God the only one who can accurately prophesy about the future?

____

3. What are three blessings for Christians that come from obeying God's Word?

____

____

____

Symbols of Revelation

Revelation 4-11; 16

Name ______________________

A **symbol** is a representation for something else. When you see a STOP, you know that it shows where a moving vehicle must stop. A ♿ symbol shows an area designated to benefit those who are disabled. Symbols are used throughout the Book of Revelation as pictures to help people understand what John saw in his vision.

Match each symbol to its description. Use the verses to check your answers.

______ 1. Since the days of Noah, this has shown God's faithfulness (Rev. 4:2-3).

______ 2. This object coming out of Christ's mouth is a symbol of His judgment (Rev. 1:16-18).

______ 3. These beings symbolize God's holy presence (Ex. 25:22).

______ 4. These symbolize the seven churches that shine as lights in a world of sin (Rev. 1:20).

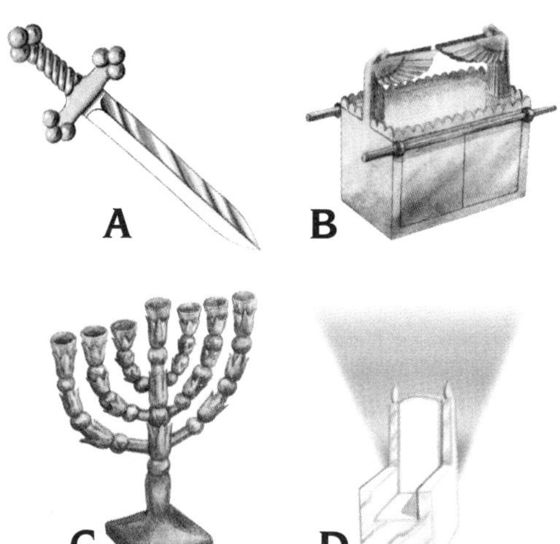

A
B
C
D

Fill in the correct letter, matching the symbol on the time line to its description.

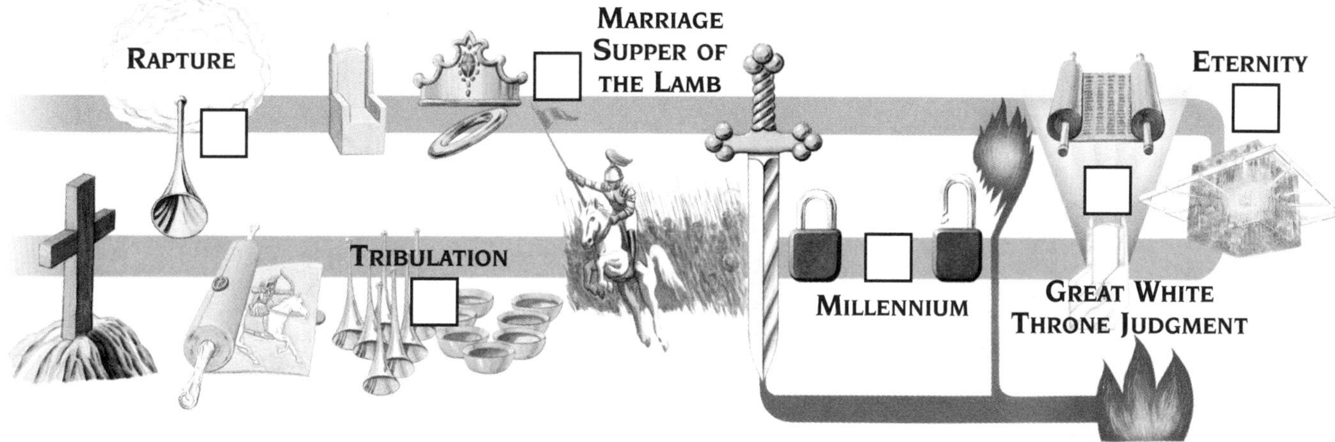

RAPTURE
MARRIAGE SUPPER OF THE LAMB
ETERNITY
TRIBULATION
MILLENNIUM
GREAT WHITE THRONE JUDGMENT

A. This thousand-year period will be a time of peace when Christ will reign over the earth.

B. This is the time without end when believers will worship Christ as their Savior and King.

C. This seven-year period will be a time of great trouble and judgment upon the earth.

D. This is Christ's imminent return for Christians, both dead and alive, preceded by a shout and the trump of God.

E. This is the time of rejoicing when the Lamb and His bride are united forever.

F. This is the place where unbelievers will be judged for their sin and sent eternally to the lake of fire.

True and Righteous Judgments

Revelation 5-6

Name ______________________

When God gave His only Son, Jesus, as a sacrifice for mankind's sins, He demonstrated His loving character. When God judges those who have rejected His gift of salvation, He will demonstrate His powerful justice. God cannot tolerate sin. It was because of sin that His Son suffered. His holiness demands that sin be punished. Jesus Christ has the authority as the slain and risen Lamb of God to execute judgment on all those who have rejected His personal sacrifice for them. Every judgment He pronounces upon sin will be righteous and just.

Use Revelation 5:1-10 to answer the questions.

1. Why was John sorrowful? ______________________
2. Who began the judgments by opening the seven-sealed scroll? ______________________
3. Why is He worthy to open the book? ______________________

Read Revelation 6:1-17; 8:1. Write the number of the seal on the correct judgment.

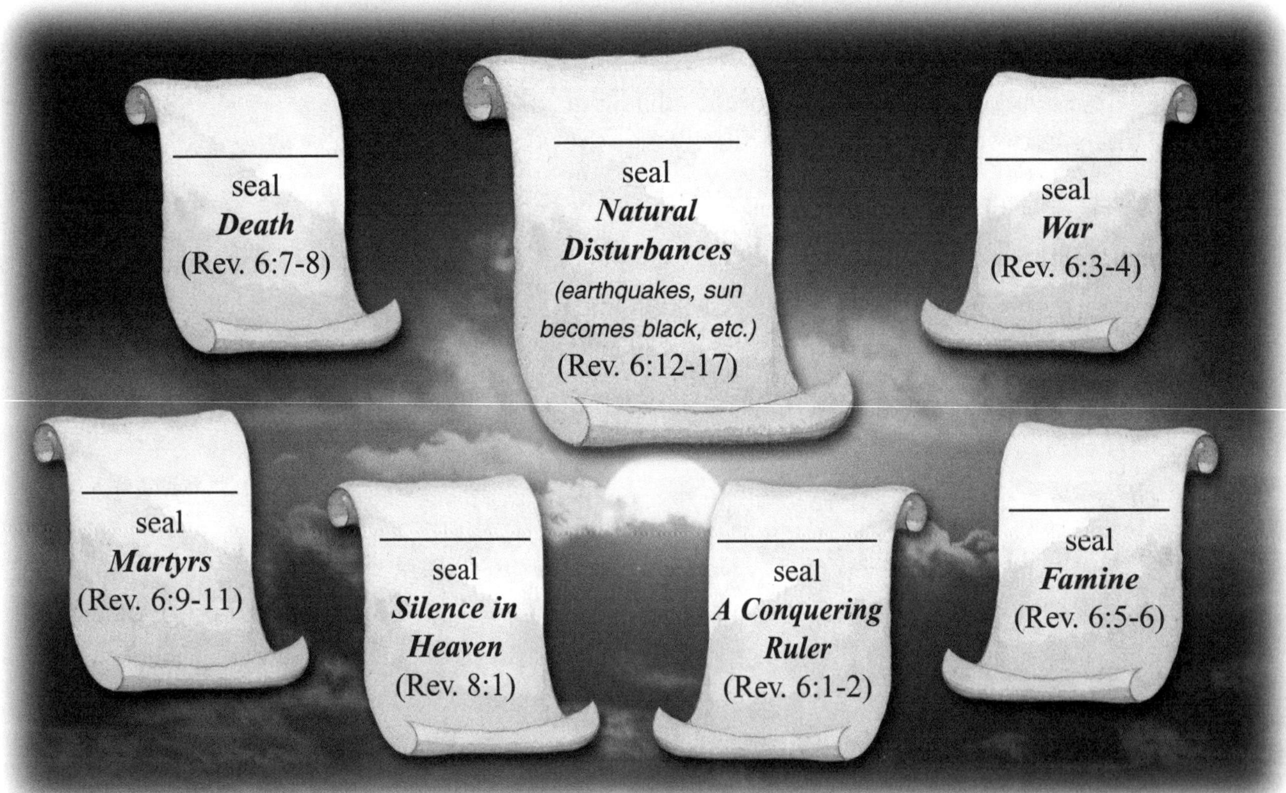

_____ seal
Death
(Rev. 6:7-8)
_____ seal
Natural Disturbances
(earthquakes, sun becomes black, etc.)
(Rev. 6:12-17)
_____ seal
War
(Rev. 6:3-4)
_____ seal
Martyrs
(Rev. 6:9-11)
_____ seal
Silence in Heaven
(Rev. 8:1)
_____ seal
A Conquering Ruler
(Rev. 6:1-2)
_____ seal
Famine
(Rev. 6:5-6)

Answer the questions.

1. What have unbelievers done to deserve these judgments? ______________________
____
2. According to Revelation 6:15-17, did the unbelievers realize what was happening to them? ______
3. Is it possible to hide your actions or whereabouts from God? ______

Holy Matrimony

Revelation 19:1-10

Name ___________________________

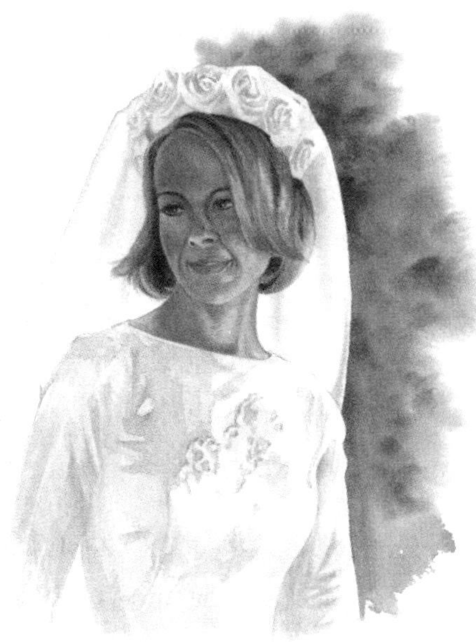

The Bible uses the beautiful picture of marriage between a man and a woman to symbolize the closeness of the bond between Christ and His church in heaven. Only those who have trusted in Christ are members of the redeemed church. These believers are called the **bride of Christ** in the Book of Revelation.

Read the verses and complete the chart to find the comparisons between earthly marriage and the marriage that will take place between Christ and His bride, the church.

Earthly Marriage	Verses	Heavenly Marriage
The husband-to-be is responsible to prepare a place for himself and his bride to live.	John 14:2-3	
The bride is traditionally married in a white dress that symbolizes her purity.	Revelation 19:7-8	
Wives are commanded to be obedient to their husbands.	Ephesians 5:22-24	
Husbands are commanded to love their wives sacrificially.	Ephesians 5:25	

THINK ABOUT IT

List several ways for a person to prepare for the events of the End Times.

I can prepare for the End Times by…

____

____

____

____

God's Protection

Name ______________________

God loves and protects His own children. He can bring them safely through the most frightening of circumstances. He can even use fearful events as a channel for bringing unsaved people to fear Him, and ultimately to salvation. God may allow Christians to experience physical persecution, but their souls are His, and they will spend eternity with Him in heaven.

Read the verses and answer the questions about God's faithful protection of His children.

1. What promise is given in Leviticus 25:18-19? ______________________
2. Psalm 4:8 says that belief in God's protection enables believers to do what? ______________________
3. What does Psalm 32:7 say God will do for Christians in times of trouble? ______________________
4. Read Psalm 121. Copy one verse from this psalm that is an encouragement to you about God's protection. ______________________

   ____

   ____
5. According to Proverbs 22:3, what is a Christian's responsibility in time of trouble?

   ____

Circle the seven synonyms for *protect.* Then unscramble the underlined letters of the synonyms to discover why God keeps His promises to His children for protection.

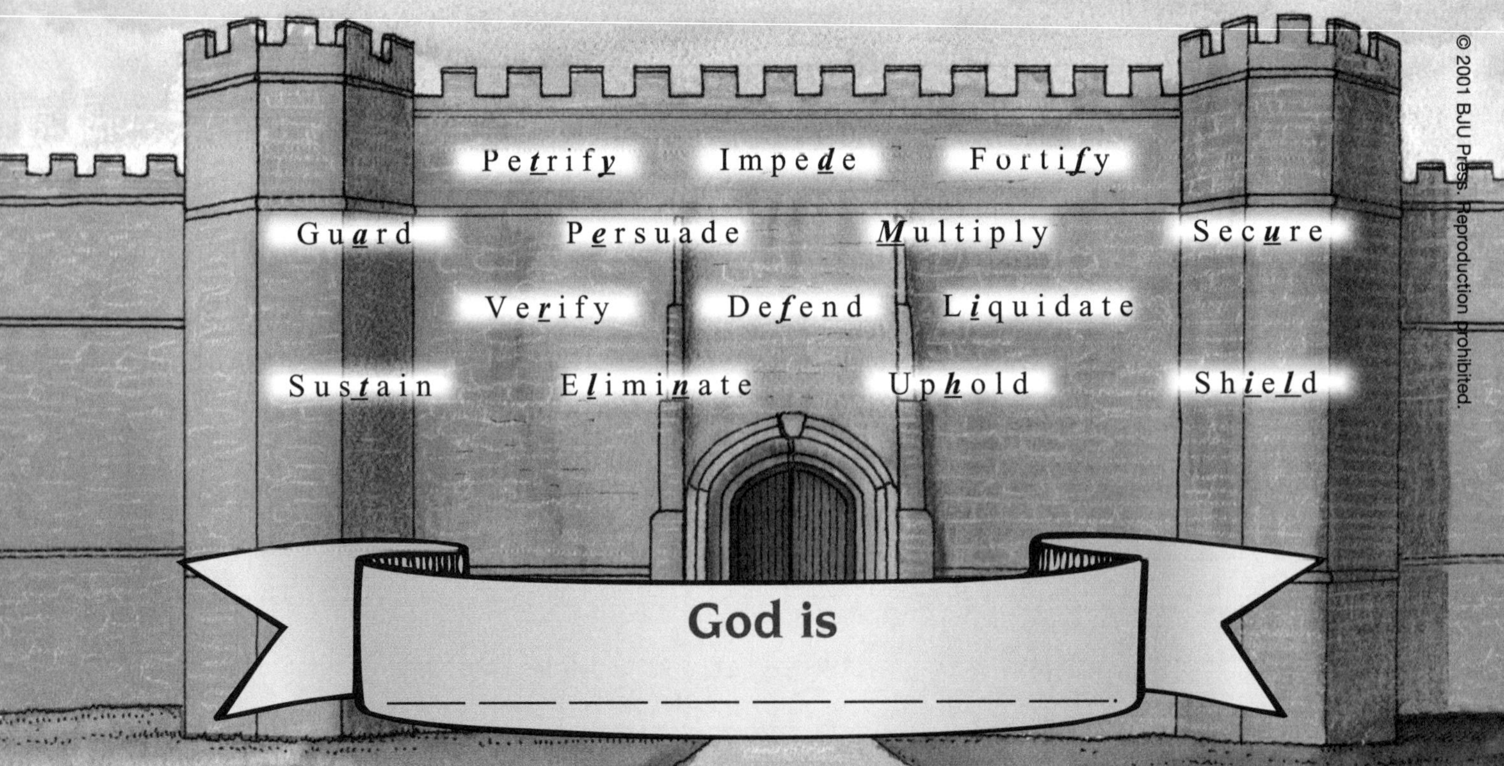
Petrify
Impede
Fortify
Guard
Persuade
Multiply
Secure
Verify
Defend
Liquidate
Sustain
Eliminate
Uphold
Shield
God is
_ _ _ _ _ _ _ _ _ _ _ _ _.

What Does God Say About My Future?

Name ______________________________

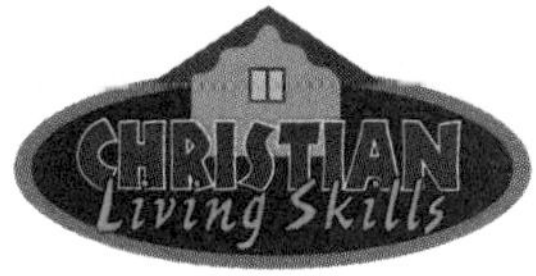
CHRISTIAN
Living Skills

The world around you is changing rapidly!

It is a challenge to keep up with the fast pace of technology, politics, and cultural issues. Much of what you hear on the news can be very discouraging and can even sound chaotic! What are you to do? As you think about these uncertainties, you have one person on whom you can depend. As a Christian, you have a heavenly Father who loves you and is surprised by nothing that is happening around you.

Read the verses and write one lesson about God taught in each verse.

Proverbs 15:3 ______________________________

Ecclesiastes 3:14 ______________________________

Malachi 3:6 ______________________________

You have an exciting future!

Christians have many wonderful promises from their heavenly Father. As you look forward to growing up, getting your driver's license, finding a job, going to college, or getting married, keep in mind that God already knows what is going to happen to you and has good plans for your life (Jer. 29:11). God loves you and promises to give you joy if you will trust Him to guide you. If you are a Christian, you can look forward to spending eternity with God.

Read the verses and fill in the blanks. Then unscramble the letters in the boxes to discover how a Christian can face the future with confidence.

Psalm 84:11 God is a sun and ___ [___] ___ ___ ___ ___. No good ___ ___ [___] ___ ___ will He withhold from me if I obey Him.

Psalm 33:11 The plans of God's heart will ___ ___ [___] ___ ___ firm forever.

Philippians 1:6 I can be ___ ___ ___ [___] ___ ___ ___ ___ [___] that God, who has started a good work in my life, will do what it takes to finish it.

As a Christian, I can have complete ______________ that God is trustworthy and in control of my future.

God is immutable!

When we refer to God's character as **immutable**, we mean that He never changes. No matter what has happened, no matter what is happening now, and no matter what will happen in the future, God's holy character is always the same. Knowing that God never changes brings great security and stability to a Christian!

Something to Think About

My Future

Name ______________________

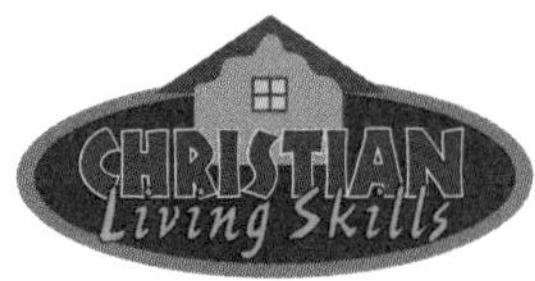
CHRISTIAN
Living Skills

Looking Back

It is a great encouragement to a Christian to see what God has already done in his life. He can see how God has protected him, provided for him, and blessed him. Seeing how God has been faithful in the past motivates the Christian to trust God to lead him in the future.

Think about how you have seen God working in your life in the past. Complete the statements.

I know that God protected me when ______________________

One thing that God has provided for me is ______________________

God has blessed me with ______________________

Living Now

You can look back at what has happened in your life, and you can look forward to what you hope will happen. *However, you are actually living right now in the present.* God has put you in this point of time for a reason. He has something He wants you to accomplish today. You have the responsibility to find out what God's perfect will is for you today. Don't get in a hurry to jump into the future. Live for God today, and soon you will find that you can meet the uncertainties of the future with confidence because you are in God's will.

Read the verses and write one sentence about each one that tells you what your responsibility is for today.

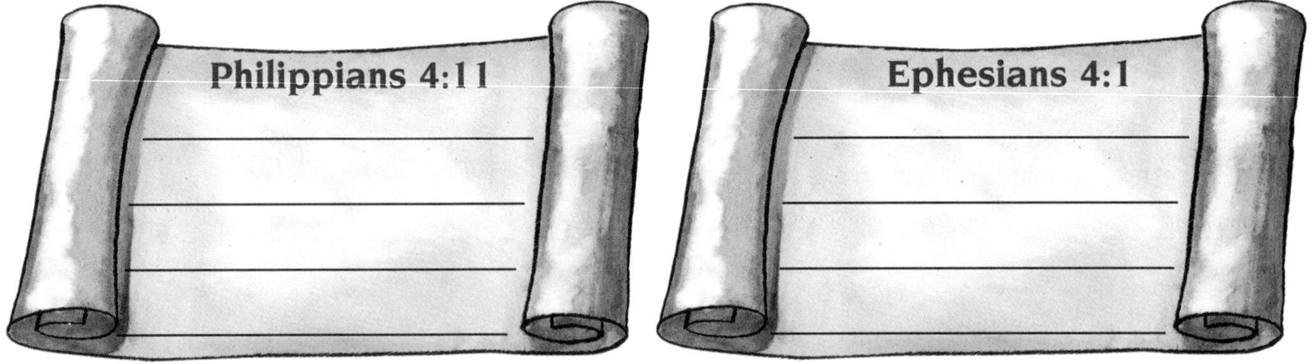
Philippians 4:11
Ephesians 4:1

What About Me?

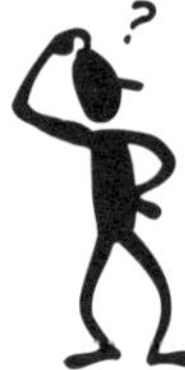

Looking Forward

Christians should have the assurance that God will be with them throughout their lives on earth, and that they will be with God for all eternity. That's definitely a future to look forward to!

Take time at home to think about your attitude toward your future. Consider the following questions.

Can I look forward to a future with God in heaven?
Am I trying to grow up too fast, and am I missing what God has for me today?
Do I have a true desire to find and do God's perfect will for my life?

Power in the Name

Revelation 19:11-21

Name ______________________

Answer the questions. You may use your Bible for help.

1. What is the name of the place where the great battle between Christ and the world's armies will take place? (Rev. 16:16) ______________________

2. Describe the leader of the armies of heaven in the Battle of Armageddon. Include the names given for Christ (Rev. 19:11-13).

____

____

____

3. What happens to the Beast and False Prophet in this battle? (Rev. 19:20)

____

4. What happens to the people who reject Christ and worship the Beast? (Rev. 19:21)

____

Believers can have full confidence in the name of Jesus (Ps. 9:10). His name is powerful and speaks of His holy character. The day is coming when unbelievers who take His name in vain and treat it lightly will be confronted with the truth of the power found in the name of Jesus.

Match the verses to the correct statement describing the power found in the name of Jesus.

_____ 1. Acts 16:18

_____ 2. Acts 9:29

_____ 3. Acts 3:6-7

_____ 4. Acts 2:38

_____ 5. John 20:31

A. Forgiveness of sins is given in His name.

B. We can have life if we believe in His name.

C. His name has the power to cast out demonic spirits.

D. His name enables His servants to preach boldly.

E. People were healed in His name.

Read Philippians 2:9-11 and answer the questions.

1. How does this passage describe the name of Jesus? ______________________

2. Who will bow at the sound of this name someday? ______________________

____

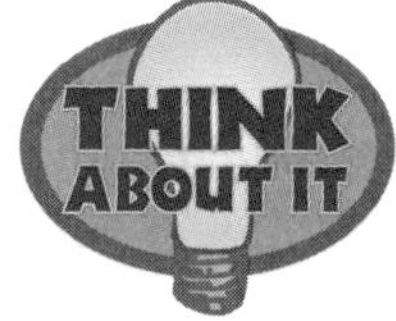
THINK
ABOUT IT

When will you bow and confess?

You have a choice either to confess this truth now and join the obedient army of Christ . . . or to wait until later, when you will be forced to bow your knee and admit that Christ is Lord. He will be victorious at last, whether you cooperate with Him or not. Christ lovingly urges you to come now, before it is too late. If you have never given Christ the control of your life, won't you do it today?

Angelic Activity

Matthew 28:1-8

Name ______________________

Angels were created by God and play very important roles in the world. They are mentioned throughout the Bible as supernatural beings who have been given specific tasks by God. While angels usually appeared to people in the form of humans, the Bible describes many different kinds of angels.

Read Isaiah 6:1-4 and follow the instructions.

1. What kind of angels did Isaiah see around the throne of God? ______________________
2. What were the angels in Isaiah's vision doing? ______________________

____

Draw a picture of what you think these angels might look like from Isaiah's description.

Read the clues and verses to discover the names of these angels.

I was given the privilege of announcing Jesus' coming birth to Mary (Luke 1:26-28).

____

I am the type of angel that was assigned to guard the Tree of Life after Adam and Eve were cast out of the Garden of Eden for their sin (Gen. 3:24).

____

I rebelled against God and was cast from heaven (Isa. 14:12-15).

____

I led God's angels in a heavenly battle against Satan and won (Rev. 12:7-9).

____

Solve the puzzle to discover the meaning of the word *angel*. Cross out every other letter beginning with the first one. Then, starting with the right side and going left, write the remaining letters of the puzzle.

A	R	L	E	P	G	W	N	M	E	O	S	K	S	N	E	R	M

Angel means ___ ___ ___ ___ ___ ___ ___ ___ ___.

Songs of Praise

Revelation 15:3-4

Name ______________________

The Bible records many instances when God's people sang praises to Him for His faithfulness to them. A grateful heart of praise is a natural response to God's goodness. Songs of praise and worship to God and the Lamb will continue throughout eternity.

Using the references and clues, write who sang or will sing these songs of praise to God.

I sang this song of praise when I was given wonderful news from God about how I would serve Him (Luke 1:46-55).

____

I sang this song of praise when God delivered me out of the hand of my enemies (II Sam. 22:1-51).

____

We sang this song of praise when God miraculously delivered us from Pharaoh's army (Exod. 15:1-19).

____

____

We will sing this new song of praise to the Lamb, who is worthy to open the sealed scroll (Rev. 5:8-10).

____

____

We will sing this song after the Tribulation when we are united with Christ (Rev. 14:3).

____

____

We will sing this song of praise and worship to the Lamb in heaven (Rev. 5:13).

____

____

Songs of praise are full of adjectives describing the works and character of God. Read Revelation 15:3-4 and list the adjectives used to describe God and His actions.

God is described as:

____

____

God's actions are described as:

____

____

____

____

Marvelous Millennium

Revelation 20

Name ______________________

The **Millennium** will be a marvelous time for God's people. Although sin will still be present in the world, Christ's righteousness will prevail.

Use Revelation 20:1-6 to answer the questions.

1. How long is the Millennium? ______________________
2. Where will Satan be during the Millennium? ______________________
3. What will the earth be like during the Millennium? ______________________
4. What will happen to the people who are beheaded because they will serve Christ and not worship the beast? ______________________

After the peaceful Millennium, Satan will be released from the bottomless pit and will go back to deceiving people. Amazingly, there will be those who reject Christ at that time even after living under His peaceful, prosperous reign.

Read Revelation 20:7-10 and answer the questions.

1. What will the people who choose to reject Christ after the Millennium attempt to do to God's people?
2. What will happen to those who go to battle against God's people?
3. What will happen to Satan?

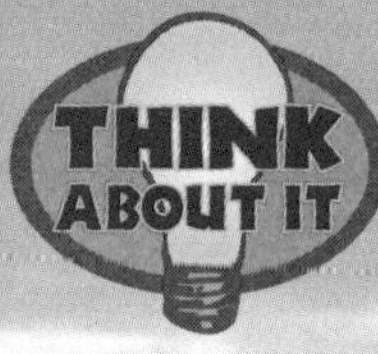
THINK
ABOUT IT

Do *you* know anyone who has never put his trust in Christ? What can you do to help that person?

In the City of God

Revelation 21

Name ______________________________

Things will be very different in the City of God! Life on this sin-filled earth will be over, and God's mighty justice will prevail over sin and death. Revelation gives a beautiful description of God's holy city. Believers can look forward to living there with great joy and anticipation.

Read the verses from Revelation to complete the chart.

Things Not Found in the New Heaven and Earth	
21:1 There will be no ____________.	**21:8** The kind of people who will not be there are . . . ______________________ ______________________ ______________________ ______________________ ______________________ ______________________
21:4 There will be no . . . ______________________ ______________________ ______________________ ______________________	
21:22 There will be no ____________.	
21:23 There will be no ____________ or ____________.	

Answer the questions.

1. What will provide light in the city? (Rev. 21:23) ______________________
2. Why do you think there will be no temple or church in the City of God? (Rev. 21:22)

   ____

Read the description of the City of God in Revelation 21:10-21. Write a paragraph describing it to someone who has not read these verses.

____

____

____

____

____

Prophet Focus

Zechariah (ca. 520 B.C.)

Name ______________________

Zechariah was given revelation from God about things to come. God showed Zechariah eight visions in the same night. Each vision was meant to teach the Israelites something about themselves, about God, or about their future. You can read about these visions in Zechariah 1-6.

God used the first two visions to show Israel that He would punish them for exalting themselves against the land of Judah and hurting His people. Zechariah's third vision revealed that God would someday restore, extend, and bless the land of Israel. In Zechariah's fourth vision, he learned that God would cleanse Israel from their sin, and his fifth vision showed him that God would raise up Zerubbabel to finish building the temple. Zechariah's sixth vision pictured God's Word and His curse on those who break His laws. His seventh and eighth visions revealed that God would remove Israel's sin, set up His kingdom, and judge the nations who had rebelled against Him and harmed Israel. Zechariah reminded the Israelites of their need to repent.

In Zechariah's writings, he refers to Christ as the Branch. Some of Zechariah's prophecies about Christ were fulfilled during Christ's earthly ministry. Many of Zechariah's prophecies will be fulfilled at Christ's Second Coming. Christ will bring peace over the whole earth during a period of time called the Millennium. People from every nation will come to Jerusalem where Christ will reign. Though Israel tried to destroy Christ, they will one day worship Him as King over all.

Use the information to complete the puzzle.

Across

3. Zechariah was given eight _____ from God.
4. Zerubbabel would be the one to finish building the _____.
6. Some of the visions were meant to teach the Israelites about their _____.
7. During the Millennium, _____ will reign from the city of Jerusalem.

Down

1. Peace will be over the whole earth during the _____.
2. Zechariah's _____ vision was about God's curse on those who break His laws.
5. Zechariah's special name for Christ is the _____.

Read the verses and complete the statements.

Zechariah 9:9 This prophecy was fulfilled when ______________________

Zechariah 14:9 This prophecy will be fulfilled when ______________________

What Does God Say About My Thoughts?

Name ______________________

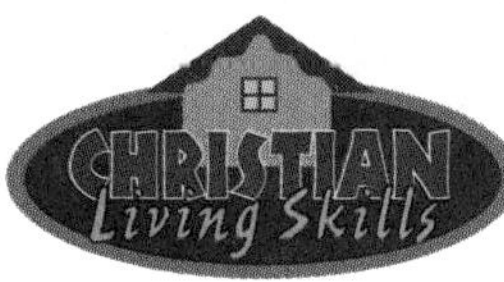
CHRISTIAN
Living Skills

God created people with the ability to think and make decisions.

Your mind is capable of imagination, memorization, and reasoning. Because thoughts have a powerful influence on emotions and actions, the Bible teaches Christians to fill their minds with God's Word so that they can make choices that are pleasing to God instead of seeking things to please themselves.

Read the verses and answer the questions.

Matthew 22:37 1. With what three parts does Jesus say a person should love God?

______________ ______________ ______________

Romans 12:2 2. What part of a Christian must be made new? For what purpose?

____

Romans 8:5-8 3. What is the difference between people who live according to their sinful nature and people who live according to the Spirit?

____

____

4. The mind controlled by the sinful nature leads to ______________.

5. The mind controlled by the Spirit leads to ______________ and ______________.

What kind of thoughts should a Christian think?

Because a Christian wants to please God, he should be careful to put right thoughts into his mind. This means that he does not allow his eyes to see or his ears to hear things that God hates. Not only does he avoid sinful things, he also daily fills his mind with the Word of God so that his mind will be ready to make right choices.

Read Philippians 4:8 to discover the kind of things Christians should think about. Circle the words in the puzzle.

I must think on things that are

true	honest
just	noble
right	pure
lovely	virtuous
excellent	

H	T	N	E	L	L	E	C	X	E	V
H	O	E	S	T	U	R	P	L	L	O
G	O	R	U	T	S	J	B	R	L	Y
H	T	N	I	R	T	O	U	S	T	L
O	T	T	E	Z	N	T	G	I	R	E
U	H	R	I	S	V	S	H	R	U	V
T	G	V	I	R	T	U	O	U	S	O
E	I	X	C	E	L	J	E	N	T	L
T	R	U	E	X	E	R	U	P	R	L

Something to Think About

My Thoughts

Name ______________________

CHRISTIAN Living Skills

How can a Christian guard his thoughts from sin?

God's Word gives Christians instructions on how to discipline their thoughts. The Bible says that every imagination of our sinful mind is evil (Gen. 8:21) and that Christians must work hard to put on a new attitude of holiness (Eph. 4:23-24).

Read the verses and complete the sentences to discover how to guard your mind from sinful thoughts.

Matthew 15:19 I must realize that evil thoughts come out of my ______________.

II Corinthians 10:5 I must take captive every ______________ and make it obedient to Christ.

Colossians 3:2 I must set my ______________________ on holy things, not on worldly things.

Philippians 4:13 I can do all things through ______________ who gives me strength.

The mind is greatly influenced by what we see and hear.
Christians are daily bombarded with sinful advertisements and worldly music. Satan will tempt you to think about sinful things that do not please God. You must be on guard!

Read each scenario and choose the answer that would please Christ.

Scenario	Which response pleased Christ?
While Derek was waiting in line to pay for the gas his mom had pumped, he noticed a magazine with sensuous pictures on the rack in front of him.	○ He continued to look at the magazine, but didn't buy it. ○ He looked away but continued to think about the picture he saw. ○ He looked away and asked God to help him think pure thoughts.
Elisa's mom dropped her off at the library with instructions to choose three good books to check out. As Elisa was looking for her books, she noticed a romance novel that she knew her mom would not approve of.	○ She looked through the book, but she didn't plan to check it out. ○ She did not pick up the book and was thankful her mom wanted her to please Christ. ○ She did not look at the book but was irritated with her mom for having strict standards.
While Ryan and Dustin were watching TV, a commercial for a violent, immoral program began.	○ They watched the commercial and talked about how bad it was. ○ They muted the sound, but continued to watch the commercial. ○ They turned the channel to avoid hearing and seeing impure things.

What About Me?

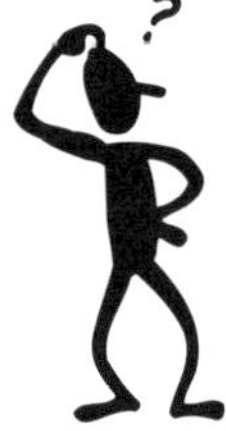

Take time at home to evaluate what you think about.

Do I give in to the temptation to think about impure things?
Do I ask God to help me fight impure thoughts?
Have I memorized God's Word to help me fight temptation?
Do I think about and watch for Christ's return?

Back to the First Love

Revelation 2:1-7

Name ______________________

Use Revelation 2:1-7 to fill in the missing information about the letter to a church, recorded by John.

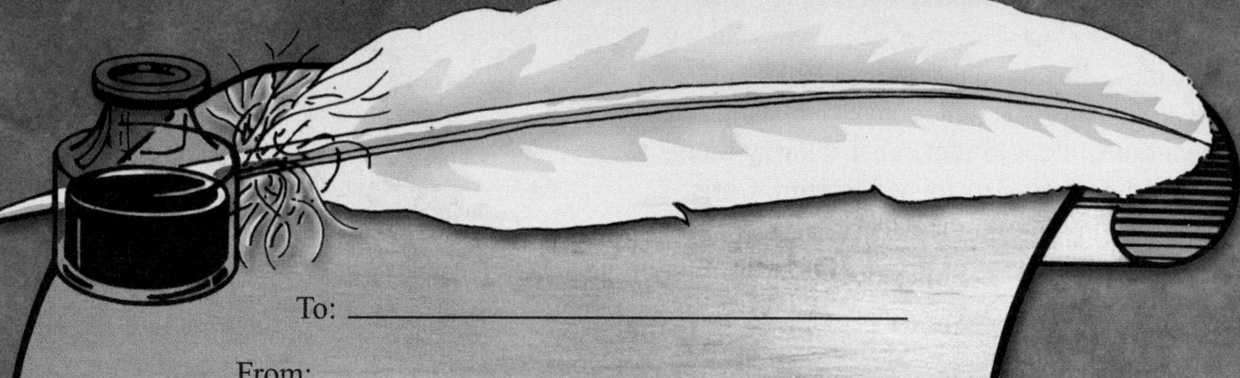

To: ______________________

From: ______________________

Dear Church:

I have several things for which to commend you. I know that you have done good works and have persevered in the faith. I also know that you will not tolerate ______________________. You have put to the test those who falsely claim to be apostles and have found them to be ______________________. You have endured many hardships for My name and have not ______________________.

However, I hold one thing against you: you have ______________________. You must remember the love you first had for Me, and you must ______________ and turn back to the way you first served Me.

I am glad that you hate the deeds of the ______________, which I also hate. Listen closely to what the ______________ is saying to the churches. If you return to your first love, I will give you the right to eat of the ______________ which is in paradise.

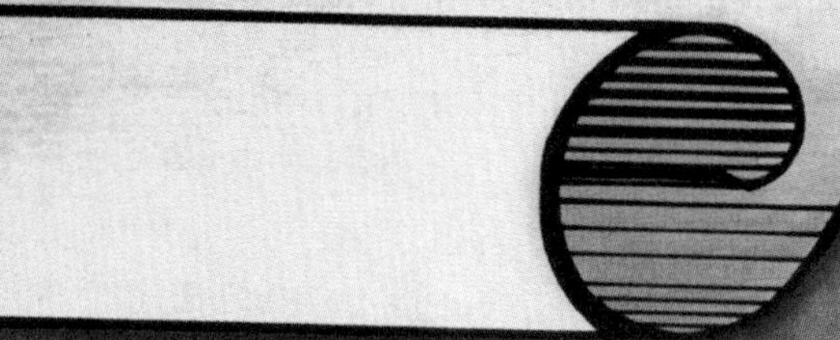

Remember His Love

Revelation 2:4-5

Name ______________________________

The people of the church in Ephesus started out their spiritual lives on the right track. They loved Christ and were committed to serving Him no matter what the cost. However, somewhere along the way, they allowed other things to take first priority. As part of Christ's rebuke to this church, He encouraged them to remember the way things had been when they first trusted in Him. Christ knew that if they turned their focus back to Him, they would remember the special relationship with Him that they were now missing.

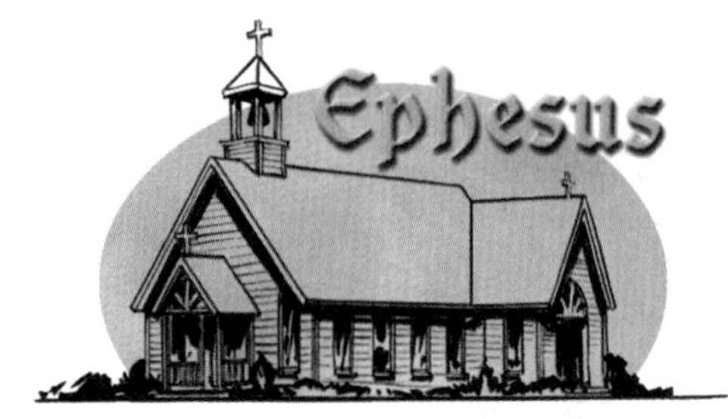
Ephesus

Read the verses and write the wonderful things Christ has done and is doing now for Christians.

Romans 5:8

____

Romans 8:34

____

Philippians 4:13

____

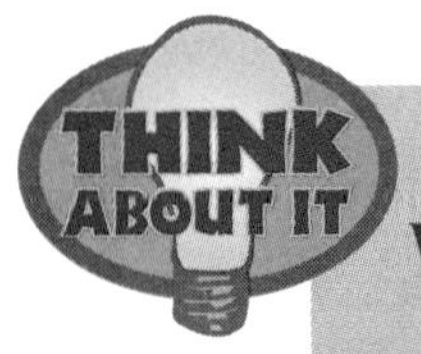
THINK ABOUT IT

Mark your answer with an *X*.

Which of the following do *you* do?	Which are wrong motives for doing these things?
_____ read the Bible daily	_____ to get the things you want
_____ attend church regularly	_____ to be noticed
_____ pray	_____ to show the Lord how much you love Him
_____ memorize Scripture verses	_____ to be praised in front of your friends
_____ help your parents	_____ to win a prize at Sunday school
_____ obey home and school rules	_____ to show God how good you are so He will in turn be good to you
	_____ to impress your friends or family members

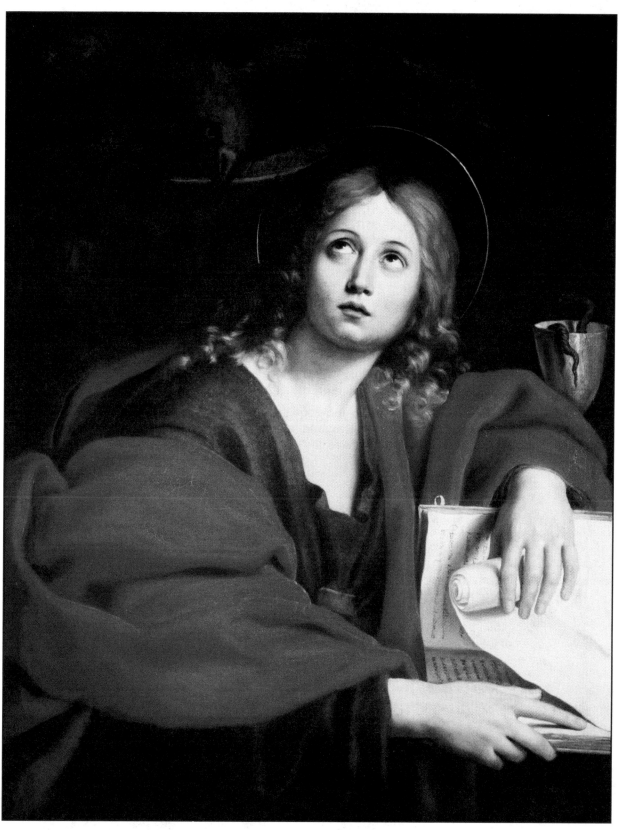

St. John the Evangelist
Domenico Zampieri

Bob Jones University Museum & Gallery, Inc.

Name ______________________

St. John the Evangelist

by Domenico Zampieri (1581-1641)

Domenico Zampieri (Dō mĕn ē´ kō Zăm pyĕr´ ē) started his education by studying with a teacher from Flanders. Later he became an apprentice in the Carracci Art Academy. The academy was a type of art school where talented young boys learned to paint. Domenico must have been a good student, because in 1602 he moved to Rome to help his teacher, Annibale Carracci, with a large commission to paint pictures on the walls and ceilings of a palace for the Farnese family. The paintings were frescoes—paintings done on the plaster of the walls while the plaster was still damp. When the paint and the plaster dried together, the result was a painting that was part of the wall. Domenico painted some of his own most famous masterpieces in fresco. In fact, paintings in oil as we see here are fairly rare for Domenico.

Domenico painted idealized human figures with perfect characteristics—better than real life, like this portrait of John, the disciple of Jesus. The pose in this picture is a typical scholar pose—a young man of pale complexion, seated with books and scrolls. This is the idealized way to represent John, a writer of one of the Gospels.

Domenico's style is very refined—showing intense emotion, but never rough. The objects in his paintings are very clear, and the colors are rich. Notice that John's robe has big folds that make it look like very thick fabric.

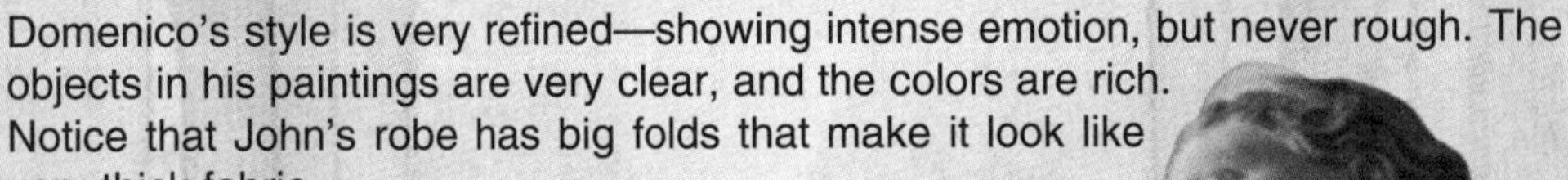

John is called the Evangelist because he wrote the Gospel of John. In the background of this painting is an eagle, one of the four animals seen by John in his vision in the Book of Revelation (Rev. 4:7). Scholars correspond these four beasts with each of the four evangelists, or the four Gospel writers. The eagle was chosen as the symbol for John because of John's "high-flying" teachings about Christ as God. Notice that the eagle holds a quill feather in its beak. It is as though John is ready to write, and the eagle is bringing his own quill for him to use as a pen.

Notice the golden cup with the snake behind John. Like many symbols used by Renaissance artists, this one is based on a legend about John's life. The story was that John was given poison to drink, and as proof of his faith in God, he survived the poison.

The Crown of Life

Revelation 2:8-11

Name ______________________

God promises special blessings to those who remain faithful to him under persecution and trials. The church in Smyrna was experiencing these kinds of trials.

Answer the questions.

1. What two kinds of trials were the Christians in Smyrna experiencing? (Rev. 2:9)
   - ______________________
   - ______________________

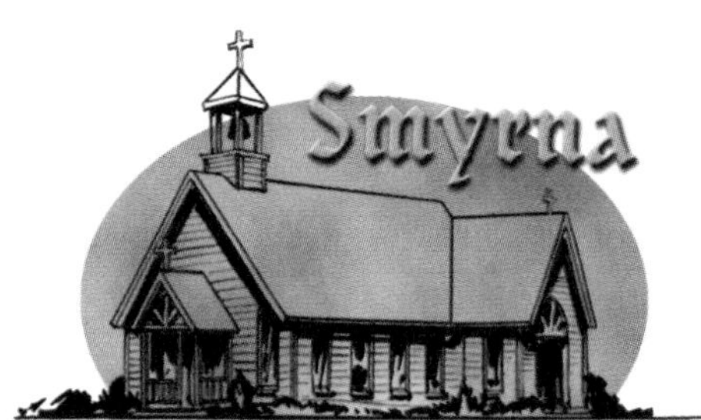
Smyrna

2. What two commands did Jesus give these Christians? (Rev. 2:10)
   - ______________________

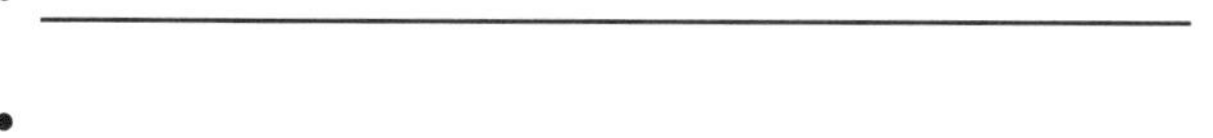

   - ______________________

3. What did Jesus promise these Christians if they were faithful? (Rev. 2:10)
   - ______________________

The Bible is full of promises for Christians who are going through severe trials. Match each verse to the correct summary.

_____ 1. Christians will not be tempted above what they are able to bear; God will make a way of escape for them.

_____ 2. When Christians are persecuted and required to speak, the Spirit of God will give them the words to say.

_____ 3. The kingdom of heaven is theirs; their reward in heaven is great.

_____ 4. If Christians have suffered along with Christ, they will be even more glad when His glory is revealed.

_____ 5. His grace is sufficient; when Christians are weak, He will give them His strength.

A. Matthew 10:17-20

B. II Corinthians 12:9-10

C. I Peter 4:12-13

D. I Corinthians 10:13

E. Matthew 5:10-12

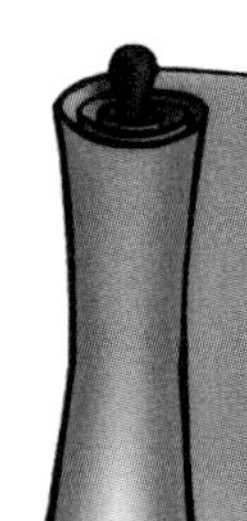

The Lord will give Christians grace for their trials when they go through them. They don't need to worry about how they are going to go through a trial that hasn't happened to them yet (Matt. 6:34).

Using a Concordance

Name ______________________

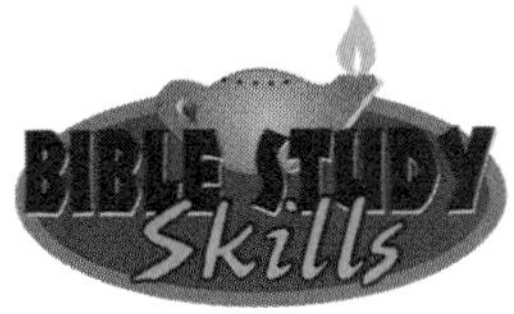
BIBLE STUDY
Skills

A **concordance** is a helpful study tool using keywords to locate verses in the Bible that contain those words. Some concordances, like the sample, also include verses about a particular topic.

Read each question below. Write a keyword that you would look for in a concordance to discover the answer. Some questions have more than one possible keyword.

1. Where can I find the story of David and Goliath? ______________
2. Where can I find out which precious stones will be included in the foundation of the New Jerusalem? ______________
3. Where can I find a verse that has the word *joy* in it? ______________

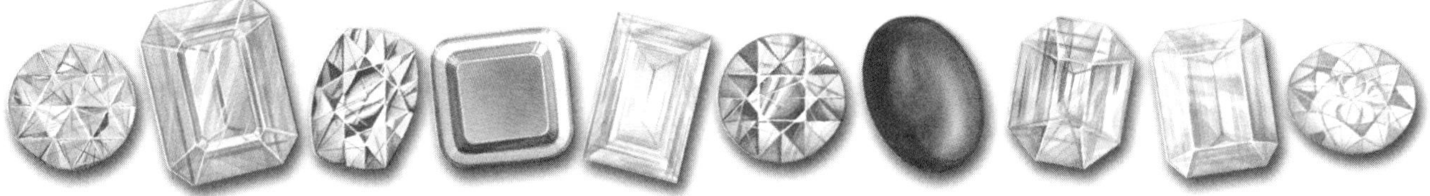

Use the concordance entry and your Bible to answer the following questions.

Which reference tells you about the marriage supper of the Lamb?

____

Who was the first martyr?

____

Which two references in Revelation talk about martyrs?

____

Which reference takes you to a verse about pressing forward for the prize?

____

MARAH, bitter waters healed there. Ex.15:23
MARANATHA, 1 Cor.16:22
MARK, Gen.4:15, the Lord set a *m* on Cain
Ps.37:37, *m* the perfect man
130:3, if thou shouldest *m* iniquities
Jer.2:22, thine iniquity is *m* before me
23:18, who hath *m* his word
Phil.3:14, I press toward the *m* for the prize
17, *m* them who walk so
MARK, evangelist. Acts 12:12
goes with Paul and Barnabas. Acts 12:25; 13:5
leaves them at Perga. Acts 13:13
contention about him. Acts 15:37
approved by Paul. 2 Tim.4:11
MARRIAGE, instituted. Gen.2:18
honorable. Ps.128; Prov.31:10; Heb.13:4
its obligations. Mt.19:4; Rom.7:2; 1 Cor.6:16; 7:10; Eph.5:31
parables concerning. Mt.22; 25
belongs to this world only. Mt.22:30; Mk.12:23
at Cana, miracle at. Jn.2
Paul's opinion of. 1 Cor.7; 1 Tim.5:14
of the Lamb, typical. Rev.19:7
unlawful marriages. Lev.18; Dt.7:3; Josh.23:12; Ezra 9; 10; Neh.13:23
MARRY, forbidding to. 1 Tim.4:3
MARS' HILL, English of Areopagus. Acts 17:22
MARTHA, instructed by Christ. Jn.11:5,21
reproved by Him. Lk.10:38
MARTYR, Stephen the first. Acts 7; 22:20. *See* Rev.2:13; 17:6
MARVEL, Mt.8:10; Mk.6:6; Lk.7:9, Jesus *m*
Mk.5:20, all men did *m*
Jn.3:7; 5:28; 1 Jn.3:13, *m* not
MARVELOUS, Job 5:9, *m* things without number
Ps.17:7, *m* loving-kindness
118:23; Mt.21:42; Mk.12:11, *m* in our eyes
Jn.9:30, here is a *m* thing
1 Pet.2:9, into his *m* light

Why are there two different entries for *MARK* in this concordance?

____

Truth and Falsehood

Revelation 2:12-29

Name ______________________________

The world is full of wrong ideas which can lead you to wrong decisions. Satan would love to deceive you into believing his lies about God, your sin, and your choice between them. Be alert! Ask God for the wisdom to recognize false teaching and the courage to condemn it. Do not allow your mind to be influenced by the deception of the world.

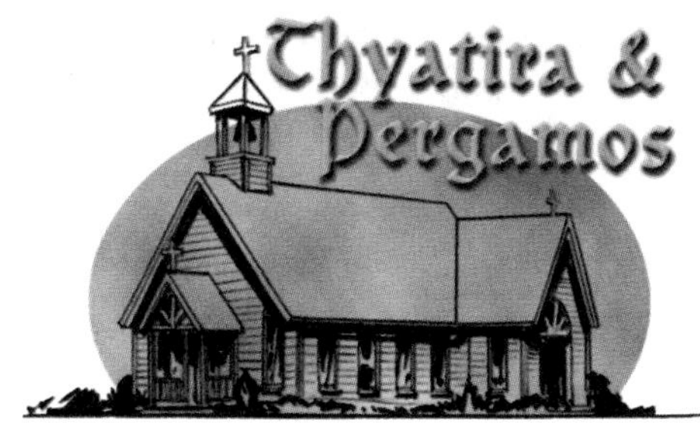
Thyatira & Pergamos

Answer the questions.

1. What was the church in Pergamos doing wrong? (Rev. 2:12-14)

   ____

2. What was the church in Thyatira doing wrong? (Rev. 2:18-20)

   ____

3. What should be the guideline for recognizing false teaching? ______________________________

Can you recognize which are false teachings that Christians should not tolerate? You have probably heard many of these ideas from the world. Mark with an *X* the seven false teachings.

_____ It is okay to tell a little lie for a good cause (Eph. 4:25).

_____ God's plan for your life is perfect (Jer. 29:11; Ps. 138:8).

_____ To be successful, you need to learn how to love yourself (Luke 9:23).

_____ Before making a decision, always consider the consequences of it (Job 4:8; Hos. 10:12).

_____ You deserve the very best in life (Luke 9:24-25).

_____ Before you blame your problems on other people, take a look at yourself (Matt. 7:3-5).

_____ Treat other people the way they treat you (Matt. 5:43-48).

_____ God loves you and wants you to know Him (John 3:16; Phil. 3:10).

_____ If you don't know what to do, trust your feelings (Prov. 3:5-6).

_____ Listen to your parents (Eph. 6:1).

_____ Since we only go through life once, we need to get all we can out of this world (I John 2:15-17).

_____ If you want to get to the top, you might have to toot your own horn or step on some other people (Matt. 5:5; Ps. 75:6-7).

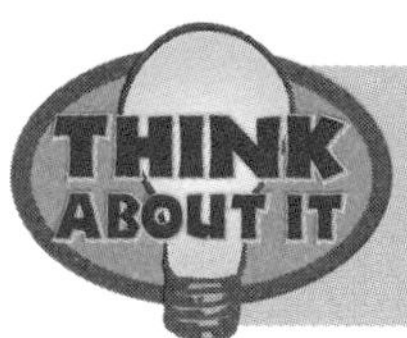
THINK ABOUT IT

What would you tell someone who tried to get you to accept one of the false ideas above? Read the verses from God's Word that support your answer. Consider memorizing them.

Singing with Understanding

"Now I Belong to Jesus" (vv. 1-3)

Name ______________________

Read verses 1-3 of the hymn on page 320 to complete the words. The left column contains a list of words from the hymn that describe a person before salvation. The right column contains a list of words that describe a person after he has been saved.

Before salvation...	After salvation...
l______________ (v. 2)	r______________ed (v. 1)
d______________ (v. 2)	j______________ (v. 3)
s______________ (v. 2)	f______________ (v. 3)
s______________ (v. 2)	r______________ed (v. 3)
e______________ (v. 3)	b____________ to Jesus (v. 1-3)

I Belong

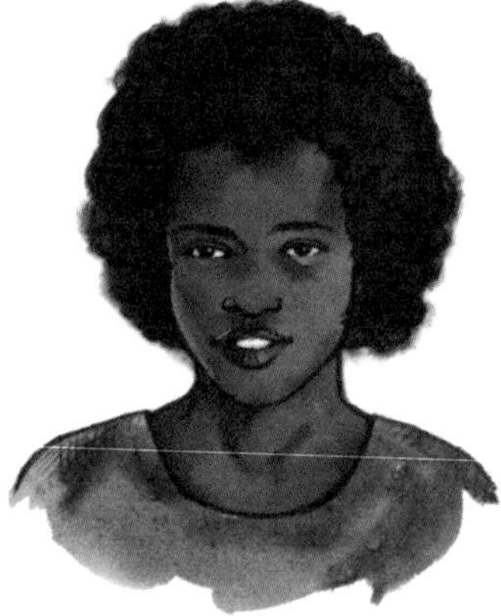

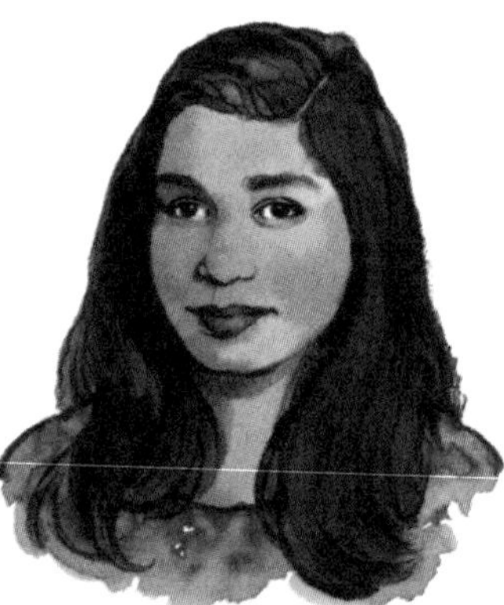

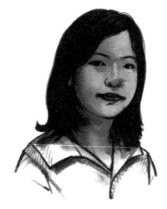

Can you think of some Scripture verses that tell how a person can know for sure that he belongs to Jesus? Write the verses on the lines below. (You may use a concordance and Bible for help.)

____

____

____

____

____

____

____

What Does God Say About My Entertainment?

Name ______________________

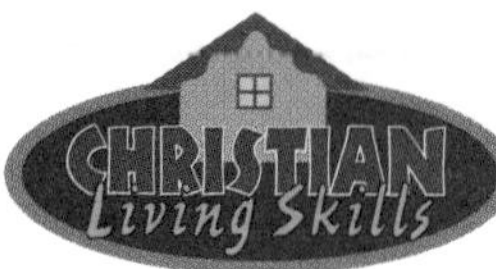
CHRISTIAN
Living Skills

People spend a great amount of money and time on entertaining themselves. What kinds of things do you do to entertain yourself? Read a book? Watch a video? Play a computer game? Hang out with friends? Go shopping? Although the young people in the Bible did not have videos, computer games, or television, God did give them instructions in His Word about how to please Him in their free time.

Read each verse. In your own words, write the Bible principle that gives you God's desires about how you choose to entertain yourself.

Psalm 101:3 ______________________

Philippians 4:8 ______________________

Proverbs 21:17 ______________________

When making your choices about what to do in your free time, consider the following questions:

1. Will this activity please God?
2. Will this activity be a stumbling block to others?
3. Will this activity please my parents?
4. Will this activity encourage me to be lazy?
5. Will this activity encourage Christian character in me?

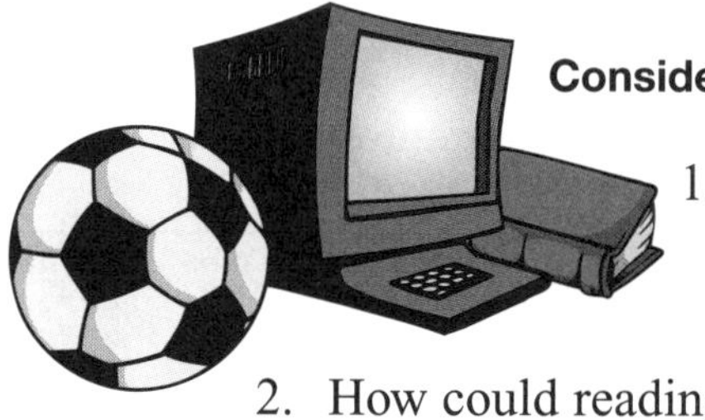

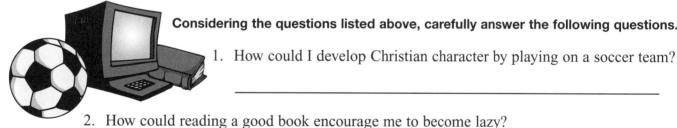

Considering the questions listed above, carefully answer the following questions.

1. How could I develop Christian character by playing on a soccer team?

____

2. How could reading a good book encourage me to become lazy?

____

3. How could playing a violent computer game be a stumbling block?

____

4. Why will my parents be displeased if I make the choice to watch television instead of doing my assignments?

____

5. Why will God be displeased when I watch a program in which the characters take His name in vain?

____

Something to Think About

My Entertainment

Name ______________________

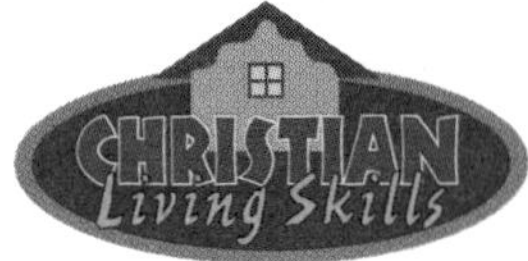
CHRISTIAN
Living Skills

God's Word gives you principles to follow about what you allow your eyes to see, what you allow your mind to think about, and how much time and money you spend on entertainment. God wants you to enjoy the blessings He has given to you. He also, however, wants you to be holy. Every Christian has the responsibility of guarding his eyes and mind from sin. Every Christian must also avoid laziness.

Read the verses. Write the correct reference that supports each principle for setting entertainment standards that please God.

I Corinthians 6:12
I Corinthians 4:2
Psalm 119:4
I Corinthians 10:24

I must choose my entertainment carefully because some activities could actually control me.

____

I must choose entertainment activities in which I can fully obey God's holy law.

____

I should choose entertainment that will not hurt my testimony to others.

____

God requires me to be responsible with the time and opportunities He has given me.

____

What About Me?

Take time at home to list the top four activities you enjoy doing in your free time for entertainment. Mark whether each activity is pleasing or displeasing to God. Complete the chart.

Activity	Pleasing to God?	Displeasing to God?	How is it pleasing to God? OR How is it displeasing to God?

Think about your answers. Are you pleasing God or yourself?

Two by Two

Name ______________________________

Christ's statements in Revelation 3:19-20 are presented in groups of two. Read the verses and answer the questions to discover the five pairs.

1. What are two proofs of God's love for you according to verse 19?

   ______________________ ______________________

2. What two things are you commanded to do in verse 19?

   ______________________ ______________________

3. What two things does Christ say He is doing in verse 20?

   ______________________ ______________________

4. What two responsibilities are given in verse 20?

   ______________________ ______________________

5. What two promises does Christ give in these verses to those who open to Him?

   ______________________ ______________________

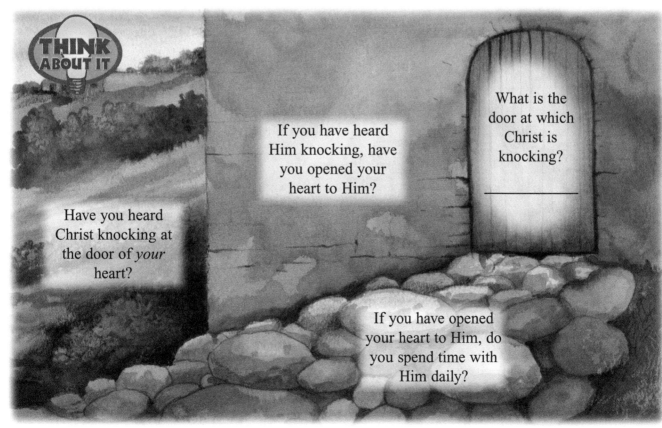

THINK ABOUT IT

Have you heard Christ knocking at the door of *your* heart?

If you have heard Him knocking, have you opened your heart to Him?

What is the door at which Christ is knocking?

____

If you have opened your heart to Him, do you spend time with Him daily?

Vital Signs

Revelation 3:1-6

Name ______________________

Answer the questions about Revelation 3.

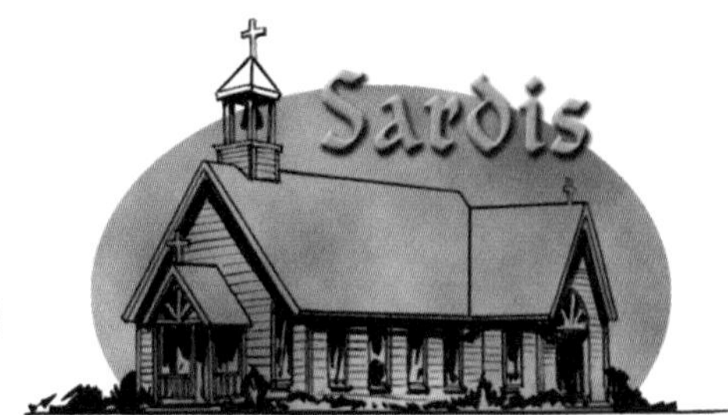
Sardis

1. What did other people think of the church in Sardis? (v. 1)

   ____

2. What was the main problem with the church in Sardis? (v. 1)

   ____

3. What did Christ tell them they needed to do? (vv. 2-3) ______________________________________

   ____

4. What might happen if they aren't alert and watching? (v. 3) ______________________________________

   ____

At the site of an emergency, the medical officials immediately examine any injured people for their vital signs. A **vital sign** is a physical indication that the person is living. Vital signs include a person's pulse rate, respiratory rate, and temperature. Checking the vital signs allows the emergency personnel to decide what actions should be taken to restore the injured person to good health. The spiritual life of a Christian also has vital signs that indicate the condition of his relationship with God. The church in Sardis looked like it was alive, but when God examined its spiritual vital signs, it was actually dead.

What about you? What do your spiritual vital signs reveal about your heart? Read the verses to discover the missing words. Then check your vital signs by asking yourself the questions.

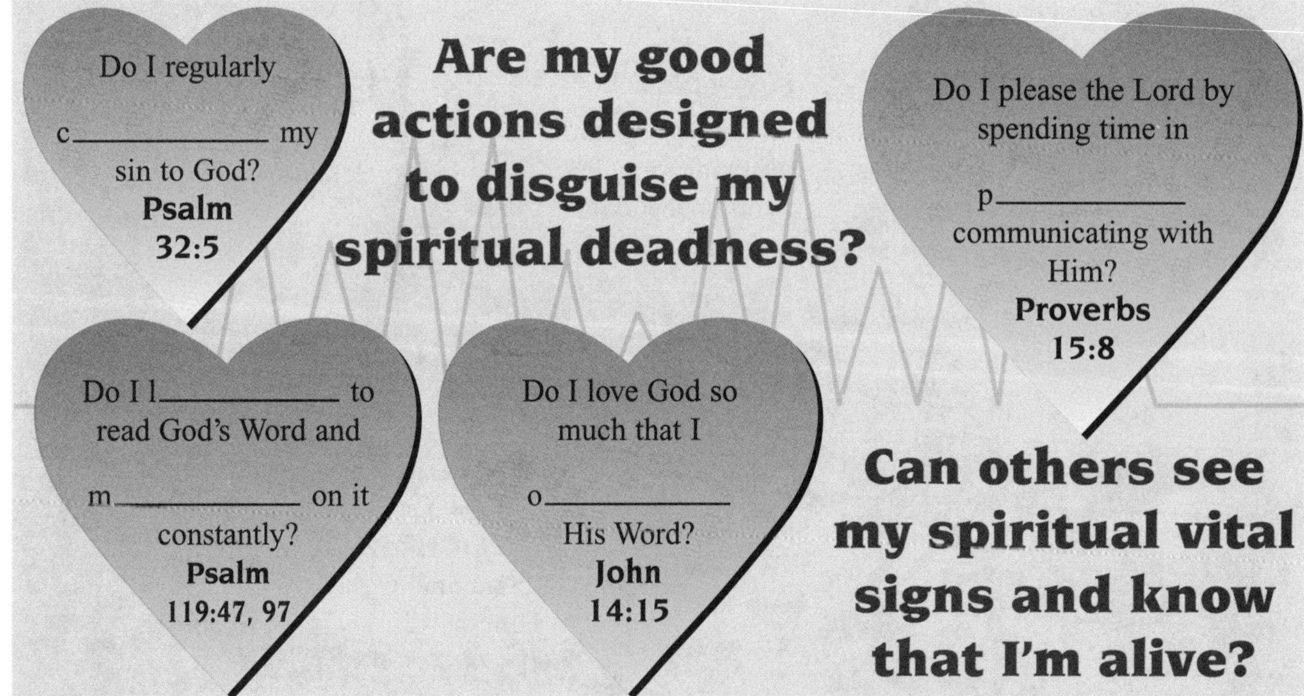
Do I regularly c__________ my sin to God? Psalm 32:5
Are my good actions designed to disguise my spiritual deadness?
Do I please the Lord by spending time in p__________ communicating with Him? Proverbs 15:8
Do I l__________ to read God's Word and m__________ on it constantly? Psalm 119:47, 97
Do I love God so much that I o__________ His Word? John 14:15
Can others see my spiritual vital signs and know that I'm alive?

Standing Firm

Revelation 3:7-13

Name ______________________

Mark whether the following statements are true or false. You may want to refer to Revelation 3:7-13 for help.

1. Christ praised the church in Philadelphia because they had remained faithful to Him. ○ True ○ False
2. Christ rebuked the church in Philadelphia because they had denied His name. ○ True ○ False
3. Christ warned that enemies of the church in Philadelphia would one day destroy the church. ○ True ○ False
4. God promised to keep the church in Philadelphia from the hour of trial and temptation. ○ True ○ False
5. God promised that those in the church who overcame would become pillars in His temple. ○ True ○ False
6. God commanded the church in Philadelphia to hold on to what they had so no one would take their golden sandals. ○ True ○ False

God allows trials to enter the lives of Christians to strengthen their character and to increase their faith. Even during these times of difficulty, God's Word remains true. God loves His children, and offers words of encouragement and motivation to stand firm for Christ.

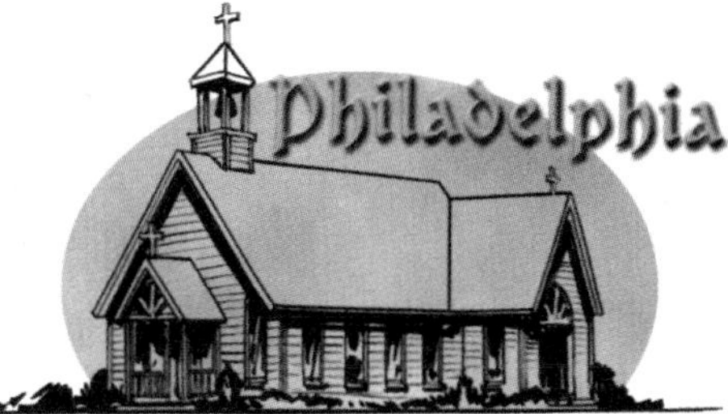
Philadelphia

Solve the puzzle to find out what God asked the church in Philadelphia to do.

% − [penny] + 7 − en + [ear] − a + e = ______________________

Read the verses and summarize the encouragement to Christians given in each verse.

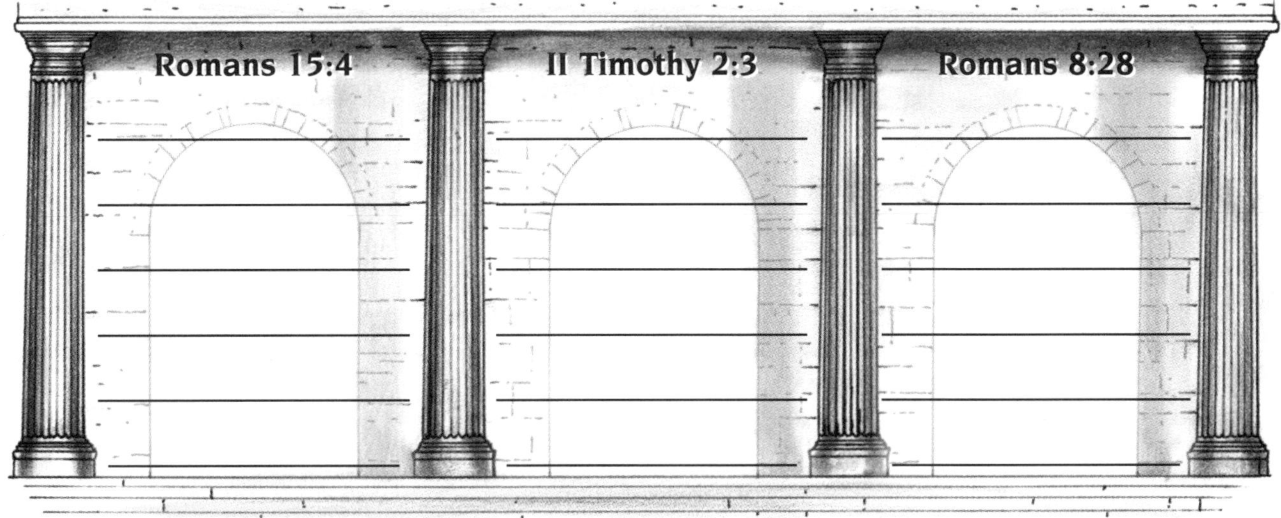
Romans 15:4
II Timothy 2:3
Romans 8:28

Hold Fast

Revelation 2:12-29

Name ______________________

Because of much false teaching in the world, Christians must be cautious and discerning about everything they hear and see. God's Word challenges Christians to hold tightly to truth.

Read the verses and write the correct reference for each challenge.

Hebrews 10:23 **Proverbs 4:13** **Revelation 3:11** **II Thessalonians 2:15**

Don't let anyone steal your crown! Hold on to what you have learned because Christ is coming soon!

____

Stand firm for the teachings of God's Word!

____

Hold on to good instruction because it guards your life!

____

Hold on to your profession of faith in Christ! God is faithful and will fulfill His promises!

____

Christians are faced with the responsibility of recognizing and rejecting false teaching. How can you do this? Use the code to find out how you can guard against Satan's deception.

1. ___ ___ ___ ___ ___ ___ ___ your sin.
   ✈ ❖ ▼ ✖ ▲ ✱ ✱

2. ___ ___ ___ God for wisdom and discernment.
   ● ✱ ❂

3. ___ ___ ___ ___ ___ ___ ___ ___ God's Word.
   ➤ ▲ ➤ ❖ ✪ ◆ ➧ ▲

4. ___ ___ ___ ___ for the Holy Spirit's guidance.
   ♥ ✪ ● ✚

A - ●	C - ✈
E - ▲	F - ✖
I - ◆	K - ❂
M - ➤	N - ▼
O - ❖	P - ♥
R - ✪	S - ✱
Y - ✚	Z - ➧

Neither Cold nor Hot

Revelation 3:14-22

Name ______________________

Answer the questions. You may use your Bible for help.

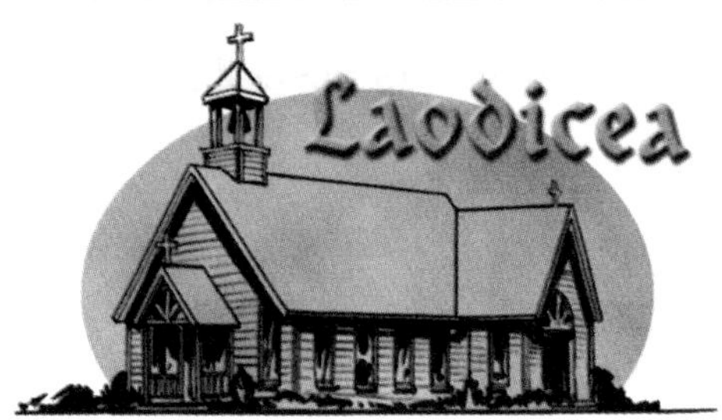
Laodicea

1. What does it mean to be lukewarm as a Christian?

   ____

   ____

2. What did the people in the church in Laodicea think about themselves? (Rev. 3:17)

   ____

3. What was really true about them? (Rev. 3:17) ______________________

   ____

4. Where could they find what they needed? (Rev. 3:18) ______________________

5. What did Christ tell them to do? (Rev. 3:19) ______________________

   Why? (Rev. 3:19) ______________________

6. What could they enjoy if they repented? (Rev. 3:20-21) ______________________

   ____

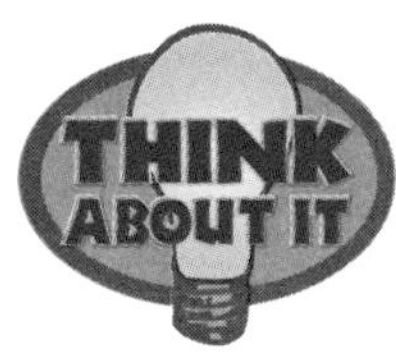
THINK
ABOUT IT

Take time at home to think about the following truths.

God sometimes uses difficult circumstances to cause Christians to repent. Because God is good, He loves you and wants to fellowship with you. Often it is only when trouble comes into your life that He can really get your attention. How might God be chastening you right now? What do you think He wants you to realize about Himself? What do you think He wants you to realize about yourself? What do you think He wants you to do in response to His chastening?

How would you describe yourself spiritually?

hot?

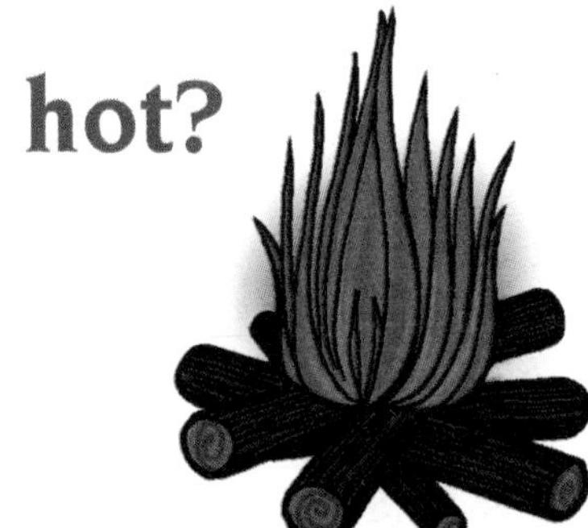

lukewarm?

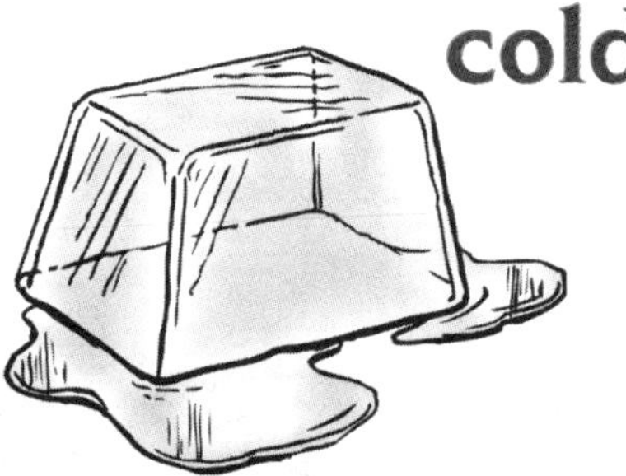

cold?

Is there a sin in your life that is keeping you from being a zealous, active, and obedient Christian?

The Seven Churches: Review

Revelation 2-3

Name ______________________

Match each fact to the correct church. You may use your Bible for help.

_____ 1. Christ rebuked this church because it was tolerating the teachings of the evil woman, Jezebel (Rev. 2:18-20).

_____ 2. Christ encouraged this church to endure suffering and persecution and to be faithful unto death (Rev. 2:8-10).

_____ 3. Christ rebuked this church for being spiritually dead even though others thought it was alive (Rev. 3:1-2).

_____ 4. Christ told this church that it was poor, blind, miserable, and wretched (Rev. 3:14-17).

_____ 5. Christ challenged this church to return to its first love (Rev. 2:1-4).

_____ 6. Christ told this church He had set before it an open door of opportunity to glorify God (Rev. 3:7-8).

_____ 7. Christ praised this church for its faithfulness to Him, but rebuked it for holding on to the false teachings of Balaam and the Nicolaitans (Rev. 2:14-16).

A. Church in Sardis
B. Church in Philadelphia
C. Church in Pergamos
D. Church in Laodicea
E. Church in Ephesus
F. Church in Smyrna
G. Church in Thyatira

Answer the questions.

1. List two things all the letters to the churches had in common.
   - ______________________________
   - ______________________________

2. What was different about the letter to the church in Philadelphia from all the other letters?

____

3. For what reason do you think Christ sent the letters to the churches?

____

____

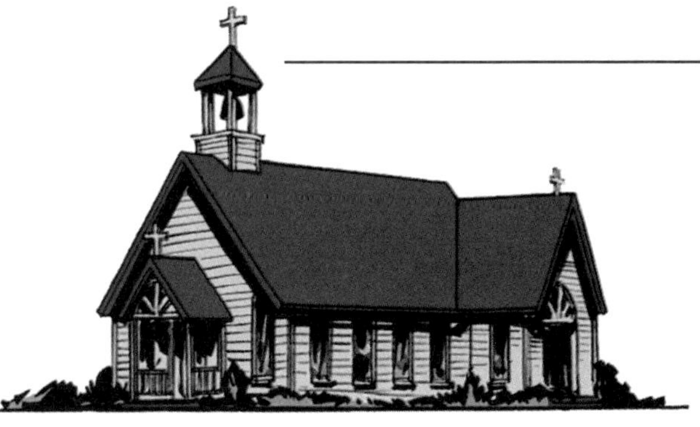

THINK ABOUT IT

Think about the spiritual condition of your heart. With which church do you most closely identify?

What Does God Say About Being Dependable?

Name ______________________________

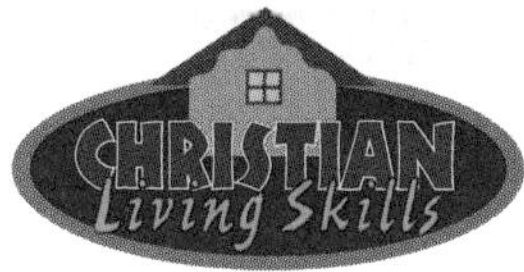
CHRISTIAN
Living Skills

Are you responsible? Trustworthy? Dependable? These three character traits can be used as synonyms to describe someone who is *reliable and able to be trusted to complete his work and make the right decision, no matter what the situation.* A dependable person proves himself to be trustworthy. A trustworthy person proves himself capable of handling more responsibilities that will bring more opportunities to serve God. Ultimately, a dependable person will experience God's blessings for his obedience.

Read the verses and fill in the blanks for the causes and effects found in each verse.

Verse	Cause	Effect
Luke 16:10	If I am responsible in the little things I do . . .	. . . then I ______________________________ ______________________________.
Matthew 25:21	If I ______________________________ ______________________________.	. . . then I will be given more responsibilities.

Beginning at the center, draw a line as you find your way through the maze. Then write the words over which you cross in order on the blanks below to discover the blessings of Christlike character that pleases God.

Desire to be like Christ

______________________________ (reliable)

______________________________ (able to be trusted)

______________________________ (able to make the right decision)

______________________________ (advantages given to you) → ______________________________ to be a good testimony

PRIVILEGES
SELFISH
DEPENDABLE
Desire to be like Christ
TRUSTWORTHY
DISOBEDIENT
RESPONSIBLE
OPPORTUNITY
LAZY
Christ-likeness

Something to Think About

Review

Name ______________________

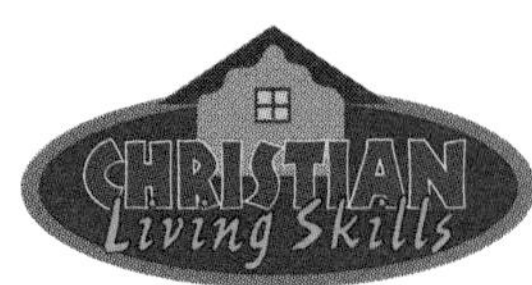
CHRISTIAN
Living Skills

God's Word has much to say about the kind of person you are becoming. You have been taught this year many ways that you can become more like Christ. Are you being responsible to make right choices about what you have learned? What changes have you made in your life because of your desire to be like Christ?

Read the verses and write God's reminder about the responsibility you have to Him.

Romans 14:12	James 4:17
______________________	______________________
______________________	______________________

What About Me?

Take time at home to think about the Christian Living Skills topics you have studied this year. Answer the following questions.

1. Write two statements about how you have learned to be more like Christ this year.

   ____

   ____

2. Write one change you have made in your actions this year to become more like Christ.

   ____

3. Describe one area in your life in which you still need to make changes to be more like Christ.

   ____

Think about your level of responsibility in the following areas. Rate yourself on a scale from 1 to 4.

Evaluation Questions	Pleasing Myself ⟷			Pleasing God
1. Am I careful to complete the details of my assignments?	1	2	3	4
2. Do I complete my assignments on time?	1	2	3	4
3. Am I diligent and hardworking?	1	2	3	4
4. Can I be trusted to make the right decision no matter what?	1	2	3	4
5. Do I tell the truth about everything?	1	2	3	4
6. Do I ever make the choice to not be lazy?	1	2	3	4
7. Do I treat my body like the temple of the Holy Spirit?	1	2	3	4
8. Is God pleased with my appearance?	1	2	3	4
9. Do I forgive others who have wronged me?	1	2	3	4
10. Am I bold to tell others about what Christ has done for me?	1	2	3	4

Hymns

O God, Our Help in Ages Past

From Psalm 90
Isaac Watts

Ascribed to William Croft
Supplement to the New Version, 1708

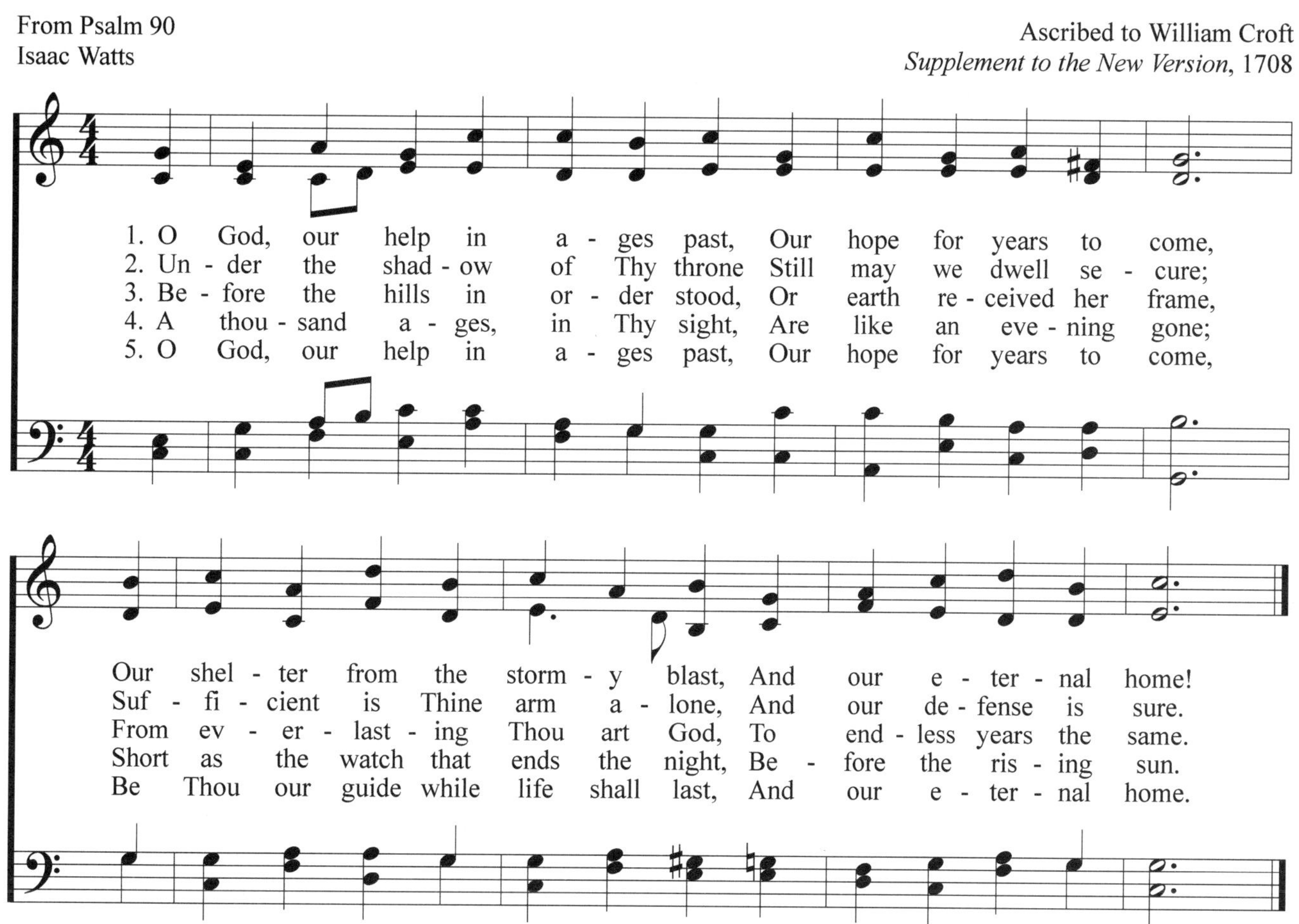
1. O God, our help in a - ges past, Our hope for years to come,
2. Un - der the shad - ow of Thy throne Still may we dwell se - cure;
3. Be - fore the hills in or - der stood, Or earth re - ceived her frame,
4. A thou - sand a - ges, in Thy sight, Are like an eve - ning gone;
5. O God, our help in a - ges past, Our hope for years to come,
Our shel - ter from the storm - y blast, And our e - ter - nal home!
Suf - fi - cient is Thine arm a - lone, And our de - fense is sure.
From ev - er - last - ing Thou art God, To end - less years the same.
Short as the watch that ends the night, Be - fore the ris - ing sun.
Be Thou our guide while life shall last, And our e - ter - nal home.

Faith of Our Fathers!

Frederick W. Faber

Henri F. Hemy
Alt. by James G. Walton

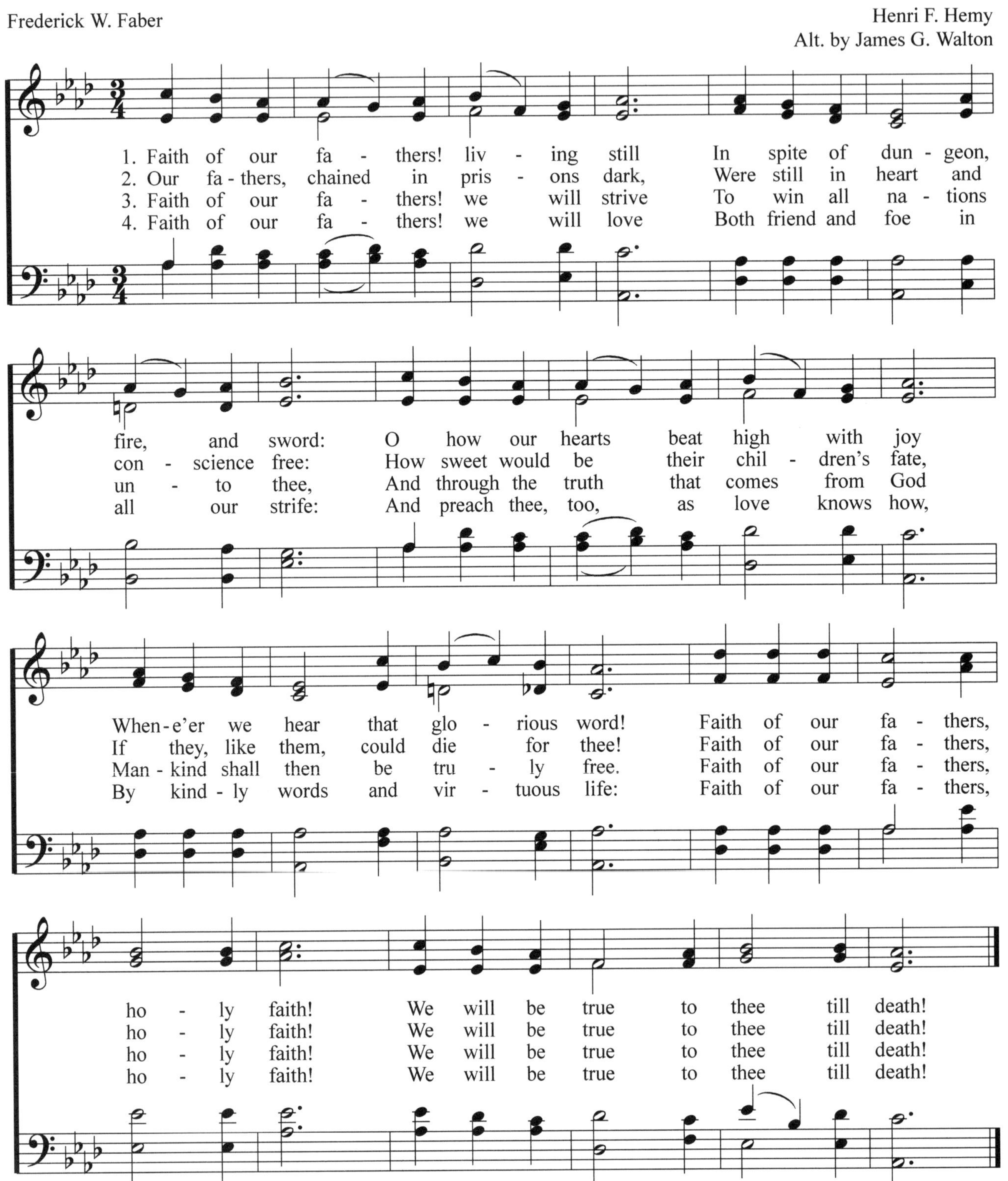
1. Faith of our fa - thers! liv - ing still In spite of dun - geon,
2. Our fa - thers, chained in pris - ons dark, Were still in heart and
3. Faith of our fa - thers! we will strive To win all na - tions
4. Faith of our fa - thers! we will love Both friend and foe in
fire, and sword: O how our hearts beat high with joy
con - science free: How sweet would be their chil - dren's fate,
un - to thee, And through the truth that comes from God
all our strife: And preach thee, too, as love knows how,
When - e'er we hear that glo - rious word! Faith of our fa - thers,
If they, like them, could die for thee! Faith of our fa - thers,
Man - kind shall then be tru - ly free. Faith of our fa - thers,
By kind - ly words and vir - tuous life: Faith of our fa - thers,
ho - ly faith! We will be true to thee till death!
ho - ly faith! We will be true to thee till death!
ho - ly faith! We will be true to thee till death!
ho - ly faith! We will be true to thee till death!

When I See the Blood

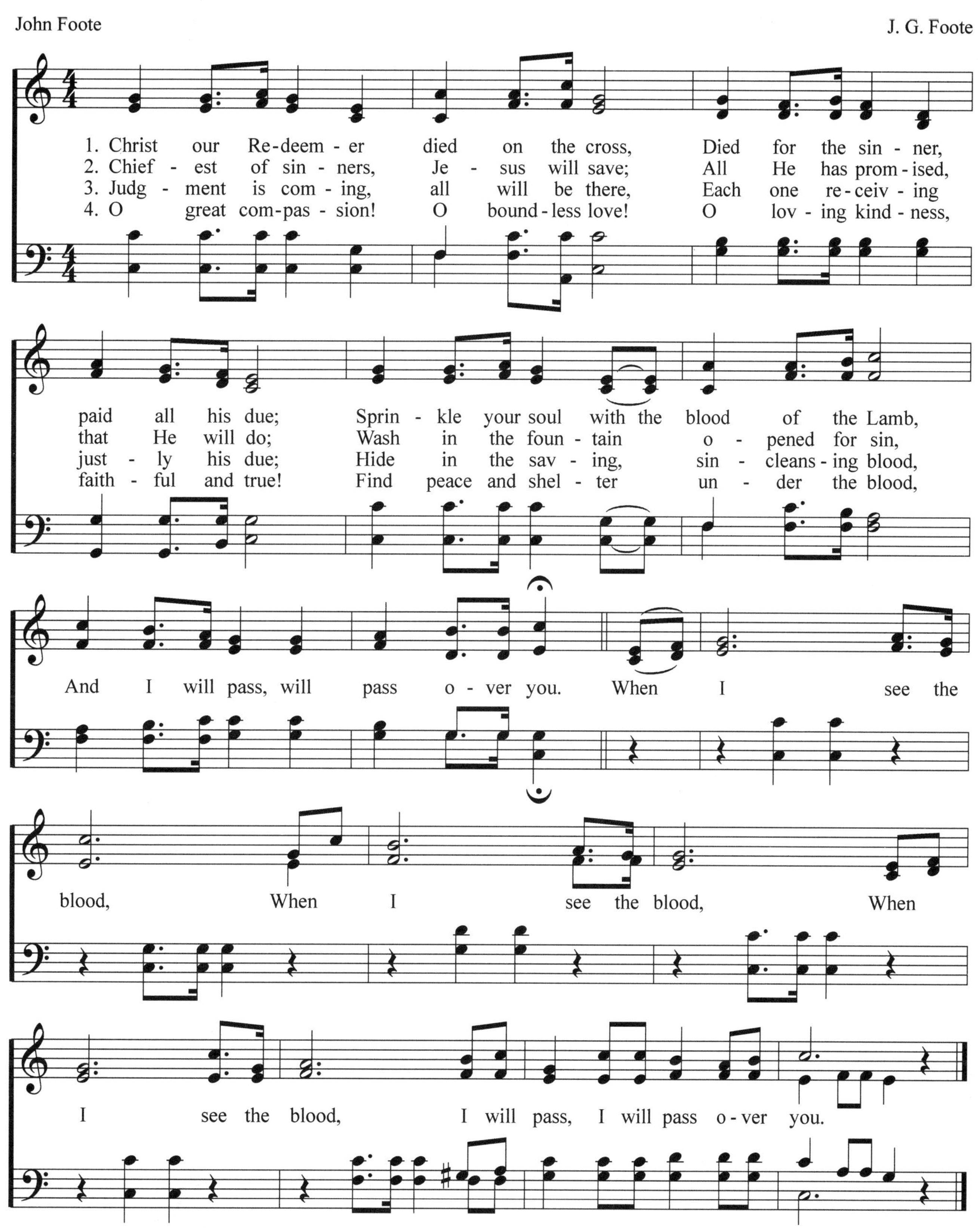
John Foote
J. G. Foote
1. Christ our Re-deem - er died on the cross, Died for the sin - ner,
2. Chief - est of sin - ners, Je - sus will save; All He has prom - ised,
3. Judg - ment is com - ing, all will be there, Each one re - ceiv - ing
4. O great com-pas - sion! O bound - less love! O lov - ing kind - ness,
paid all his due; Sprin - kle your soul with the blood of the Lamb,
that He will do; Wash in the foun - tain o - pened for sin,
just - ly his due; Hide in the sav - ing, sin - cleans - ing blood,
faith - ful and true! Find peace and shel - ter un - der the blood,
And I will pass, will pass o - ver you. When I see the
blood, When I see the blood, When
I see the blood, I will pass, I will pass o - ver you.

O Come, O Come, Emmanuel

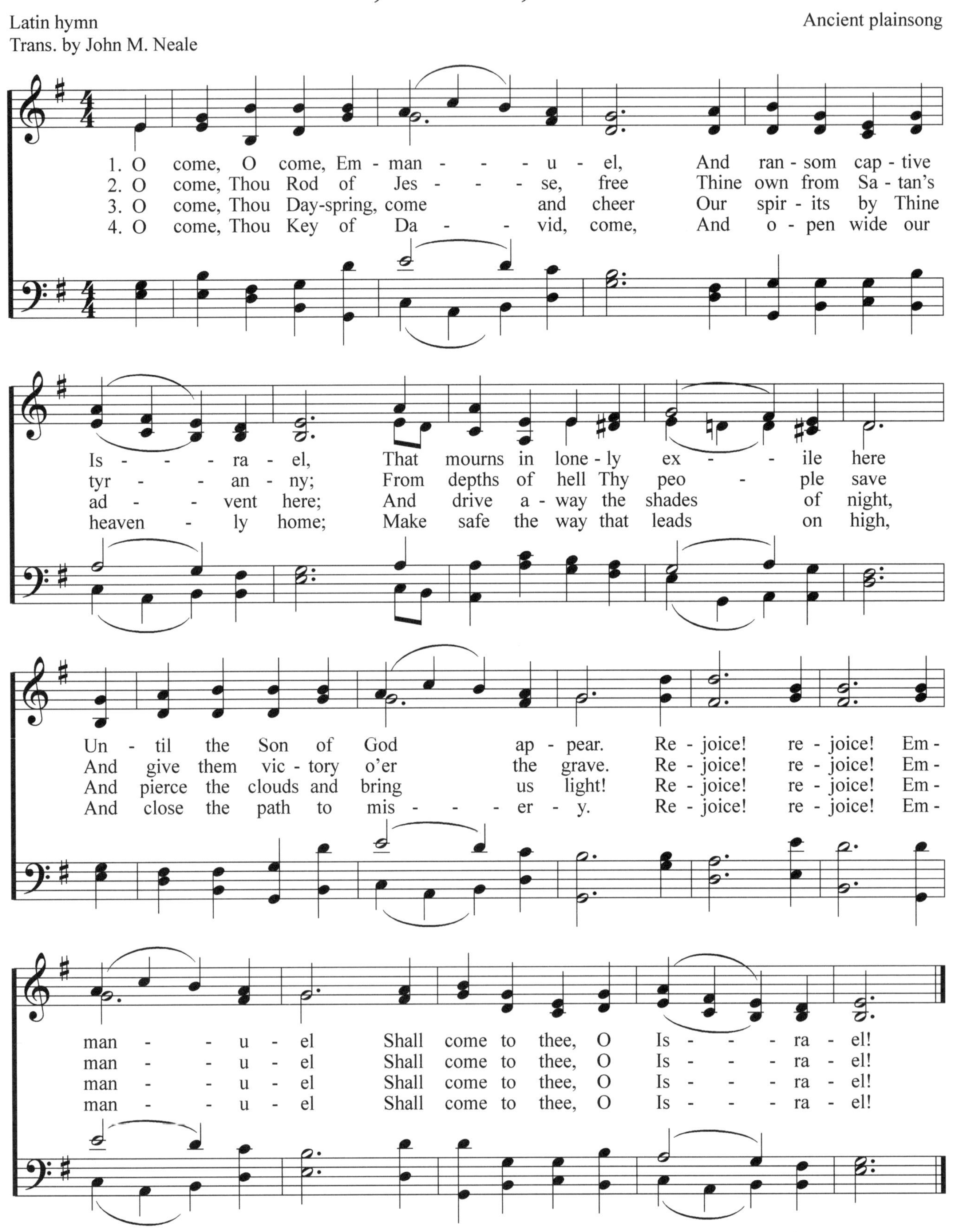

Latin hymn
Trans. by John M. Neale
Ancient plainsong
1. O come, O come, Em - man - - - u - el, And ran - som cap - tive
2. O come, Thou Rod of Jes - - - se, free Thine own from Sa - tan's
3. O come, Thou Day-spring, come and cheer Our spir - its by Thine
4. O come, Thou Key of Da - - vid, come, And o - pen wide our
Is - - - ra - el, That mourns in lone - ly ex - - ile here
tyr - - an - ny; From depths of hell Thy peo - ple save
ad - - vent here; And drive a - way the shades of night,
heaven - ly home; Make safe the way that leads on high,
Un - til the Son of God ap - pear. Re - joice! re - joice! Em -
And give them vic - tory o'er the grave. Re - joice! re - joice! Em -
And pierce the clouds and bring us light! Re - joice! re - joice! Em -
And close the path to mis - - - - er - y. Re - joice! re - joice! Em -
man - - u - el Shall come to thee, O Is - - - - ra - el!
man - - u - el Shall come to thee, O Is - - - - ra - el!
man - - u - el Shall come to thee, O Is - - - - ra - el!
man - - u - el Shall come to thee, O Is - - - - ra - el!

Great Is Thy Faithfulness

Thomas O. Chisholm William M. Runyan

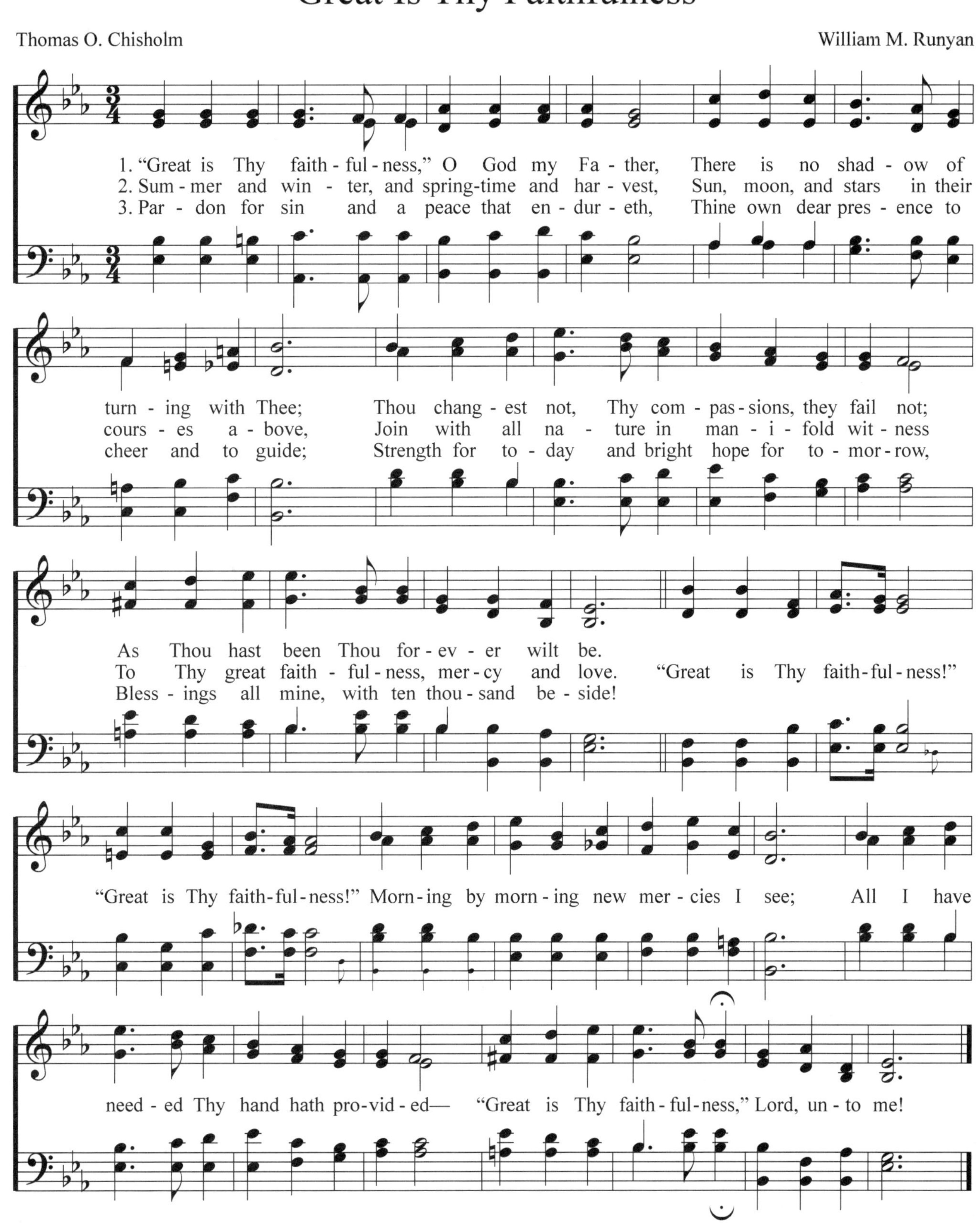
1. "Great is Thy faith - ful - ness," O God my Fa - ther, There is no shad - ow of
2. Sum - mer and win - ter, and spring-time and har - vest, Sun, moon, and stars in their
3. Par - don for sin and a peace that en - dur - eth, Thine own dear pres - ence to
turn - ing with Thee; Thou chang - est not, Thy com - pas - sions, they fail not;
cours - es a - bove, Join with all na - ture in man - i - fold wit - ness
cheer and to guide; Strength for to - day and bright hope for to - mor - row,
As Thou hast been Thou for - ev - er wilt be.
To Thy great faith - ful - ness, mer - cy and love. "Great is Thy faith-ful - ness!"
Bless - ings all mine, with ten thou - sand be - side!
"Great is Thy faith-ful-ness!" Morn-ing by morn - ing new mer - cies I see; All I have
need - ed Thy hand hath pro-vid - ed— "Great is Thy faith - ful - ness," Lord, un - to me!

GREAT IS THY FAITHFULNESS
Words: Thomas O. Chisholm
Music: William M. Runyan

Standing on the Promises

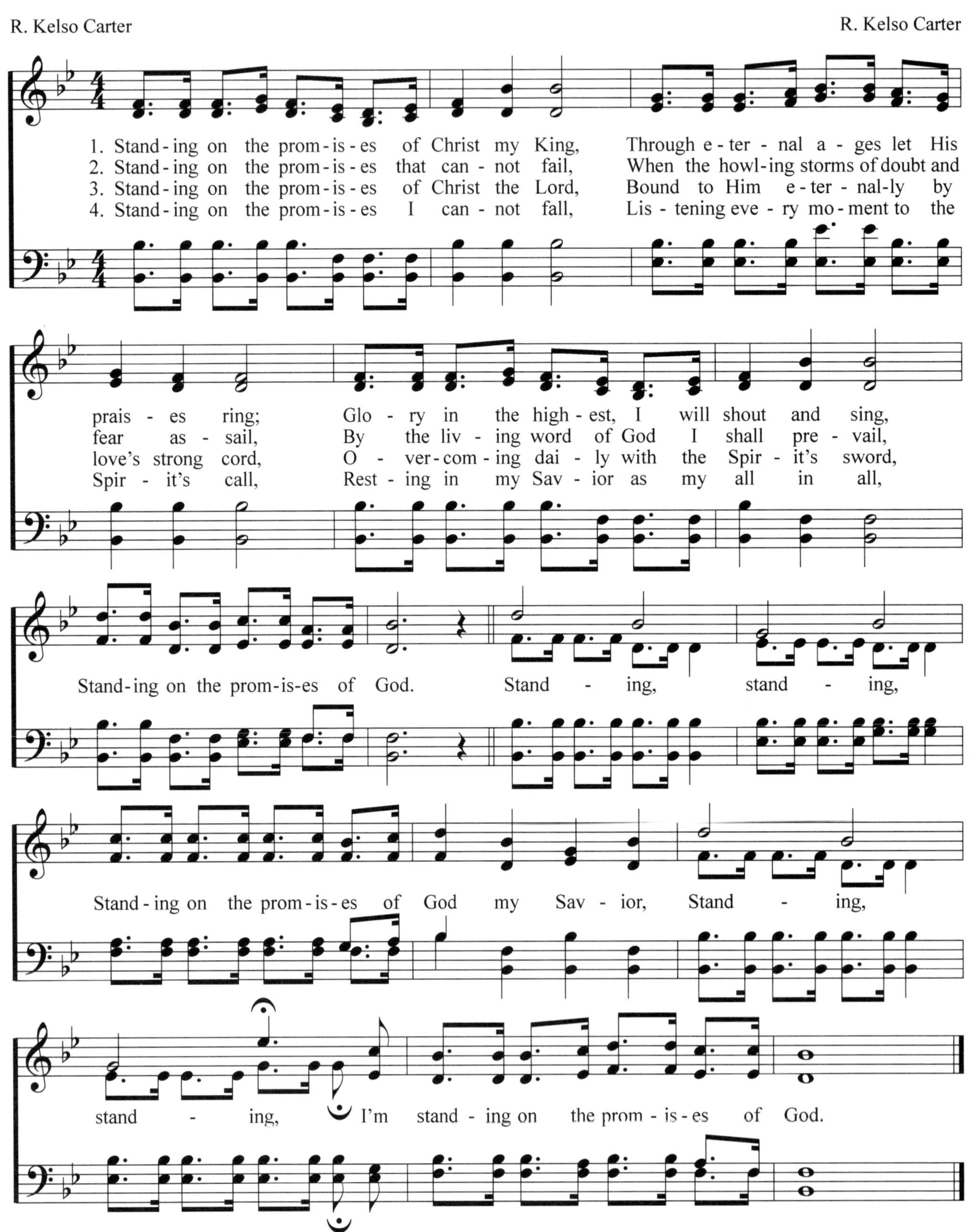
R. Kelso Carter
R. Kelso Carter
1. Stand-ing on the prom-is-es of Christ my King, Through e-ter-nal a-ges let His prais-es ring; Glo-ry in the high-est, I will shout and sing,
2. Stand-ing on the prom-is-es that can-not fail, When the howl-ing storms of doubt and fear as-sail, By the liv-ing word of God I shall pre-vail,
3. Stand-ing on the prom-is-es of Christ the Lord, Bound to Him e-ter-nal-ly by love's strong cord, O-ver-com-ing dai-ly with the Spir-it's sword,
4. Stand-ing on the prom-is-es I can-not fall, Lis-tening eve-ry mo-ment to the Spir-it's call, Rest-ing in my Sav-ior as my all in all,
Stand-ing on the prom-is-es of God.
Stand-ing, stand-ing,
Stand-ing on the prom-is-es of God my Sav-ior, Stand-ing,
stand-ing, I'm stand-ing on the prom-is-es of God.

Our Great Savior

J. Wilbur Chapman

Rowland H. Prichard
Arr. by Robert Harkness

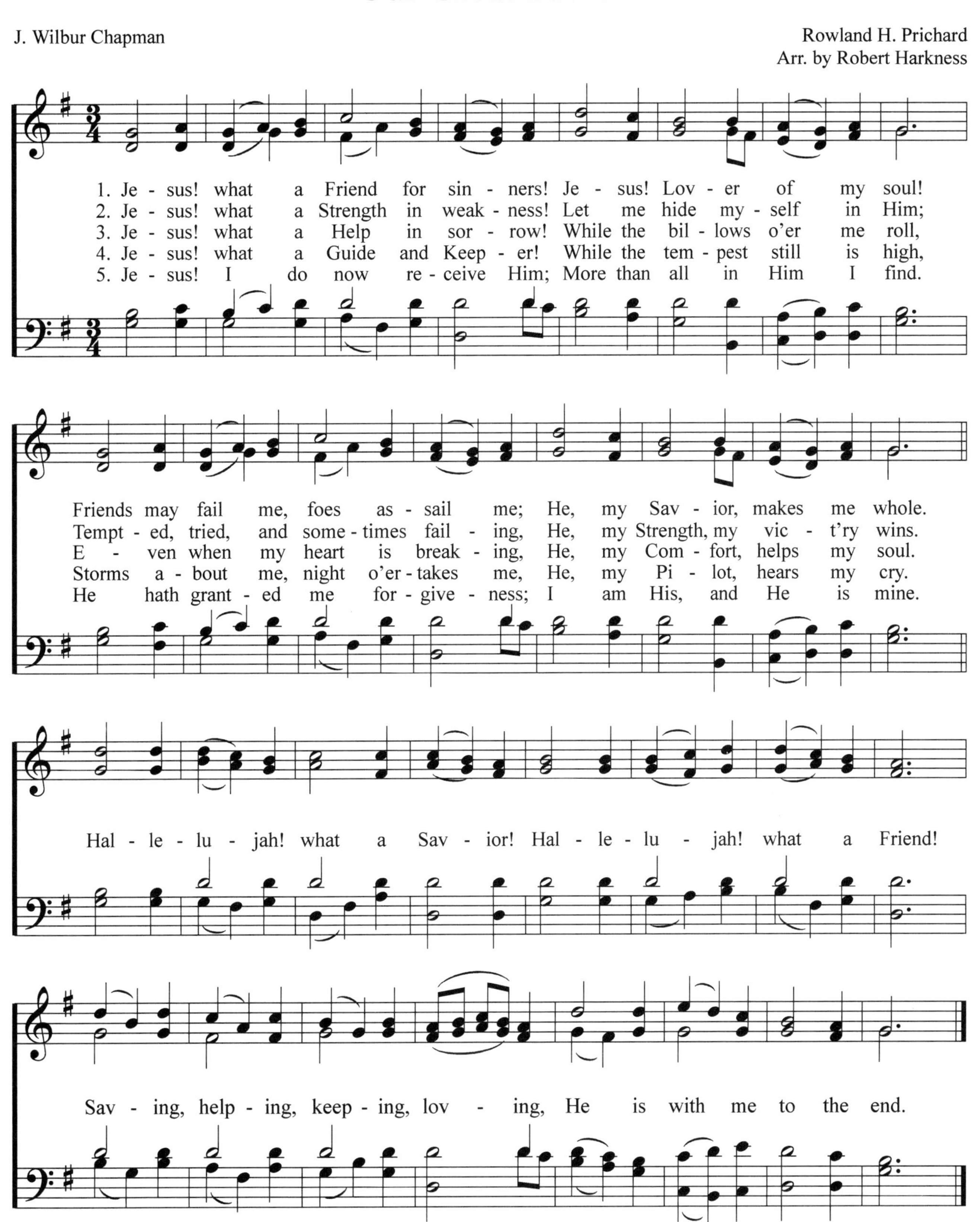
1. Je - sus! what a Friend for sin - ners! Je - sus! Lov - er of my soul!
2. Je - sus! what a Strength in weak - ness! Let me hide my - self in Him;
3. Je - sus! what a Help in sor - row! While the bil - lows o'er me roll,
4. Je - sus! what a Guide and Keep - er! While the tem - pest still is high,
5. Je - sus! I do now re - ceive Him; More than all in Him I find.
Friends may fail me, foes as - sail me; He, my Sav - ior, makes me whole.
Tempt - ed, tried, and some - times fail - ing, He, my Strength, my vic - t'ry wins.
E - ven when my heart is break - ing, He, my Com - fort, helps my soul.
Storms a - bout me, night o'er - takes me, He, my Pi - lot, hears my cry.
He hath grant - ed me for - give - ness; I am His, and He is mine.
Hal - le - lu - jah! what a Sav - ior! Hal - le - lu - jah! what a Friend!
Sav - ing, help - ing, keep - ing, lov - ing, He is with me to the end.

Christ the Lord Is Risen Today

Charles Wesley

From *Lyra Davidica*

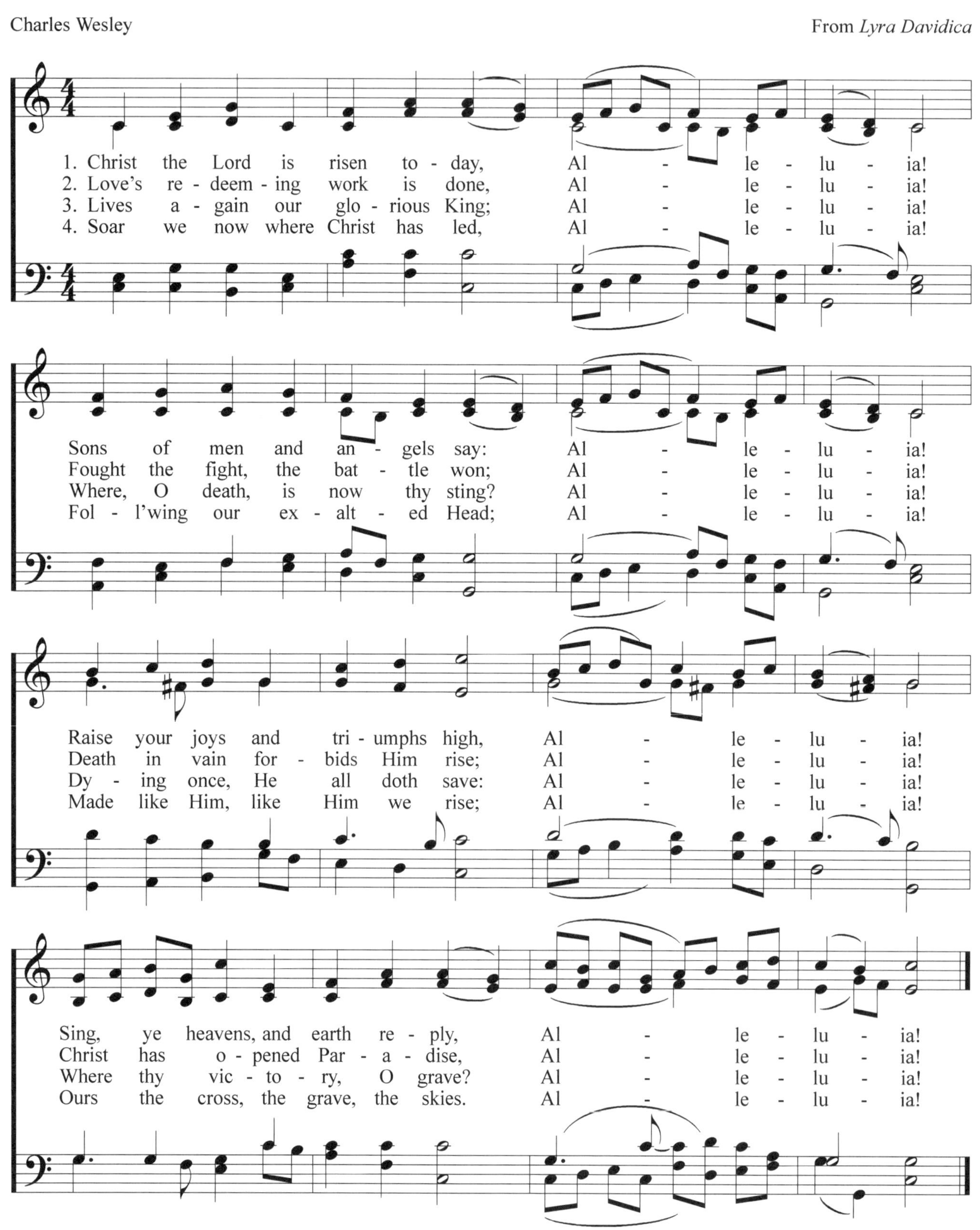
1. Christ the Lord is risen to - day, Al - le - lu - ia!
2. Love's re - deem - ing work is done, Al - le - lu - ia!
3. Lives a - gain our glo - rious King; Al - le - lu - ia!
4. Soar we now where Christ has led, Al - le - lu - ia!
Sons of men and an - gels say: Al - le - lu - ia!
Fought the fight, the bat - tle won; Al - le - lu - ia!
Where, O death, is now thy sting? Al - le - lu - ia!
Fol - l'wing our ex - alt - ed Head; Al - le - lu - ia!
Raise your joys and tri - umphs high, Al - le - lu - ia!
Death in vain for - bids Him rise; Al - le - lu - ia!
Dy - ing once, He all doth save: Al - le - lu - ia!
Made like Him, like Him we rise; Al - le - lu - ia!
Sing, ye heavens, and earth re - ply, Al - le - lu - ia!
Christ has o - pened Par - a - dise, Al - le - lu - ia!
Where thy vic - to - ry, O grave? Al - le - lu - ia!
Ours the cross, the grave, the skies. Al - le - lu - ia!

Footprints of Jesus

Mary B. C. Slade

Asa B. Everett

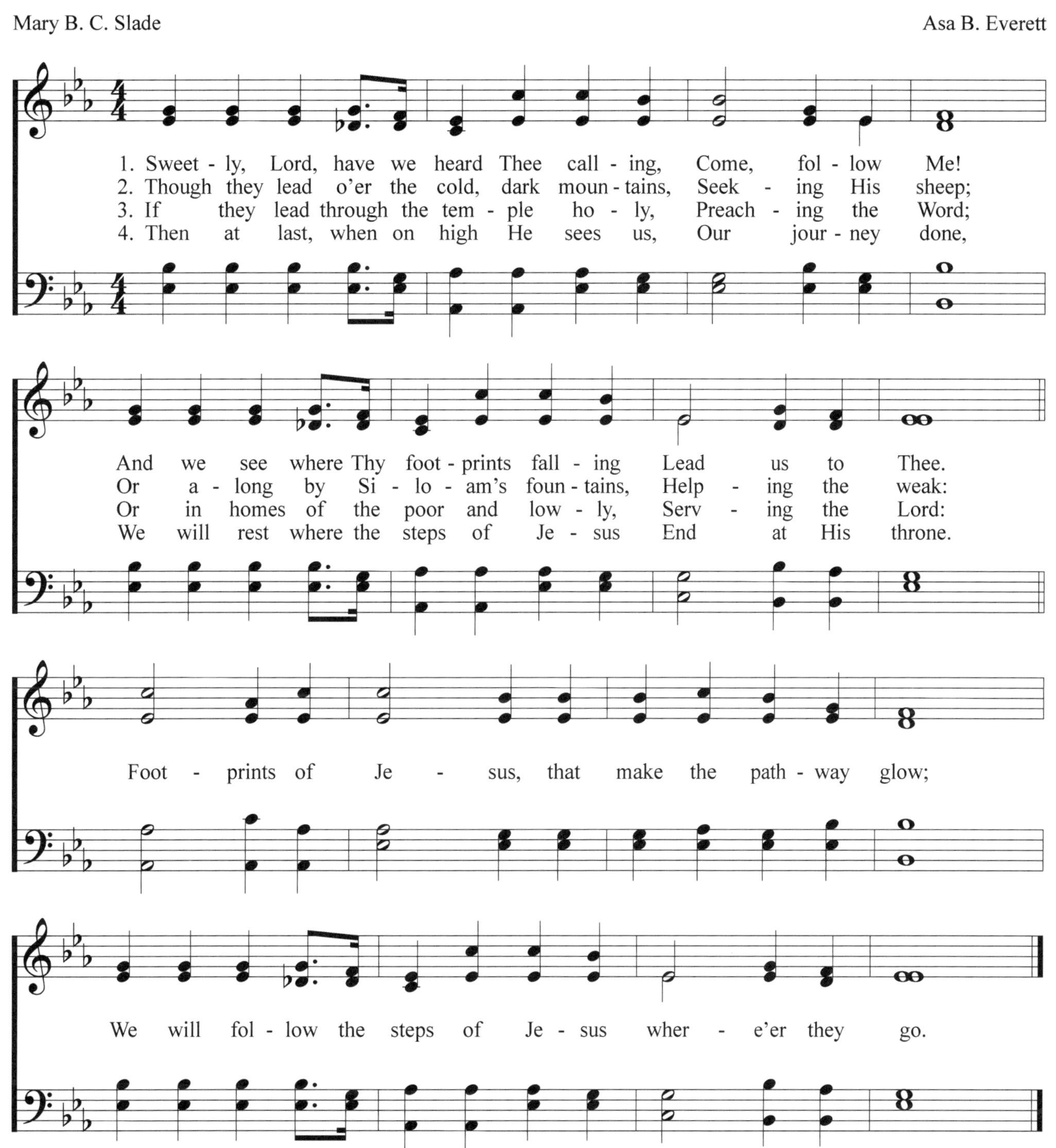
1. Sweet - ly, Lord, have we heard Thee call - ing, Come, fol - low Me!
2. Though they lead o'er the cold, dark moun - tains, Seek - ing His sheep;
3. If they lead through the tem - ple ho - ly, Preach - ing the Word;
4. Then at last, when on high He sees us, Our jour - ney done,
And we see where Thy foot - prints fall - ing Lead us to Thee.
Or a - long by Si - lo - am's foun - tains, Help - ing the weak:
Or in homes of the poor and low - ly, Serv - ing the Lord:
We will rest where the steps of Je - sus End at His throne.
Foot - prints of Je - sus, that make the path - way glow;
We will fol - low the steps of Je - sus wher - e'er they go.

Now I Belong to Jesus

Norman J. Clayton

Norman J. Clayton

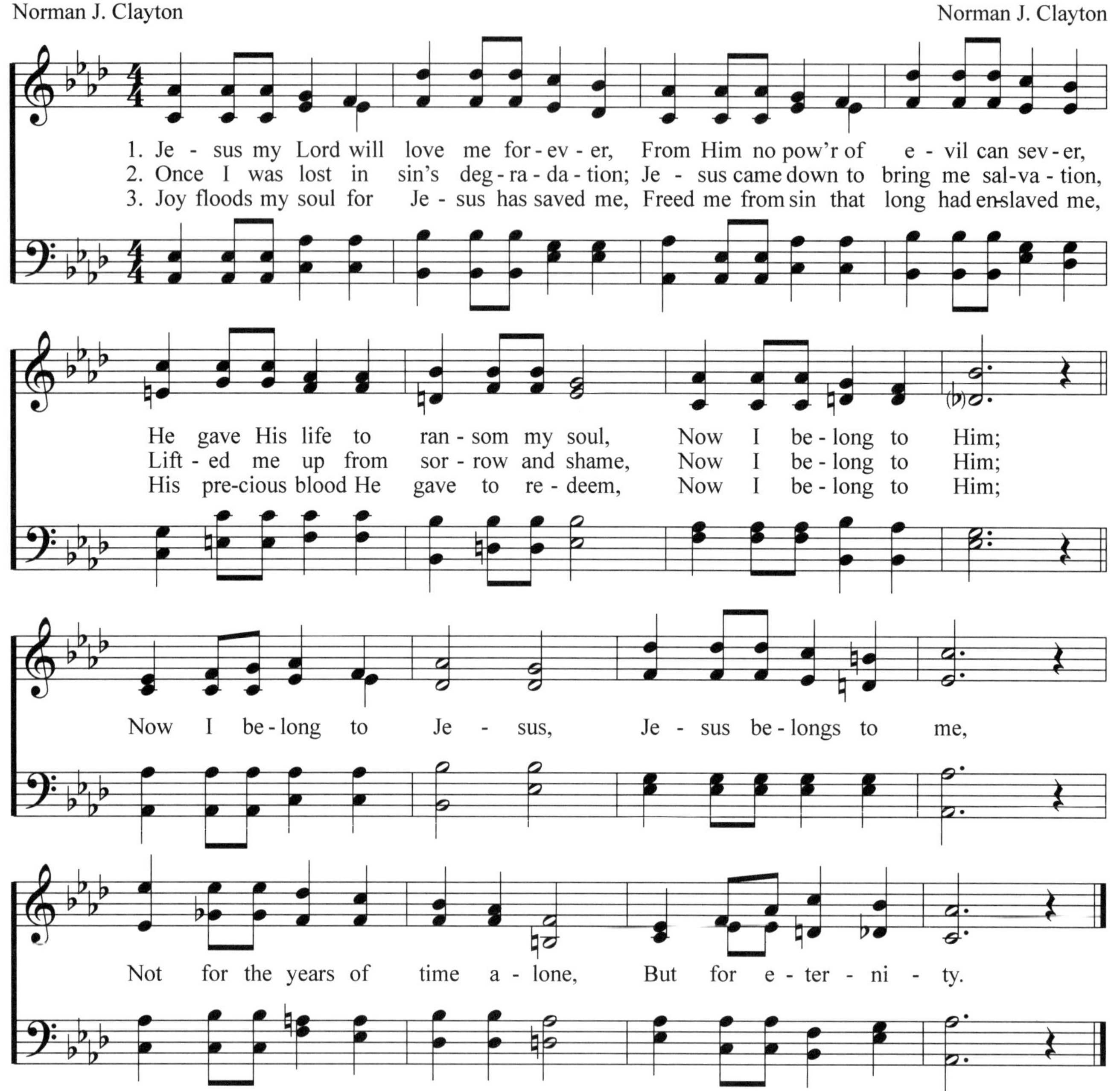
1. Je - sus my Lord will love me for - ev - er, From Him no pow'r of e - vil can sev - er,
2. Once I was lost in sin's deg - ra - da - tion; Je - sus came down to bring me sal - va - tion,
3. Joy floods my soul for Je - sus has saved me, Freed me from sin that long had en-slaved me,
He gave His life to ran - som my soul, Now I be - long to Him;
Lift - ed me up from sor - row and shame, Now I be - long to Him;
His pre-cious blood He gave to re - deem, Now I be - long to Him;
Now I be - long to Je - sus, Je - sus be - longs to me,
Not for the years of time a - lone, But for e - ter - ni - ty.

God's Word Charts

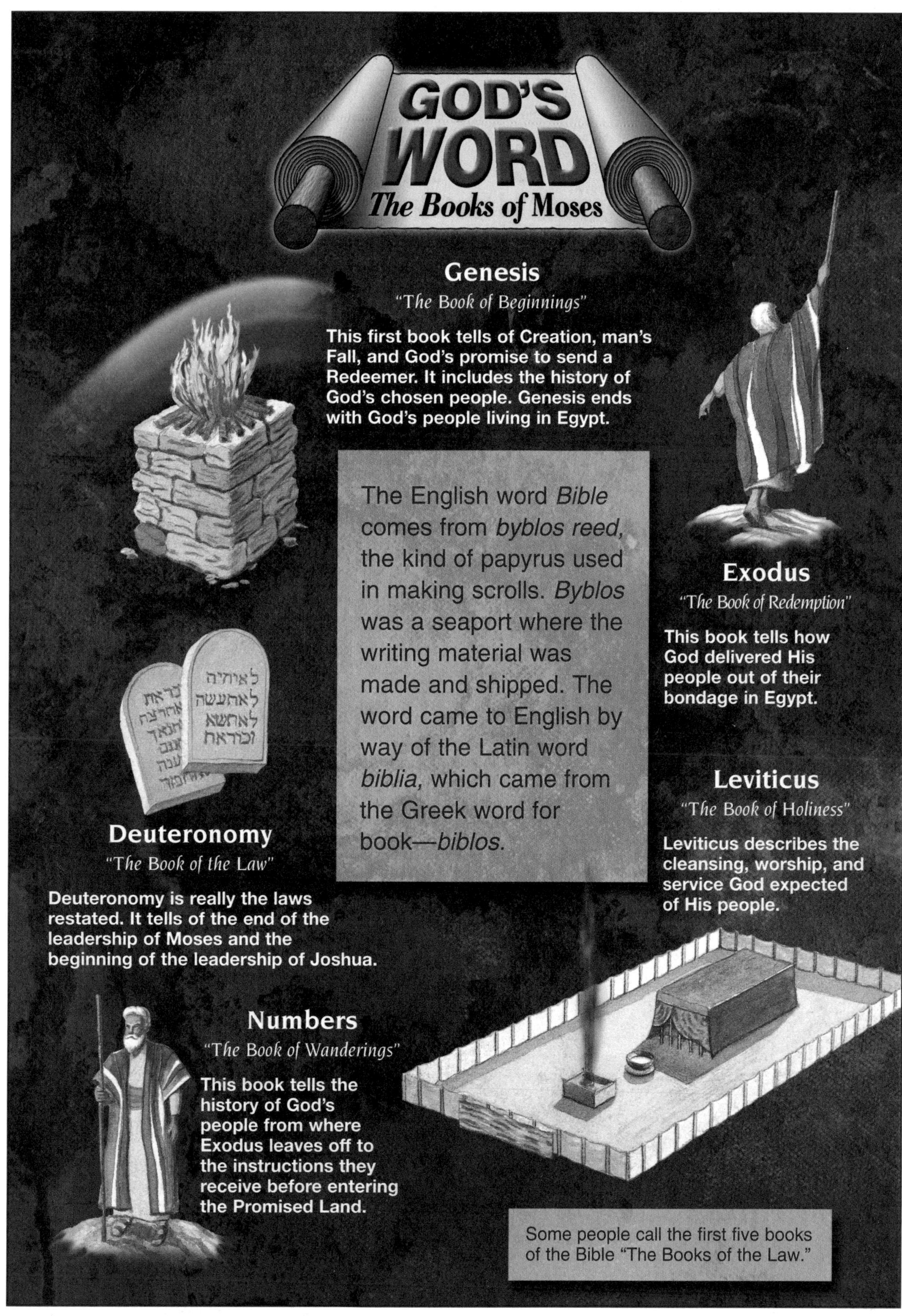
GOD'S WORD
The Books of Moses
Genesis
"The Book of Beginnings"
This first book tells of Creation, man's Fall, and God's promise to send a Redeemer. It includes the history of God's chosen people. Genesis ends with God's people living in Egypt.
The English word *Bible* comes from *byblos reed,* the kind of papyrus used in making scrolls. *Byblos* was a seaport where the writing material was made and shipped. The word came to English by way of the Latin word *biblia,* which came from the Greek word for book—*biblos.*
Exodus
"The Book of Redemption"
This book tells how God delivered His people out of their bondage in Egypt.
Leviticus
"The Book of Holiness"
Leviticus describes the cleansing, worship, and service God expected of His people.
Deuteronomy
"The Book of the Law"
Deuteronomy is really the laws restated. It tells of the end of the leadership of Moses and the beginning of the leadership of Joshua.
Numbers
"The Book of Wanderings"
This book tells the history of God's people from where Exodus leaves off to the instructions they receive before entering the Promised Land.
Some people call the first five books of the Bible "The Books of the Law."

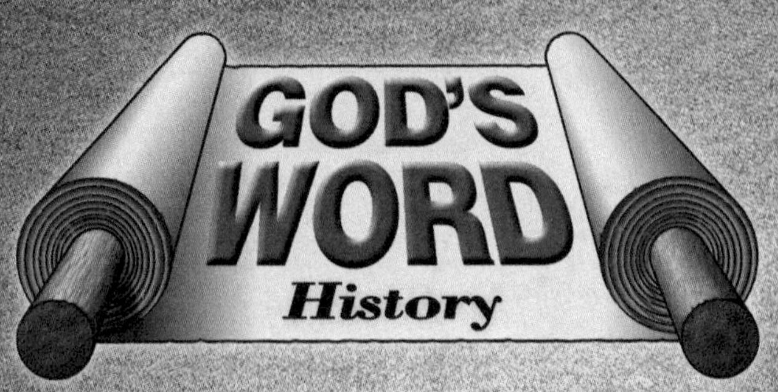
GOD'S
WORD
History

Joshua

"Conflict and Conquest"

God faithfully guided His people under the leadership of Joshua as they fought for and won the Promised Land.

Judges

"Oppression and Deliverance"

For three hundred years, from the death of Joshua to the time of Samuel, the Israelites were in a cycle of sin, punishment, confession, and deliverance from their enemies.

Ruth

"The Romance of Redemption"

God worked through the personal and family history of Ruth, an ancestor of Jesus Christ.

I and II Samuel

"Kingdom Established"

Samuel guided Israel wisely and well. He anointed two kings: Saul, who failed to please God, and David, who was a man after God's heart.

I and II Kings

"Kingdom Divided"

From David to the time of the Babylonian captivity, God's people were led by kings who turned their hearts toward God and kings who turned them away. The land split into two kingdoms, Israel and Judah.

I and II Chronicles

"Israel's Worship"

Throughout the time of Samuel and Israel's first two kings, priests led Israel in worshiping God.

Ezra

"Return from Captivity"

Ezra led a group of God's people back from Babylon and, along with Nehemiah, encouraged them to rebuild the temple and rededicate themselves.

Nehemiah

"Jerusalem Rebuilt"

God used Nehemiah to plan the rebuilding of the walls of Jerusalem and to lead His people in finishing this huge task.

Esther

"The Providence of God"

God ordered events to place Esther as a queen so that she could be used to save His people from destruction in the land of their captivity.

IN GOD'S HANDS

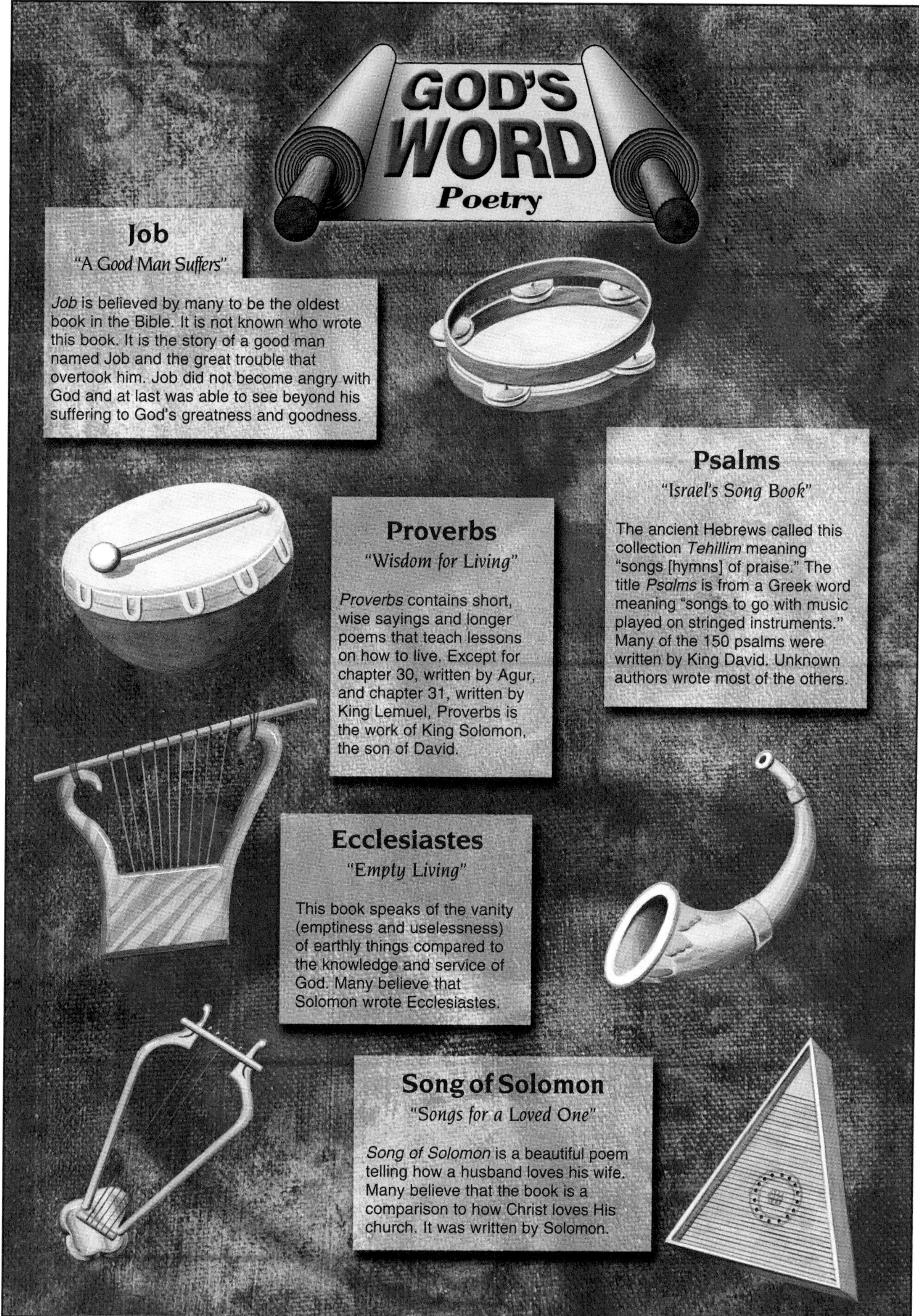
GOD'S WORD
Poetry
Job
"A Good Man Suffers"
Job is believed by many to be the oldest book in the Bible. It is not known who wrote this book. It is the story of a good man named Job and the great trouble that overtook him. Job did not become angry with God and at last was able to see beyond his suffering to God's greatness and goodness.
Psalms
"Israel's Song Book"
The ancient Hebrews called this collection *Tehillim* meaning "songs [hymns] of praise." The title *Psalms* is from a Greek word meaning "songs to go with music played on stringed instruments." Many of the 150 psalms were written by King David. Unknown authors wrote most of the others.
Proverbs
"Wisdom for Living"
Proverbs contains short, wise sayings and longer poems that teach lessons on how to live. Except for chapter 30, written by Agur, and chapter 31, written by King Lemuel, Proverbs is the work of King Solomon, the son of David.
Ecclesiastes
"Empty Living"
This book speaks of the vanity (emptiness and uselessness) of earthly things compared to the knowledge and service of God. Many believe that Solomon wrote Ecclesiastes.
Song of Solomon
"Songs for a Loved One"
Song of Solomon is a beautiful poem telling how a husband loves his wife. Many believe that the book is a comparison to how Christ loves His church. It was written by Solomon.

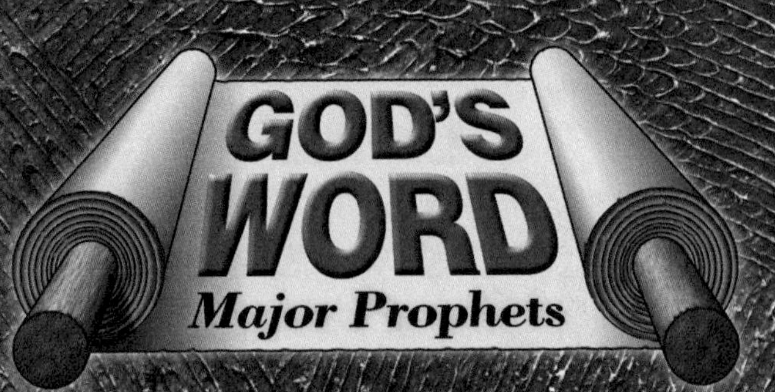
GOD'S
WORD
Major Prophets

Isaiah

"The Messianic Prophet"

Isaiah was sent to turn Judah back to the Lord. He predicted the fall of the nation and the return of a small number of godly people. He wrote of the power, suffering, rejection, death, and judgment of Jesus Christ.

These books are called the Major Prophets because of their length and position among Bible books. They are not more important than the rest of the prophetic books.

Jeremiah

"The Weeping Prophet"

Jeremiah was sent to the people of Jerusalem to tell them to turn from sin to avoid punishment. When they would not listen, he cried over their stubbornness.

Lamentations

"Sorrow for God's People"

To lament means "to weep or to mourn." Lamentations was written by Jeremiah. He wrote the sad story of Jerusalem's downfall, but he also gave hope of God's mercy in the future.

Ezekiel

"The Watchman Prophet"

Ezekiel was taken prisoner when the Babylonians took Judah. God used him to comfort and encourage the other prisoners. He warned of more punishment if the people continued to do wrong.

Daniel

"The Consistent Prophet"

Daniel was taken into exile in Babylon. He never gave up worshiping God in this pagan nation. His prophecies spoke of the visions he saw of the sinful last times on earth, the Second Coming of Christ, the resurrection, and judgments.

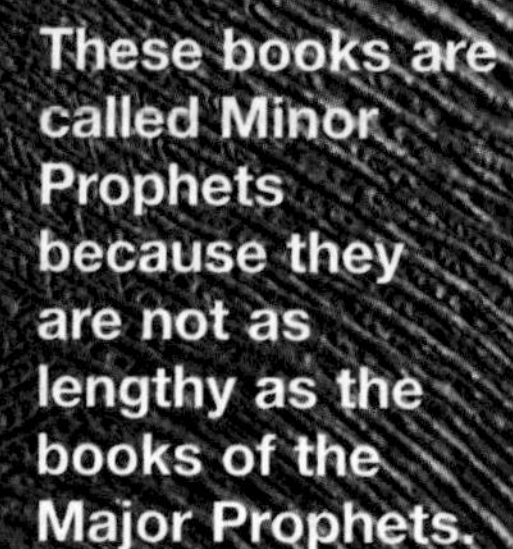

These books are called Minor Prophets because they are not as lengthy as the books of the Major Prophets.

GOD'S WORD

Minor Prophets

Hosea
"God's Love for His People"

Joel
"The Day of the Lord"

Amos
"Prepare to Meet God"

Obadiah
"God Judges the Pride of Edom"

Jonah
"God's Mercy"

Micah
"The Coming Kingdom"

Nahum
"God Judges Apostasy"

Habakkuk
"God Is Holy"

Zephaniah
"No Hope After Judgment"

Haggai
"Doing God's Work"

Zechariah
"Christ Will Reign Supreme"

Malachi
"Our Unchanging God"

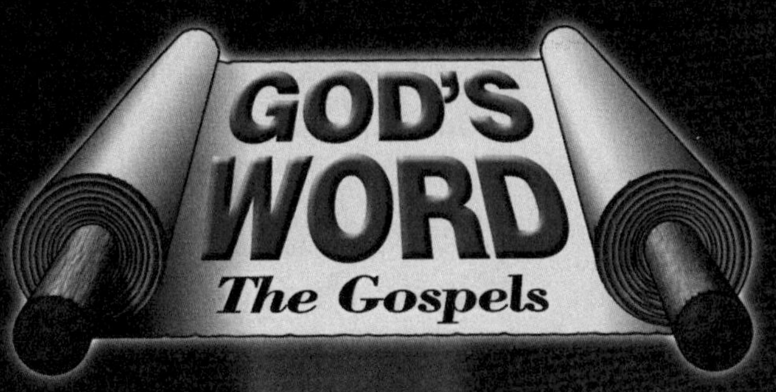
GOD'S
WORD
The Gospels

The word *gospel* comes from *godspel,* an Anglo-Saxon word meaning "good message" or "good news."

Matthew

tells of *Christ the Promised King.* Some people believe Matthew wrote this book in Aramaic rather than Greek.

Mark

shows *Christ the Obedient Servant.* It was written in Rome by John Mark before he traveled to Egypt to teach others of Christ in that country.

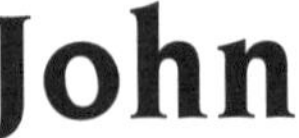

Luke

relates the story of *Christ the Perfect Man.* It was written by Luke probably when he was in Caesarea with Paul.

John

reveals *Christ the Son of God.* It was written before John was exiled to Patmos.

The Gospels have been called "Four Portraits of Jesus."

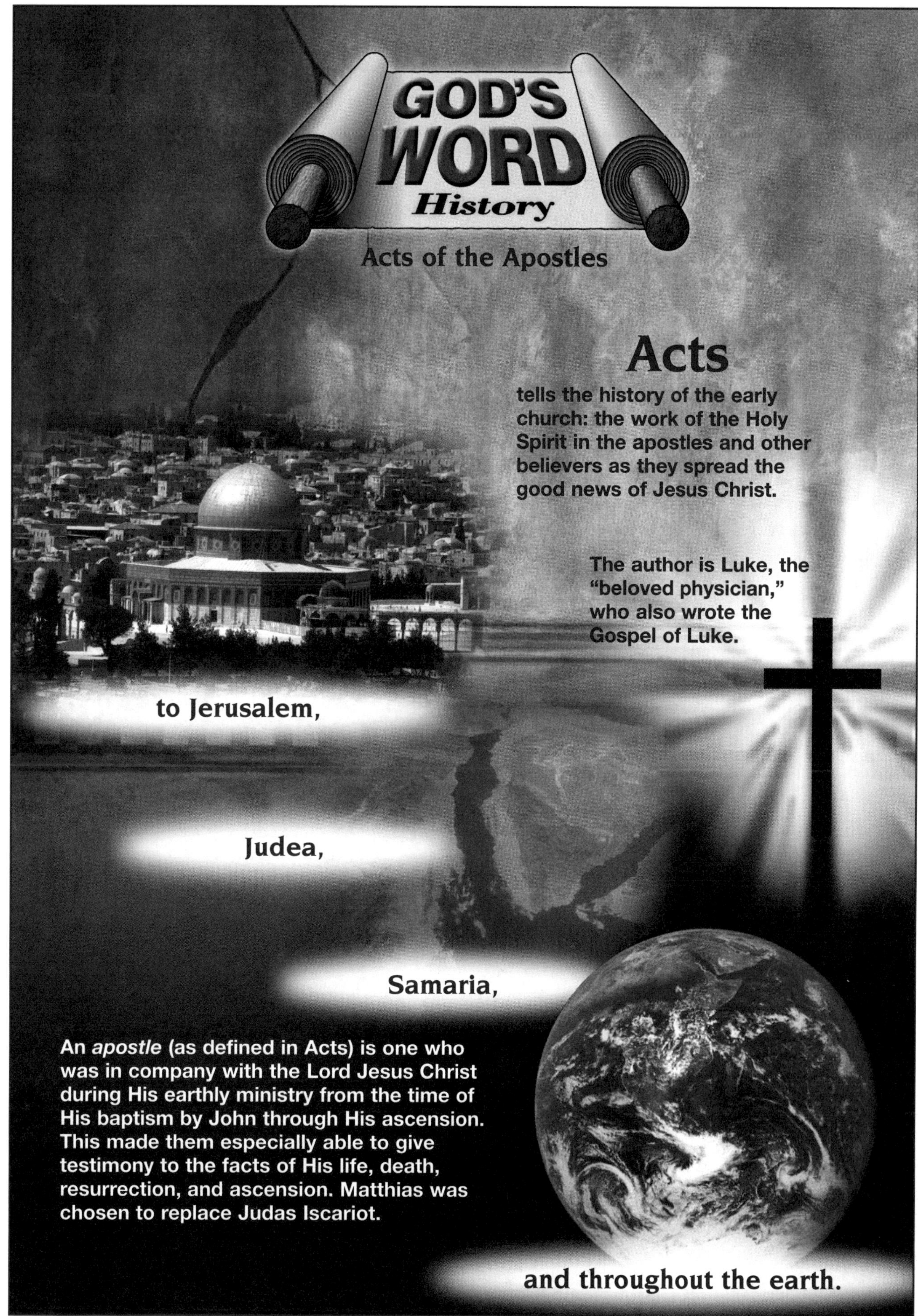
GOD'S
WORD
History
Acts of the Apostles
Acts
tells the history of the early church: the work of the Holy Spirit in the apostles and other believers as they spread the good news of Jesus Christ.
The author is Luke, the "beloved physician," who also wrote the Gospel of Luke.
to Jerusalem,
Judea,
Samaria,
An *apostle* (as defined in Acts) is one who was in company with the Lord Jesus Christ during His earthly ministry from the time of His baptism by John through His ascension. This made them especially able to give testimony to the facts of His life, death, resurrection, and ascension. Matthias was chosen to replace Judas Iscariot.
and throughout the earth.

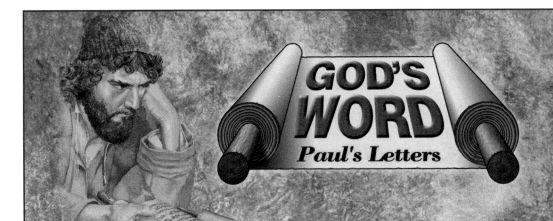
GOD'S
WORD
Paul's Letters

Romans: *The Righteousness of God* (To the church in Rome)

I Corinthians: *Conduct in the Church* (To the church in Corinth)

II Corinthians: *The Heart of Paul* (To the church in Corinth)

Galatians: *Law or Grace?* (To the church in Galatia)

Ephesians: *Blessings in Christ* (To the church in Ephesus)

Philippians: *Joy in Christ* (To the church in Philippi)

Colossians: *Life in Christ* (To the church in Colosse)

I Thessalonians: *Christ Will Come for His Saints* (To the church in Thessalonica)

II Thessalonians: *Christ Will Come a Second Time to Judge Sinners* (To the church in Thessalonica)

I Timothy: *Guard the Truth* (To Timothy)

II Timothy: *Preach the Truth* (To Timothy)

Titus: *Live the Truth* (To Titus)

Philemon: *Forgiveness* (To Philemon)

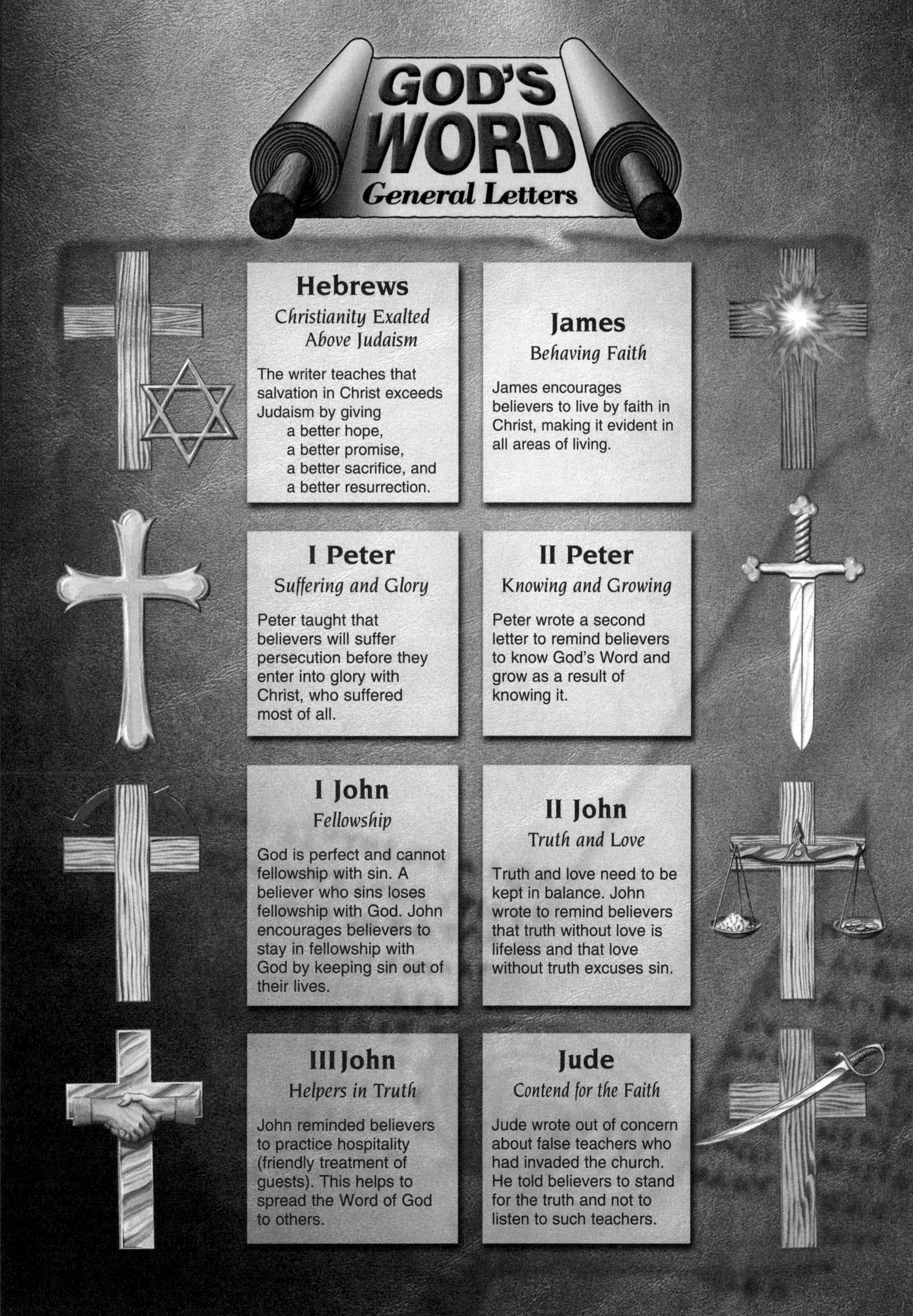
GOD'S WORD
General Letters
Hebrews
Christianity Exalted Above Judaism
The writer teaches that salvation in Christ exceeds Judaism by giving
a better hope,
a better promise,
a better sacrifice, and
a better resurrection.
James
Behaving Faith
James encourages believers to live by faith in Christ, making it evident in all areas of living.
I Peter
Suffering and Glory
Peter taught that believers will suffer persecution before they enter into glory with Christ, who suffered most of all.
II Peter
Knowing and Growing
Peter wrote a second letter to remind believers to know God's Word and grow as a result of knowing it.
I John
Fellowship
God is perfect and cannot fellowship with sin. A believer who sins loses fellowship with God. John encourages believers to stay in fellowship with God by keeping sin out of their lives.
II John
Truth and Love
Truth and love need to be kept in balance. John wrote to remind believers that truth without love is lifeless and that love without truth excuses sin.
III John
Helpers in Truth
John reminded believers to practice hospitality (friendly treatment of guests). This helps to spread the Word of God to others.
Jude
Contend for the Faith
Jude wrote out of concern about false teachers who had invaded the church. He told believers to stand for the truth and not to listen to such teachers.

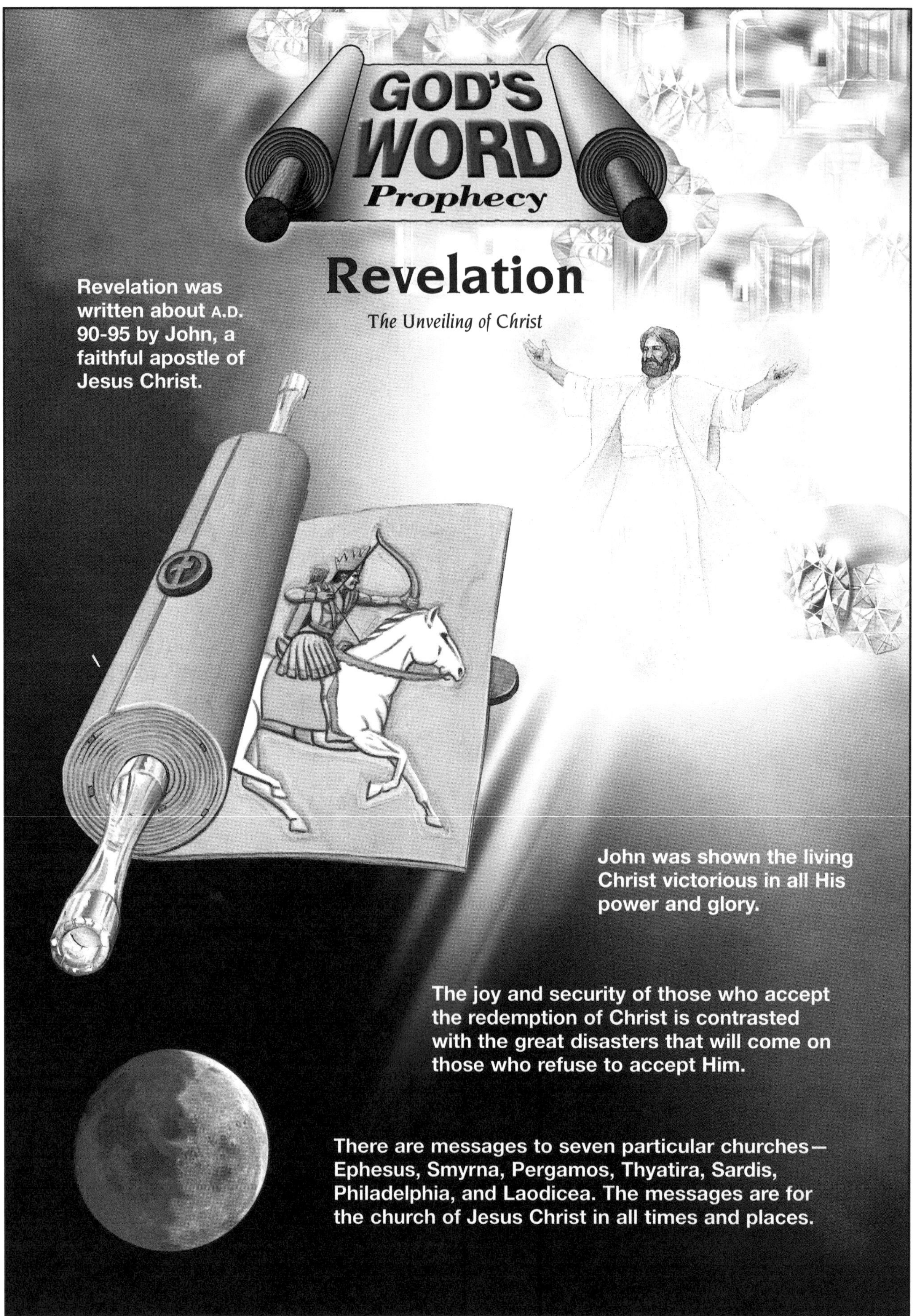
GOD'S
WORD
Prophecy
Revelation
The Unveiling of Christ
Revelation was written about A.D. 90-95 by John, a faithful apostle of Jesus Christ.
John was shown the living Christ victorious in all His power and glory.
The joy and security of those who accept the redemption of Christ is contrasted with the great disasters that will come on those who refuse to accept Him.
There are messages to seven particular churches—Ephesus, Smyrna, Pergamos, Thyatira, Sardis, Philadelphia, and Laodicea. The messages are for the church of Jesus Christ in all times and places.

Maps

World Map

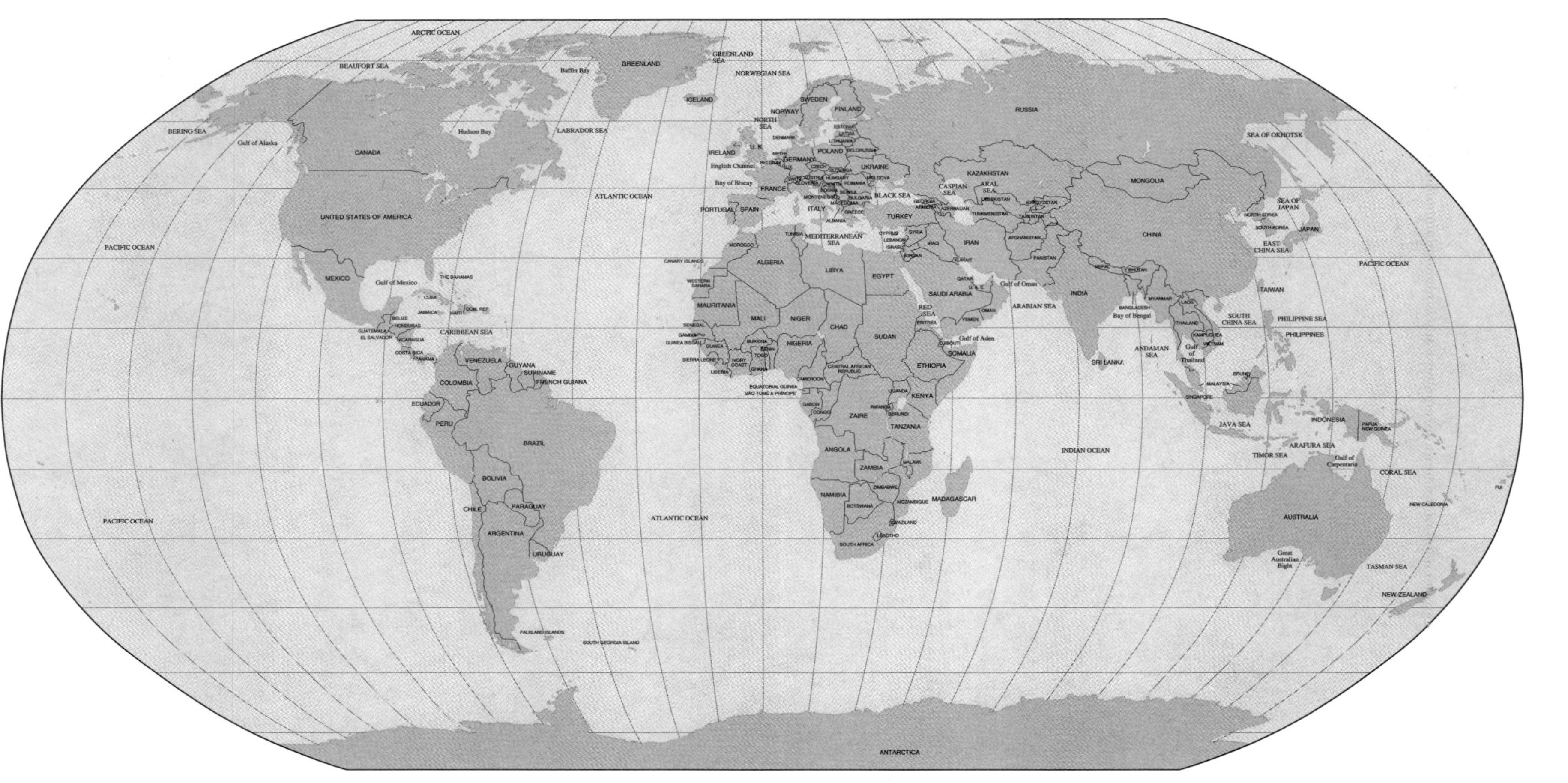
ARCTIC OCEAN
BEAUFORT SEA
BERING SEA
Gulf of Alaska
CANADA
Hudson Bay
Baffin Bay
GREENLAND
LABRADOR SEA
GREENLAND SEA
NORWEGIAN SEA
ICELAND
UNITED STATES OF AMERICA
PACIFIC OCEAN
MEXICO
Gulf of Mexico
CARIBBEAN SEA
VENEZUELA
GUYANA
SURINAME
FRENCH GUIANA
COLOMBIA
ECUADOR
PERU
BRAZIL
BOLIVIA
CHILE
PARAGUAY
ARGENTINA
URUGUAY
ATLANTIC OCEAN
SWEDEN
NORWAY
FINLAND
NORTH SEA
U.K.
IRELAND
English Channel
GERMANY
POLAND
UKRAINE
Bay of Biscay
FRANCE
PORTUGAL
SPAIN
ITALY
BLACK SEA
TURKEY
MEDITERRANEAN SEA
RUSSIA
KAZAKHSTAN
CASPIAN SEA
ARAL SEA
MONGOLIA
CHINA
IRAN
ALGERIA
LIBYA
EGYPT
SAUDI ARABIA
RED SEA
Gulf of Oman
ARABIAN SEA
INDIA
Bay of Bengal
MAURITANIA
MALI
NIGER
CHAD
SUDAN
NIGERIA
ETHIOPIA
Gulf of Aden
SOMALIA
KENYA
ZAIRE
TANZANIA
ANGOLA
ZAMBIA
NAMIBIA
MADAGASCAR
SRI LANKA
ANDAMAN SEA
INDIAN OCEAN
SEA OF OKHOTSK
SEA OF JAPAN
JAPAN
EAST CHINA SEA
TAIWAN
SOUTH CHINA SEA
PHILIPPINE SEA
PHILIPPINES
PACIFIC OCEAN
JAVA SEA
INDONESIA
ARAFURA SEA
TIMOR SEA
Gulf of Carpentaria
CORAL SEA
AUSTRALIA
Great Australian Bight
TASMAN SEA
NEW ZEALAND
ANTARCTICA

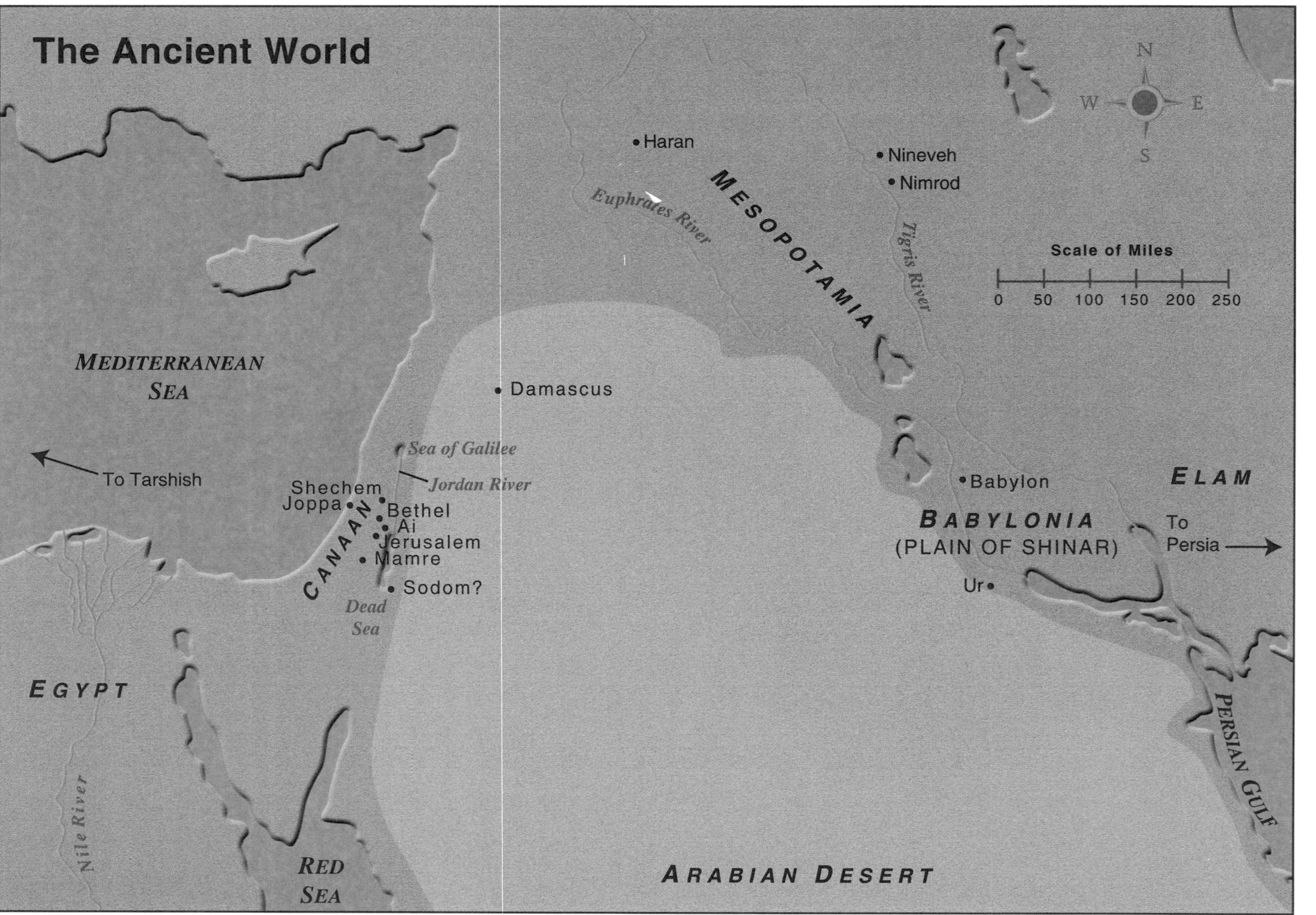

The Ancient World
N
W
E
S
Haran
Euphrates River
MESOPOTAMIA
Nineveh
Nimrod
Tigris River
Scale of Miles
0 50 100 150 200 250
MEDITERRANEAN SEA
Damascus
Sea of Galilee
To Tarshish
Jordan River
Shechem
Joppa
Bethel
Ai
Jerusalem
Mamre
Sodom?
CANAAN
Dead Sea
Babylon
ELAM
BABYLONIA
(PLAIN OF SHINAR)
To Persia
Ur
EGYPT
Nile River
RED SEA
PERSIAN GULF
ARABIAN DESERT

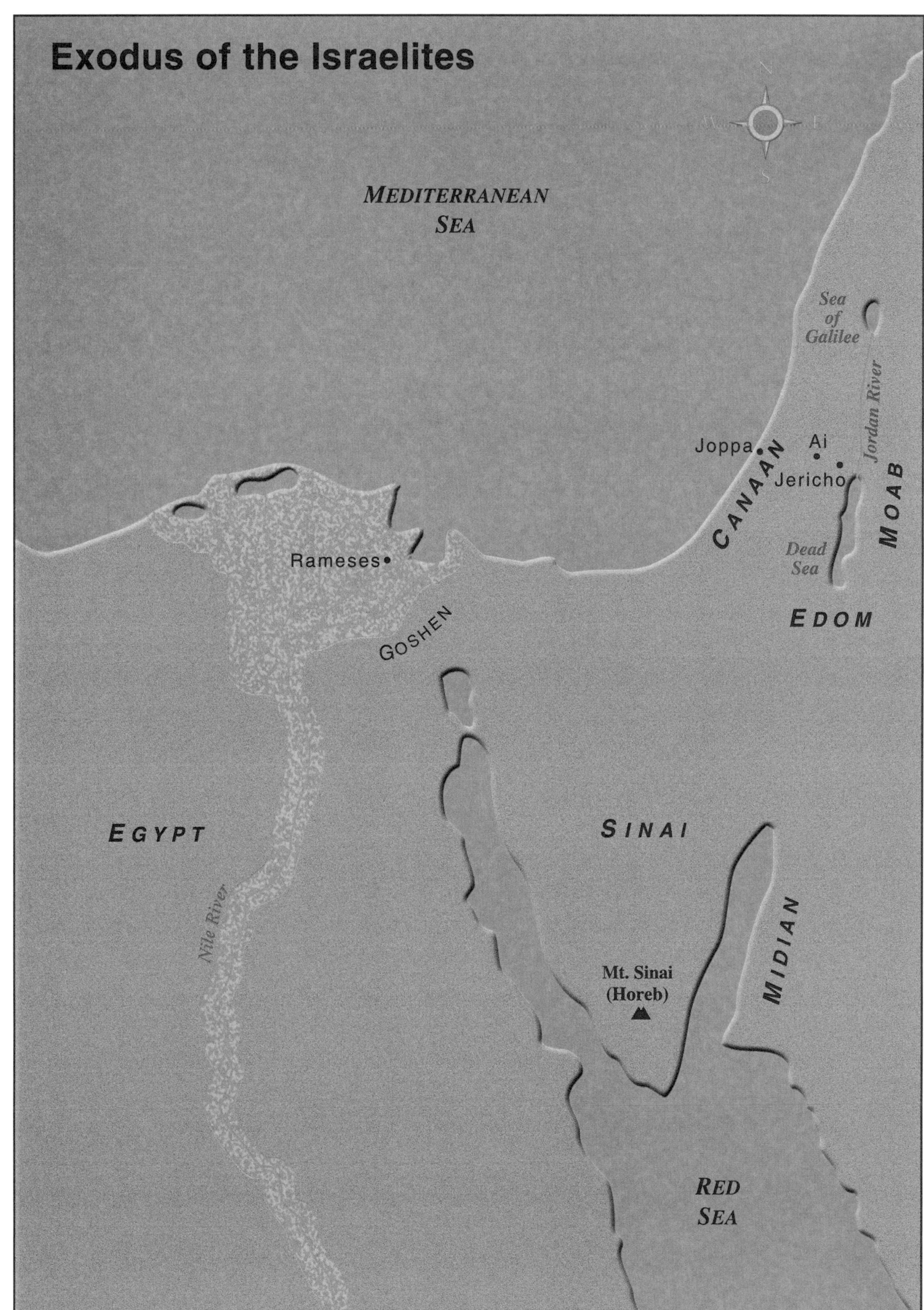
Exodus of the Israelites
N
S
W
E
MEDITERRANEAN
SEA
Sea
of
Galilee
Jordan River
Joppa
Ai
Jericho
CANAAN
MOAB
Dead
Sea
EDOM
Rameses
GOSHEN
EGYPT
SINAI
Nile River
MIDIAN
Mt. Sinai
(Horeb)
RED
SEA

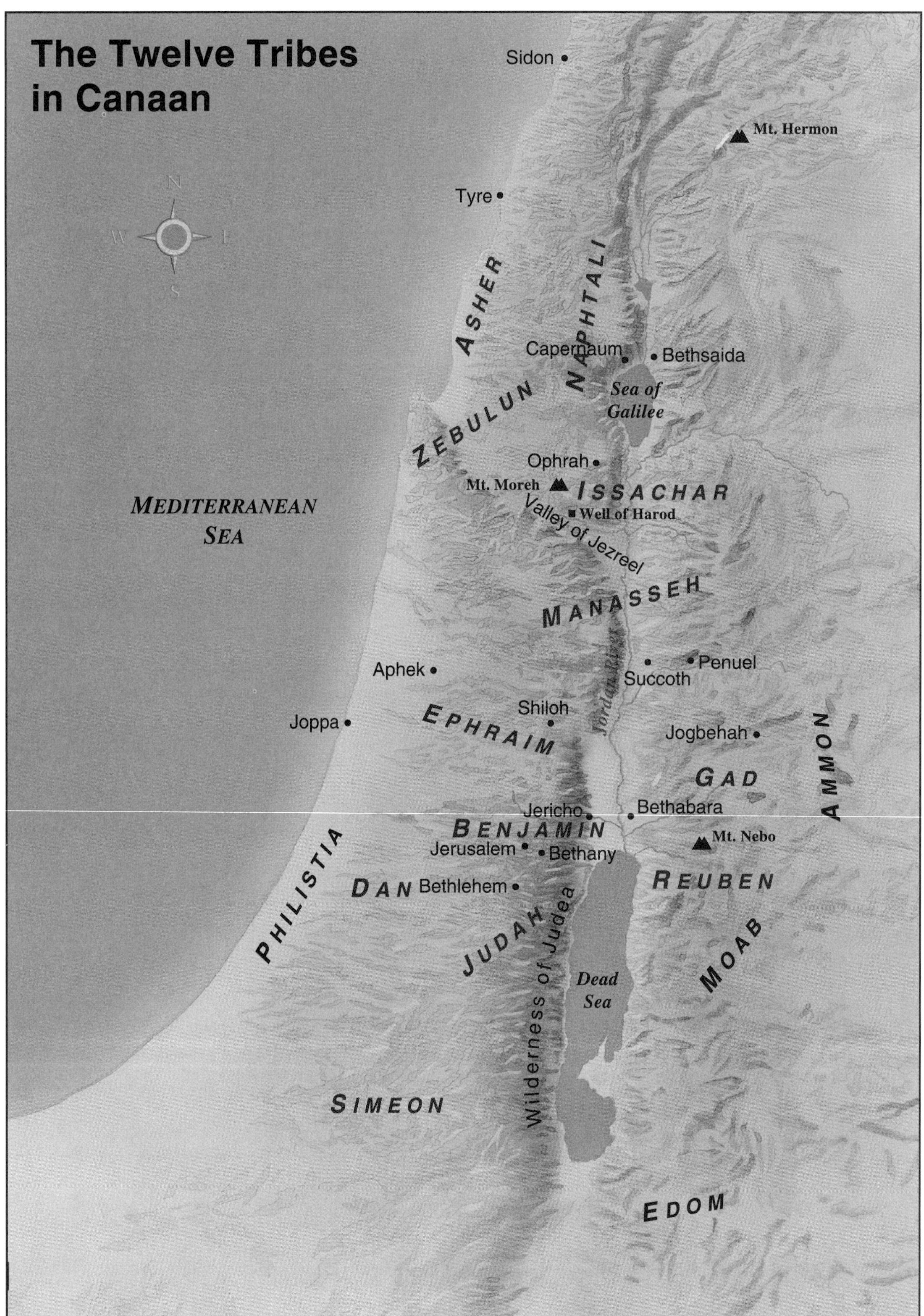
The Twelve Tribes in Canaan
Sidon
Mt. Hermon
Tyre
N
W
E
S
ASHER
NAPHTALI
Capernaum
Bethsaida
Sea of Galilee
ZEBULUN
Ophrah
Mt. Moreh
ISSACHAR
Well of Harod
Valley of Jezreel
MEDITERRANEAN SEA
MANASSEH
Aphek
Penuel
Succoth
Jordan River
Shiloh
Joppa
EPHRAIM
Jogbehah
GAD
AMMON
Jericho
Bethabara
BENJAMIN
Mt. Nebo
Jerusalem
Bethany
PHILISTIA
DAN
Bethlehem
REUBEN
JUDAH
Wilderness of Judea
MOAB
Dead Sea
SIMEON
EDOM

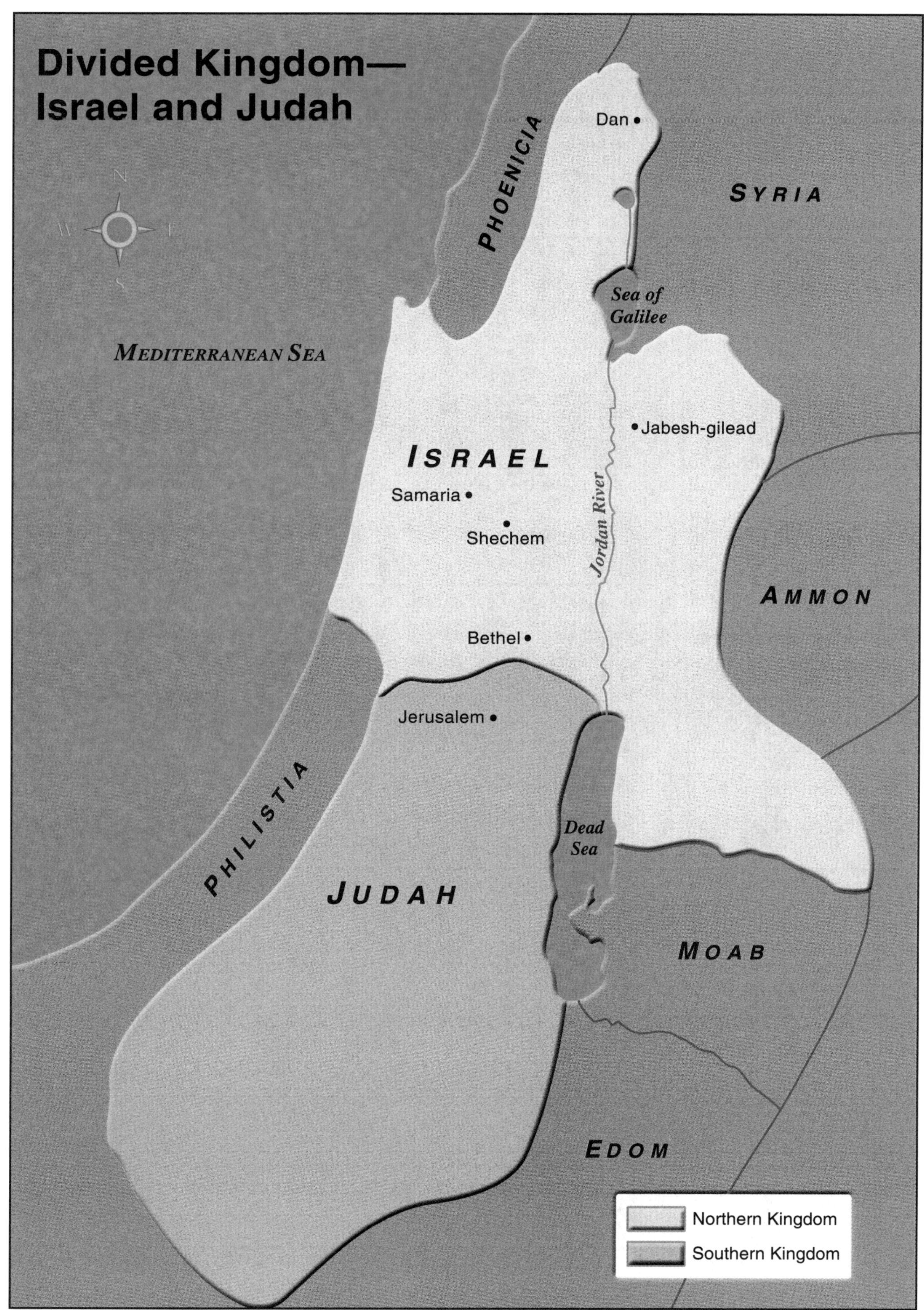

Divided Kingdom—
Israel and Judah
Dan
PHOENICIA
SYRIA
Sea of Galilee
MEDITERRANEAN SEA
Jabesh-gilead
ISRAEL
Samaria
Shechem
Jordan River
AMMON
Bethel
Jerusalem
PHILISTIA
Dead Sea
JUDAH
MOAB
EDOM
Northern Kingdom
Southern Kingdom

Palestine and Beyond

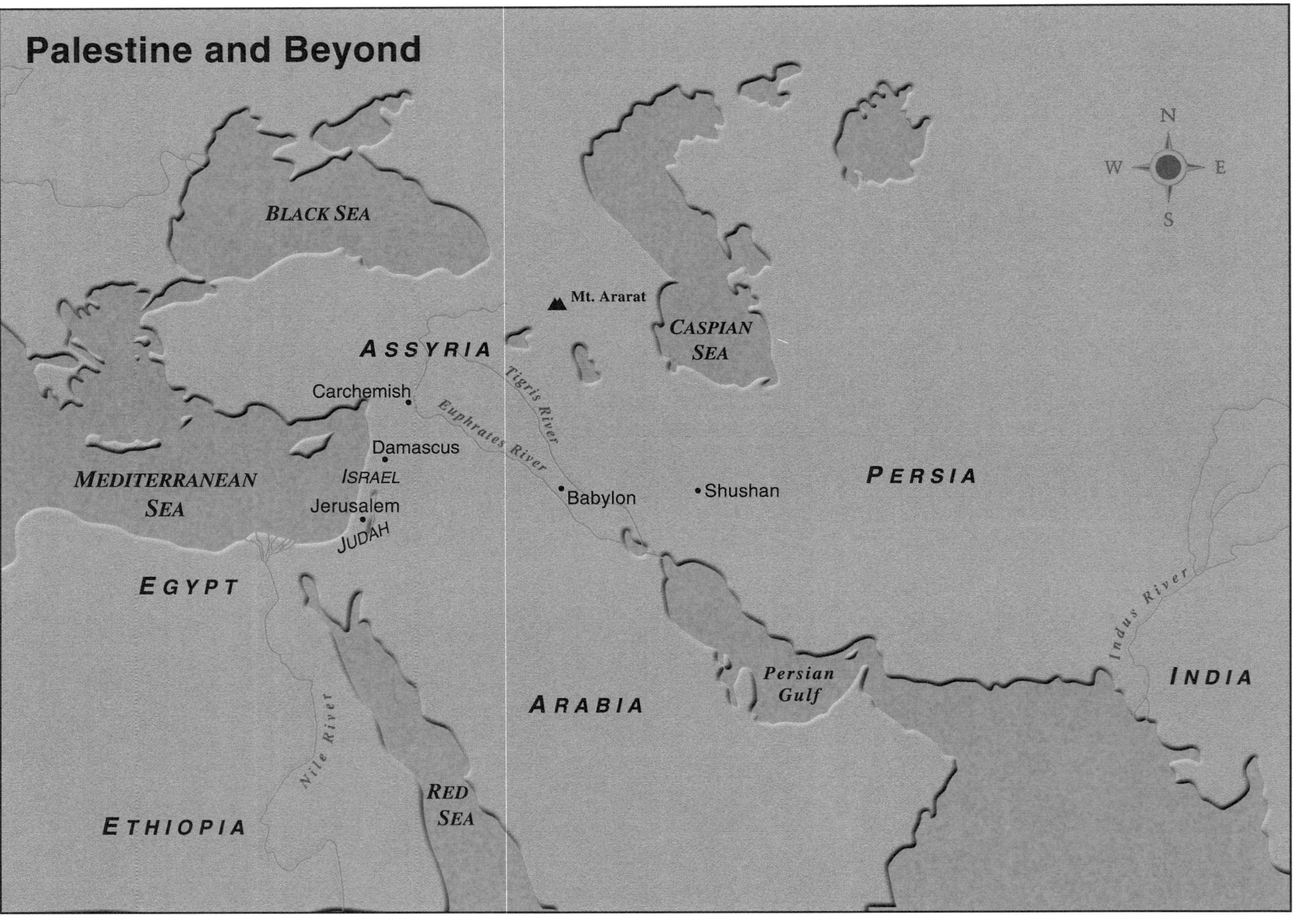

N
W
E
S
BLACK SEA
Mt. Ararat
CASPIAN SEA
ASSYRIA
Tigris River
Carchemish
Euphrates River
Damascus
ISRAEL
MEDITERRANEAN SEA
Jerusalem
JUDAH
Babylon
Shushan
PERSIA
EGYPT
Indus River
INDIA
Persian Gulf
ARABIA
Nile River
RED SEA
ETHIOPIA

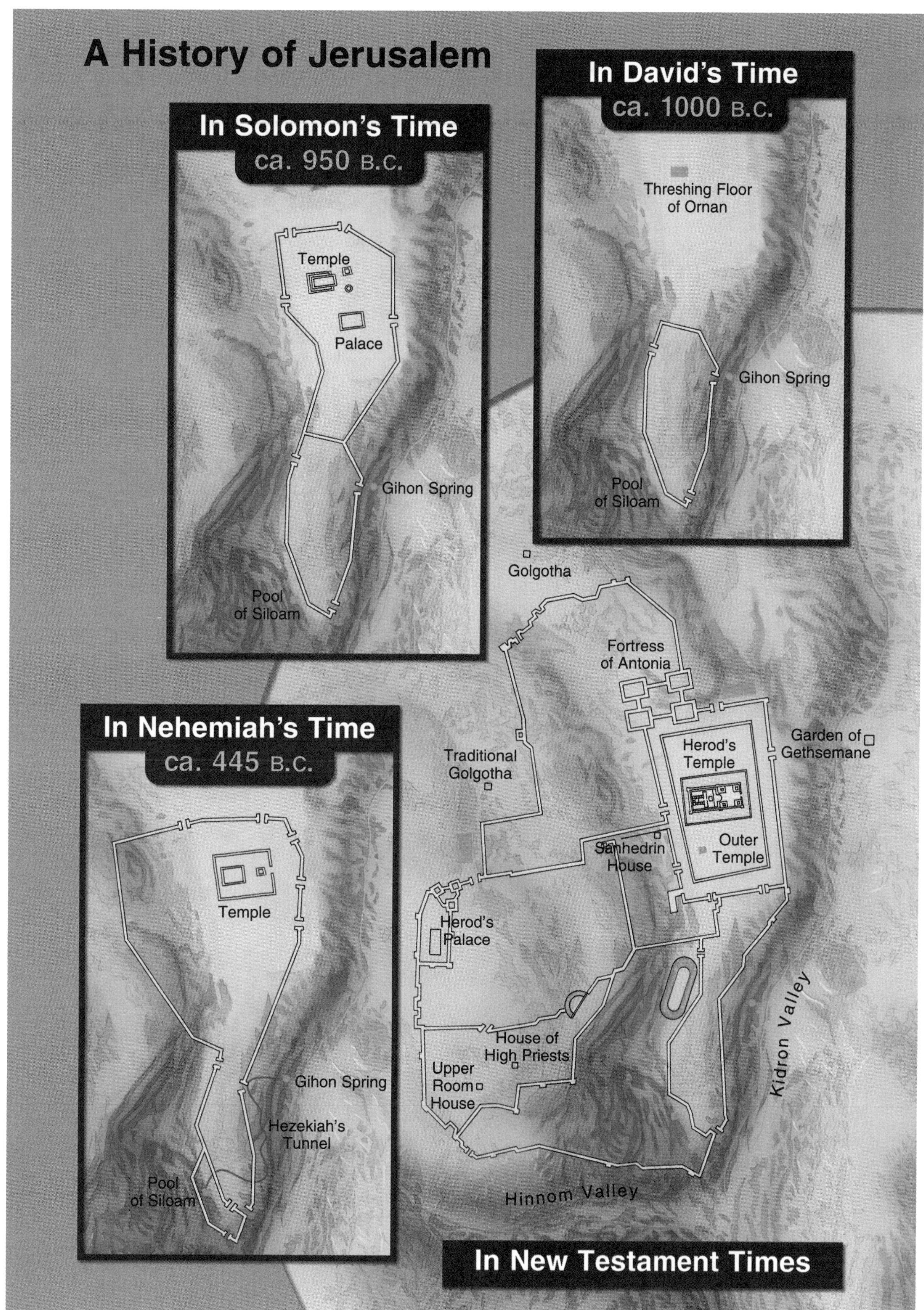
A History of Jerusalem
In Solomon's Time
ca. 950 B.C.
Temple
Palace
Gihon Spring
Pool of Siloam
In David's Time
ca. 1000 B.C.
Threshing Floor of Ornan
Gihon Spring
Pool of Siloam
In Nehemiah's Time
ca. 445 B.C.
Temple
Gihon Spring
Hezekiah's Tunnel
Pool of Siloam
Golgotha
Fortress of Antonia
Traditional Golgotha
Herod's Temple
Garden of Gethsemane
Sanhedrin House
Outer Temple
Herod's Palace
House of High Priests
Upper Room House
Kidron Valley
Hinnom Valley
In New Testament Times

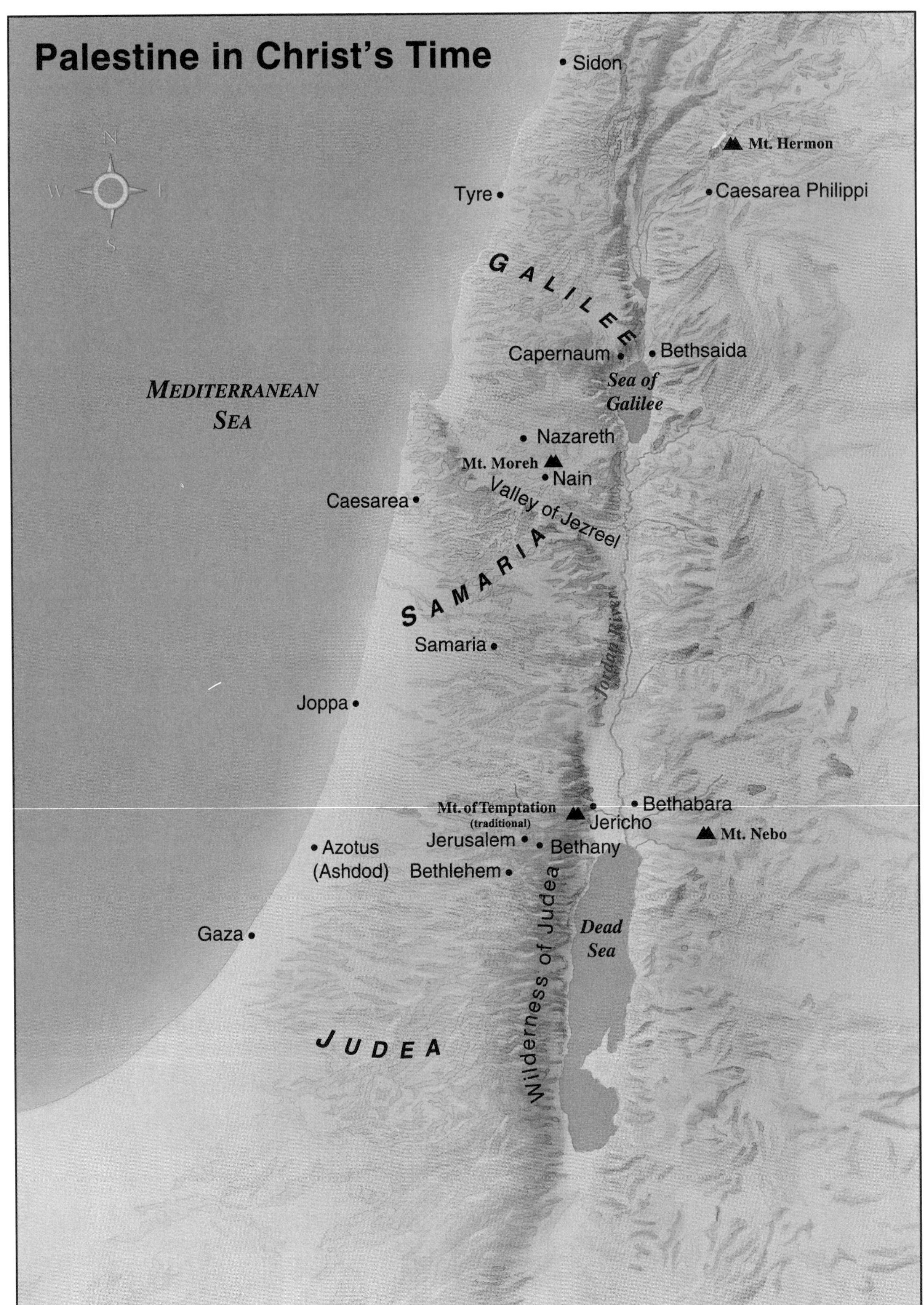
Palestine in Christ's Time
Sidon
Mt. Hermon
Tyre
Caesarea Philippi
GALILEE
Capernaum
Bethsaida
Sea of Galilee
MEDITERRANEAN SEA
Nazareth
Mt. Moreh
Nain
Caesarea
Valley of Jezreel
SAMARIA
Jordan River
Samaria
Joppa
Mt. of Temptation (traditional)
Bethabara
Jericho
Mt. Nebo
Azotus (Ashdod)
Jerusalem
Bethany
Bethlehem
Gaza
Dead Sea
Wilderness of Judea
JUDEA

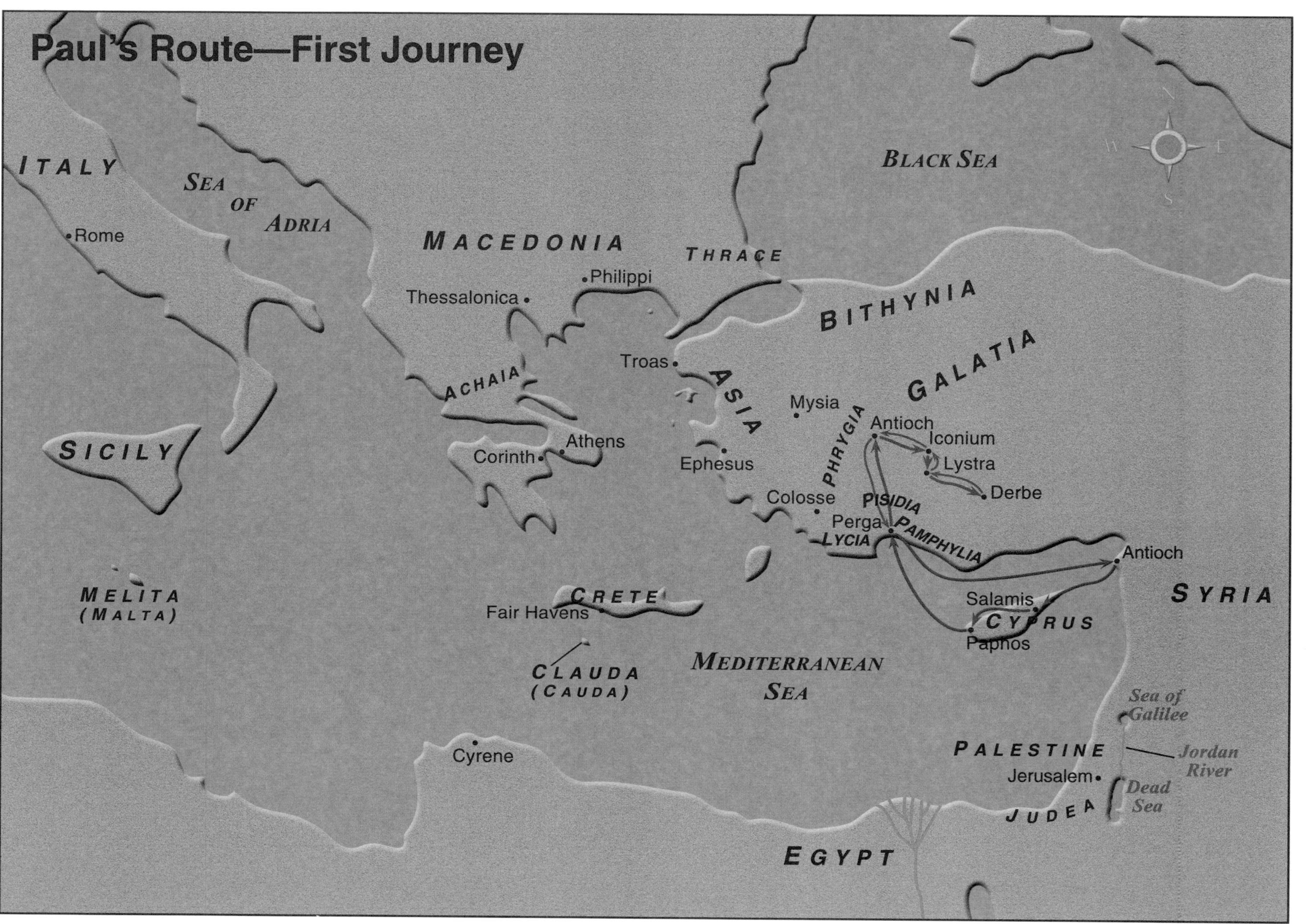
Paul's Route—First Journey
ITALY
Rome
SEA OF ADRIA
SICILY
MELITA (MALTA)
MACEDONIA
Thessalonica
Philippi
THRACE
ACHAIA
Corinth
Athens
BLACK SEA
BITHYNIA
GALATIA
Troas
ASIA
Ephesus
Mysia
PHRYGIA
Antioch
Iconium
Lystra
Derbe
Colosse
PISIDIA
Perga
PAMPHYLIA
LYCIA
Antioch
SYRIA
CRETE
Fair Havens
CLAUDA (CAUDA)
MEDITERRANEAN SEA
Salamis
CYPRUS
Paphos
Sea of Galilee
PALESTINE
Jordan River
Jerusalem
Dead Sea
JUDEA
Cyrene
EGYPT

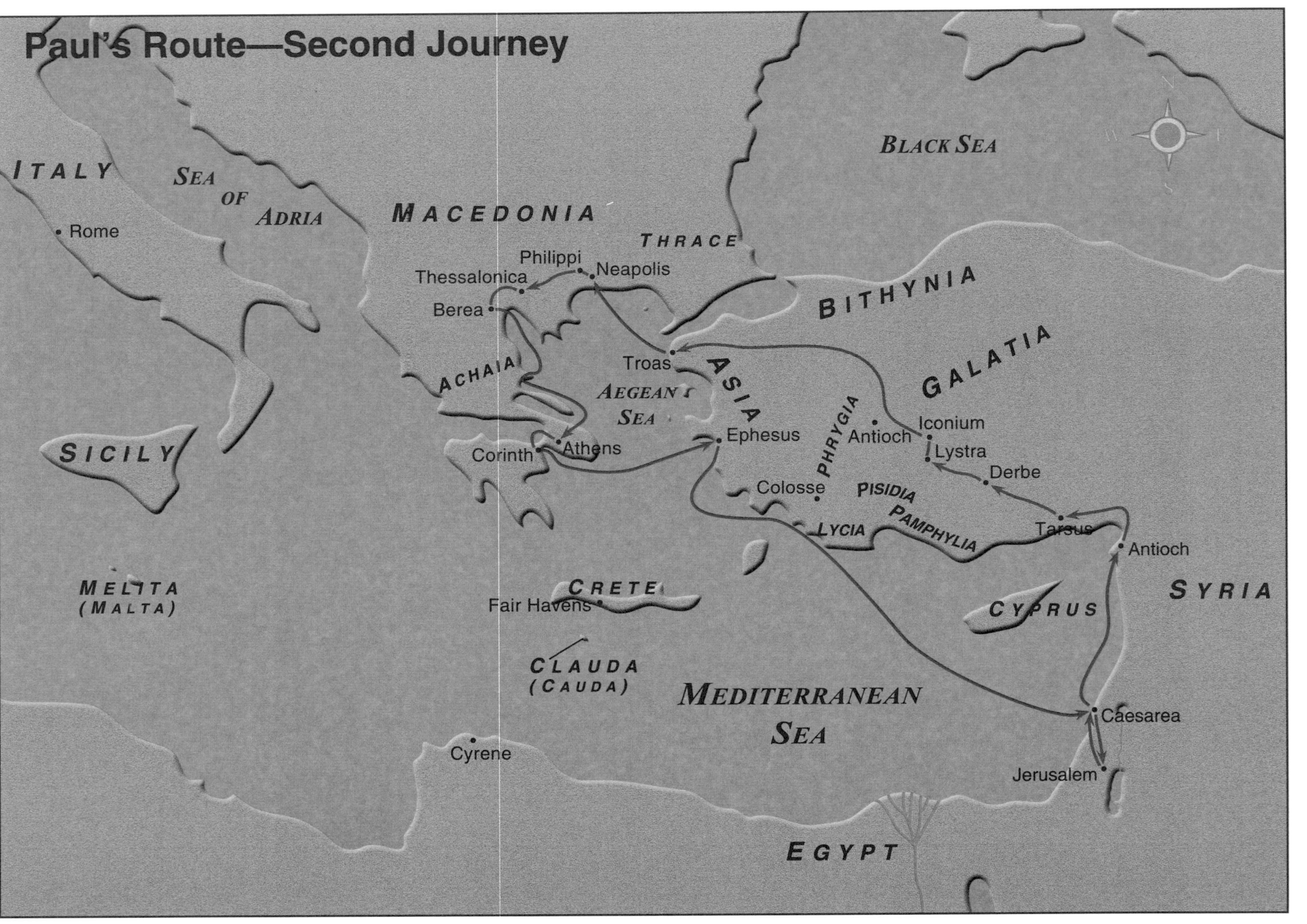
Paul's Route—Second Journey
ITALY
Rome
SEA OF ADRIA
SICILY
MELITA
(MALTA)
MACEDONIA
THRACE
Philippi
Neapolis
Thessalonica
Berea
ACHAIA
Corinth
Athens
AEGEAN SEA
Troas
ASIA
Ephesus
BLACK SEA
BITHYNIA
GALATIA
PHRYGIA
Antioch
Iconium
Lystra
Derbe
Colosse
PISIDIA
PAMPHYLIA
LYCIA
Tarsus
Antioch
SYRIA
CYPRUS
CRETE
Fair Havens
CLAUDA
(CAUDA)
MEDITERRANEAN SEA
Caesarea
Jerusalem
Cyrene
EGYPT

Paul's Route—Third Journey

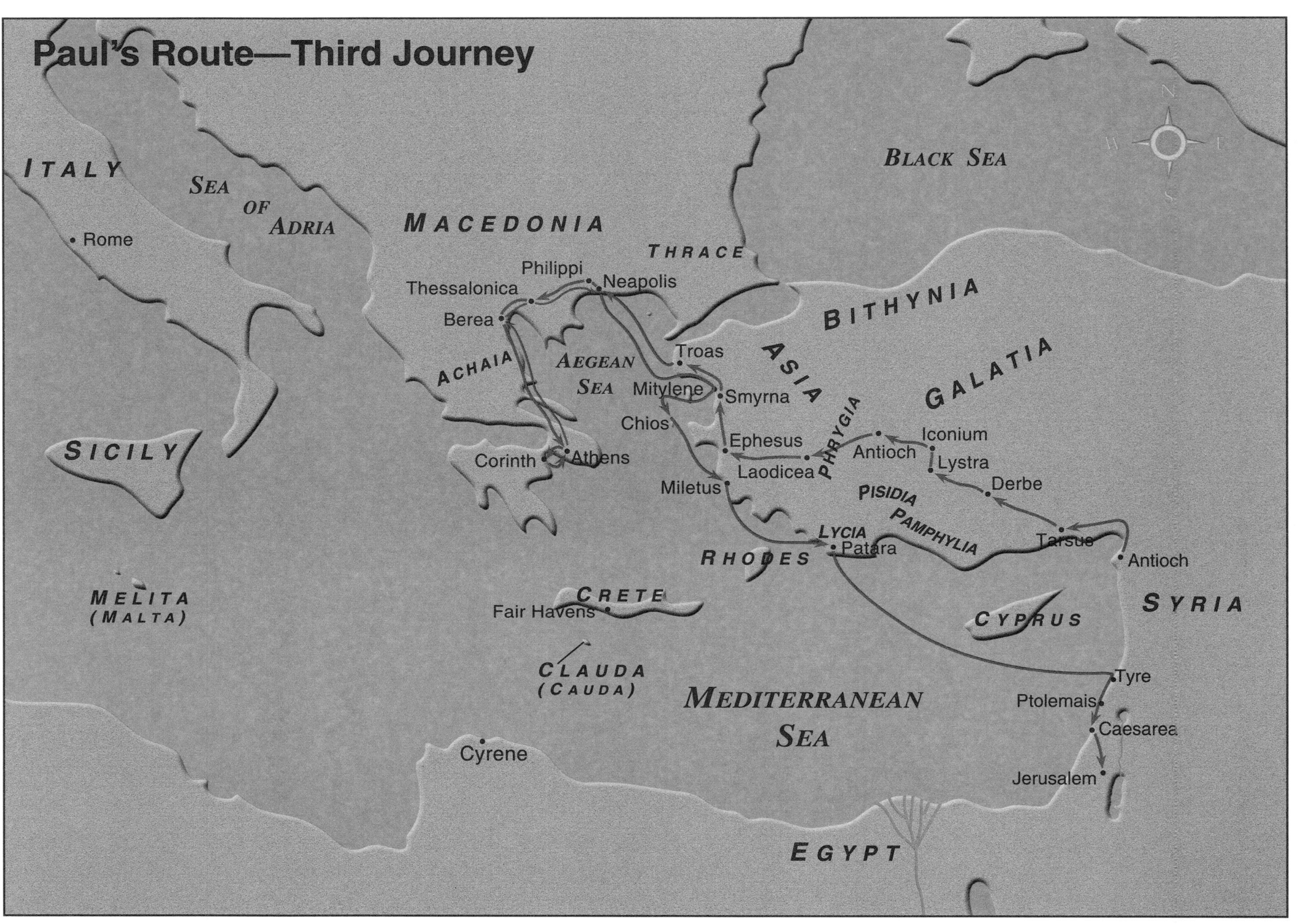
ITALY
SEA OF ADRIA
Rome
MACEDONIA
THRACE
Philippi
Neapolis
Thessalonica
Berea
ACHAIA
AEGEAN SEA
SICILY
Corinth
Athens
Troas
Mitylene
Chios
Smyrna
Ephesus
Laodicea
Miletus
ASIA
BITHYNIA
BLACK SEA
N
S
E
W
GALATIA
PHRYGIA
Antioch
Iconium
Lystra
Derbe
PISIDIA
PAMPHYLIA
LYCIA
Patara
RHODES
Tarsus
Antioch
SYRIA
CYPRUS
MELITA (MALTA)
CRETE
Fair Havens
CLAUDA (CAUDA)
MEDITERRANEAN SEA
Tyre
Ptolemais
Caesarea
Jerusalem
Cyrene
EGYPT

The Seven Churches in Revelation

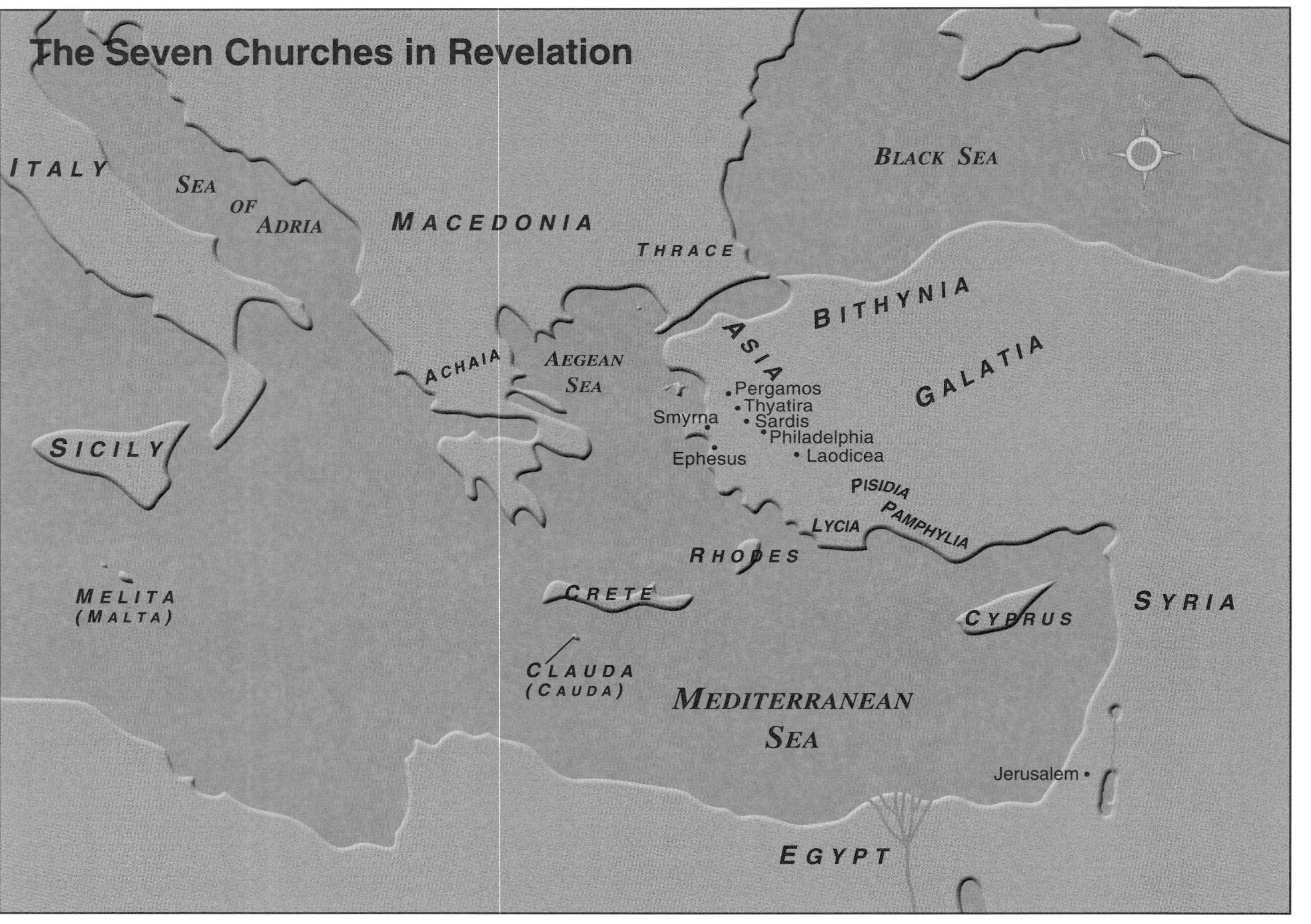
ITALY
SEA OF ADRIA
MACEDONIA
THRACE
BLACK SEA
BITHYNIA
ASIA
GALATIA
ACHAIA
AEGEAN SEA
Pergamos
Thyatira
Sardis
Smyrna
Philadelphia
Ephesus
Laodicea
PISIDIA
PAMPHYLIA
LYCIA
RHODES
SICILY
MELITA (MALTA)
CRETE
CYPRUS
SYRIA
CLAUDA (CAUDA)
MEDITERRANEAN SEA
Jerusalem
EGYPT

Heroes of the Faith

Hero of the Faith

Charles Spurgeon A.D. 1834-1892

Name ______________________________

Charles Haddon Spurgeon came from a large family. His parents could not afford to keep him, so they sent him to live with his grandparents until he was six years old. His grandfather taught him the principle that became one of his life themes—Do right no matter what.

God used a substitute preacher in a small church to lead Spurgeon to Christ. After that, Spurgeon began to take every opportunity to speak to others of his Lord. Charles Spurgeon gave himself competely to God, and God used him to bring thousands to Himself.

Spurgeon was a writer as well as a preacher. Joseph Passmore, a printer and a member of Spurgeon's church, recognized Spurgeon's gift of preaching and knew that others could also benefit from his sermons. This resulted in Spurgeon writing out his sermons for Passmore to print as a method of reaching people that could not or would not attend the church services. Spurgeon's ministry continues today through his printed works.

Spurgeon loved children and spent time with them in the orphanage he had helped develop. He had a very busy schedule, but he would visit the children, tell them stories, and bring them gifts. Only God truly knows how many children are in heaven because Spurgeon gave himself completely to Christ.

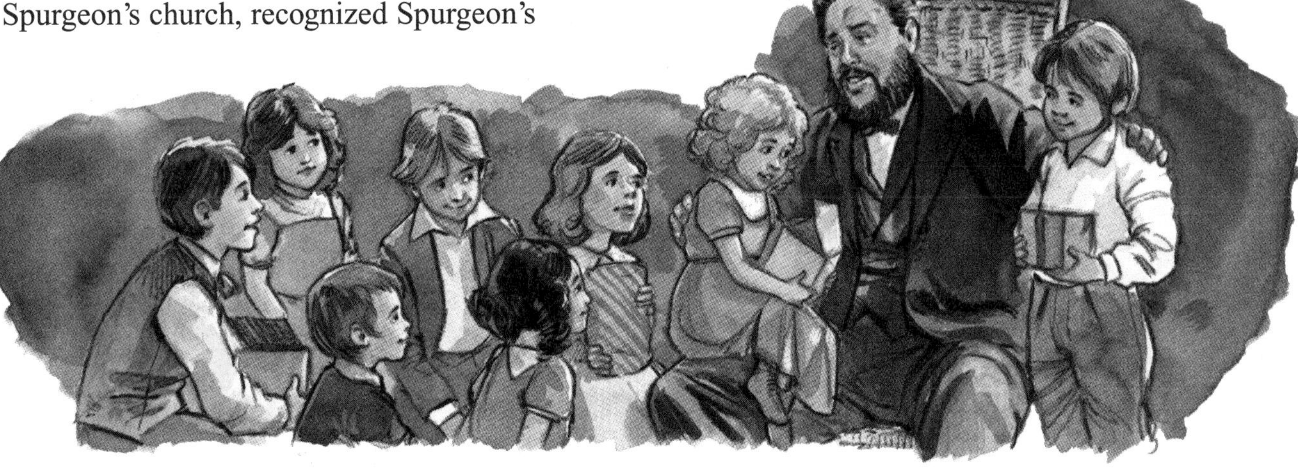

Answer the questions.

1. In what ways did God use Spurgeon to affect others for Christ?

____

2. Why do you think that Spurgeon was so effective?

____

3. How can you give your life to Christ?

____

____

Hero of the Faith

Polycarp ca. A.D. 61-147

Name ______________________________

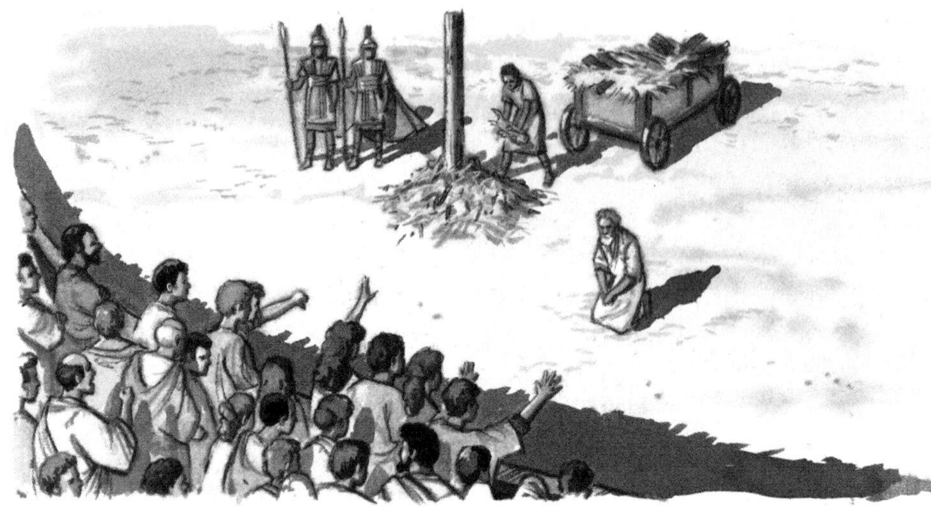

A **martyr** is a person who has given his life for his faith; a martyr dies rather than renounce what he believes.

Polycarp was a student of the apostle John. Polycarp himself became a teacher to others, and he told about his conversations with the apostle John and with others who had seen Christ.

Polycarp could not teach openly. Religious leaders of his day persecuted him and tried to persuade him to deny his faith in Christ. He had determined to please his Lord. Polycarp would sacrifice everything—even his life—for God.

When Polycarp's enemies found him hidden in a little village, he invited the soldiers in for something to eat and drink. Before they took him away, he asked if he could pray without interruption. Permission was granted, and he prayed for every man he had ever known. Some of the soldiers repented of the evil they were planning on doing to Polycarp, a true man of God.

Polycarp did not hesitate to claim Christ even when his persecutors threatened to throw him to the wild beasts or to burn him at the stake. Polycarp never shied away from being called a Christian. Before he was to be burned, he asked permission to pray. After he prayed, his tormentors prepared to fasten him to a stake. He asked that they leave him to stand without being secured. He knew that God would give him the strength to remain there while he suffered. Because he refused to deny Christ, he was burned at the stake as a martyr.

Christians have the same responsibility as Polycarp did. In most countries, God's children have His Word in their language. They have a greater responsibility because they have all of His teaching available. Polycarp left Christians an example to help them obey Christ faithfully even if it costs them their lives!

Describe what you think would happen if every Christian had to wear a label that said he believed in Christ.

____

____

____

Hero of the Faith

Isaac Watts A.D. 1674-1748

Name ______________________________

As a young child, Isaac Watts loved to read and write. The young Isaac saw the need for worship through music in the church. At his church, a deacon would read a line, and the congregation would sing that same line. People found it dull. Isaac's father encouraged him to do something about it, so Isaac Watts wrote a new hymn for every Sunday for the next two years. His hymns affected many lives and continue to do so to this day.

Isaac Watts never married, but he loved children. He wrote the first hymnal ever produced for children. When Spurgeon was a boy, his grandmother gave him an English penny for every Watts hymn he learned. Spurgeon memorized so many that his grandmother had to reduce the amount she gave him.

Fanny Crosby, a blind poet, was saved after hearing Watts's hymn "Alas! and Did My Savior Bleed." Five thousand native South Sea Islanders thanked God by singing Watts's hymn "Jesus Shall Reign" when their king changed the words in their constitution to Christ-honoring statements.

Watts wrote "O God, Our Help in Ages Past" shortly before Queen Anne's death. God used this song based on Psalm 90 to comfort many. Watts's hymns are still sung in churches today.

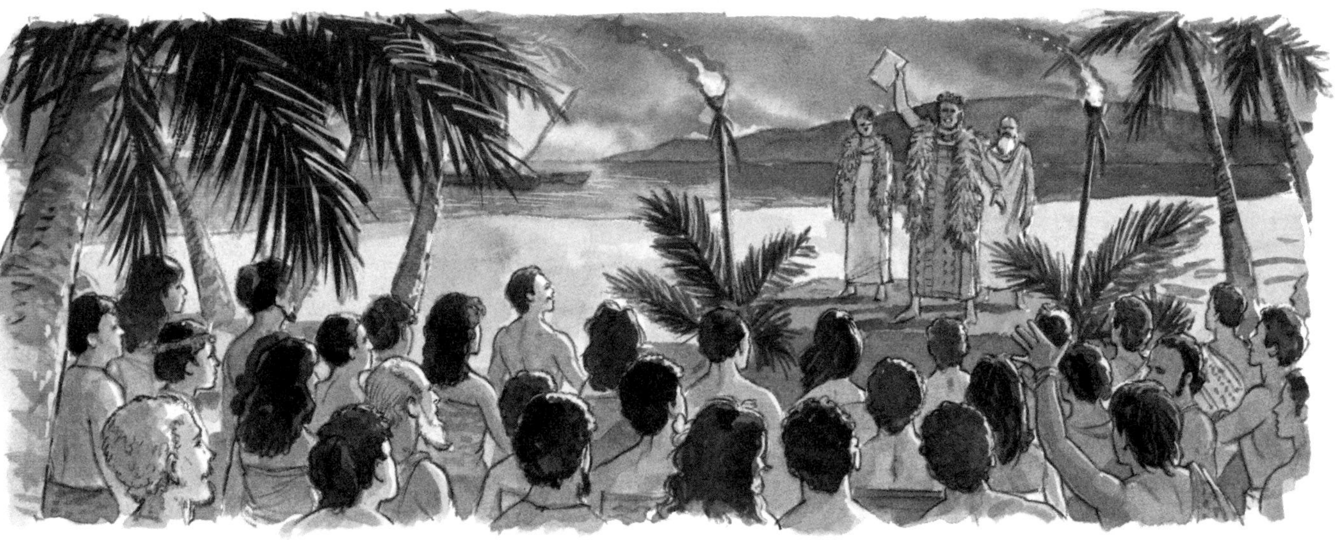

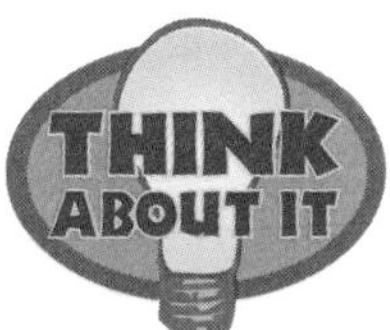
THINK
ABOUT IT

What talent has God given you?
How can you use that talent for Him?

____

____

____

Hero of the Faith

David Livingstone A.D. 1813-1873

Name ______________________________

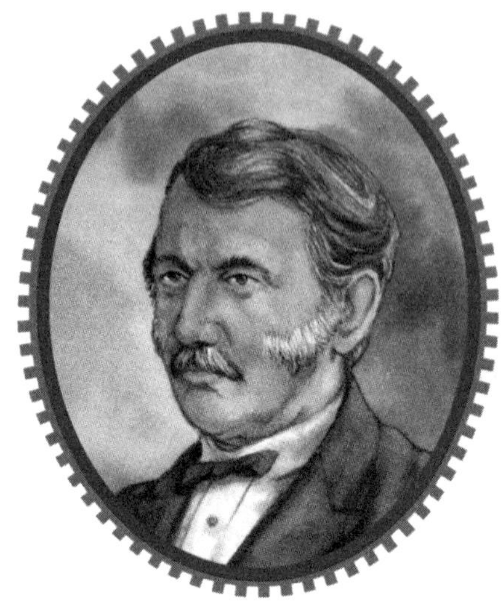

> *I have seen the smoke of a thousand villages where the Gospel has not yet been proclaimed.*—Robert Moffat

David Livingstone grew up in the midst of poverty. Though he lived with little, he learned to work hard and to make the best of difficult situations. At the age of twenty, he knew that God wanted him to be a doctor on the mission field. After hearing Robert Moffat, a missionary to Africa, Livingstone became burdened for the African people.

Livingstone knew how to work hard. When he went to Africa, some of the Africans thought that he was weak because he was very thin. But he could outlast the Africans on rigorous walks. Once he put his life in danger to kill a lion that was too near the villages. Livingstone's left arm was seriously injured, but the Africans knew that he courageously loved them.

When his wife died, he was saddened, but Livingstone continued serving the Lord. His own health was not good, but he would not quit. He never discovered the source of the Nile River, and he did not end the slave trade. He did travel 29,000 miles in Africa, charting about a million square miles and adding many lakes to the maps. He spent over half of his life taking the gospel to the Africans and caring for their physical needs. One African man described Livingstone as "a man who knew the way to the hearts of all."

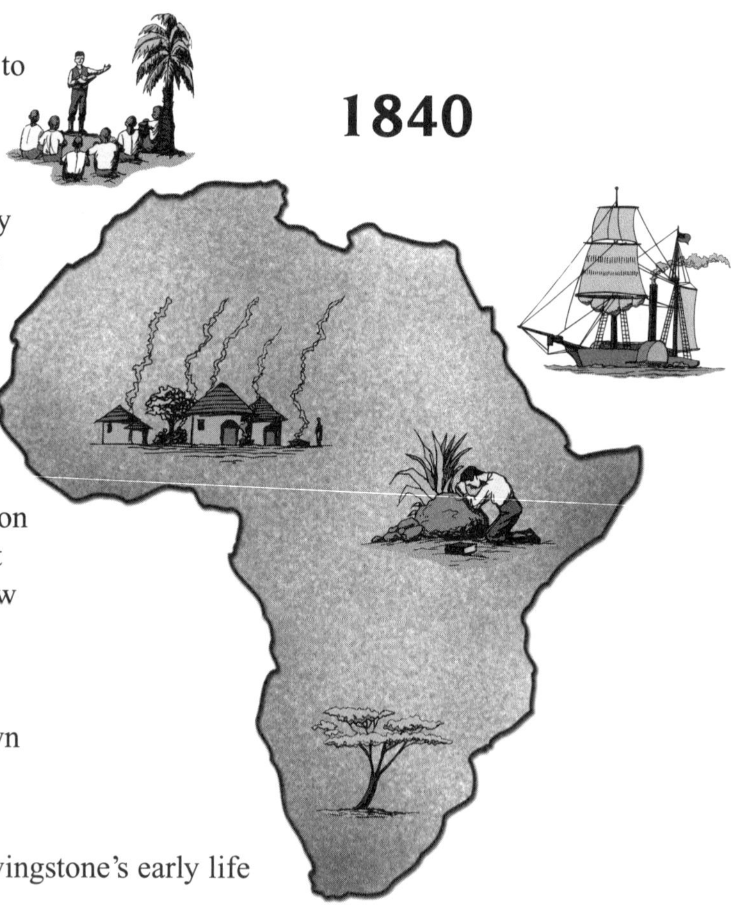
1840

Answer the questions.

1. What were some characteristics of David Livingstone's early life that later helped him on the mission field?

____

2. How can you prepare yourself for the task or place to which God might lead you?

____

Name ____________________

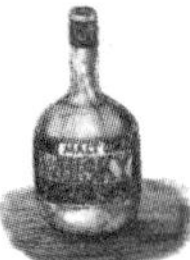

From Darkness into Light

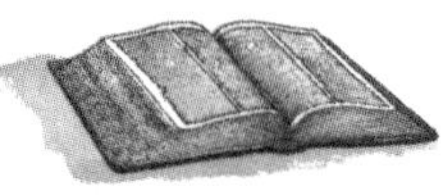

When Samson Occom was seventeen, he wanted to learn as much as he could about God and His Word, but he faced many obstacles. He was Mohegan—a Native American, and the English-speaking people did not readily accept him.

Reverend Eleazar Wheelock believed that he could civilize Native Americans through education. Occom studied under Wheelock, but after four years, he had to stop his studies because of poor eyesight. In spite of his handicap, Occom went as a missionary to other Native Americans.

Occom ministered to the Montauk Native Americans for over twelve years. He served the Montauk as their preacher, teacher, counselor, doctor, and judge. Many times he barely had enough finances to feed his family. He had to hunt, fish, and make wooden spoons and pails to bring in a meager income.

Samson Occom hcard about a Native American church that was in need of a pastor among the Oneidas in New York. While traveling to the church, a smallpox epidemic prevented him from going further. Occom observed the people in New York City coming and going—filling the day with busyness. Drunkards staggered in the streets. People cursed—profaning God's holy name. He had never seen such wickedness among English people. Occom determined to always be an example of Christ's love to everyone he met.

Samson Occom suffered to serve Native Americans, but he was able to reach many with the gospel. He was the first Native American to speak to a European congregation, to write hymns, and to write for publication. He paved the way for acceptance of Native Americans among European Americans.

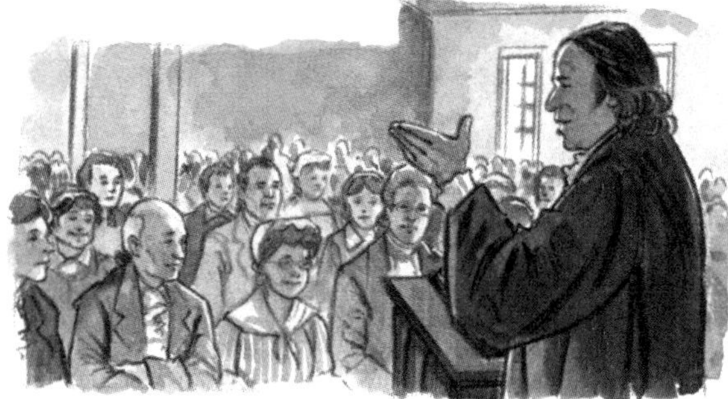

Answer the questions.

1. What did Samson Occom do when his plans to pastor a church in New York among the Oneidas were blocked?

   ____

   ____

2. What should you do when your plans to serve God seem to be blocked?

   ____

   ____

3. How can you be an example of Christ's love?

   ____

Hero of the Faith

Martin Luther A.D. 1483-1546

Name ______________________

Martin Luther was persecuted for his faith in Jesus Christ. While a devout Catholic, he found that good works can not gain peace with God. Through his testimony, princes, monks, and nuns were saved. Many religious leaders sought to rid themselves of Luther.

Luther was given a promise of safety to come before the emperor of Germany at the Diet of Worms. Many tried to persuade Luther to renounce the truth he had written. Luther refused to agree with the sale of indulgences, which deceived people into thinking their sins were forgiven. The religious leaders called Luther a heretic and asked that his promise of safety be annulled.

Luther left the city of Worms with friends who promised to protect him. After several days of travel they came to a forest. As they were riding in the forest, armed and masked horsemen seized Luther and left his friends. The men continually changed course through the forest until dark when they headed toward the castle of Wartburg.

Throughout the land his enemies rejoiced in his capture, and his friends mourned. Luther was a prisoner. His clothes were changed, his beard grew, and he was called "Knight George." But Luther was safe. Frederick, the elector of Saxony, had planned Luther's abduction to protect him from religious enemies. Luther lived at the castle for almost a year. During this time, he wrote letters and books, and translated the New Testament into German. The following year, a complete Bible in German was published.

Throughout the last years of his life, Martin Luther preached and wrote, and he spoke at religious meetings. He wrote hymns and books of theology. Several hymns have been translated into English, such as "A Mighty Fortress Is Our God." On a monument in Luther's memory, these words testify of his life: "If it is of God, it will last; if it is of man, it will pass."

Answer the questions.

1. How did Martin Luther react to being told to renounce his writings? ______________________

   ____

2. What types of ministries did Luther contribute to during his lifetime, and which ministry seemed to affect the most people?

   ____

   ____

3. Why was Luther persecuted?

   ____

   ____

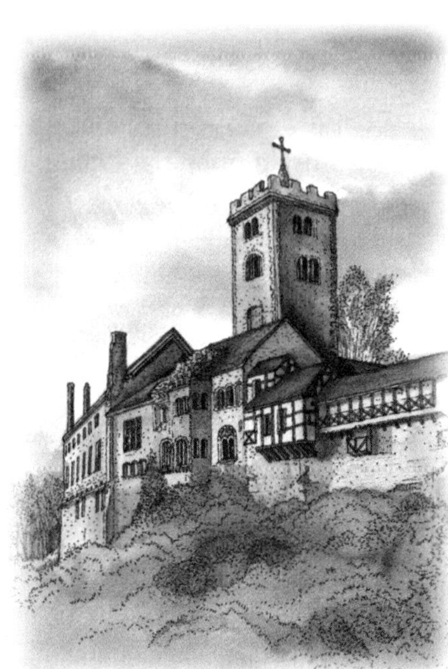

Stuart's Run to Faith

The application novel *Stuart's Run to Faith,* by Sharon Hambrick, is used in teaching lessons in Unit 3. Stuart is unsaved, and he dislikes attending the Christian school. During the school year, he learns the value of true friends and—finally—accepts God's love for himself.

It is suggested that the students have a copy of the book so that they can read the chapters silently before the teacher discusses the story with them. (*Note:* The teacher may choose to read the book aloud to the students.) Worktext pages 355-363 are designed to accompany the teaching of the story.

Stuart's Run to Faith may be purchased through BJU Press. For more information, call 1-800-845-5731 or look for the catalog at www.bjup.com.

Stuart's Run to Faith

Chapters 1-2

Name ______________________

You can tell that Stuart values sports by the way that he decorated his room using pictures from cereal boxes. Stuart's goal is to one day have his picture appear on the front of a cereal box as a gold medalist in running.

Write one of your goals on the box on page 357. Under *Ingredients,* list character traits that would help you accomplish your goal. Illustrate yourself making the goal or glue a picture of yourself onto the box.

Put the box together.

1. **Cut out the box on page 357 on the heavy black lines.**
2. **Fold the tabs on the dotted lines.**
3. **Glue or tape the A tabs to the inside of the B tabs.**
4. **Glue or tape the C tabs to the inside of the B tabs.**
5. **Glue or tape the D tab to the inside of the E tab.**

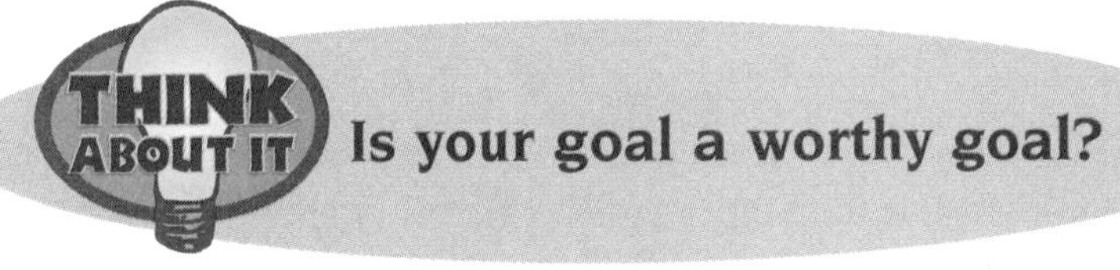
THINK ABOUT IT
Is your goal a worthy goal?

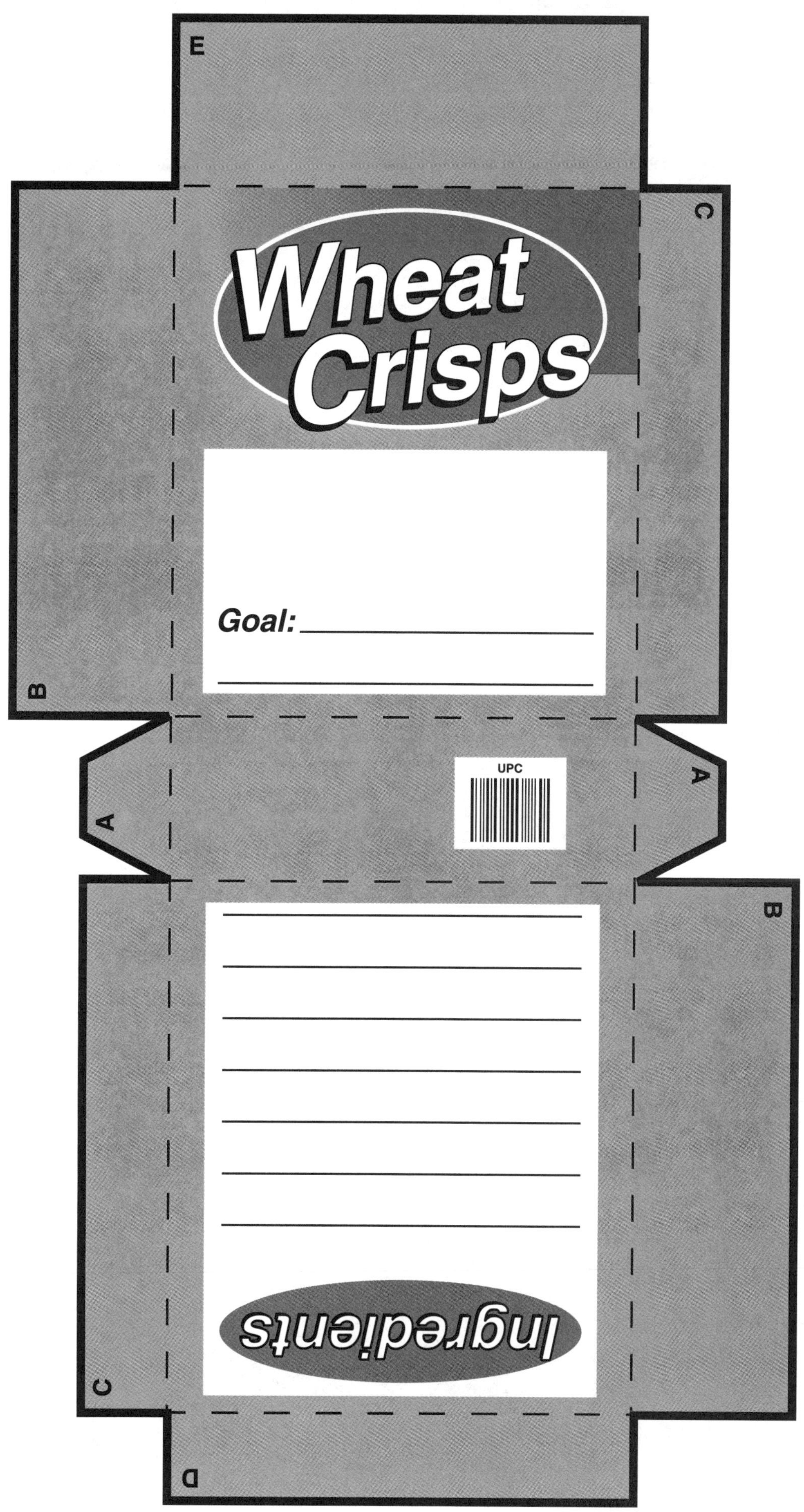
E
C
Wheat Crisps
Goal:
B
UPC
A
A
B
Ingredients
C
D

Stuart's Run to Faith

Chapters 3-5

Name ______________________

Read the verses. Choose the word or phrase that best completes the comparison.

evidence of salvation **faith** **the gospel** **the Word**

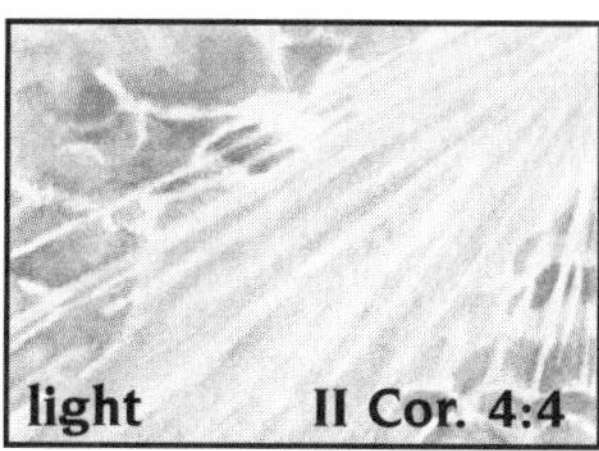
light II Cor. 4:4

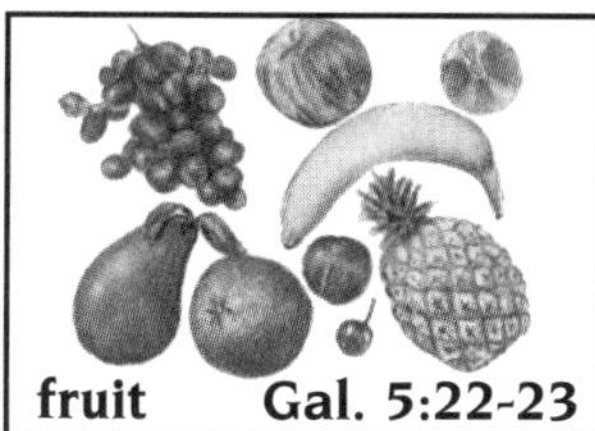
fruit Gal. 5:22-23

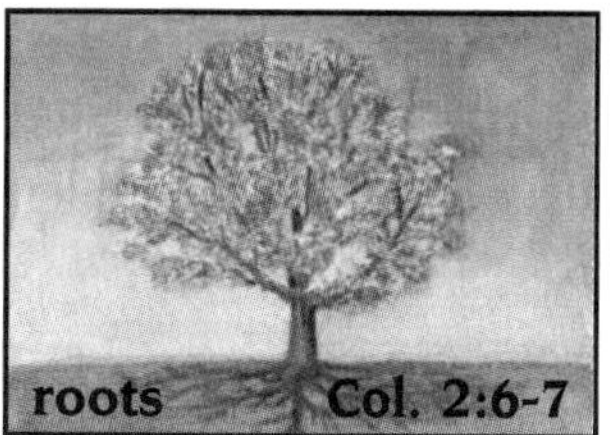
roots Col. 2:6-7

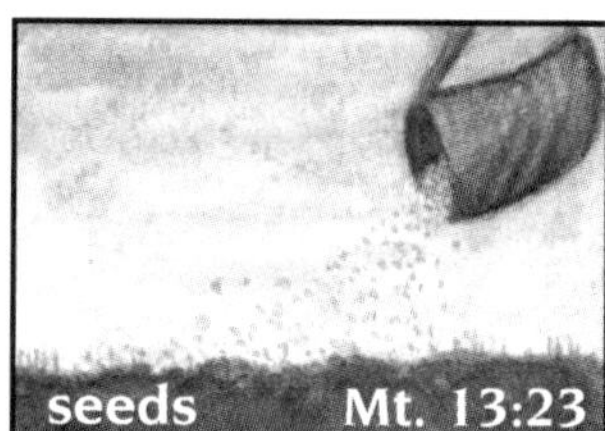
seeds Mt. 13:23

______________ ______________ ______________ ______________

Write the names of the people influencing Stuart for the Lord in the correct boxes.

Philip Baltz
Patricia Baltz
Grandma Ellie
Arby Jenkins
Coach Pickering
Mr. Hogan
Mr. Thompson
Mr. Watson

1. Who first shared the gospel with Stuart?

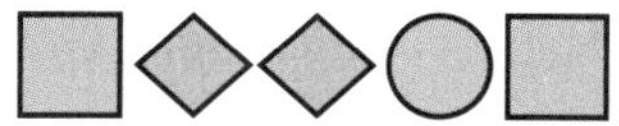

2. Which five people are also influencing Stuart for salvation?

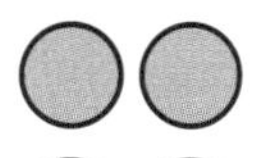 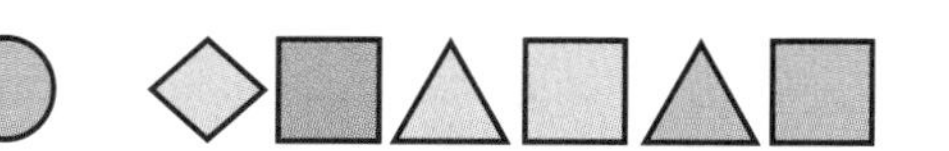

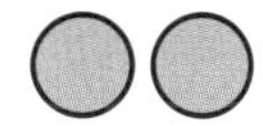 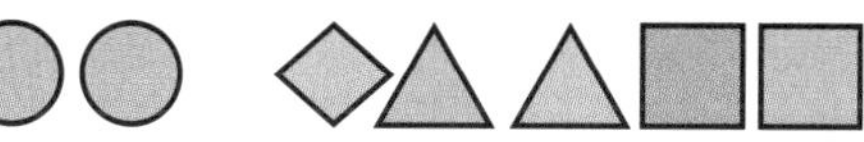

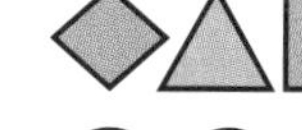 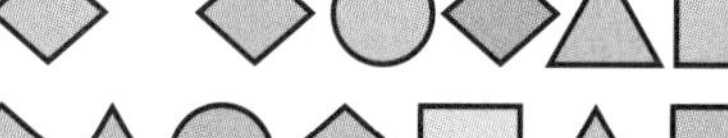

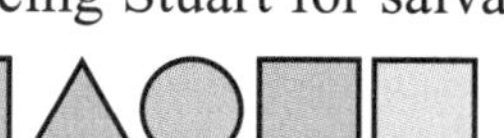

Use the color code to find the message from I Corinthians 3:6-8.

Paul 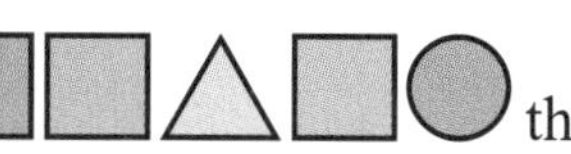 the gospel seed, 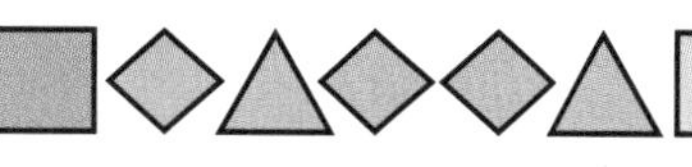 watered it,

but 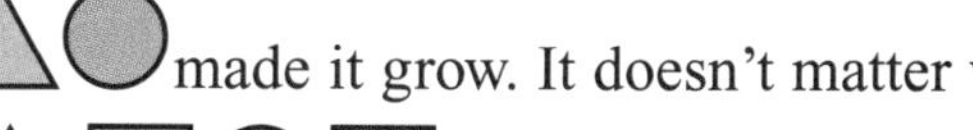 made it grow. It doesn't matter who 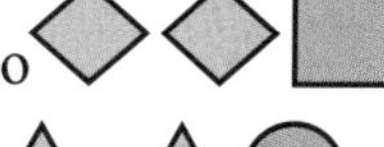 the seed or who

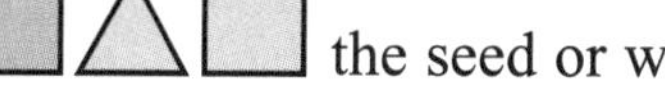 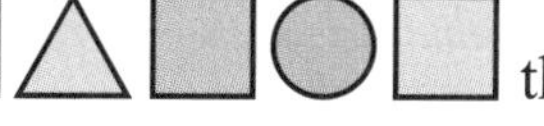 the seed, because it is 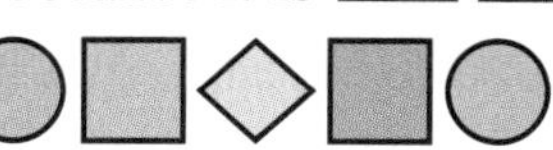 who makes it grow. The ones who

plant and water the seed will each be 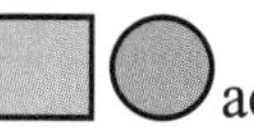 according to their works.

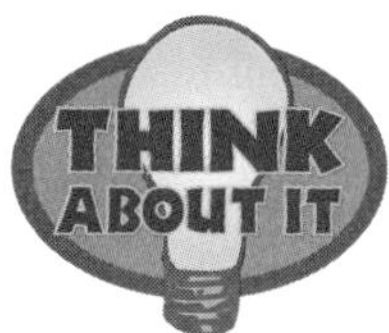
THINK
ABOUT IT

Are you working to draw others to the Lord? Who are your fellow laborers?

____

Stuart's Run to Faith

Chapters 8-9

Name ____________________

Use the letters on the web to fill in the blanks to complete the comparisons. The first number tells the location on the side of the web. If the second number is a *1,* the letter is located on the inner spiral. If the second number is a *2,* the letter is found on the outer spiral. For example *5,1* is the letter *L.*

It is truly frightening to fall into the hands of the L___ ___ ___ ___ ___ God. (Heb. 10:31)
5,1 2,1 1,2 2,1 6,2 7,1

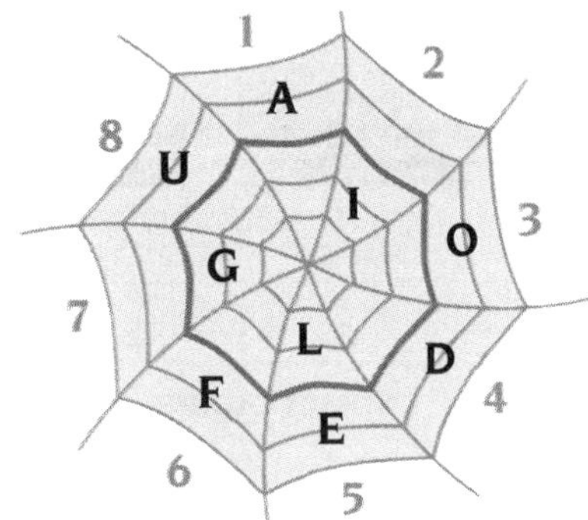
1
2
3
4
5
6
7
8
A
U
I
O
G
L
D
F
E

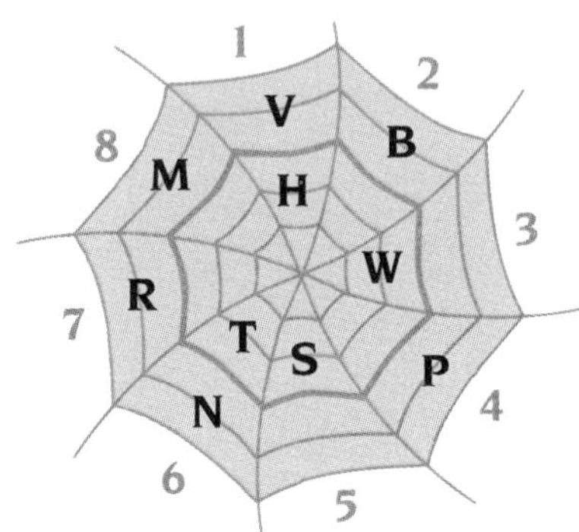
1
2
3
4
5
6
7
8
V
B
M
H
W
R
T
S
P
N

In his famous sermon "Sinners in the Hands of an Angry God" Jonathan Edwards compares the sinner to an ugly creeping ___ ___ ___ ___ ___ ___. Just as a spider's web
5,1 4,2 2,1 4,2 5,2 7,2

cannot break the fall of a ___ ___ ___ ___ ___, a sinner's good deeds cannot keep
5,1 6,1 3,2 6,2 5,2

him from falling into hell. Notice the illustration from Job 8:13-14. Those who

___ ___ ___ ___ ___ ___ God have no ___ ___ ___ ___. What they put their
6,2 3,2 7,2 7,1 5,2 6,1 1,1 3,2 4,2 5,2

trust in is as fragile as a spider's ___ ___ ___.
3,1 5,2 2,2

Jonathan Edwards made other comparisons in his famous sermon. Psalm 7:11-13 tells us that

God is a ___ ___ ___ ___ ___ ___ ___ ___ ___ Judge and is angry with the
7,2 2,1 7,1 1,1 6,1 5,2 3,2 8,2 5,1

wicked continually. If the wicked do not repent, God will sharpen His ___ ___ ___ ___ ___;
5,1 3,1 3,2 7,2 4,2

His bow is bent and ready. He has prepared His ___ ___ ___ ___ ___ ___.
1,2 7,2 7,2 3,2 3,1 5,1

God's wrath on the sinner is also compared to a destructive storm and a furnace.

Isaiah prophesies that the Lord will come with ___ ___ ___ ___, and with His
6,2 2,1 7,2 5,2

chariots like a whirlwind, to show His fierce anger and to rebuke with

___ ___ ___ ___ ___ ___ of fire.
6,2 5,1 1,2 8,2 5,2 5,1

Stuart's Run to Faith

Chapters 10-12

Name ______________________

Some songs Stuart heard in chapel were written in a question and answer format. See how much you know about the work of Christ by filling in the blanks below. You may use the catechism section "Do I Know About the Work of Christ?" on pages 378-80.

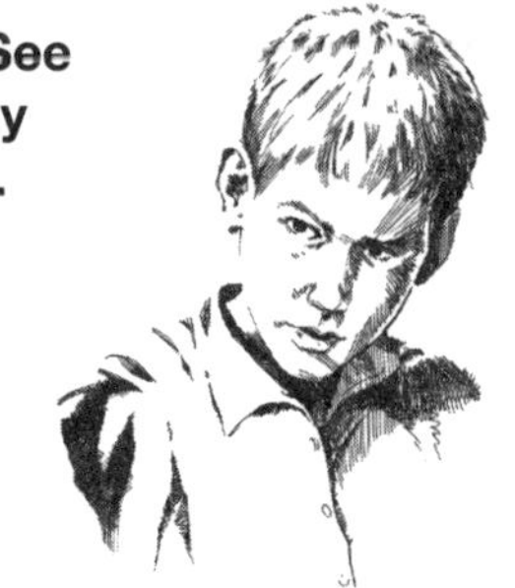

behavior	believes	heart	holy
justice	living	No one	penalty
perfectly	repents	sinners	Spirit

What can wash away my sin? What is the work of Christ?	*Nothing but the blood of Jesus.* The work of Christ is to __________ keep the law of God and to suffer the __________ for our sins.
What can make me whole again? What does God require of man before he can go to heaven?	*Nothing but the blood of Jesus.* No one can enter heaven unless his ______ is changed.
Nothing can for sin atone— What is meant by atonement?	*Nothing but the blood of Jesus.* The atonement is Christ's satisfying of divine __________ by His sufferings and death in the place of __________.
Naught of good that I have done— Can anyone be saved by his own works?	*Nothing but the blood of Jesus.* __________ can be saved by his own works.
Would you be free from your burden of sin? Who will be saved?	*There's pow'r in the blood, pow'r in the blood.* Whoever __________ and __________ on the Lord Jesus Christ will be saved.
Would you o'er evil a victory win? Who can change a sinner's heart?	*There's wonderful pow'r in the blood.* The Holy ________ can change a sinner's heart.
Would you do service for Jesus your King? What is sanctification?	*There's pow'r in the blood, pow'r in the blood.* Sanctification is God's making me ________ in heart and __________.
Would you live daily His praises to sing? What are the two parts of sanctification?	*There's wonderful pow'r in the blood.* The two parts of sanctification are dying to sin and __________ to righteousness.

Stuart's Run to Faith

Chapters 16-18

Name ______________________

Stuart trusts God for his salvation, but he struggles with trusting Him for day to day events. For each sentence that shows a character trusting in self, shade the letter below that corresponds to that sentence number. If the sentence reveals how a character is trusting God, leave the corresponding letter blank.

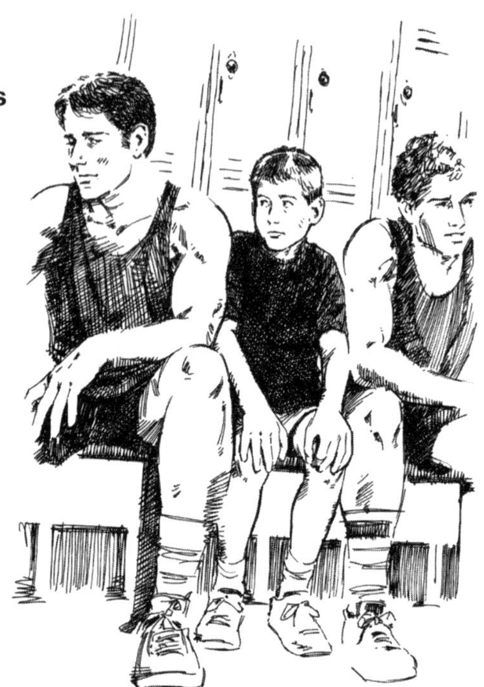

1. Stuart is scared about going to Hamilton Junior High School.
2. Stuart requests prayer about his school situation during his world history class.
3. Miss Ward prays for Stuart's school situation.
4. Ray thinks everyone can work to keep Stuart at GCA.
5. Stuart asks his mom if he can work his way through school.
6. Stuart thinks Mr. Hogan will find a way to keep him at GCA.
7. Mr. Hogan advises Stuart to accept his mom's decision and to consider that the Lord might use him in the new environment.

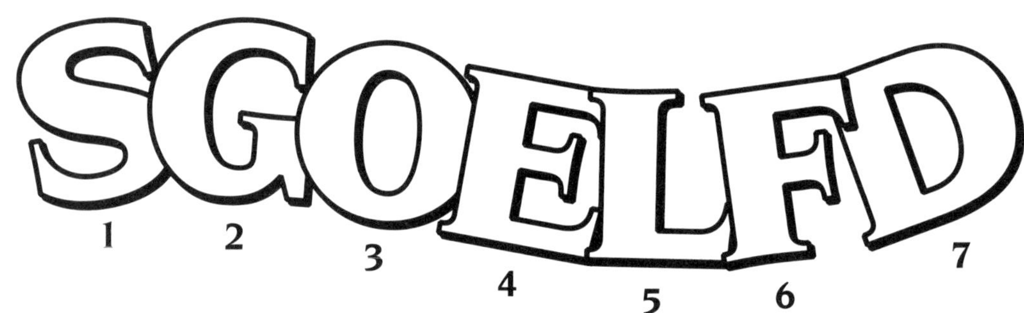

SGOELFD
1 2 3 4 5 6 7

Look at the shaded letters and answer the question.

What should our trust not be in? ___ ___ ___ ___

Read each verse. What else does the Bible say that men trust in? Write the item or person mentioned in each verse. Rearrange the circled letters to answer the last question.

Psalm 44:6 ___ ___ ___ or ___ ___ ___ ___ ___

Psalm 118:8-9 ___ ___ ___ or ___ ___ ___ ___ ___ ___ ___

Proverbs 3:5-6 our own ___ ___ ___ ___ ___ ___ ___ ___ ___ ___ ___ ___ ___

I Timothy 6:17 ___ ___ ___ ___ ___ ___

Whom should we put our trust in? ___ ___ ___

Stuart's Run to Faith

Chapters 19-20

Name ______________________

Read II Corinthians 5:17 and answer the questions.

1. When someone is "in Christ" (saved) does his life change? ______________

2. What does someone become when he gets saved? ______________

3. How does Stuart's life change when he accepts Jesus Christ as his Savior?

____

____

Living a life separated to God results in a life separated from sin. A Christian will change from an unsaved lifestyle to a lifestyle that pleases God. This is the result of the Holy Spirit working in a believer's heart day by day to conform him to the image of Jesus Christ. Although salvation occurs in an instant, sanctification is a lifelong process. It requires submitting to the Holy Spirit's control to have the mind (attitude) of Christ and not the world's outlook.

When Paul wrote to the Christians at Corinth, he asked them about their outlook on the world and the things of God. In each question, he listed several things that cannot go together because they are absolutely opposite in nature and character.

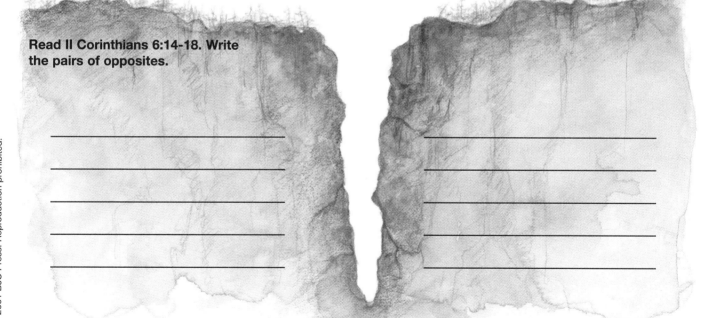

Read II Corinthians 6:14-18. Write the pairs of opposites.

______________ ______________

______________ ______________

______________ ______________

______________ ______________

______________ ______________

THINK ABOUT IT Just as the people of Corinth needed to think about their lives, you need to think about yours. Are you a believer in Christ? Are you doing right in the sight of God? Are you walking in light?

Are you daily asking the Holy Spirit to change you into the image of Christ? As you grow in Christ, the chasm between you and the world's attitudes, values, and actions will also grow.

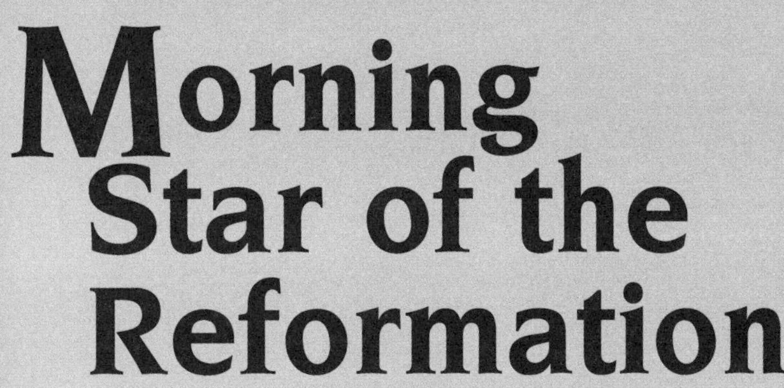

Morning Star of the Reformation

The historical novel *Morning Star of the Reformation,* by Andy Thomson, is used in teaching lessons in Unit 7. The book is about John Wycliffe, an important leader in church history. He is remembered for translating the Bible from Latin into English so that the common people could read the Bible themselves.

It is suggested that the teacher read the chapters aloud before discussing the story with the students. Worktext pages 365-372 are designed to accompany the teaching of the story.

Morning Star of the Reformation may be purchased through BJU Press. For more information, call 1-800-845-5731 or look for the catalog at www.bjup.com.

Morning Star of the Reformation

Chapters 1-3

Name ______________________

Fill in the circle next to the correct answer.

1. What was pinned to the dead thief's clothing?
   - ○ an indulgence
   - ○ directions for his burial
2. What is an indulgence?
   - ○ a list of a person's sins
   - ○ a false pardon of sins so that a person thinks he or someone else is forgiven of sin
3. How does a person obtain an indulgence?
   - ○ purchased from the church
   - ○ received as a gift from God

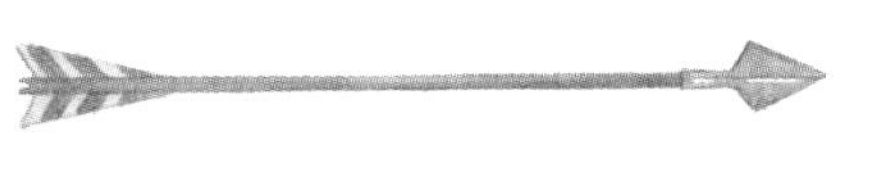

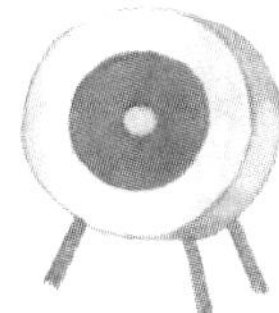

Read Luke 5:20-24 and answer the questions.

4. Of what did the scribes and Pharisees accuse Jesus?

   (v. 21) ______________________

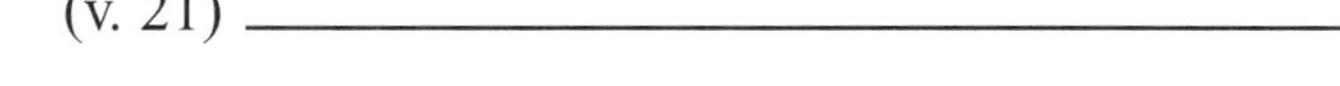

5. What question did they ask? (v. 21) ______________________
6. Why did Jesus heal the man? (v. 24) ______________________

   ____
7. Does man have power or authority to forgive sins? ______________________
8. If a man claims to have power to forgive sins, what sin is he committing? ______________________

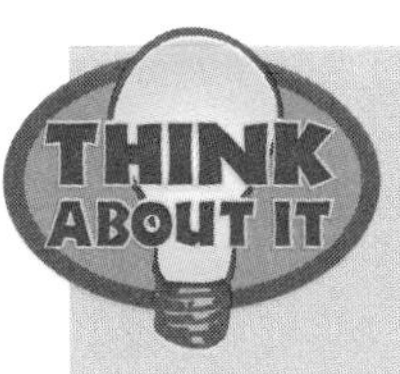
THINK
ABOUT IT

How would you explain why the selling of pardons (indulgences) is not a scriptural practice?

____

____

Morning Star of the Reformation

Chapters 7-9

Name ______________________________

One of the skills the students learned at Oxford University was solid **argumentation.** Being able to explain what you believe to others is important. However, you must also learn to defend what you believe. Both Fleet Nigel and John Wycliffe were able to perform this skill well.

Read the points of Fleet Nigel's and John Wycliffe's arguments about the Bible. Identify which man used each point in his argument.

Poor, ignorant men and women cannot be trusted to interpret the Bible accurately.
____

Everyone is responsible to care for the state of his eternal soul.
____

Common people do not know and cannot understand how to care for their eternal souls.
____

Men and women alike should have the opportunity to hear the Scriptures taught in plain English.
____

The interpretation of the church fathers is equal to that of the Scripture.
____

The church fathers were imperfect men capable of making errors.
____

Scripture alone is perfect, and it alone can be trusted to show the way of salvation.
____

The church fathers can be trusted to show the way of salvation.
____

Answer the questions.

1. Based on the above arguments, with which man do you agree? ______________________
2. Explain why you agree with the man you chose. ______________________

____

Another form of argument the young scholars learned at Oxford was called **disputation.** This method breaks down each part of a question and defines it for the purpose of clear explanation.

Practice the skill of disputation by reading the question and writing your own definition for each word.

Question:
Is the Word of God perfect?

Word ______________________

God ______________________

perfect ______________________

Rewrite the question using your definitions.

____

____

Morning Star of the Reformation

Chapters 12-13

Name ______________________________

John Wycliffe's great desire was that people would understand that Scripture pointed the way to true salvation, not the church. He was grieved and concerned because the church of his day deceived people by teaching salvation by trusting in works rather than Christ alone. He made every effort to point out that nothing—no person, no church, no tradition, no desire—should come between God and man.

Draw a line connecting the statements to the correct description of what is coming between these people and the truth of salvation found in God's Word.

"I have been a pretty good person. I go out of my way to be nice to everybody. God must be pleased with that!"

"My neighborhood friends might laugh at me if I become a Christian."

"I know I'll have to give up my rock music if I become a Christian."

Other people

Worldly entertainment

Good works

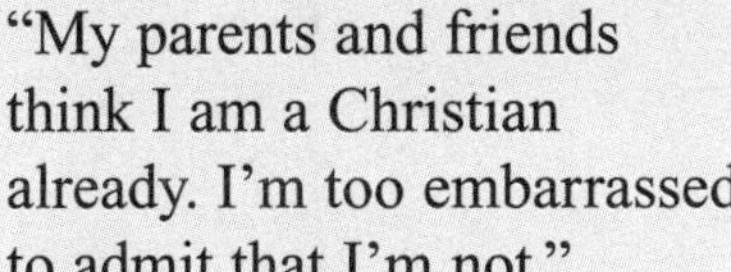

"My parents and friends think I am a Christian already. I'm too embarrassed to admit that I'm not."

"I'm scared God will call me to be a missionary in Africa or something if I become a Christian."

"I believe in God, but I just want to do my own thing and live my life the way I want to live it right now."

Fear of the unknown

Pride

Selfishness

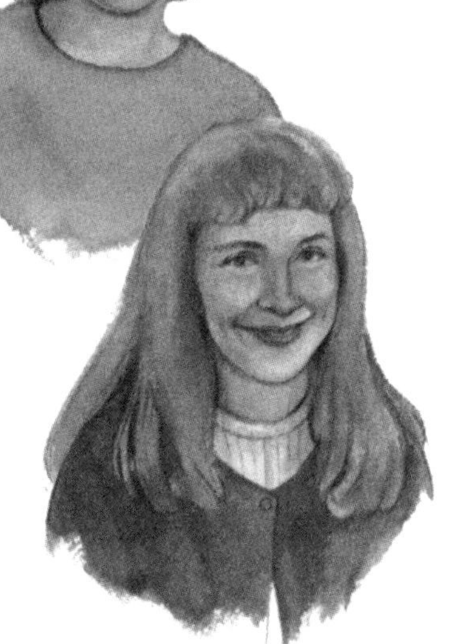

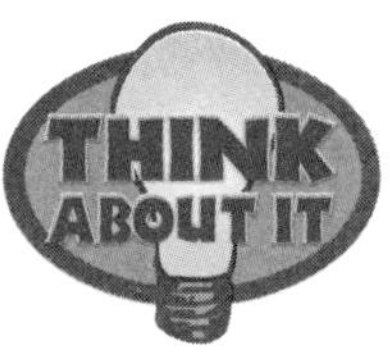
THINK
ABOUT IT

Can you think of anything else that might come between a person's heart and the truth of God's Word?

Is there anything coming between YOU and the truth of God's Word?

Morning Star of the Reformation
Chapters 14-16

Name ____________________

Write II Timothy 2:2 in the center circle. Write the correct names on the lines. Each name will be used twice.

John → **Sebastian** → **William** →

______ helps ______ study Latin.

______ helps ______ translate the Bible from Latin into English.

II Timothy 2:2

____

____

____

____

____

____

____

____

______________ teaches his son ______________ Latin.

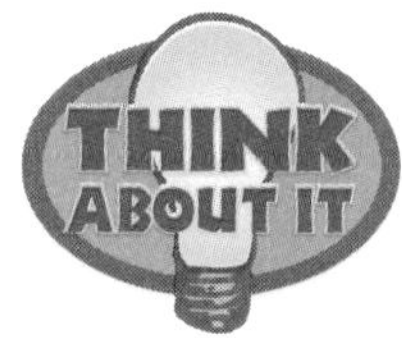
THINK
ABOUT IT

How does II Timothy 2:2 apply to the lives of these men?

____

____

Morning Star of the Reformation

Chapters 17-19

Name ______________________

Read each Scripture verse to find the true path from Oxford to London. Color all the references and color only the statements proven true with Scripture.

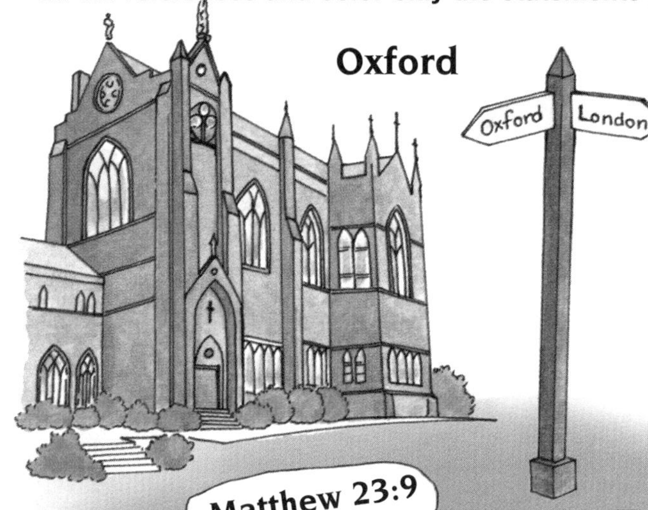

Oxford
Oxford
London

John Wycliffe was able to travel from Oxford to London to defend his teachings because he had studied the Scripture and had a solid foundation for his beliefs. He was walking in the truths of Scripture.

Matthew 23:9

A preacher or pope should be called by God the Father's name.

Spiritually speaking, the name *Father* is for God alone.

Psalm 86:5

A person needs only to call on the Lord to receive forgiveness.

A person needs to confess to a preacher or priest and do penance.

I Timothy 2:5

Jesus Christ is the only mediator between man and God the Father.

The priest is the mediator between man and God the Father.

Do you know Scripture well enough to tell others?

I Peter 2:21-24

Christ's suffering is the Christian's example for doing penance.

Christ suffered in the place of sinners. Repentance needs no penance.

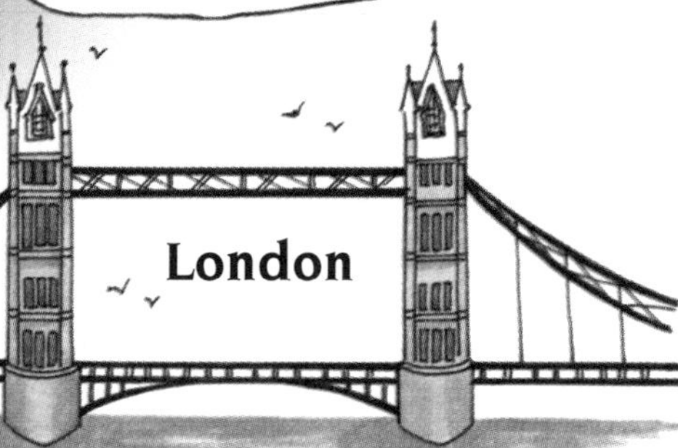

London

Morning Star of the Reformation

Chapters 20-23

Name ______________________

Complete the sentences. To read God's promise about His Word, hold your page up to a mirror.

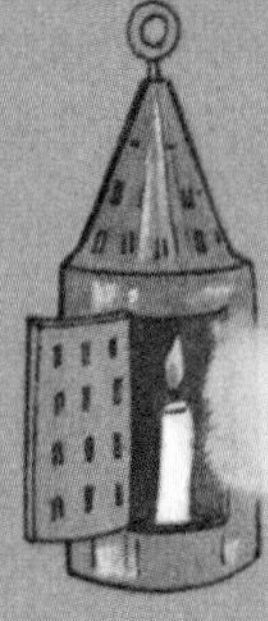

Jesus referred to Himself as the __________ of the world. Those who follow Him will not walk in ______________ (John 8:12).

God's Word is a ____________ and a __________ (Ps. 119:105).

The Lord is our ___________. He will lighten our _______________ (II Sam. 22:29).

You are the _________ of the world (Matt. 5:14).

Let your __________ ___________ before men that they may see your good works and glorify your Father in Heaven (Matt. 5:16).

You were once in ______________. Now you are ____________ in the Lord. Walk as children of _________ (Eph. 5:8).

John Wycliffe led others to the Lord by pointing them to the Word of God.

He reflected the Lord Jesus in his life and was a light in the darkness around him.

Isaiah 55:11
So shall my word
be that goeth forth
out of my mouth: it
shall not return
unto me void, but
it shall accomplish
that which I please,
and it shall
prosper in the
thing whereto I
sent it.

Who can you be a light to today? Think of someone with whom you can share the glorious light of the gospel.

Catechism

Do I Know About God?

1. **Who is God?**
   God is a spirit and does not have a body like man (John 4:24).

2. **What is God like?**
   God is infinite, eternal, and unchangeable (Psalms 139:7-10; 90:2; Malachi 3:6).

3. **Where is God?**
   God is everywhere (Psalm 139:7-12; Proverbs 15:3).

4. **Can you see God?**
   No, I cannot see God, but He always sees me (Jeremiah 23:23-24; John 1:18).

5. **Does God know all things?**
   Yes, nothing can be hidden from God (Job 34:21).

6. **Can God do all things?**
   Yes, God can do all His holy will (Matthew 19:26).

7. **Does God ever do evil?**
   No, God is always good (Exodus 34:6; Psalm 86:5).

8. **Are there more gods than one?**
   No, there is only one God (Isaiah 45:6; I Timothy 2:5).

9. **In how many persons does this one God exist?**
   God exists in three persons (Matthew 3:16-17; II Corinthians 13:14).

10. **Who are the three persons of God?**
    The three persons of God are the Father, the Son, and the Holy Spirit (Matthew 28:19).

11. **Who made God?**
    Nobody made God (Psalm 90:2).

12. **Has God ever had a beginning?**
    No, God has always been (Psalm 90:2; Revelation 4:8).

13. **Will God ever die?**
    No, God lives forever (Psalm 90:2).

14. **What is God's attitude toward us?**
    God loves us unconditionally (John 3:16; Romans 5:8).

Do I *Know About God's Creation*?

1. **Who made you?**
   God made me (Genesis 1:27; Job 33:4).

2. **What else did God make?**
   God made all things (Genesis 1:1-31; John 1:3).

3. **Why did God make you and all things?**
   God made me and all things for His own glory (Romans 11:36; I Corinthians 6:20).

4. **How can you glorify God?**
   I can glorify God by loving Him and doing what He commands (Micah 6:8; I John 5:3).

5. **Why ought you to glorify God?**
   I ought to glorify God because He made me and takes care of me (Psalm 146:5-10).

6. **Where do you learn how to love and obey God?**
   I learn how to love and obey God in the Bible alone (Deuteronomy 30:11-16; Joshua 1:8).

7. **Who wrote the Bible?**
   Holy men who were taught by the Holy Spirit wrote the Bible (II Peter 1:21).

8. **Who were our first parents?**
   Adam and Eve were our first parents (Genesis 2:7, 18-22).

9. **Of what were our first parents made?**
   God made the body of Adam out of the dust of the ground and formed Eve from the body of Adam (Genesis 2:7, 21-22).

10. **Whom did God make Adam to be like?**
    God made Adam after His own image (Genesis 1:27; 9:6).

11. **What did God give Adam and Eve besides bodies?**
    God gave them souls that could never die (Genesis 2:7).

12. **Do you have a soul as well as a body?**
    Yes, I have a soul that can never die (Ecclesiastes 12:7; I Thessalonians 5:23).

13. **How do you know that you have a soul?**
    God tells me so in Genesis 2:7, "And the Lord God formed man of the dust of the ground, and breathed into his nostrils the breath of life; and man became a living soul" (Genesis 2:7).

14. **In what condition did God make Adam and Eve?**
    God made them holy and happy (Genesis 1:27-31).

Do I Know What God Says About Sin?

1. **What is a covenant?**
   A covenant is an agreement between two or more persons (Genesis 9:11-17).

2. **What was Adam's part in the covenant in order to stay in the Garden of Eden?**
   Adam was required to obey God perfectly (Genesis 2:15-17).

3. **Did Adam obey God?**
   No, Adam chose to disobey God (Genesis 3:6).

4. **Did Adam's sin affect himself alone?**
   No, Adam's sin made all men lose communion with God and become sinful in nature and subject to God's wrath (Romans 5:14; 6:23; Ephesians 2:3).

5. **How did God punish Adam's disobedience?**
   Adam's punishment was death and separation from God (Genesis 3:17-24).

6. **What is sin?**
   Sin is the transgression of the law of God (I John 3:4).

7. **What is meant by transgression?**
   Transgression is failing to do what God commands or doing what God forbids (Psalm 25:6-7; Matthew 15:3-6).

8. **What was the sin of our first parents?**
   Adam and Eve disobeyed God and ate the fruit that God told them not to eat (Genesis 2:17; 3:6).

9. **Who tempted Adam and Eve to sin?**
   Satan tempted Eve, and she gave the fruit to Adam (Genesis 3:1-6).

10. **What happened to our first parents when they had sinned?**
    Instead of being holy and happy, they became sinful and miserable (Genesis 3:8-24).

11. **What effect did Adam's sin have on all mankind?**
    Because of Adam's sin, every man is born with a sinful nature that wants to do evil and has no fellowship with God (Romans 5:12).

12. **What is that sinful nature we inherit from Adam called?**
    Our corrupt nature is called original sin (Psalm 51:5; Romans 5:12).

13. **What does every sin deserve?**
    Every sin deserves the wrath and curse of God (Psalm 89:30-32; Galatians 3:10).

Do I Know About Angels and Satan?

1. **Did God make anyone before Adam and Eve?**
   Yes, God made angels (Job 38:7; Genesis 3:24).

2. **What do angels do?**
   They serve God (Hebrews 1:14).

3. **Are all angels good?**
   No, some angels are holy, while others are evil (Matthew 25:31; Revelation 12:9).

4. **Who is Satan?**
   Satan is an evil spirit who is the enemy of God and all Christians (John 8:44; I Peter 5:8).

5. **Was Satan ever good?**
   Yes, Satan was once one of God's greatest angels (Isaiah 14:12-15).

6. **What was Satan's name when he was one of God's angels?**
   Satan's name was Lucifer (Isaiah 14:12).

7. **Why is Lucifer not one of God's angels today?**
   Lucifer became jealous of God and wanted to be as great as He, so God cast him out of heaven (Isaiah 14:12-15; Revelation 12:7-9).

8. **What is Lucifer now called?**
   Lucifer is now called Satan or the Devil (Luke 10:18; I John 3:8).

9. **Who is stronger, God or Satan?**
   God is stronger (I John 3:8; 4:4).

10. **Does Satan want God's will to be done?**
    No, Satan always wants people to do the opposite of what God wants them to do (I Chronicles 21:1; Ephesians 6:11-12, 16).

Do I Know About the Work of Christ?

1. **Who can save us?**
   The only Savior of men is the Lord Jesus Christ (John 14:6; Acts 4:12).

2. **What does God require of man before he can go to heaven?**
   No one can enter heaven unless his heart is changed (John 3:3, 16; Acts 4:12).

3. **What is this change of heart called?**
   This change of heart is called regeneration (Ezekiel 36:26-27; Titus 3:5-6).

4. **Who can change a sinner's heart?**
   The Holy Spirit can change a sinner's heart (Titus 3:5).

5. **How is a heart changed?**
   A heart is changed by the Holy Spirit because of the grace of God shown in the work of Christ (Titus 3:4-7).

6. **What is grace?**
   Grace is God's kindness to us when we deserve punishment (Deuteronomy 7:6-9; Ephesians 2:8-9).

7. **What is the work of Christ?**
   The work of Christ is to keep perfectly the law of God and to suffer the penalty for our sins (II Corinthians 5:21; Hebrews 9:11-14).

8. **Can anyone be saved by his own works?**
   No one can be saved by his own works (Ephesians 2:8-9; Titus 3:4-7).

9. **Did Christ ever sin?**
   No, Christ was holy, sinless, and undefiled (II Corinthians 5:21; Hebrews 7:26).

10. **How could the Son of God suffer?**
    Christ, the Son of God, became man that He might obey and suffer in our nature (Philippians 2:7-8; Hebrews 2:9).

11. **What is meant by atonement?**
    The atonement is Christ's satisfying divine justice by His sufferings and death in the place of sinners (Romans 5:8-11).

12. **What do we gain from the work of Christ?**
    God regenerates, justifies, and sanctifies those who believe in Christ (I Corinthians 6:11; Titus 3:5-7).

13. **What is justification?**
    Justification is God's forgiving me and treating me just as if I had never sinned (Romans 3:24-25; II Corinthians 5:19, 21).

14. **How am I justified?**
    I am justified by faith in the work of Christ and on the grounds of His righteousness (Romans 3:25-28).

15. **What is sanctification?**
Sanctification is God's making me holy in heart and behavior (I Corinthians 6:19-20).

16. **What are the two parts of sanctification?**
The two parts of sanctification are dying to sin and living to righteousness (Romans 8:13; Galatians 2:20).

17. **For whom did Christ obey and suffer?**
Christ obeyed and suffered for sinners (Romans 5:8).

18. **What kind of death did Christ die?**
Christ died the painful and shameful death of being nailed to a cross (Luke 23:33-38; Philippians 2:8).

19. **Who will be saved?**
Whoever repents and believes on the Lord Jesus Christ will be saved (Isaiah 55:7; John 3:16).

20. **What does it mean to repent?**
To repent is to be sorry for sin and to hate and forsake it because it is displeasing to God (II Chronicles 7:14; II Corinthians 7:9).

21. **What is saving faith in Christ?**
Saving faith is believing that Christ died for my sins, that He was buried, and that He rose again according to the Scriptures (I Corinthians 15:1-4).

22. **Can you repent and believe in Christ by your own power?**
No, I cannot repent and believe in Christ without the help of God's Holy Spirit (John 3:5-6; Titus 3:5).

23. **Does Christ care for little children?**
Yes, for He says in Mark 10:14, "Suffer the little children to come unto me, and forbid them not: for of such is the kingdom of God" (Mark 10:14).

24. **How long has it been since Christ died?**
Christ died nearly 2,000 years ago.

25. **How were people saved before the coming of Christ?**
People were saved by believing in a Savior to come (Hebrews 11:13).

26. **How did people show their faith before the coming of Christ?**
People showed their faith by offering sacrifices on God's altar (Hebrews 11:4).

27. **What did the sacrifices represent?**
The sacrifices represented Christ, the Lamb of God, who was to die for sinners (John 1:29, 36; Hebrews 9:11-14).

28. **How many offices does Christ have?**
Christ has three offices (Acts 3:22; Hebrews 5:5-6; Revelation 19:16).

29. What are Christ's offices?
Christ's offices are prophet, priest, and king (Acts 3:22; Hebrews 5:5-6; Revelation 19:16).

30. How is Christ a prophet?
Christ teaches us the will of God (Luke 4:18; John 15:15).

31. How is Christ a priest?
Christ died for our sins and pleads with God for us (Romans 3:26; Hebrews 7:25-27).

32. How is Christ a king?
Christ rules over us, defends us, and will establish His kingdom on earth (Isaiah 33:22; I Corinthians 15:25).

Do I *Know About the* Resurrection?

1. **On which day of the week do Christians worship?**
   Christians worship on the first day of the week, called the Lord's Day (Acts 20:7; I Corinthians 16:1-2).

2. **Why is it called the Lord's Day?**
   On that day Christ rose from the dead (Matthew 28:1-6; Mark 16:1-6).

3. **How should the Lord's Day be spent?**
   The Lord's Day should be spent in prayer and praise, in hearing and reading God's Word, and in doing good to our fellow man (Luke 13:10-13; Acts 15:21; 16:13).

4. **Did Christ remain in the tomb after His crucifixion?**
   No, Christ rose bodily from the tomb on the third day after His death (Matthew 16:21; 28:1-6; I Corinthians 15:3-4).

5. **Where is Christ now?**
   Christ is in heaven, interceding for us (Acts 1:9; Ephesians 1:19-21; Hebrews 4:14-16; 7:25).

Do I Know About God's Ordinances?

1. **What is an ordinance?**
   An ordinance is a way of remembering Christ's death and resurrection (Romans 6:3-10; I Corinthians 11:23-26).

2. **How many ordinances are there in the Bible?**
   There are two ordinances in the Bible (Matthew 28:19; I Corinthians 11:23-26).

3. **What are the two ordinances?**
   The two ordinances are baptism and the Lord's Supper (Matthew 26:26-28; 28:19).

4. **Who appointed these ordinances?**
   The Lord Jesus Christ appointed them (Matthew 26:26-28; 28:18-19).

5. **Why did Christ appoint these ordinances?**
   Christ appointed these ordinances to distinguish His disciples from the world and to comfort and strengthen them (Acts 2:38-41; Romans 6:4).

6. **What sign is used in baptism?**
   The sign used in baptism is water (Matthew 3:6, 11, 14-17).

7. **What does baptism mean?**
   Baptism is an outward sign of our union with Christ and our decision to follow Him (Romans 6:3-11; Galatians 3:27).

8. **In whose name are we baptized?**
   We are baptized in the name of the Father and of the Son and of the Holy Spirit (Matthew 28:19).

9. **What is the Lord's Supper?**
   The Lord's Supper is a remembrance of Christ's death for us on the cross and a looking forward to His return (Matthew 26:26-28; I Corinthians 11:23-26).

10. **Who is to partake of the Lord's Supper?**
    All those who have trusted Christ as their Savior and are living for Him may partake of the Lord's Supper (I Corinthians 11:28, 29).

11. **What are the elements used in the Lord's Supper?**
    The elements used in the Lord's Supper are bread and the fruit of the vine (Matthew 26:26-28; Mark 14:22-25).

12. **What do the bread and fruit of the vine symbolize?**
    The bread symbolizes Christ's body which was crucified for us, and the cup symbolizes His blood which was shed for us (Matthew 26:26-28; Mark 14:22-25; Luke 22:17-20).

Do I Know About God's Commandments?

1. **How many commandments did God give on Mount Sinai?**
   God gave ten commandments (Exodus 20:1-17).

2. **What are the Ten Commandments sometimes called?**
   They are called the Decalogue.

3. **What does *Decalogue* mean?**
   The word *Decalogue* means "ten words."

4. **What do the first four commandments teach?**
   The first four commandments teach our duty to God (Exodus 20:1-11; Matthew 22:37-38).

5. **Is God pleased with those who love and obey Him?**
   Yes, for He says in Proverbs 8:17, "I love them that love me; and those that seek me early shall find me" (Proverbs 8:17).

6. **Is God displeased with those who do not love and obey Him?**
   Yes, for He says in Psalm 7:11, "God judgeth the righteous, and God is angry with the wicked every day" (Psalm 7:11).

7. **What is the first commandment?**
   The first commandment is "Thou shalt have no other gods before me" (Exodus 20:3).

8. **What does the first commandment teach us?**
   The first commandment teaches us to worship God alone (Matthew 4:10).

9. **What is the second commandment?**
   The second commandment is "Thou shalt not make unto thee any graven image, or any likeness of any thing that is in heaven above, or that is in the earth beneath, or that is in the water under earth" (Exodus 20:4-6).

10. **What does the second commandment teach us?**
    The second commandment teaches us to worship God in a proper manner and to avoid idolatry (Exodus 20:23; Deuteronomy 6:13-18).

11. **What is the third commandment?**
    The third commandment is "Thou shalt not take the name of the Lord thy God in vain; for the Lord will not hold him guiltless that taketh his name in vain" (Exodus 20:7).

12. **What does the third commandment teach us?**
    The third commandment teaches us to reverence God's name, Word, and works (Psalms 29:2; 107:21-22; 138:2).

13. **What is the fourth commandment?**
    The fourth commandment is "Remember the sabbath day, to keep it holy" (Exodus 20:8-11).

14. **What does the fourth commandment teach us?**
The fourth commandment teaches us that one day of the week is God's special day (Leviticus 19:30; Deuteronomy 5:12).

15. **What do the last six commandments teach?**
The last six commandments teach our duty to our fellow man (Exodus 20:12-17; Matthew 22:39).

16. **What is the fifth commandment?**
The fifth commandment is "Honour thy father and thy mother: that thy days may be long upon the land which the Lord thy God giveth thee" (Exodus 20:12).

17. **What does the fifth commandment teach us?**
The fifth commandment teaches us that God blesses those that love and obey their parents (Romans 13:1; Ephesians 6:1-3).

18. **What is the sixth commandment?**
The sixth commandment is "Thou shalt not kill" (Exodus 20:13).

19. **What does the sixth commandment teach us?**
The sixth commandment teaches us to avoid anger and injury to others (Genesis 9:6; I John 3:15).

20. **What is the seventh commandment?**
The seventh commandment is "Thou shalt not commit adultery" (Exodus 20:14).

21. **What does the seventh commandment teach us?**
The seventh commandment teaches us to be pure in heart, language, and conduct (I Corinthians 7:2; Ephesians 4:29; 5:3-4).

22. **What is the eighth commandment?**
The eighth commandment is "Thou shalt not steal" (Exodus 20:15).

23. **What does the eighth commandment teach us?**
The eighth commandment teaches us to respect the property of others and to be honest and industrious (Romans 12:11, 17; Ephesians 4:28; II Thessalonians 3:10-12).

24. **What is the ninth commandment?**
The ninth commandment is "Thou shalt not bear false witness against thy neighbour" (Exodus 20:16).

25. **What does the ninth commandment teach us?**
The ninth commandment teaches us to tell the truth (Proverbs 14:5; Zechariah 8:16; I Peter 3:16).

26. **What is the tenth commandment?**
The tenth commandment is "Thou shalt not covet thy neighbour's house, thou shalt not covet thy neighbour's wife, nor his manservant, nor his maidservant, nor his ox, nor his ass, nor any thing that is thy neighbour's" (Exodus 20:17).

27. What does the tenth commandment teach us?
The tenth commandment teaches us to be content with what we have (Galatians 5:26; Philippians 4:11).

28. Of what use are the Ten Commandments to us?
They teach us how God wants us to live and show us our need of a Savior (Joshua 1:7-8; Galatians 5:26; Philippians 4:11).

29. What commandments does God command us to obey first of all?
God commands us to obey the two great commandments (Matthew 22:37-40).

30. What is the first great commandment?
The first great commandment says in Matthew 22:37, "Thou shalt love the Lord thy God with all thy heart, and with all thy soul, and with all thy mind" (Matthew 22:37).

31. What is the second great commandment?
The second great commandment says in Matthew 22:39, "Thou shalt love thy neighbour as thyself" (Matthew 22:39).

32. Who is your neighbor?
All my fellow men are my neighbors (Luke 10:25-37; Galatians 6:10).

Do I Know About Prayer?

1. **What is prayer?**
   Prayer is talking to God (Psalm 10:17; Philippians 4:6).

2. **In whose name should we pray?**
   We should pray only in the name of Christ, our intercessor (John 16:23).

3. **What guide has Christ given us to teach us how to pray?**
   Christ has given us the Lord's Prayer (Matthew 6:9-13).

4. **How should we pray?**
   We should pray after this manner: "Our Father which art in heaven, Hallowed be thy name. Thy kingdom come. Thy will be done in earth, as it is in heaven. Give us this day our daily bread. And forgive us our debts, as we forgive our debtors. And lead us not into temptation, but deliver us from evil: For thine is the kingdom, and the power, and the glory, for ever. Amen" (Matthew 6:9-13).

5. **How many petitions are there in the Lord's Prayer?**
   There are six petitions in the Lord's Prayer (Matthew 6:9-13).

6. **What is the first petition?**
   The first petition is "Hallowed be thy name" (Matthew 6:9).

7. **What do we pray for in the first petition?**
   We tell God He is holy and we want to honor Him (Psalm 145:1-13; Romans 11:36).

8. **What is the second petition?**
   The second petition is "Thy kingdom come" (Matthew 6:10).

9. **What do we pray for in the second petition?**
   We pray that God's Kingdom may be established on earth (Psalm 67:1-3; Romans 10:1).

10. **What is the third petition?**
    The third petition is "Thy will be done in earth, as it is in heaven" (Matthew 6:10).

11. **What do we pray for in the third petition?**
    We pray that the will of God be done in the life of every one on earth (Psalm 103:22; Romans 12:2).

12. **What is the fourth petition?**
    The fourth petition is "Give us this day our daily bread" (Matthew 6:11).

13. **What do we pray for in the fourth petition?**
    We pray that God would give us all things needful (Proverbs 30:8; Philippians 4:19).

14. **What is the fifth petition?**
    The fifth petition is "And forgive us our debts, as we forgive our debtors" (Matthew 6:12).

15. **What do we pray for in the fifth petition?**
We pray that God would pardon our sins for Christ's sake and enable us to forgive those who have injured us (Psalm 51:1; Matthew 6:14-15).

16. **What is the sixth petition?**
The sixth petition is "And lead us not into temptation, but deliver us from evil" (Matthew 6:13).

17. **What do we pray for in the sixth petition?**
We pray that God will keep us from being tempted and will keep us from sin when we are tempted (Psalm 51:10, 12; Matthew 26:41).

Do I Know What God Says About the Future?

1. **Will Christ come again?**
   Yes, Christ has promised to return to take us to be with Him (John 14:1-3; Acts 1:11).

2. **When will Christ return?**
   No one knows when Christ will return (Matthew 24:42, 50; 25:13).

3. **What are the two parts of the Second Coming?**
   The Second Coming consists of the Rapture and the glorious appearing (I Corinthians 15:51-52; Revelation 19:11-16).

4. **What will happen at the Rapture?**
   At the Rapture Christ will bring to life all Christians who have died, change those who are living, and give them an incorruptible body (I Corinthians 15:51-52; I Thessalonians 4:15-17).

5. **What will happen at the glorious appearing?**
   Christ will return to earth, remove all the wicked, and establish His Kingdom (II Thessalonians 1:7-10; Revelation 19:11-16).

6. **What becomes of man at death?**
   The body returns to dust, and the soul goes either to heaven or hell (Genesis 3:19; Romans 6:23).

7. **What will become of the wicked in the day of judgment?**
   The wicked will be cast into the lake of fire (Psalm 9:17; Revelation 20:11-15).

8. **What is hell?**
   Hell is a place of dreadful and endless torment (Matthew 25:41; Mark 9:43; Luke 16:19-26; Revelation 20:10, 13-15).

9. **What will become of the righteous?**
   The righteous will be taken to heaven (Matthew 5:11-12; 25:46; John 10:28; 14:1-3; Colossians 3:4).

10. **What is heaven?**
    Heaven is a glorious and happy place where the saved will be forever with the Lord.

Glossary

A

almighty all-powerful; one of God's names

angel heavenly messenger sent by God to earth; spirit who lives with God in heaven

apostasy a complete turning away from God

apostle man chosen by Jesus to see the events of His life and His resurrection and to tell others of Him

ark large boat built by Noah

ark of the covenant the sacred box in which the Ten Commandments, a pot of manna, and Aaron's rod were kept

ascension Christ's going upward into heaven forty days after His resurrection

assurance condition of knowing for sure; certainty

atone to give a satisfactory payment for a sin, wrongdoing, or injury

B

baptize to wash with water as a sign of a believer's following after Christ

begotten being the child of

beseech to beg or plead with

blasphemy attributing evil to God; denying good that should be attributed to God; giving God's attributes to something or someone other than God

blessed holy; having God's favor

blessing a gift from God

born again referring to one who has experienced the new birth (see *new birth*)

Bread of Heaven a name for Christ, who provides physical and spiritual food

burnt offering Old Testament offering to God that was burned on an altar

C

caesar a title given to Roman emperors

Calvary "the place of a skull"; the place near Jerusalem where Jesus was crucified; Golgotha

Canaan the land that God promised to give to the Israelites in the Old Testament; a name symbolizing heaven

carnal worldly; describes thoughts, ideas, and actions that reflect the heart of unbelievers in rebellion against God's standards

centurion Roman commander of about one hundred soldiers

charity love

cherubim more than one angel of the class called cherubs

Christian a person who believes in and accepts Christ as his Savior

church all of those who believe in Christ and are saved

cleanseth frees from guilt; purges or clears

Comforter the Holy Spirit

commandment an order

commend to give to someone for safekeeping

compassion deep feeling for another person's problems or sorrows; sympathy

condemn to declare guilty of wrongdoing

confess to admit to doing wrong; to admit one's guilt; saying what God says about sin

corrupt evil and dirty; wicked; sinful

countenance expression of a person's face; the face itself

covenant promise or agreement made between two or more persons

covet to have a great want for something belonging to someone else; to wish something was yours

create to make something from nothing

creator one that makes something new; Creator God

crucify to put to death by nailing or binding to a cross

D

Day of Atonement a day once a year when the high priest entered the holy of holies to offer sacrifices as payment for the people's sins

death separation of the body and spirit; separation from God

dedicate to set aside for a holy purpose

demon an evil spirit

descend to come down; to pass down from parent to child

devil an evil spirit; a demon; another name for Satan

disciple one who follows and serves Jesus; a follower of a certain belief

divine having to do with God; holy and sacred

doctrine what a certain group of people believes and teaches; a belief or principle

draught drawing in of fish in a net

E

edify to build up spiritually

Elohim a Hebrew name for God indicating His power and authority

Emmanuel a name of Jesus, meaning "God with us"

epistle letter or written work

eternal without end

eternity time without beginning or end

eunuch man in charge of a royal household

evangelize to spread the gospel

everlasting without end; going on forever

exalt to speak highly of; to praise and glorify

exhort to try to convince

F

faith trust in God; firm belief without physical proof

false prophet man who preaches or teaches religious ideas against those found in God's Word; deceiver

fellowship being together as friends; enjoying each other's company

firmament sky between the heavens and the earth

fisher of men person who leads others to be saved

follower one who serves another; one who believes and lives by another's teachings; disciple

foreknowledge knowledge of something before it exists or happens

forerunner person who goes before to prepare the way for another or to tell of another's coming

foretold predicted; told about future happenings

forgiveness act of excusing or pardoning someone for a wrongdoing

fornication immoral or evil behavior; idolatry

frankincense gum from certain trees that gives off a spicy, sweet odor when burned

fruit anything yielded or produced

furlough period of time off from one's regular job or duties

G

genealogy record of ancestral descent; family tree

generation all the people born in a certain time period

Gentile any person who is not Jewish

girdle belt worn at the waist around a loose fitting thigh-length shirt

glorify to praise or worship

godliness devotion toward God which results in obeying God's laws and following God's will

Good Shepherd a name for Christ showing He leads and guides us

gospel the truth of the good news of Christ's coming to earth, dying for our sins, and rising from the tomb

grace God's kindness to us even though we do not deserve it

Great Commission Christ's command to His disciples to teach the gospel (Matthew 28:19-20)

guilty having done wrong and deserving punishment

H

harlot bad or immoral woman

heart innermost center of the natural condition of man; center of man's thought life and emotions

heathen person who does not know of or believe in God

heaven glorious and happy place where God and His angels live; where saved people will live eternally

Hebrew Jewish language; Jewish person

hell place of dreadful and endless torment where the unsaved are punished after death

high priest head or chief of the Jewish priests with the responsibility of overseeing the temple and administering religious ceremonies

holy attribute of God: sinless, perfect, and righteous

holy of holies the holiest place; place in the tabernacle where the ark of the covenant was kept

Holy Spirit the third Person of the Trinity who lives in the hearts of Christians; the Holy Ghost

homage special respect shown to honor someone

honor *n.* glory and praise; honesty; *vb.* to treat with love, admiration, and respect

hospitality kind or friendly treatment of guests; the art of being friendly and generous to others

household of faith believers born into the family of God through faith in Jesus Christ; born-again Christians

humble not proud of oneself or boastful; meek or modest

humility state of being without self-pride and boastfulness

I

I Am one of the names for God showing His eternal existence "apart from" creation

idol statue worshiped as a god; person or thing loved more than God

image likeness; something that is like another in form or nature; idol

impute to transfer (righteousness or guilt) from one person to another

incarnate the Son of God in human flesh

incense substance that gives off a sweet smell when it is burned

incorruptible clean and perfect; without error

inerrant without error or mistake

infallible incapable of error; perfect

infinite very great; without boundary; endless

iniquity sin and wickedness

inspiration God's breathing (of the Scriptures) into holy men

intercede to plead on behalf of another

interpret to explain the meaning of

Israel God's chosen people; the Jews; the land of the Jews

J

Jehovah the personal name of God in the Old Testament, meaning "the Eternal One who reveals Himself"

Jew a person of the Hebrew race, God's chosen people

Jubilee Year a celebration the Jews observed every fifty years

judgment act of hearing and deciding a case; decision given by a judge

just right, fair, and honest; good and righteous

justify to declare righteous

K

knowledge understanding gained through experience and study

L

Lamb name used for Jesus Christ; it shows that by His death He paid the sacrifice for our sins just as a lamb was sacrificed in the Old Testament for the sins of the Israelites

laver large bowl used in washing sacrifices in the Jewish tabernacle or temple

law rule made by God or human authority

leaven substance such as yeast that causes dough to rise; often considered a symbol of sin in the Bible

leper person who has leprosy

leprosy skin disease that attacks the nerves, causes weakening and wasting away of muscles, and is characterized by white, scaly scabs; a picture of sin

Levite member of the tribe of Levi from which the Jewish priests were chosen

longsuffering patience in pain or trouble

Lord God; Jesus Christ

Lord's Supper communion; a church service by which we remember Christ's sacrifice on the cross; the last meal that Jesus had with His disciples

lots (to cast) using bits of paper or wood to decide the outcome or determine the portion of something given to each person

Lucifer Satan's name before he was cast out of heaven

M

magistrate officer of a government, such as a judge or president.

malefactor one who does evil; criminal

Man of Sorrows a name for Jesus, showing His sorrow and suffering for the sins of the world

mediator person who acts as a go-between

mercy God's witholding of the punishment we deserve

mercy seat the gold plate covering the ark of the covenant on which the high priest sprinkled the blood for a sin offering; the throne of God

Messiah the Old Testament name for the promised Redeemer; Christ

might power

Millennium period of one thousand years on earth following the Tribulation when Christ will reign

millstone one of two round, flat stones used for grinding grain

miracle supernatural event done by the power of God that shows His works

missionary person who goes out to tell the story of Jesus and God's plan of salvation

moneychanger person who exchanges one kind of money for another kind

myrrh fragrant extract from the wood and bark of a common Palestinian bush

N

Nazarene a person from Nazareth; another name for Jesus

Nazarite a Hebrew who had taken certain religious vows; he could not drink wine, cut his hair, or touch an unclean thing

new birth occasion, upon confession and belief in the gospel, that God gives eternal life to a sinner

new heaven and new earth future heaven and earth that will be created by God

O

obey to do what one is told to do

observance act of keeping customs, laws, or religious ceremonies

offering giving of something as an act of worship to God

omnipotent all-powerful; almighty

omnipresent always present; existing everywhere at the same time

omniscient all-knowing; having complete knowledge of everything

ordinance rule, especially one given by God; a way of remembering Christ's death and resurrection

P

palsy loss of power to feel or move

parable short story that teaches a lesson; earthly story with a heavenly meaning

paradise heaven; dwelling place of God and His angels, and where the saved will dwell in eternity

pardon forgiveness

Passover the death angel's passing over the Hebrew homes that had blood sprinkled on the doorpost (Exodus 12:13)

Passover Feast an eight-day Jewish feast in remembrance of the Israelites' escape from Egypt

patriarch father, ruler, or founder of a family, tribe, or group

Pentecost a Jewish celebration (feast) held fifty days after Passover to remember the harvest and the giving of the Ten Commandments; the giving of the Holy Spirit to the apostles and early Christians

persecution harmful or cruel treatment

perseverance the quality of never giving up; determination to stick to a purpose or goal; patience

pharaoh title given to the kings of ancient Egypt

Pharisee member of a Jewish group that was strict in keeping Jewish law

Philistines enemies of the Jews who lived in the Holy Land during Old Testament times

plague suffering or trouble sent from God; rapid spreading of a deadly disease

potter's field cemetery for poor or friendless people

praise to express the worth or value of something through words or songs

prayer act of speaking to God

precept a teaching; a rule of behavior

predestine to determine destiny beforehand

priest Old Testament servant of God chosen by God to offer sacrifices

proclaim to make known to the public

prodigal wasteful and careless

prophecy the telling of future events

prophesy to tell about future events; to proclaim God's will

prophet a Bible preacher who told of God's will and future events

propitiation act of appeasing wrath; our means of salvation through Christ's death

proud feeling pleased over something done, made, or owned; honored; dignified

providence divine acts of God in making all things to work out His purpose and plan

province section of a kingdom or an empire; in Roman times, a section of the empire ruled by a governor

psalm religious song, poem, or hymn of praise to God

publican tax collector of ancient Rome

pure not mixed with anything else; not having fault or guilt; clean

R

rabbi "teacher" or "master"; a Jewish religious leader

ram's horn trumpet made of a curly horn from a male sheep

ransom price paid to free captives

Rapture taking of the saved to heaven when Christ returns

reconcile to bring together again in peace and friendship after being separated

redeemer one who buys back something that was lost; one who saves or sets free; Jesus Christ

redemption act of being rescued or freed from sin; our salvation

regeneration act of receiving a new spiritual life; salvation; new birth

remission forgiveness of sin

repent to be sorry for and ask forgiveness for sin

repentance act of being sorry for, asking forgiveness for, and turning away from sin, or a change of mind about sin

resurrection act of coming to life again

revelation what God has made known to man

right correct; true; just

righteous doing that which is right in the sight of God; hating sin and loving good

S

Sabbath the seventh day of the week; the biblical day used for worship and rest

sackcloth rough cloth made from the hair of goats and camels and worn as a sign of sadness

sacrifice offering to God for the forgiveness of sin

Sadducees group of Jews who did not believe in angels or resurrection

saint person who is saved

salvation God's saving us from the punishment of sin

salvific capable of providing salvation or redemption

sanctification making holy in heart and behavior by God and the Holy Spirit after salvation

sanctuary holy place set apart for the worship of God

Sanhedrin the Jews' seventy-member supreme court for religious and government cases

Satan another name for the Devil; an evil spirit who is the enemy of God and of all Christians

saved description of one who has believed the gospel and asked forgiveness for sins; set free from sin and its results

savior one who saves others from trouble or disaster

Savior Jesus Christ our Lord

scapegoat one who takes the blame for others; in Old Testament times a goat was taken into the wilderness every year, symbolically taking the blame for the sins of the people; Jesus took the blame for our sins

Scripture holy writings of God; the Bible

separation being set apart; living differently from the unsaved in a total and noticeable way

sepulchre or **sepulcher** tomb or cave used for burial

seraph angel of important position described in Isaiah 6:2 as having six wings and believed to lead in the worship of God

servant person who works for someone else

Sheol a Hebrew name for hell

shofar or **shophar** ancient Hebrew trumpet made of a ram's horn and used for giving signals

sin disobedience to the law of God

slothful lazy

smite to hit or slap; to destroy or kill

sojourn to stay in one place for a time

soothsayer one who tells the future, or pretends to; a fortuneteller

sorcerer person who practices magic and claims to have the help of evil spirits

soul part of the person that thinks, acts, feels, and lives forever

sow to spread or plant seed

surety person who agrees to be responsible for the debts or faults of another

swaddling clothes strips of cloth used to wrap around a newborn baby

synagogue Jewish congregation or a place to meet for worship

T

tabernacle tent used by the Israelites as a place of worship while they were wandering in the wilderness

tablet small flat sheet of stone used for writing

talent unit of weight for gold or silver; ability to do something well

tares harmful weeds that grow in grain fields

temperance the control of one's actions and speech

temple building used for the worship of God or of false gods

temptation act of trying to make a person do something wrong; attraction

Ten Commandments the ten rules for living that God gave to Moses on Mt. Sinai (Exodus 20)

testament will or promise; divisions of the Bible

testify to give evidence for; to tell about what one has seen or heard

testimony open statement of one's beliefs or faith in God

thresh to separate the grain or seeds from a plant such as wheat

till to plow or cultivate the ground

tithe small part; small tax; offering to God of one-tenth of all that a person earns

transfiguration the changed appearance of Christ on the mountain (Matthew 17:1-13)

transform to change the appearance, shape, or nature of a thing

transgression sin; act of doing what God forbids

translate to take to heaven without death; to make something understandable in another language

trespass to disobey; to sin

tribe any one of the twelve groups of the Hebrews, each of which descended from one of the sons of Jacob

Tribulation a period of seven years of great trouble and misery on earth during the End Times

tribute tax; expression of thanks or respect

Trinity God the Father, God the Son, and God the Holy Spirit, in one divine nature

trust *n.* firm, unchanging belief in the power, love, or truthfulness of a person or thing; faith and confidence; *vb.* to have faith in

twinkling quick wink of the eye; very short time; moment

U

unbelief lack of thinking that something is true

undefiled clean and pure; not corrupted or made dirty

unfaithful not keeping one's promises

ungodly sinful and wicked

unrighteousness wickedness; sinfulness

V

vainglory great pride in oneself; boastful display or "showing off"; arrogance; opposite of humility

vengeance punishment or injury in return for a wrong

vessel large boat or ship; container for holding liquids; person made or used for some purpose

viper type of poisonous snake

virgin pure, unmarried female

virtue moral goodness and excellent behavior; purity

W

watchtower high tower or high place from which to watch for enemy ships, forces, etc.

wayside side of a path or road

wilderness region of land with no people; dry, bare land

wise men men who gain knowledge, especially from the heavens; the men who followed the star from the East to Bethlehem where Jesus was born

witness *n.* person who tells about an event he has seen; *vb.* to tell others about Christ and the way of salvation

Word the way God speaks to man; in Scripture, referring to both the Bible (the written Word) and Jesus Christ (the living Word)

world the earth; all the people who live on earth; a large amount; the plans, ideas, theories, fads, music, fashions, and entertainment of society that do not reflect God's holiness and turn people's hearts against God

worship to show honor, love, and respect

Y

yoke wooden frame that fastens two oxen or horses together for pulling a plow or heavy load; a burden

Z

Zion heaven; a name for Jerusalem; a hill in Jerusalem that represents the whole city

Index

Illustration Credits

The following individuals have contributed to the illustrations included in this textbook.

Illustrators
Paula Cheadle
Johanna Ehnis
Preston Gravely Jr.
Jim Hargis
Del Thompson
John Roberts

Contributing Illustrators
©1999-2001 www.arttoday.com
John Bjerk
Justin Gerard
Jeremy Jantz
Stefanie Kubina
Joel Leineweber
Mary Ann Lumm
John Muessen
Keith Neely
Duane Nichols
Kathy Pflug
Lynda Slattery
Melissa Smith
Noelle Snyder
Stephanie True
Sanela Tutaris
Joe Tyrpak
Dan Van Leeuwen
Julie Yang

God's Word Charts Designer
Joel Leineweber

Photograph Credits

The following agencies and individuals have furnished materials to meet the photographic needs of this textbook. We wish to express our gratitude to them for their important contribution.

©1999-2001 www.arttoday.com
Corel
Dawn L. Watkins
Digital Stock
Dr. Stewart Custer
Gene Fisher
German Information Center
Joyce Landis
Moody Press
Museum of Printing History
NASA
Oxford University Press, Inc.
Photodisc, Inc.
Suzanne Altizer
Tara Swaney
Unusual Films

Masterworks
Bob Jones University Museum and Gallery, Inc.

Michael Overcoming Satan by Jose Antolinez 25
Jacob Shown the Coat of Joseph by Giovanni Battista Carlone 63
Preparing to Depart for Canaan by Leandro Bassano 81
The Flight into Egypt by Domenico Fiasella 111
The Destruction of the Army of Sennacherib by Ilario Spolverini 137
Esther Before Ahasuerus by Claude Vignon 171
Raising of Lazarus by Francesco Granacci 201
The Mocking of Christ by a Northern Follower of Caravaggio 223
The Ascension by Gustave Doré 239
St. John the Evangelist by Domenico Zampieri 293

Cover and Title Page
Dawn L. Watkins; PhotoDisc, Inc.

Unit 1
NASA 3; Digital Stock 9, 12; PhotoDisc, Inc. 14, 17 (all), 23; taken from *The New Scofield Reference Bible, KJV* ©1967, by Oxford University Press, Inc. 24 (both); Bob Jones University Museum and Gallery, Inc. 25; Corel 26

Unit 2
Digital Stock 38, 51; PhotoDisc, Inc. 43, 53 (both), 54; Corel 55 (left, right middle); ©1999-2001 www.arttoday.com 55 (left middle, middle, right); taken from *The New Scofield Reference Bible, KJV* ©1967, by Oxford University Press, Inc. 44, 56; Bob Jones University Museum and Gallery, Inc. 63; Corel 64

Unit 3
PhotoDisc, Inc., 76 (background); taken from *New Unger's Bible Dictionary* ©1988, by Moody Press 76; Tara Swaney 77, 91; Bob Jones University Museum and Gallery, Inc. 81; Corel 82; Digital Stock 85; ©1999-2001 www.arttoday.com 86

Unit 4

Digital Stock 107; taken from *The New Scofield Reference Bible, KJV* ©1967, by Oxford University Press, Inc. 110; Bob Jones University Museum and Gallery, Inc. 111; Corel 112; Gene Fisher 113; Tara Swaney 116 (all), 118; PhotoDisc, Inc. 117

Unit 5

Taken from *Williams Complete Bible Commentary* by George Williams 122; PhotoDisc, Inc. 125, 126, 141, 145, 149; ©1999-2001 www.arttoday.com 128; Suzanne Altizer 131; Bob Jones University Museum and Gallery, Inc. 137; Corel 138; Tara Swaney 148

Unit 6

PhotoDisc, Inc. 157 (all), 164, 165, 166, 179, 183; Tara Swaney 160; Bob Jones University Museum and Gallery, Inc. 171; Corel 172; taken from *The New Scofield Reference Bible, KJV* ©1967, by Oxford University Press, Inc. 174, 177

Unit 7

Digital Stock 190; Unusual Films 192, 215; Bob Jones University Museum and Gallery, Inc. 201; Corel 202; PhotoDisc, Inc. 203, 209; Museum of Printing History 207; German Information Center 208; Joyce Landis 210

Unit 8

Taken from *The New Scofield Reference Bible, KJV* ©1967, by Oxford University Press, Inc. 219; Bob Jones University Museum and Gallery, Inc. 223; Corel 224; ©1999-2001 www.arttoday.com 229

Unit 9

Bob Jones University Museum and Gallery, Inc. 239; Corel 240; Taken from *Witness to Christ: A Commentary on —Acts* by Stewart Custer, Ph.D. 242; Brian Johnson 243; PhotoDisc, Inc. 261, 262 (bottom), 264, 266 (bottom); Tara Swaney 262 (top); Joyce Landis 266 (top left)

Unit 10

PhotoDisc, Inc. 278, 286, 287, 291, 294, 304; Bob Jones University Museum and Gallery, Inc. 293; Corel 294; taken from *The New Scofield Reference Bible, KJV* ©1967, by Oxford University Press, Inc. 296

God's Word Charts

PhotoDisc, Inc. 323-332

Teacher's Visual Packet for Use with Bible 6 Truths

God's Word Charts—Photodisc, Inc. and Corel Corporation

Paintings—Bob Jones University Museum and Gallery, Inc.

Prayer Journal

Date ________________

Prayer Request ________________

How It Was Answered ________________

Date ________________

Prayer Request ________________

How It Was Answered ________________

Date ________________

Prayer Request ________________

How It Was Answered ________________

Date ________________

Prayer Request ________________

How It Was Answered ________________

Date ________________

Prayer Request ________________

How It Was Answered ________________

Date ________________

Prayer Request ________________

How It Was Answered ________________

Prayer Journal

Date ____________

Prayer Request ____________

How It Was Answered ____________

Date ____________

Prayer Request ____________

How It Was Answered ____________

Date ____________

Prayer Request ____________

How It Was Answered ____________

Date ____________

Prayer Request ____________

How It Was Answered ____________

Date ____________

Prayer Request ____________

How It Was Answered ____________

Date ____________

Prayer Request ____________

How It Was Answered ____________

Prayer Journal

Date ____________________

Prayer Request ____________________

How It Was Answered ____________________

Date ____________________

Prayer Request ____________________

How It Was Answered ____________________

Date ____________________

Prayer Request ____________________

How It Was Answered ____________________

Date ____________________

Prayer Request ____________________

How It Was Answered ____________________

Date ____________________

Prayer Request ____________________

How It Was Answered ____________________

Date ____________________

Prayer Request ____________________

How It Was Answered ____________________

Prayer Journal

Date ____________

Prayer Request ____________

How It Was Answered ____________

Date ____________

Prayer Request ____________

How It Was Answered ____________

Date ____________

Prayer Request ____________

How It Was Answered ____________

Date ____________

Prayer Request ____________

How It Was Answered ____________

Date ____________

Prayer Request ____________

How It Was Answered ____________

Date ____________

Prayer Request ____________

How It Was Answered ____________

Prayer Journal

Date ________________

Prayer Request ____

How It Was Answered ____

Date ________________

Prayer Request ____

How It Was Answered ____

Date ________________

Prayer Request ____

How It Was Answered ____

Date ________________

Prayer Request ____

How It Was Answered ____

Date ________________

Prayer Request ____

How It Was Answered ____

Date ________________

Prayer Request ____

How It Was Answered ____

Prayer Journal

Date ____________

Prayer Request ____________

How It Was Answered ____________

Date ____________

Prayer Request ____________

How It Was Answered ____________

Date ____________

Prayer Request ____________

How It Was Answered ____________

Date ____________

Prayer Request ____________

How It Was Answered ____________

Date ____________

Prayer Request ____________

How It Was Answered ____________

Date ____________

Prayer Request ____________

How It Was Answered ____________

Prayer Journal

Date ____________

Prayer Request ____________

How It Was Answered ____________

Date ____________

Prayer Request ____________

How It Was Answered ____________

Date ____________

Prayer Request ____________

How It Was Answered ____________

Date ____________

Prayer Request ____________

How It Was Answered ____________

Date ____________

Prayer Request ____________

How It Was Answered ____________

Date ____________

Prayer Request ____________

How It Was Answered ____________

JONES & BARTLETT LEARNING INFORMATION SYSTEMS SECURITY & A

LABORATORY MANUAL TO ACCOMPANY

Auditing IT Infrastructures for Compliance

VERSION 2.0

VLAB SOLUTIONS

Powered by vLab Solutions

JONES & BARTLETT LEARNING

World Headquarters
Jones & Bartlett Learning
5 Wall Street
Burlington, MA 01803
978-443-5000
info@jblearning.com
www.jblearning.com

Jones & Bartlett Learning books and products are available through most bookstores and online booksellers. To contact Jones & Bartlett Learning directly, call 800-832-0034, fax 978-443-8000, or visit our website, www.jblearning.com.

Substantial discounts on bulk quantities of Jones & Bartlett Learning publications are available to corporations, professional associations, and other qualified organizations. For details and specific discount information, contact the special sales department at Jones & Bartlett Learning via the above contact information or send an email to specialsales@jblearning.com.

Production Credits

Chief Executive Officer: Ty Field
President: James Homer
Chief Product Officer: Eduardo Moura
SVP, Curriculum Solutions: Christopher Will
Director of Sales, Curriculum Solutions: Randi Roger
Author: vLab Solutions, LLC, David Kim, President
Editorial Management: High Stakes Writing, LLC, Lawrence J. Goodrich, President
Copy Editor, High Stakes Writing: Katherine Dillin
Developmental Editor, High Stakes Writing: Dee Hayes
Associate Program Manager: Rainna Erikson
Production Manager: Susan Beckett
Rights & Photo Research Associate: Lauren Miller
Manufacturing and Inventory Control Supervisor: Amy Bacus
Senior Marketing Manager: Andrea DeFronzo
Cover Design: Scott Moden
Cover Image: © ErickN/ShutterStock, Inc.
Printing and Binding: Edwards Brothers Malloy
Cover Printing: Edwards Brothers Malloy

ISBN: 978-1-284-05918-2

6048

Printed in the United States of America

18 17 16 15 14 10 9 8 7 6 5 4 3 2 1

© Rodolfo Clix/Dreamstime.com

Contents

Ethics and Your Personal Responsibilities

The material presented in this course is designed to give you a real-life look at the use of various tools and systems that are at the heart of every cybersecurity practitioner's daily responsibilities. During this course, you will have access to software and techniques used by professionals to investigate and test the security of critical infrastructures and information technology systems and devices. With this access come certain ethical responsibilities:

1. Do not exceed your authorized level of access. This includes remaining within your authorized level of access when using lab-provided software tools to scan or attack computers and software applications as directed within the lab procedures.
2. Do not attempt to use your authorized access for unauthorized purposes either inside or outside of the VSCL environment.
3. Do not attempt to attack or otherwise compromise the confidentiality, integrity, or availability of *any* IT systems, services, or infrastructures outside of the VSCL.
4. Comply with your academic institution's *Code of Student Conduct* and all other applicable policies and regulations.
5. Comply with applicable federal, state, and local laws regarding the use and misuse of information technology systems and services.
6. Comply with applicable laws regarding intellectual property rights, including patents and trademarks and copyrights.

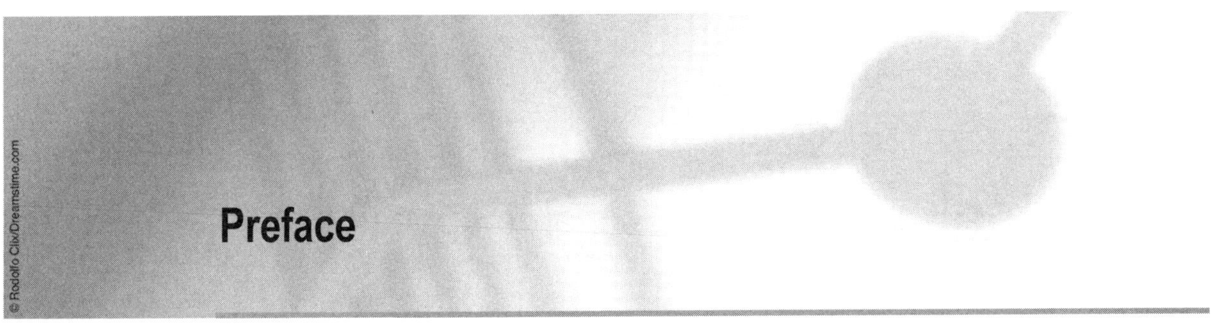
Preface

Welcome! This lab manual is your step-by-step guide to completing the laboratory exercises for this course. You will have an opportunity to gain valuable hands-on experience with professional-grade tools and techniques as you work through the lab activities and answer the lab questions found at the end of each lab.

How to Use This Lab Manual

This lab manual features step-by-step instructions for completing the following hands-on lab exercises:

Lab #	Lab Title
1	Assessing the Impact of Sarbanes-Oxley (SOX) Compliance Law on Enron
2	Aligning Auditing Frameworks for a Business Unit Within DoD
3	Defining a Process for Gathering Information Pertaining to a HIPAA Compliance Audit
4	Aligning an IT Security Assessment—Risks, Threats, and Vulnerability—to Achieve Compliance
5	Defining a Process for Gathering Information Pertaining to a GLBA Compliance Audit
6	Auditing the Workstation Domain for Compliance
7	Auditing the LAN-to-WAN Domain for Compliance
8	Auditing the Remote Access Domain for Compliance
9	Auditing the System/Application Domain for Compliance
10	Charting Your Career Path—Professional Certifications

Step-by-Step Instructions

For each lab, you are provided with detailed, step-by-step instructions and screen captures showing the results of key steps within the lab. All actions that you are required to take are shown in **bold** font. The screen captures will also help you identify menus, dialog boxes, and input locations.

Deliverables

As you work through each lab, you will be instructed to record specific information or take a screen capture to document the results you obtained by performing specific actions. The deliverables are designed to test your understanding of the information, and your successful completion of the steps and functions of the lab. All of these documentation tasks should be pasted into a single file (MS Word .doc, .docx, or other compatible format) and submitted for grading by your instructor.

You will create two deliverable files for each lab:

- *Lab Report file* (including screen captures taken at specific steps in the lab)
- *Lab Assessment file* (including answers to questions posed at the end of each lab)

You may use either Microsoft® Word or any other compatible word processing software for these deliverables. For specific information on deliverables, refer to the Deliverables section in each lab.

Lab Assessment File

At the end of each lab, there is a set of questions which are to be answered and submitted for grading in the Lab Assessment file. (Your instructor may provide alternate instructions for this deliverable.) For some questions, you may need to refer to your Lab Report file to obtain information from the lab. For other questions, you may need to consult a textbook or other authoritative source to obtain more information.

Web References

URLs for Web resources listed in this laboratory manual are subject to change without prior notice. These links were last verified on April 13, 2014. Many times, you can find the required resource by using an Internet search engine and a partial URL or keywords. You may also search the Internet Archives (also referred to as the "Wayback Machine") for a given URL that is no longer available at the original Web site (http://www.archive.org).

Technical Support

If you need help completing a lab in this manual, contact the Jones & Bartlett Learning Help Desk using the information below. Remember to include the name of your institution and reference the course name and number in your ticket details

Phone: 1-866-601-4525

Online: http://www.jblcourses.com/techsupport

Monday-Thursday:	8AM – 10PM
Friday:	8AM – 8PM
Saturday:	8AM – 5PM
Sunday:	10AM – 11PM

(All hours are EST)

If you need help outside of these hours, submit an online ticket or leave a message on our toll-free phone line, and someone from the help desk will get back to you as soon as possible.

Credits

Adobe Reader is a registered trademark of Adobe Systems Incorporated in the United States and/or other countries. Active Directory, Excel, Microsoft, Windows, and Windows Server are registered trademarks of Microsoft Corporation in the United States and/or other countries. Linux is a registered trademark of Linus Torvalds. Citrix is a trademark of Citrix Systems, Inc. and/or one or more of its subsidiaries, and may be registered in the United States Patent and Trademark Office and in other countries. FileZilla is a registered trademark of Tim Kosse. Firefox is a registered trademark of the Mozilla Foundation. Nessus is a registered trademark of Tenable Network Security. Nmap Security Scanner and Zenmap are either registered trademarks or trademarks of Insecure.com LLC. Wireshark is a registered trademark of the Wireshark Foundation. pfSense is a federally registered trademark of Electric Sheep Fencing LLC. Debian is a registered trademark of Software in the Public Interest, Inc. Openswan is an unregistered trademark of Xelerance.

All other product names are the property of their respective owners.

Lab 1: Assessing the Impact of Sarbanes-Oxley (SOX) Compliance Law on Enron

Introduction

The Sarbanes-Oxley (SOX) Act of 2002, also known as Sarbox or SOX, is a U.S. federal law. First proposed by Senator Paul Sarbanes and Representative Michael Oxley, it is the result of the Public Company Account Reform and Investor Protection Act and Corporate Accountability and Responsibility Act. Sarbanes-Oxley dramatically changed how public companies do business.

The bill stems from the fraud and accounting debacles at companies such as Enron and WorldCom. Former President George W. Bush characterized the act "as the most far-reaching reforms of American business practices since the time of Franklin Delano Roosevelt." The act's primary purpose was to restore public confidence in the financial reporting of publicly traded companies. As a result, the act mandated many reforms to enhance corporate responsibility, enhance financial disclosures, and prevent fraud.

In this lab, you will research the Enron fraud case and the SOX compliance law's requirements, you will provide references documenting your findings, and you will identify other compliance laws that have been drafted as a result of Enron and other industries. In addition, you will write an executive summary describing the Enron fraud case's impact and the U.S. government's reaction to it.

Learning Objectives

Upon completing this lab, you will be able to:

- Use the Internet to complete research on the Enron fraud case and provide three references documenting your findings.
- Research SOX requirements and provide three references documenting your findings.
- List the key elements of fraud committed by Enron that led to the Sarbanes-Oxley (SOX) compliance law.
- Identify other compliance laws in the United States that have been drafted for other vertical industries as a result of Enron's issues.
- Draft an executive summary describing the Enron fraud case's impact and the U.S. government's reaction to this and other industry compliance needs.

Deliverables

Upon completion of this lab, you are required to provide the following deliverables to your instructor:

1. Lab Report file;
2. Lab Assessments file.

Hands-On Steps

▶ Note:
This is a paper-based lab. To successfully complete the deliverables for this lab, you will need access to Microsoft® Word or another compatible word processor. For some labs, you may also need access to a graphics line drawing application, such as Visio or PowerPoint. Refer to the Preface of this manual for information on creating the lab deliverable files.

1. On your local computer, **create** the **lab deliverable files**.
2. **Review** the **Lab Assessment Worksheet**. You will find answers to these questions as you proceed through the lab steps.
3. **Review** the following information about the Enron Corporation:

   Enron Corporation was an energy company that, at one point, was the seventh largest company in the United States and the largest trader of natural gas and electricity in the country. Enron started in the mid '80s and, by the '90s, the company was involved with trading and ownership in electric, coal, steel, paper, water, and broadband capacity. In 2001, Enron filed for bankruptcy, making it the largest bankruptcy in history at the time. An accounting scandal caused the company's collapse. Thousands of Enron's employees were laid off. Employees lost their life savings because of the loss of the company's stock. Shareholders lost $11 billion.

"Too Big to Fail"
It's important to appreciate how large a company Enron was just before the accounting scandal broke. Both powerful and with a diverse holding, Enron today would be considered "too big to fail."

4. On your local computer, **open** a new **Internet browser window**.
5. Using your favorite search engine, **search for more information** on the following topics regarding the Enron fraud case:
   - Early history of the investigation
   - Misleading financial accounts
   - Accounting scandal of 2001
   - California's deregulation and subsequent energy crisis

Crafting Law
Like other significant pieces of legislation, SOX also wasn't crafted perfectly from the start or without negative consequences.

6. In your Lab Report file, **summarize** your findings and **cite** at least three sources.

7. Using your favorite search engine, **search for more information** on the following topics regarding the requirements of Sarbanes-Oxley:

   - Incidents that led to passage of SOX
   - Chronology of SOX passage from bill proposal through signing into law
   - Pros and cons of Sarbanes-Oxley
   - Sarbanes-Oxley Section 302
   - Sarbanes-Oxley Section 401
   - Sarbanes-Oxley Section 404
   - Section 404's consequences for small businesses
   - Sarbanes-Oxley Section 802
   - Sarbanes-Oxley Section 1107

8. In your Lab Report file, **summarize** your findings and **cite** at least three sources.

9. In your Lab Report file, **describe** the elements of the fraud Enron committed that led to the creation of SOX.

The Erosion of Public Trust

Media coverage of the Enron scandal was nonstop. When the public learned that former Enron employees had lost their retirement savings, people understood they could not automatically trust companies to act in employees' or shareholders' best interests. Public trust in the stock market eroded, resulting in significant losses outside of Enron. The Enron scandal was key in a demand for compliance legislation for publicly traded companies.

10. In your Lab Report file, **identify** the other U.S. compliance laws that have been drafted as a result of the Enron case.

11. In your Lab Report file, **write an executive summary** describing the impact of Enron's fraud case and the U.S. government's reaction to it and other industry compliance needs.

▶ Note:

This completes the lab. **Close** the **Web browser**, if you have not already done so.

Evaluation Criteria and Rubrics

The following are the evaluation criteria for this lab that students must perform:

1. Use the Internet to complete research on the Enron fraud case and provide three references documenting your findings. – **[20%]**
2. Research SOX requirements and provide three references documenting your findings. – **[20%]**
3. List the key elements of fraud committed by Enron that led to the Sarbanes-Oxley (SOX) compliance law. – **[20%]**
4. Identify other compliance laws in the United States that have been drafted for other vertical industries as a result of Enron's issues. – **[20%]**
5. Draft an executive summary describing the Enron fraud case's impact and the U.S. government's reaction to this and other industry compliance needs. – **[20%]**

Lab #1 - Assessment Worksheet

Assessing the Impact of Sarbanes-Oxley (SOX) Compliance Law on Enron

Course Name and Number: ______________________________

Student Name: ______________________________

Instructor Name: ______________________________

Lab Due Date: ______________________________

Overview

In this lab, you researched the Enron fraud case and the SOX compliance law's requirements, you provided references documenting your findings, and you identified other compliance laws that have been drafted as a result of Enron and other industries. In addition, you wrote an executive summary describing the Enron fraud case's impact and the U.S. government's reaction to it.

Lab Assessment Questions & Answers

1. What section of the SOX compliance law requires proper controls and, hence, security controls to ensure the confidentiality and integrity of financial information and recordkeeping within an IT infrastructure? Explain the information contained in this section.

2. Who is Richard Scrushy and why is he relevant to SOX?

3. Who, under SOX, is legally accountable for certifying and approving the integrity of the company and its financial reporting to the Securities and Exchange Commission (SEC) and other financial organizations?

4. Where would someone go to find the quarterly and annual reports for a publicly traded company?

5. What are some of the criminal penalties for falsifying documents or covering up information related to financial matters and SOX?

6. What is the link between SOX compliance law and information systems security?

7. What sections within SOX compliance law pertain to needing proper internal controls?

8. Explain how the sections within SOX compliance law require proper security controls as they relate to having internal controls.

9. Why are vice presidents and other executive managers who are privy to financial performance data considered insiders to a publicly traded company as defined by the Securities and Exchange Commission (SEC)?

10. True or false: SOX compliance law now holds CEOs and CFOs of publicly traded companies accountable for their actions as officers in a publicly traded company.

Lab 2: Aligning Auditing Frameworks for a Business Unit Within DoD

Introduction

Business units in the Department of Defense (DoD) have auditing frameworks that provide baseline requirements and hardening guidelines to business units that a government network must meet.

The primary benefit of utilizing an audit framework is having a standardized and structured way to base security policy. An audit then helps the organization determine how well it is adhering to its security policies. When an audit is combined with a risk assessment, the organization is equipped to identify present gaps. The organization can take steps to narrow or eliminate those gaps, mitigating its IT risk.

In this lab, you will identify the requirements and hardening guides that provide a frame to which a government network and business should adhere, you will assess the available sites under the Department of Defense (DoD) and identify agencies in charge of providing security guidelines, and you will review the hardening and best practice guidelines provided by DoD's Defense Information Systems Agency (DISA), National Institute of Standards and Technology (NIST), and Information Assurance Support Environment (IASE).

Learning Objectives

Upon completing this lab, you will be able to:

- Identify the minimum baseline requirements and hardening guidelines that provide a framework to which a government network and business unit should adhere.
- Assess all the available sites under the Department of Defense (DoD) and identify the agencies in charge of providing security guidelines and best practices for federal entities.
- Review all the hardening and best practice guidelines provided by DoD's Defense Information Systems Agency (DISA), Information Assurance Support Environment (IASE), and NIST 800-53 series.
- Draft an executive summary identifying and explaining the two auditing frameworks or hardening guidelines/security checklists used by DoD.

Deliverables

Upon completion of this lab, you are required to provide the following deliverables to your instructor:

1. Lab Report file;
2. Lab Assessments file.

Hands-On Steps

▶ Note:
This is a paper-based lab. To successfully complete the deliverables for this lab, you will need access to Microsoft® Word or another compatible word processor. For some labs, you may also need access to a graphics line drawing application, such as Visio or PowerPoint. Refer to the Preface of this manual for information on creating the lab deliverable files.

1. On your local computer, **create** the **lab deliverable files**.
2. **Review** the **Lab Assessment Worksheet**. You will find answers to these questions as you proceed through the lab steps.
3. **Consider** the following scenario:

   You work for a governmental unit of DoD and your manager has asked you to write a brief paper outlining the importance of having the proper DoD-approved frameworks in place when an organization wants to conduct business with a governmental unit. Your task is to evaluate all the available DoD, IASE, and National Institute of Standards and Technology (NIST) hardening guides on the Internet and to write a brief analysis of the technical controls and hardening guides that should be implemented as a minimum guideline for divisions of government agencies such as yours.

Frameworks as a Guide

Frameworks are, in general, a set of ideas or rules to guide you, whether the rules apply to how to administer IT equipment, how to manage your daily work, or how to drive a car. The framework does not detail the manner in which you conduct yourself hour by hour, but only the general rules you should avoid breaking. The DoD-approved frameworks you research will provide these rules in the form of controls.

Controls can either describe or prescribe "best practices" to secure your IT environment. It is also these controls that grant auditors the ability to measure whether the IT environment following that framework is staying compliant, that is, keeping within these rules.

4. On your local computer, **open** a new **Internet browser window**.
5. In the address box of your Internet browser, **type** the URL **http://www.defense.gov/RegisteredSites/RegisteredSites.aspx** and **press Enter** to open the Web site.
6. **Review** the DoD list of registered Web sites, and **review** the content of some of the information assurance sites.

▶ Note:
At first glance, the voluminous list of DoD Web sites is daunting. It begins with dozens upon dozens of links under the "A" heading alone. Tips to make your review more efficient include using the Search bar. Do not merely search "information assurance," but use terms such as information, security, and assurance.

7. In your Lab Report file, **list** three of the DoD-registered Web sites that provide guidelines and documents related to information assurance.

▶ Note:
Each office, agency, and department might showcase its own range of products, toolkits, standards, etc. Do not be overwhelmed with searching and surfing links. The object of this lab step is to gain a general appreciation of the available Web sites as well as identify some of those providing security guidelines and best practices for federal entities.

8. In the address box of your Internet browser, **type** the URL **http://www.disa.mil/** and **press Enter** to open the Web site.
9. **Review** the Defense Information Systems Agency (DISA) Web site, focusing on the agency's services and capabilities. **Evaluate** which services and capabilities are relevant to the task of formulating a framework for secure government operations.

▶ Note:
By reading the Standard Features section of each individual service from the DISA Service Catalog (accessible through the "Service Catalog" link toward the top of DISA's homepage at *http://www.disa.mil/*), you might become aware of more relevant capabilities than initially apparent from the Service Catalog's listings.

In browsing internal links on pages from the DISA Service Catalog, you might be prompted for a DoD-approved public key infrastructure (PKI) client certificate to access the linked page. Without the certificate, your browsing will end there. A DoD-approved PKI client certificate is not required to complete this lab.

10. In the address box of your Internet browser, **type** the URL **http://iase.disa.mil/index2.html** and **press Enter** to open the Web site.
11. **Review** DISA's Information Assurance Support Environment.
12. **Click** the link for **Security Technical Implementation Guides (STIGs)** in the left-hand column on the page. **Review** the STIGs available, focusing on the following topics:
    - Network Hardening Guides
    - Secure Remote Computing
    - Windows® Operating Systems
    - Application Security

13. In the address box of your Internet browser, **type** the URL **http://csrc.nist.gov/publications/PubsSPs.html** and **press Enter** to open the Web site.

14. **Review** the NIST list of Special Publications (800 Series), and **review** the contents of the guides related to **Security Controls for Federal Information Systems and Organizations** (800-53 and 800-53 A titles).

15. In your Lab Report file, **write an executive summary** identifying two common auditing frameworks used for DoD. **Describe** these and be sure to include a discussion of the hardening guidelines and security checklists used by DoD.

> ▶ **Note:**
> This completes the lab. **Close** the **Web browser**, if you have not already done so.

Evaluation Criteria and Rubrics

The following are the evaluation criteria for this lab that students must perform:

1. Identify the minimum baseline requirements and hardening guidelines that provide a framework to which a government network and business unit should adhere. – **[25%]**
2. Assess all the available sites under the Department of Defense (DoD) and identify the agencies in charge of providing security guidelines and best practices for federal entities. – **[25%]**
3. Review all the hardening and best practice guidelines provided by DoD's Defense Information Systems Agency (DISA), Information Assurance Support Environment (IASE), and NIST 800-53 series. – **[25%]**
4. Draft an executive summary identifying and explaining the two auditing frameworks or hardening guidelines/security checklists used by DoD. – **[25%]**

Lab #2 - Assessment Worksheet

Aligning Auditing Frameworks for a Business Unit Within DoD

Course Name and Number: ______________________________

Student Name: ______________________________

Instructor Name: ______________________________

Lab Due Date: ______________________________

Overview

In this lab, you identified the requirements and hardening guides that provide a frame to which a government network and business should adhere, you assessed the available sites under the Department of Defense (DoD) and identified agencies in charge of providing security guidelines, and you reviewed the hardening and best practice guidelines provided by DoD's Defense Information Systems Agency (DISA), National Institute of Standards and Technology (NIST), and Information Assurance Support Environment (IASE).

Lab Assessment Questions & Answers

1. What is the difference between DITSCAP and DIACAP?

2. What is DCID 6/3, and why would you use DCID 6/3 as opposed to DIACAP for certification and accreditation of a system?

3. What is C&A, and what are the following acronyms that are related to the C&A process: DISN, GIG, PAA, DAA, and DISA?

4. What is the Defense Industrial Base Sector?

5. Who develops the configuration and validation requirements for IT products and services within DoD?

6. What is DoDD 8570.01?

7. Find a copy of the DoDD 8570.01-M revision dated April 2010. What professional certifications comply with the 8570.01-M specification and workforce development program as defined by the DoD?

8. What is the current, working URL for the DISA Military STIGs unclassified homepage?

9. Which DISA STIGs are currently available on the DISA Military STIGs unclassified homepage?

10. Why does the updated version of NIST 800-53a call for continuous monitoring?

Lab 3: Defining a Process for Gathering Information Pertaining to a HIPAA Compliance Audit

Introduction

It's important for health care companies to understand the Health Insurance Portability and Accountability Act of 1996 (HIPAA) and its Privacy and Security rules. The act applies not only to doctors and hospitals but to all health care providers and researchers who are able to share patient information that's classified as private. HIPAA was designed to protect the consumer, not the health care providers. It's important to understand HIPAA's primary aspects and how it impacts and defines an audit scope.

In this lab, you will gather information about the health care industry that addresses the requirements a health care organization must comply with. You will relate the HIPAA Privacy and Security rules to National Institute of Standards and Technology (NIST) standards and encryption technologies to ensure confidentiality of electronic protected health information (ePHI) transmission. You will evaluate HIPAA requirements and identify what ePHI data consists of and apply HIPAA Privacy and Security rules to ensure confidentiality, integrity, and availability. Finally, you will relate the security requirements for protected heath information (PHI) to an overall privacy and security strategy for a health care organization.

Learning Objectives

Upon completing this lab, you will be able to:

- Relate the Health Insurance Portability and Accountability Act (HIPAA) Privacy and Security rules to NIST standards and encryption technologies to ensure confidentiality of ePHI transmission.
- Evaluate the requirements for a health care organization to become compliant with the Health Insurance Portability and Accountability Act of 1996 (HIPAA).
- Identify what ePHI data consists of and apply HIPAA Privacy and Security rules to ensure its confidentiality, integrity, and availability.
- Relate the security requirements for protected health information (PHI) to an overall privacy and security strategy for a health care organization.
- Draft an executive summary that defines a process for obtaining and addressing HIPAA compliancy for a health care organization.

Deliverables

Upon completion of this lab, you are required to provide the following deliverables to your instructor:

1. Lab Report file;
2. Lab Assessments file.

Hands-On Steps

> **▶ Note:**
> This is a paper-based lab. To successfully complete the deliverables for this lab, you will need access to Microsoft® Word or another compatible word processor. For some labs, you may also need access to a graphics line drawing application, such as Visio or PowerPoint. Refer to the Preface of this manual for information on creating the lab deliverable files.

1. On your local computer, **create** the **lab deliverable files**.
2. **Review** the **Lab Assessment Worksheet**. You will find answers to these questions as you proceed through the lab steps.
3. **Review** the following scenario:

   Your manager has asked you to identify information and resources in the health care industry that address what laws, rules, and guidelines your health care organization needs to follow. Your health care organization is to have an audit so you need to gather information for the upcoming audit, which will be more stringent than any that have been done before. The health care organization that employs you believes it is necessary to conduct a review of its HIPAA compliance (or lack of compliance) and put the gathered information into a report to show all the requirements the organization faces. Your manager has asked you to perform this function knowing that your work has been above reproach. He expects a summary of the HIPAA requirements the organization needs to comply with and any financial regulatory acts for which it might also be held liable. You will need to dig deep into the Health Insurance Portability and Accountability Act of 1996 (HIPAA) Privacy Rule and Security Rule. You can use resources from *HHS.gov*, the U.S. Department of Health and Human Services' Web site, to evaluate the HIPAA Privacy and Security rules.

> **Scope Creep**
> Your job is to define the audit's scope and objectives prior to the audit. As you start this assignment, be sure you know what the audit goals are and then define what the audit scope includes and does not include. Every experienced auditor knows that an audit without a properly defined scope and goals is an audit in risk of "scope creep" or an ever-increasing effort beyond what is necessary.

4. On your local computer, **open** a new **Internet browser window**.
5. In the address box of your Internet browser, **type** the URL **http://www.himss.org/ASP/index.asp** and **press Enter** to open the Healthcare Information and Management Systems Society (HIMSS) Web site. **Review** the Web site.
6. At the top of the HIMSS Web site, **click** the **About HIMSS link**.

7. On the left side of the HIMSS Web site, **click** on the **FAQs link**. **Review** the information you find.

> **▶ Note:**
> Reading through the history of HIMSS will provide insight on how HIMSS progressed. This history is available by clicking on the left sidebar link titled "History of HIMSS."

8. Then, in the Search box in the upper right corner of the screen, **type** the words **Health Information Technology** and **press Enter**. **Review** the information you find.

9. In your Lab Report file, **note** what you learn about the HIMSS Web site and how it helps companies and organizations address health care issues.

10. In the address box of your Internet browser, **type** the URL **http://csrc.nist.gov/news_events/HIPAA-May2010_workshop/presentations/2-3-logging-auditing-mcmillan-cynergistek.pdf** and **press Enter** to open the Web site.

11. **Review** the following sections:

    - Logging & Audit Requirements
    - Privacy vs. Security
    - Challenges & Barriers

12. In your Lab Report file, **note** the information you can gather from these sections of the document.

13. In the address box of your Internet browser, **type** the URL **http://healthit.hhs.gov/portal/server.pt?open=512&objID=1147&parentname=CommunityPage&parentid=8&mode=2&in_hi_userid=11673&cached=true** and **press Enter** to open the Web site.

14. **Browse** the **Privacy and Security section** of The Office of the National Coordinator for Health Information Technology, and **review** the available information and resources provided.

> **▶ Note:**
> The Privacy and Security section of The Office of the National Coordinator for Health Information Technology Web page also provides students with both historical rationale behind HIPAA as well as valuable toolkits for conducting assessments and employing best practices.

15. In your Lab Report file, **note** the types of information you can gather from The Office of the National Coordinator for Health Information Technology.

16. In the address box of your Internet browser, **type** the URL **www.HHS.gov** and **press Enter** to open the Web site.

17. Using the Search box in the upper right corner of the Web page, **search** the Health and Human Services Web site for information on HIPAA's main points and requirements.

18. In your Lab Report file, **discuss** these requirements.

> **▶Note:**
> The HIPAA Security Information Series is an educational series that provides information about all of HIPAA's administrative, physical, and technical safeguards as well as HIPAA's main requirements. You can access this information through Health IT's Privacy and Security section, which you visited in step 13, by typing the URL *http://healthit.hhs.gov/portal/server.pt?open=512&objID=1147&parentname=CommunityPage&parentid=8&mode=2&in_hi_userid=11673&cached=true*. **Click** on the **HIPAA and Health IT link** in the left-hand column. Then look for the **HIPAA Security Information Series hyperlink** about halfway down the page.

19. In the address box of your Internet browser, **type** the URL **http://www.hhs.gov/ocr/privacy/hipaa/understanding/srsummary.html** and **press Enter** to open the Web site.

20. **Review** the HIPAA Security Rule.

21. In your Lab Report file, **discuss** these topics:

- Who is covered by the Security Rule?
    - Health plans
    - Health care clearinghouses
    - Any health care provider who transmits health information in electronic form in connection with a transaction for which the secretary of HHS has adopted standards under HIPAA
- What information is protected?
    - Protected health information (PHI)
    - De-identified health information
- General rules
- Risk analysis and management
- Administrative, physical, and technical safeguards
    - Security management process
    - Facility access and control
    - Access, audit, and integrity controls
    - Transmission security
- Policies, documentation, and penalty enforcements

Privacy Rule Versus Security Rule

Unlike the HIPAA Privacy Rule, the Security Rule applies only to electronic protected health information (ePHI). Both the Privacy Rule and the Security Rule seek to ensure information confidentiality, but the Security Rule makes specific use of administrative, technical, and physical safeguards to protect any electronic form.

22. In the address box of your Internet browser, **type** the URL **http://www.hhs.gov/ocr/privacy/hipaa/understanding/summary/index.html** and **press Enter** to open the Web site.

23. **Review** the HIPAA Privacy Rule.

24. In your Lab Report file, **discuss** these topics:

- General principle for uses and disclosures
- Permitted vs. authorized uses and disclosures to the individual
  - Treatment, payment, health care operations
  - Opportunity to agree or object
  - Incidental use and disclosure
  - Public interest
- Limiting disclosure and notifications
- Policies, documentation, and penalty enforcements
  - For violations occurring prior to 2/18/2009
  - Penalty amount: Up to $100 per violation
  - For violations occurring on or after 2/18/2009
  - Calendar year cap respectively: $25,000 and $1,500,000

HIPAA's Final Rule

It wasn't until 2006 that HIPAA's Final Rule was enacted. The Final Rule focuses on enforcement of HIPAA. The Final Rule, called the Enforcement Rule, was created as a result of violations and noncompliance. The Enforcement Rule details investigation procedures as well as penalties and procedures with which to deal with HIPAA violations.

25. In your Lab Report file, **write an executive summary** that defines a process for obtaining and documenting information needed to perform a HIPAA compliancy audit.

▶Note:

This completes the lab. **Close** the **Web browser**, if you have not already done so.

Evaluation Criteria and Rubrics

The following are the evaluation criteria for this lab that students must perform:

1. Relate the Health Insurance Portability and Accountability Act (HIPAA) Privacy and Security rules to NIST standards and encryption technologies to ensure confidentiality of ePHI transmission. – **[20%]**
2. Evaluate the requirements for a health care organization to become compliant with the Health Insurance Portability and Accountability Act of 1996 (HIPAA). – **[20%]**
3. Identify what ePHI data consists of and apply HIPAA Privacy and Security rules to ensure its confidentiality, integrity, and availability. – **[20%]**
4. Relate the security requirements for protected health information (PHI) to an overall privacy and security strategy for a health care organization. – **[20%]**
5. Draft an executive summary that defines a process for obtaining and addressing HIPAA compliancy for a health care organization. – **[20%]**

Lab #3 - Assessment Worksheet

Defining a Process for Gathering Information Pertaining to a HIPAA Compliance Audit

Course Name and Number: ____

Student Name: ____

Instructor Name: ____

Lab Due Date: ____

Overview

In this lab, you gathered information about the health care industry that addresses the requirements a health care organization must comply with. You related the HIPAA Privacy and Security rules to National Institute of Standards and Technology (NIST) standards and encryption technologies to ensure confidentiality of electronic protected health information (ePHI) transmission. You evaluated HIPAA requirements and identified what ePHI data consists of and applied HIPAA Privacy and Security rules to ensure confidentiality, integrity, and availability. Finally, you related the security requirements for protected heath information (PHI) to an overall privacy and security strategy for a health care organization.

Lab Assessment Questions & Answers

1. What are the four parts of the administrative simplification requirements of HIPAA?

2. Name three factors used to determine whether you need to comply with HIPAA.

3. What are the three categories of entities affected by HIPAA Medical Privacy Regulations?

4. What would business associates of covered entities consist of as it pertains to HIPAA's regulation?

5. Who/what is covered by the HIPAA Privacy Rule? Give some examples.

6. What information is protected in HIPAA?

7. Describe the Basic Principle and Required Disclosures of HIPAA.

8. Is a health information organization (HIO) covered by the HIPAA Privacy Rule?

9. Does the HIPAA Privacy Rule inhibit electronic health information exchange across different states or jurisdictions?

10. How should a covered entity respond to any HIPAA Privacy Rule violation of a health information organization (HIO) acting as its business associate?

11. True or false: As a patient, your doctor must have you sign a HIPAA Consent and Release Form to share your ePHI or PHI with insurance providers who pay your medical bills. This is part of the HIPAA Privacy Rule.

12. After the patient provides consent and permission to the medical practice or covered entity, what agreement is needed between the medical practice and its downstream medical insurance claims processor or downstream medical specialist that requires the patient's ePHI?

13. Why is security awareness training for all employees within a health care organization a major component of HIPAA compliance?

14. Under the HIPAA Security Rule, it is a requirement for a health care organization to have a security incident response plan and team to handle potential security incidents and breaches. Why is this a requirement?

15. True or false: It is a requirement for a health care organization to secure the transmission of ePHI through the public Internet.

Lab 4: Aligning an IT Security Assessment—Risks, Threats, and Vulnerability—to Achieve Compliance

Introduction

In general, security assessments are more technical, more focused, and, in the case of penetration testing, more targeted than an audit. Comparatively speaking, the auditor takes the broader, holistic view. Nevertheless, an auditor still needs to gather reliable and relevant evidence to measure compliance. What happens when the auditor lacks the technical skills to gather that evidence? An auditor can employ other experts, given proper permission is granted, to conduct testing such as a security assessment. If that is the case, it is important that the assessment is aligned with the audit's objectives.

In this lab, you will review the vulnerability life cycle and explain the different types of disclosure to mitigate different risk factors. You will identify risks that attacks, vulnerabilities, malicious code phishing, underground economies, and spam have on organizations. You will look at the risks caused by zero-day vulnerabilities, HTTP Client versus Server Side attacks, Malicious JavaScript, PHP Remote File Include, botnets, and PDF attacks on organizations. You will also look at the practices of vulnerability management to prevent threats from old or previously performed attacks on known vulnerabilities within the seven domains of a typical IT infrastructure.

Learning Objectives

Upon completing this lab, you will be able to:

- Review the vulnerability life cycle and explain the different types of disclosure to mitigate different risk factors, such as nondisclosure, full disclosure, limited disclosure, and responsible disclosure.
- Identify the risks that attacks, vulnerabilities, malicious code phishing, underground economies, and spam have on organizations.
- Mitigate the risks caused by zero-day vulnerabilities, HTTP Client versus Server Side attacks, Malicious JavaScript, PHP Remote File Include, botnets, and PDF attacks on organizations.
- Align best practices in vulnerability management to prevent threats from old or previously performed attacks on known vulnerabilities within the seven domains of a typical IT infrastructure.
- Draft an executive summary explaining how security assessments performed on the seven domains of a typical IT infrastructure can be used to help achieve compliance for an organization.

Deliverables

Upon completion of this lab, you are required to provide the following deliverables to your instructor:

1. Lab Report file;
2. Lab Assessments file.

Hands-On Steps

> **▶ Note:**
> This is a paper-based lab. To successfully complete the deliverables for this lab, you will need access to Microsoft® Word or another compatible word processor. For some labs, you may also need access to a graphics line drawing application, such as Visio or PowerPoint. Refer to the Preface of this manual for information on creating the lab deliverable files.

1. On your local computer, **create** the **lab deliverable files**.
2. **Review** the **Lab Assessment Worksheet**. You will find answers to these questions as you proceed through the lab steps.
3. **Review** the following scenario:

   Your organization is a governmental agency that serves a vital role in homeland security functions. In fact, your hiring took longer than you would have liked because it seemed as though the organization's managers wanted to know a lot about you before they gave you clearance to work. After a year at the job, your manager feels your progress has come a long way, so she is giving you more responsibility and has asked you to analyze the benefits of reporting risks, threats, and vulnerabilities in an IT assessment that is under way. Your manager would like for you to conduct research and report your findings about the type of vulnerabilities that require disclosure and when it is lawful or unlawful to conceal information produced by vulnerability assessments. She would also like for you to include some trends on current security threats and the types of responsible disclosure being performed by other organizations.

4. On your local computer, **open** a new **Internet browser window**.
5. In the address box of your Internet browser, **type** the URL **http://www.sans.org** and **press Enter** to open the Web site.
6. In the Custom Search box on the Web page's upper right corner, **search** for "**How do we define Responsible Disclosure?**"
7. On the search results page, **click** on the top link labeled "**How do we define Responsible Disclosure?**" to open the PDF article. **Read** about the following topics:
   - Vulnerability Life Cycle
   - Types of Disclosure
   - Nondisclosure
   - Full Disclosure
   - Limited Disclosure
   - Responsible Disclosure
   - Existing Policies and Proposals

▶ Note:
When reading through the different types of disclosure, consider how the consequences differ from type to type. For example, a company's nondisclosure policy about a vulnerability means little-to-no public knowledge. The consequence might mean the black hat (hacker) community has limited or no knowledge of the vulnerability. Consider also how a company's reputation changes as it handles disclosure. And lastly, consider how too much or too little disclosure can jeopardize a company's ability to manage vulnerabilities.

8. In your Lab Report file, **note** one relevant point about each section.

9. In the address box of your Internet browser, **type** the URL **http://eval.symantec.com/mktginfo/enterprise/white_papers/b-whitepaper_internet_security_threat_report_xv_04-2010.en-us.pdf** and **press Enter** to open the document "Symantec Global Internet Security Threat Report" provided by Symantec Corporation.

10. **Review** the **Highlights section** of the document that discusses the main concepts in each section. Then, **review** the following topics in the document:

    - Threat Activity Trends
    - Vulnerability Trends
    - Malicious Code Trends
    - Phishing, Underground Economy Servers, and Spam Trends

11. In your Lab Report file, **note** one relevant point about each section.

▶ Note:
After noting the relevant points from the Symantec report in step 11, examine "Appendix A—Symantec Best Practices," which is evenly divided between "enterprise" and "consumer" best practices.

12. In the address box of your Internet browser, **type** the URL **http://www.zerodayinitiative.com/advisories/published/** and **press Enter** to open the Web site.

13. **Review** some of the links on the page provided by the respected security experts at TippingPoint DVLabs and others.

▶ Note:
The "Symantec Global Internet Security Threat Report" contains several case studies that discuss zero-day vulnerabilities. As the name "zero-day" suggests, you have little lead time to be proactive. Even so, you can go on the offense by properly managing your company's assets and possibly subscribing to an alerting service.

14. **Research** other available resources (Internet resources, your textbook, and so on) to validate how performing periodic security assessments throughout the seven domains of a typical IT infrastructure can help an organization achieve compliance.

15. In your Lab Report file, **explain** how performing periodic security assessments throughout the seven domains of a typical IT infrastructure can help an organization achieve compliance.

16. In your Lab Report file, **write an executive summary** describing how security assessments throughout the seven domains of a typical IT infrastructure can help organizations achieve compliance by mitigating risks and threats.

▶ Note:
This completes the lab. **Close** the **Web browser**, if you have not already done so.

Evaluation Criteria and Rubrics

The following are the evaluation criteria for this lab that students must perform:

1. Review the vulnerability life cycle and explain the different types of disclosure to mitigate different risk factors, such as nondisclosure, full disclosure, limited disclosure, and responsible disclosure. – **[20%]**
2. Identify the risks that attacks, vulnerabilities, malicious code phishing, underground economies, and spam have on organizations. – **[20%]**
3. Mitigate the risks caused by zero-day vulnerabilities, HTTP Client versus Server Side attacks, Malicious JavaScript, PHP Remote File Include, botnets, and PDF attacks on organizations. – **[20%]**
4. Align best practices in vulnerability management to prevent threats from old or previously performed attacks on known vulnerabilities within the seven domains of a typical IT infrastructure. – **[20%]**
5. Draft an executive summary explaining how security assessments performed on the seven domains of a typical IT infrastructure can be used to help achieve compliance for an organization. – **[20%]**

Lab #4 - Assessment Worksheet

Aligning an IT Security Assessment—Risks, Threats, and Vulnerability—to Achieve Compliance

Course Name and Number: ______________________________

Student Name: ______________________________

Instructor Name: ______________________________

Lab Due Date: ______________________________

Overview

In this lab, you reviewed the vulnerability life cycle and explained the different types of disclosure to mitigate different risk factors. You identified risks that attacks, vulnerabilities, malicious code phishing, underground economies, and spam have on organizations. You looked at the risks caused by zero-day vulnerabilities, HTTP Client versus Server Side attacks, Malicious JavaScript, PHP Remote File Include, botnets, and PDF attacks on organizations. You also looked at the practices of vulnerability management to prevent threats from old or previously performed attacks on known vulnerabilities within the seven domains of a typical IT infrastructure.

Lab Assessment Questions & Answers

1. What is a PHP Remote File Include (RFI) attack, and why are these prevalent in today's Internet world?

2. What country is the top host of Structured Query Language (SQL) injection and SQL Slammer infections? Why can't the U.S. government do anything to prevent these injection attacks and infections?

3. What does it mean to have a policy of nondisclosure in an organization?

4. What trends were tracked when it came to malicious code in 2009 by the Symantec Report researched during this lab?

5. What is phishing? Describe what a typical phishing attack attempts to accomplish.

6. What is the Zero Day Initiative? Do you think this is valuable, and would you participate if you were the managing partner in a large firm?

7. What is a Server Side Include (SSI)? What are the ramifications if an SSI exploit is successful?

8. According to the TippingPoint Report researched in this lab, how do Server Message Block (SMB) attacks measure up to Hypertext Transfer Protocol (HTTP) attacks in the recent past?

9. According to the TippingPoint Report, what are some of the PHP RFI payload effects DVLabs has detected?

10. Explain the steps it takes to execute a malicious PDF attack as described in the TippingPoint Report?

11. What is a Zero Day attack and how does this relate to an organization's vulnerability window?

12. How can you mitigate the risk from users and employees clicking on an embedded URL link or e-mail attachment from unknown sources?

13. When auditing an organization for compliance, what role do IT security policies and an IT security policy framework play in the compliance audit?

14. When performing a security assessment, why is it a good idea to examine compliance in separate compartments such as the seven domains of a typical IT infrastructure?

15. True or false: Auditing for compliance and performing security assessments to achieve compliance require a checklist of compliance requirements.

Lab 5: Defining a Process for Gathering Information Pertaining to a GLBA Compliance Audit

Introduction

A financial institution is like any other business in that it aims to maintain or raise its profits. It is safe to assume that some financial institutions—faced with the choice between safeguarding an individual's information and safeguarding the institution's overhead costs—would lean toward lowering costs. Once the Gramm-Leach-Bliley Act (GLBA) was enacted in 1999, such choices were no longer an option.

Available online are several cases of documented abuse of customer trust that predate GLBA. On *http://epic.org/privacy/glba* are cases such as a bank which sold a list of its customers' credit card numbers to an adult Web site, which fraudulently invoiced the bank's clients for online "services they did not request." Those invoiced included customers with no online access. In another case, a bank shared customer information with a subsidiary. The subsidiary preyed upon low-risk customers to purchase high-risk investments, resulting in massive losses. Still other cases describe banks sharing customer information with telemarketing firms.

Once GLBA was enacted, including Title V detailing the protection of financial information, banks have since faced strict limitations on information-sharing without the customer's knowledge and consent. Protecting nonpublic information is a requirement of GLBA compliance.

In this lab, you will identify the Gramm-Leach-Bliley Act (GLBA) requirements for implementing the administrative, technical, and physical controls necessary to protect nonpublic personal information, you will define what financial information and personal information are impacted by the Privacy and Safeguards rules of GLBA, you will assess the requirements for handling nonpublic personal information and comprehend the GLBA guidelines regarding the proper security for this data, and you will investigate how GLBA has impacted controls to protect nonpublic personal information and financial information.

Learning Objectives

Upon completing this lab, you will be able to:

- Identify the Gramm-Leach-Bliley Act (GLBA) requirements for implementing the administrative, technical, and physical controls necessary to protect nonpublic personal information.
- Define what financial information and personal information are impacted by the Privacy and Safeguards rules of GLBA.
- Determine the requirements for handling nonpublic personal information and understand the GLBA guidelines on how to properly secure this data.
- Investigate how GLBA has impacted security controls for protecting nonpublic personal information and financial information.
- Draft an executive summary that defines a process for obtaining and addressing GLBA compliancy information for a financial organization's audit.

Deliverables

Upon completion of this lab, you are required to provide the following deliverables to your instructor:

1. Lab Report file;
2. Lab Assessments file.

Hands-On Steps

▶ Note:

This is a paper-based lab. To successfully complete the deliverables for this lab, you will need access to Microsoft® Word or another compatible word processor. For some labs, you may also need access to a graphics line drawing application, such as Visio or PowerPoint. Refer to the Preface of this manual for information on creating the lab deliverable files.

1. On your local computer, **create** the **lab deliverable files**.
2. **Review** the **Lab Assessment Worksheet**. You will find answers to these questions as you proceed through the lab steps.
3. On your local computer, **open** a new **Internet browser window**.
4. In the address box of your Internet browser, **type** the URL **http://en.wikipedia.org/wiki/Gramm%E2%80%93Leach%E2%80%93Bliley_Act** and **press Enter** to open a Wikipedia summary of GLBA.

GLBA's Scope

It's critical to understand GLBA's reach. The rules and protections granted to the individual by GLBA define the auditor's scope. Only by understanding GLBA, can the auditor align the audit goals and objectives to a defined scope.

5. **Review** the GLBA using Wikipedia's summary. For each of the following areas—many listed in Wikipedia's outline—**note** the most relevant information in your Lab Report file:
   - Legislative history
   - Changes caused by the act
   - Remaining restrictions
   - Financial Privacy Rule
     - Financial institutions defined
     - Consumer vs. customer defined
     - Consumer/client privacy rights
   - Safeguards Rule
   - Pretexting protection
   - Information Security Safeguards, including Guidelines for Providing Secure Data Transmission and Guidelines for Secure Disposal of Customer Information
6. Using your favorite search engine, **search for more information** on financial activities that are covered by GLBA.

When GLBA Applies

In the most general sense, if the financial activity is between any individual and a financial institution (such as a bank, brokerage house, or any company that offers a financial service or product), then GLBA applies.

7. Using your favorite search engine, **search for more information** on how to handle nonpublic personal information (NPI) and the GLBA guidelines regarding the proper security for this data. Examples of NPI include:

   - Social Security number (SSN)
   - Financial account numbers
   - Credit card numbers
   - Date of birth
   - Name, address, and phone numbers when collected with financial data
   - Details of any financial transactions

8. In your Lab Report file, **describe** the requirements for handling nonpublic personal information and the GLBA guidelines regarding the proper security for this data.

9. Using your favorite search engine, **search for more information** on the enforcement of GLBA, including:

   - The Federal Trade Commission (FTC) may bring an administrative enforcement action against any financial institution for noncompliance with the Safeguards Rule.
   - Penalties for violating the Safeguards Rule would likely include equitable damages caused by the loss of privacy, for example, a breach of security resulting in an identity theft.

An Audit's Key Points

When auditing an organization, remember that an audit means you're checking compliance against a known, expected environment. Therefore, at a bare minimum, the auditor should review the organization's written policies. Other key elements for the auditor to review include systems documentation, procedures, vendor agreements, and network documentation. If any prior audits were performed, those reports would be very helpful. In short, any documentation to better understand the organization and how it conducts business is helpful to the auditor.

10. In your Lab Report file, **write an executive summary** that summarizes how you would go about gathering and obtaining information needed to perform a GLBA Financial Privacy and Safeguards rules compliance audit for the seven domains of a typical IT infrastructure.

▶ Note:

This completes the lab. **Close** the **Web browser**, if you have not already done so.

Evaluation Criteria and Rubrics

The following are the evaluation criteria for this lab that students must perform:

1. Identify the Gramm-Leach-Bliley Act (GLBA) requirements for implementing the administrative, technical, and physical controls necessary to protect nonpublic personal information. – **[20%]**
2. Define what financial information and personal information are impacted by the Privacy and Safeguards rules of GLBA. – **[20%]**
3. Determine the requirements for handling nonpublic personal information and understand the GLBA guidelines on how to properly secure this data. – **[20%]**
4. Investigate how GLBA has impacted security controls for protecting nonpublic personal information and financial information. – **[20%]**
5. Draft an executive summary that defines a process for obtaining and addressing GLBA compliancy information for a financial organization's audit. – **[20%]**

Lab #5 - Assessment Worksheet

Defining a Process for Gathering Information Pertaining to a GLBA Compliance Audit

Course Name and Number: ______________________________

Student Name: ______________________________

Instructor Name: ______________________________

Lab Due Date: ______________________________

Overview

In this lab, you identified the Gramm-Leach-Bliley Act (GLBA) requirements for implementing the administrative, technical, and physical controls necessary to protect nonpublic personal information, you defined what financial information and personal information are impacted by the Privacy and Safeguards rules of GLBA, you assessed the requirements for handling nonpublic personal information and comprehended the GLBA guidelines regarding the proper security for this data, and you investigated how GLBA has impacted controls to protect nonpublic personal information and financial information.

Lab Assessment Questions & Answers

1. GLBA repealed parts of an act. Name the act and explain why that was significant for financial institutions and insurance companies.

2. What is another name for obtaining information under false pretenses, and what does that have to do with GLBA? What is an example of a safeguard pertinent to this requirement?

3. How does GLBA impact information systems security and the need for information systems security practitioners and professionals?

4. If your organization is a financial institution or insurance company that is also publicly traded, what other compliance law must you comply with?

5. Which one of these things does GLBA *not* require financial institutions to do?:
   a. The law requires these institutions to explain how they use and share your personal information.
   b. The law requires financial institutions to provide customers with their internal security policy.
   c. The law also allows you to stop or "opt out" of certain information sharing.
   d. The law requires that financial institutions describe how they will protect the confidentiality and security of your information.

6. Which U.S. government organization is responsible for enforcing GLBA?

7. For each of the seven domains of a typical IT infrastructure, what process or procedures would you perform to obtain information about security controls and safeguards?

8. How can a data classification standard be used within a GLBA security plan for GLBA compliance?

9. What are some examples of safeguards throughout the seven domains of a typical IT infrastructure that can be considered part of GLBA compliance?

10. If a bank or insurance company accepts credit card payments, what other standard must this organization comply with? What must an organization do to be compliant?

11. True or false: Banks that perform credit card transaction processing must be PCI DSS-compliant.

12. True or false: GLBA provides consumers with a false sense of security.

13. What is one strategy for communicating pretexting and social engineering to employees and consumers?

14. True or false: GLBA allows insurance companies to become banks and banks to become insurance companies. Now a complete portfolio of financial and insurance products and services is provided to customers.

15. PCI DSS v2.0 requires organizations to have annual security awareness training for all employees and authorized users of the organization's IT infrastructure. Why is this an important compliance requirement?

Lab 6: Auditing the Workstation Domain for Compliance

Introduction

A company's security policies and applicable legislation apply to the whole environment, from the Wide Area Network (WAN) to the servers, all the way to the end user. And as end users typically interface with the company through their workstations, this domain is no less at risk than the others.

In this lab, you will learn to recognize the risks, threats, and vulnerabilities commonly found in the Workstation Domain, you will identify known vulnerabilities and exploits on the Common Vulnerabilities & Exposures (CVE) database listing, you will describe how risks, threats, and vulnerabilities or misconfigurations at the operating system level in the Workstation Domain might expose that workstation, and you will identify steps to harden the Workstation Domain operating system and applications installed on the user's workstation for compliance and safeguarding of sensitive data and access to that data. Finally, you will apply Department of Defense (DoD) guidelines for securing the Workstation Domain, including the review and assessment of Windows 7 and Windows 2008 security guidelines.

Learning Objectives

Upon completing this lab, you will be able to:

- Recognize risks, threats, and vulnerabilities commonly found in the Workstation Domain.
- Identify Workstation Domain-known vulnerabilities and exploits on the CVE database listing of common vulnerabilities and exploits.
- Describe how risks, threats, and vulnerabilities or misconfigurations at the operating system level in the Workstation Domain might expose that workstation.
- Identify steps to harden the Workstation Domain operating system and applications installed on the user's workstation for compliance and safeguarding of sensitive data and access to that data.
- Apply DoD guidelines for securing the Workstation Domain, including the review and assessment of Windows 7 and Windows 2008 security guidelines.

Deliverables

Upon completion of this lab, you are required to provide the following deliverables to your instructor:

1. Lab Report file;
2. Lab Assessments file.

Hands-On Steps

▶ Note:
This is a paper-based lab. To successfully complete the deliverables for this lab, you will need access to Microsoft® Word or another compatible word processor. For some labs, you may also need access to a graphics line drawing application, such as Visio or PowerPoint. Refer to the Preface of this manual for information on creating the lab deliverable files.

1. On your local computer, **create** the **lab deliverable files**.
2. **Review** the **Lab Assessment Worksheet**. You will find answers to these questions as you proceed through the lab steps.
3. **Consider** the following scenario:

   You are a security consultant for an information systems security firm and have a new health care provider client under Health Insurance Portability and Accountability Act (HIPAA) compliance. Your new client wants to know the requirements and business drivers for securing the Workstation Domain in its health care environment. Your new client requires compliance with HIPAA. Similarly, your firm has a U.S. government DoD client that also wants you to perform a Workstation Domain compliance audit per DoD workstation hardening guidelines and baseline requirements.
4. On your local computer, **open** a new **Internet browser window**.
5. If you're unfamiliar with HIPAA, **complete** this step. Otherwise, **proceed** to step 6:
   a. In the address box of your Internet browser, **type** the URL **http://www.hhs.gov/ocr/privacy/hipaa/understanding/** and **press Enter** to open the Web site.
   b. **Review** to learn more about HIPAA and health information privacy.
6. In your Lab Report file, **discuss** how the compliance law requirements and business drivers for the health care provider's Workstation Domain might differ from the DoD's Workstation Domain security compliance requirements.
7. In the address box of your Internet browser, **type** the URL **http://cve.mitre.org/about/faqs.html** and **press Enter** to open the Web site.
8. **Browse** the site.
9. In your Lab Report file, **identify** the risks, threats, and vulnerabilities commonly found in the Workstation Domain.
10. In the address box of your Internet browser, **type** the URL **http://iase.disa.mil/stigs/index.html** and **press Enter** to open the Web site.

11. **Review** the Security Technical Implementation Guides (STIGs) available and the proper implementation of security based on DoD's workstation/desktop hardening guidelines.
12. In your Lab Report file, **discuss** three STIGs and the DoD's workstation/desktop hardening guidelines.

> **▶ Note:**
> You are writing about the STIGs to not only familiarize yourself with STIG formatting and nomenclature, but so you're also made aware of the available resource and its limitations.

13. In the address box of your Internet browser, **type** the URL **http://iase.disa.mil/stigs/downloads/pdf/unclassified_DesktopApplicationsGeneral_V4R1_STIG.pdf** and **press Enter** to open the PDF document from the Information Assurance Support Environment/Defense Information Systems Agency (IASE/DISA) Web site.
14. **Review** the **Desktop Applications General Version 4, Release 1** document.
15. In your Lab Report file, **discuss** this document's significant points.
16. **Review** the following concepts from this overarching DoD standards document for desktop hardening, and in your Lab Report file, **discuss** the significant points of **two** of these topics:
    - Appropriate backup strategy does not exist
    - Public instant message clients are installed
    - Peer to Peer clients or utilities are installed
    - Execution Restricted File Type Properties
    - Open-restricted File Type Properties

> **▶ Note:**
> For the two topics (referred to as "titles" in the PDF) that you choose to discuss, ask yourself the following questions: How well does the STIG identify and categorize the title? How adequately does the title identify a "finding" (vulnerability positively identified)? For example, for "Peer to Peer clients or utilities are installed," are you checking for any peer-to-peer utility, or just a particular client known at the time of its writing?

17. In the address box of your Internet browser, **type** the URL **http://iase.disa.mil/stigs/os/index.html#** and **press Enter** to open the Web site.
18. **Review** the Windows operating system (OS) security guidelines by **clicking** the +Windows tab toward the top of the page, **clicking** on Windows 7 and Windows 2008, and then **clicking** on the Guidance Documents tabs.
19. **Determine** which technical controls are appropriate for Windows 7 and Windows 2008.
20. **Note** these technical controls in your Lab Report file.
21. On the left side of the Web site, **click** the **STIGs Master List (A to Z) link**.

22. **Scroll down** the list to **locate** and then **download** the following Windows OS security guideline documents/ZIP files:

    - Windows 7 STIG (you will see several Windows 7 STIG options; **click** the one with *only* a Version number and a Release number after STIG)
    - Windows 2008 STIG (you will see a couple of Windows 2008 STIG options; **click** the one with *only* a Version number and a Release number after STIG)

> **▶ Note:**
> If a STIG version and release number is followed by "*PKI," that denotes the requirement for a DoD public key infrastructure (PKI) certificate for downloading. Examples of STIGs requiring the DoD PKI certificate include those for For Official Use Only (FOUO) systems. Customarily, lab students would not possess a DoD PKI certificate.

23. Once you've downloaded the **Windows 7 STIG ZIP file** to your desktop, **double-click** the ZIP file to extract the Windows 7 STIG folder.
24. **Double-click** the folder to open it.
25. **Double-click** the Windows 7 Manual STIG ZIP file to extract the Windows 7 Manual STIG folder.
26. **Double-click** the folder to open it.
27. **Double-click** the Windows 7 STIG Manual XML file to open it.
28. **Review** some of the following concepts. In your Lab Report file, **list** each of these and **discuss** a significant point about each:

    - Display Shutdown Button
    - Clear System Pagefile
    - Removable media devices
    - Halt on Audit Failure
    - Security Configuration Tools

29. Next, you will work with the **Windows 2008 STIG ZIP file** on your desktop. **Double-click** the ZIP file to extract the Windows 2008 STIG folder.
30. **Double-click** the folder to open it.
31. **Double-click** the Windows 2008 DC Manual STIG ZIP file to extract the Windows 2008 DC Manual STIG folder.
32. **Double-click** the folder to open it.
33. **Double-click** the Windows 2008 DC STIG Manual XML file to open it.

34. **Review** some of the following concepts and vulnerabilities for configuring and hardening Windows 2008 Domain Controllers. In your Lab Report file, **list** each of these and **discuss** a significant point about each:

    - System Recovery Backups
    - Caching of Logon Credentials
    - Dormant Accounts
    - Recycle Bin Configuration
    - Password Uniqueness
    - Printer Share Permissions

35. In the address box of your Internet browser, **type** the URL **http://cve.mitre.org/** and **press Enter** to open the Web site.

36. **Review** the National Cyber Security Division of the U.S. Homeland Security Department's **CVE listing** hosted by the Mitre Corporation. To access the CVE listing, **click CVE List** in the left-hand column to reach the CVE List Main Page.

37. In your Lab Report file, **discuss** how Workstation Domain OS and application software vulnerabilities are housed in the CVE listing.

38. **Click** the **National Vulnerability Database link** on the CVE homepage or CVE List Main Page. In your Lab Report file, **discuss** how vulnerabilities are housed in the National Vulnerability Database. **Discuss** how this is both a security control tool and an attack tool used by hackers.

39. In your Lab Report file, **write an executive summary** to summarize the top Workstation Domain risks, threats, and vulnerabilities, and include a description of the risk mitigation tactics you would perform to audit the Workstation Domain for compliance. Use the U.S. DoD workstation hardening guidelines as your example for a baseline definition for compliance.

> ▶**Note:**
> This completes the lab. **Close** the **Web browser**, if you have not already done so.

Evaluation Criteria and Rubrics

The following are the evaluation criteria for this lab that students must perform:

1. Recognize risks, threats, and vulnerabilities commonly found in the Workstation Domain. – **[20%]**
2. Identify Workstation Domain-known vulnerabilities and exploits on the CVE database listing of common vulnerabilities and exploits. – **[20%]**
3. Describe how risks, threats, and vulnerabilities or misconfigurations at the operating system level in the Workstation Domain might expose that workstation. – **[20%]**
4. Identify steps to harden the Workstation Domain operating system and applications installed on the user's workstation for compliance and safeguarding of sensitive data and access to that data. – **[20%]**
5. Apply DoD guidelines for securing the Workstation Domain, including the review and assessment of Windows 7 and Windows 2008 security guidelines. – **[20%]**

Lab #6 - Assessment Worksheet

Auditing the Workstation Domain for Compliance

Course Name and Number: ______________________________

Student Name: ______________________________

Instructor Name: ______________________________

Lab Due Date: ______________________________

Overview

In this lab, you learned to recognize the risks, threats, and vulnerabilities commonly found in the Workstation Domain, you identified known vulnerabilities and exploits on the Common Vulnerabilities & Exposures (CVE) database listing, you described how risks, threats, and vulnerabilities or misconfigurations at the operating system level in the Workstation Domain might expose that workstation, and you identified steps to harden the Workstation Domain operating system and applications installed on the user's workstation for compliance and safeguarding of sensitive data and access to that data. Finally, you applied Department of Defense (DoD) guidelines for securing the Workstation Domain, including the review and assessment of Windows 7 and Windows 2008 security guidelines.

Lab Assessment Questions & Answers

1. What are some risks, threats, and vulnerabilities commonly found in the Workstation Domain that must be mitigated through a layered security strategy?

2. File-sharing utilities and client-to-client communication applications can provide the capability to share files with other users (for instance, peer-to-peer networking or sharing). What risks and/or vulnerabilities are introduced with these applications?

3. Explain how confidentiality can be achieved in the Workstation Domain with security controls and security countermeasures.

4. Explain how data integrity can be achieved in the Workstation Domain with security controls and security countermeasures.

5. Explain how availability can be achieved in the Workstation Domain with security controls and security countermeasures.

6. Although users of desktop applications might not create mission-critical data, all of their data represents a resource that, if lost, can result in a permanent loss of information or productivity. Explain what countermeasures and best practices should be implemented to avoid this potential disaster.

7. What is the purpose of the Microsoft® Windows Security Configuration and Analysis snap-in? Explain.

8. How would you go about updating the Windows Security Options File? Explain how this option can help mitigate risk in the Workstation Domain.

9. What does the Microsoft® Windows executable GPResult.exe do and what general information does it provide? Explain how this application helps mitigate the risks, threats, and vulnerabilities commonly found in the Workstation Domain.

10. What is the risk involved in caching logon credentials on a Microsoft® Windows system?

11. What is the current URL for the location of the DISA Military STIGs on Microsoft® Windows 7 operating systems?

12. Within the Windows 7 Security Technical Implementation Guide (STIG), what are the three Vulnerability Severity Code Definitions defined?

13. DumpSec is a tool used by system administrators performing information assurance on a Microsoft® Windows 7 workstation. What is the purpose of this tool?

14. From the Windows 7 Security Technical Implementation Guide (STIG), where can Windows 7 File & Registry Settings be reviewed and audited on a Windows 7 workstation?

15. As per DoD and information assurance procedures, who must be notified if any exceptions to DoD STIGs standards for workstation configurations are to be implemented?

Lab 7: Auditing the LAN-to-WAN Domain for Compliance

Introduction

Today, networks are no longer isolated, with only the most purposeful exceptions. Virtually every local network possesses a path to the Internet and/or some external network. Apart from the smallest of businesses, office networks are segmented across oceans or only streets, connecting multiple Local Area Networks (LANs) alongside a span of other networks. The need to secure those Local Area Network-to-Wide Area Network (LAN-to-WAN) connections is critical to the security of the LANs.

In this lab, you will learn how to audit the LAN-to-WAN Domain. You will identify common risks, threats, and vulnerabilities found in the LAN-to-WAN Domain, you will assess common risks, threats, and vulnerabilities found in the LAN-to-WAN Domain, you will identify network and security policies needed to properly secure the LAN-to-WAN portion of the network infrastructure, you will audit and assess implementation of security controls within the LAN-to-WAN domain, and you will recommend LAN-to-WAN Domain hardening solutions by implementing proper security controls at the Internet ingress/egress point within an IT infrastructure.

Learning Objectives

Upon completing this lab, you will be able to:

- Identify common risks, threats, and vulnerabilities found in the LAN-to-WAN Domain that require proper security controls for mitigation.
- Apply proper security controls and configuration standards for configuration of network firewalls and intrusion detection system/intrusion prevention system (IDS/IPS) devices per Department of Defense (DoD) standards.
- Identify network and security policies needed to properly secure the LAN-to-WAN portion of the network infrastructure.
- Audit and assess implementation of security controls within the LAN-to-WAN Domain.
- Recommend LAN-to-WAN Domain hardening solutions by implementing proper security controls at the Internet ingress/egress point within an IT infrastructure.

Deliverables

Upon completion of this lab, you are required to provide the following deliverables to your instructor:

1. Lab Report file;
2. Lab Assessments file.

Hands-On Steps

> **▶ Note:**
> This is a paper-based lab. To successfully complete the deliverables for this lab, you will need access to Microsoft® Word or another compatible word processor. For some labs, you may also need access to a graphics line drawing application, such as Visio or PowerPoint. Refer to the Preface of this manual for information on creating the lab deliverable files.

1. On your local computer, **create** the **lab deliverable files**.
2. **Review** the **Lab Assessment Worksheet**. You will find answers to these questions as you proceed through the lab steps.
3. **Consider** the following scenario:

   You are a security consultant for an information systems security firm and have a new health care provider client under Health Insurance Portability and Accountability Act (HIPAA) compliance. Your new client wants to know the requirements and business drivers for securing the LAN-to-WAN Domain in its health care environment, which requires compliance with HIPAA. Similarly, your firm has a U.S. government DoD client who also wants you to perform a LAN-to-WAN Domain compliance audit per the DoD LAN and network hardening guidelines and baseline requirements. Both organizations want you to focus on the LAN-to-WAN Domain only, and you are to use DoD-provided frameworks and Security Technical Implementation Guides (STIGs) to summarize a network infrastructure hardening strategy (for more information, refer to the Auditing the Workstation Domain for Compliance lab in this lab manual).
4. On your local computer, **open** a new **Internet browser window**.
5. In the address box of your Internet browser, **type** the URL **http://iase.disa.mil/stigs/net_perimeter/index.html#** and **press Enter** to open the Web site.
6. **Review** the DoD network hardening guidelines and other National Institute of Standards and Technology (NIST) standards identified in the Defining a Process for Gathering Information Pertaining to a HIPAA Compliance Audit lab in this lab manual.
7. In the address box of your Internet browser, **type** the URL **http://www.sans.org** and **press Enter** to open the Web site.
8. In the Search box in the upper right corner of the screen, **type** the words **LAN to WAN** and **press Enter**.
9. **Research** the links you find to **identify** the risks, threats, and vulnerabilities commonly found in the LAN-to-WAN Domain.
10. **List** these risks, threats, and vulnerabilities in your Lab Report file.

11. Using information learned in the Aligning Auditing Frameworks for a Business Unit Within DoD lab in this lab manual and the Internet, **identify** and **review** the documents available for hardening network infrastructure and the LAN-to-WAN Domain as per DoD standards.

12. **List** these in your Lab Report file.

13. In the address box of your Internet browser, **type** the following URLs from the Information Assurance Support Environment/Defense Information Systems Agency (IASE/DISA) Web site and **press Enter** to **find** the STIGs for routers and switches, network policy, firewalls and IDS/IPS, and other network devices:

    - **http://iase.disa.mil/stigs/net_perimeter/network_infra/routers_switches.html**
    - **http://iase.disa.mil/stigs/net_perimeter/network_infra/policy.html**
    - **http://iase.disa.mil/stigs/net_perimeter/network_infra/firewall.html**
    - **http://iase.disa.mil/stigs/net_perimeter/network_infra/other.html**

14. **Download** the available ZIP files from the URLs listed in the previous step, including:

    - Network Infrastructure Router L3 Switch
    - Network Perimeter Router L3 Switch
    - Network L2 Switch
    - Network Policy
    - Network Firewall
    - Network IDS/IPS
    - Network Other Devices

> **▶ Note:**
> The list above provides a comprehensive coverage of network devices relevant to a LAN-to-WAN audit, but only at the hardware level. It is important to also consider factors not included, such as the administrative documentation, physical access, environmental, etc.

15. **Extract** the **Overview PDFs** from each of the ZIP files listed in the previous step. This PDF is the summary document that supports all of the XML files.

16. **Review** the following concepts from this overarching DoD standards document for network infrastructure:

    - ENCLAVE PERIMETER
    - Enclave Protection Mechanisms
    - Network Infrastructure Diagram
    - External Connections
    - Leased Lines
    - Approved Gateway/Internet Service Provider Connectivity
    - Backdoor Connections
    - IPv4 Address Privacy
    - FIREWALL

- Packet Filters
- Bastion Host
- Stateful Inspection
- Firewalls with Application Awareness
- Deep Packet Inspection
- Application-Proxy Gateway
- Hybrid Firewall Technologies
- Dedicated Proxy
- Layered Firewall Architecture
- Content Filtering
- Perimeter Protection
- Tunnels

17. Briefly **discuss** these in your Lab Report file.

18. **Extract** the **Switch Cisco Manual XML file** from the **Network L2 Switch ZIP file**.

19. **Review** some of the following concepts and vulnerabilities for configuring and hardening Cisco switches:

    - Non-registered or unauthorized IP addresses
    - In-band Mgt not configured to timeout in 10 min
    - Exclusive use of privileged and non-privileged
    - Assign lowest privilege level to user accounts
    - Log all in-band management access attempts

20. Briefly **discuss** these in your Lab Report file.

> **▶Note:**
> When discussing these concepts in your Lab Report file, consider the potential consequences of each, if they were not hardened.

21. Extract the **Perimeter Router Cisco XML file** from the **Network Perimeter Router L3 Switch ZIP file**.

22. **Review** some of the following concepts and vulnerabilities for configuring and hardening Cisco routers:

    - A log or syslog statement does not follow all deny statements
    - DNS servers must be defined for client resolver
    - Running and startup configurations are not synchronized

23. Briefly **discuss** these in your Lab Report file.

24. **Extract** the **Firewall Cisco PIX ASA XML file** from the **Network Firewall ZIP file**. **Review** at least three of the concepts and vulnerabilities for configuring and hardening Cisco firewalls as performed previously for switches and routers. **Discuss** these in your Lab Report file.

25. **Extract** the **IDS-IPS Manual XML file** from the **Network IDS/IPS ZIP file**.

26. **Review** at least three of the concepts and vulnerabilities for configuring and hardening IDS/IPS devices as performed previously for switches and routers.

> **▶ Note:**
> If an IDS/IPS were not sufficiently protected, an intruder would not only be able to penetrate the network, but would also be able to cover his/her tracks, for example, compromise an IDS to thwart and bypass detection.

27. **Discuss** these in your Lab Report file.

28. **Extract** the **Network Policy Manual XML file** from the **Network Policy ZIP file**.

29. **Review** at least three of the concepts and vulnerabilities for configuring and hardening network policy as performed previously for switches and routers.

30. **Discuss** these in your Lab Report file.

31. In your Lab Report file, **write an executive summary** summarizing the top LAN-to-WAN Domain risks, threats, and vulnerabilities and include a description of the risk mitigation tactics you would perform to audit the LAN-to-WAN Domain for compliance. Use the DoD LAN-to-WAN hardening guidelines as your example for a baseline definition for compliance.

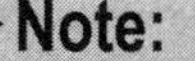

> This completes the lab. **Close** the **Web browser**, if you have not already done so.

Evaluation Criteria and Rubrics

The following are the evaluation criteria for this lab that students must perform:

1. Identify common risks, threats, and vulnerabilities found in the LAN-to-WAN Domain that require proper security controls for mitigation. – **[20%]**
2. Apply proper security controls and configuration standards for configuration of network firewalls and intrusion detection system/intrusion prevention system (IDS/IPS) devices per Department of Defense (DoD) standards. – **[20%]**
3. Identify network and security policies needed to properly secure the LAN-to-WAN portion of the network infrastructure. – **[20%]**
4. Audit and assess implementation of security controls within the LAN-to-WAN Domain. – **[20%]**
5. Recommend LAN-to-WAN Domain hardening solutions by implementing proper security controls at the Internet ingress/egress point within an IT infrastructure. – **[20%]**

Lab #7 - Assessment Worksheet

Auditing the LAN-to-WAN Domain for Compliance

Course Name and Number: _______________________________

Student Name: _______________________________

Instructor Name: _______________________________

Lab Due Date: _______________________________

Overview

In this lab, you learned how to audit the LAN-to-WAN Domain. You identified common risks, threats, and vulnerabilities found in the LAN-to-WAN Domain, you assessed common risks, threats, and vulnerabilities found in the LAN-to-WAN Domain, you identified network and security policies needed to properly secure the LAN-to-WAN portion of the network infrastructure, you audited and assessed implementation of security controls within the LAN-to-WAN Domain, and you recommended LAN-to-WAN Domain hardening solutions by implementing proper security controls at the Internet ingress/egress point within an IT infrastructure.

Lab Assessment Questions & Answers

1. What are some common risks, threats, and vulnerabilities found in the LAN-to-WAN Domain that must be mitigated through a layered security strategy?

2. What is an access control list (ACL), and how is it useful in a layered security strategy?

3. What is a Bastion Host? Provide an example of when a Bastion Host should be used and how.

4. Provide at least two examples of how the enclave requirement to place a firewall at the perimeter can be accomplished.

5. What is the difference between a traditional IP stateful firewall and a deep packet inspection firewall?

6. How would you monitor for unauthorized management access attempts to sensitive systems?

7. What is the significance of VLAN 1 traffic in a Cisco Catalyst LAN switch? Describe the vulnerabilities associated with it if it traverses across an unnecessary trunk.

8. At what logging level should the syslog service be configured on a Cisco router, switch, or firewall device?

9. As defined in the Network Infrastructure Technology Overview, describe the three layers that can be found in the DISA Enclave Perimeter layered security solution for Internet ingress/egress connections (for instance, Demilitarized Zone [DMZ] or Component Flow).

10. Which device in the Enclave Protection Mechanism Component Flow helps mitigate risks from users violating acceptable use and unwanted Web sites and URL links?

11. True or false: The Enclave Protection Mechanism includes both an internal IDS and external IDS when connecting a closed network infrastructure to the public Internet.

12. True or false: Securing the enclave requires only perimeter security and firewalls.

13. What is the primary objective of the Network Infrastructure STIG as it relates to DoD network infrastructures?

Lab 8: Auditing the Remote Access Domain for Compliance

Introduction

Beyond the relatively controlled network perimeter are the most dangerous threats and risks. However, there is a consistent requirement for access into the protected network from the outside. Permitting users and systems the remote access demands a prudent combination of policies and technology. Keeping the Remote Access Domain secure is essential to maintaining security in the other, closer domains.

In this lab, you will learn how to audit the Remote Access Domain. You will identify common risks, threats, and vulnerabilities found in the Remote Access Domain, you will assess common risks, threats, and vulnerabilities found in the Remote Access Domain, you will identify network and security policies needed to properly secure the Remote Access Domain portion of the network infrastructure, and you will audit and assess the implementation of security controls in the Remote Access Domain.

Learning Objectives

Upon completing this lab, you will be able to:

- Identify common risks, threats, and vulnerabilities found in the Remote Access Domain that require proper security controls for mitigation.
- Apply proper security controls and configuration standards for configuration of a secure Remote Access Domain as per Department of Defense (DoD) remote access standards.
- Identify network and security policies needed to properly secure the Remote Access Domain portion of the network infrastructure.
- Audit and assess implementation of security controls in the Remote Access Domain.
- Draft an executive summary recommending Remote Access Domain hardening solutions by implementing proper security controls at the Internet ingress/egress point within an IT infrastructure.

Deliverables

Upon completion of this lab, you are required to provide the following deliverables to your instructor:

1. Lab Report file;
2. Lab Assessments file.

Hands-On Steps

> **▶ Note:**
> This is a paper-based lab. To successfully complete the deliverables for this lab, you will need access to Microsoft® Word or another compatible word processor. For some labs, you may also need access to a graphics line drawing application, such as Visio or PowerPoint. Refer to the Preface of this manual for information on creating the lab deliverable files.

1. On your local computer, **create** the **lab deliverable files**.
2. **Review** the **Lab Assessment Worksheet**. You will find answers to these questions as you proceed through the lab steps.
3. **Consider** the following scenario:

   You are a security consultant for an information systems security firm and have a new health care provider client under Health Insurance Portability and Accountability Act (HIPAA) compliance. Your new client wants to know the requirements and the business drivers for securing the Remote Access Domain in a health care environment because it requires compliance with HIPAA. Similarly, your firm has a U.S. government DoD client that also wants you to perform a Remote Access Domain compliance audit per DoD remote access hardening guidelines and baseline requirements. Both organizations want you to focus on the Remote Access Domain only, and you are to use DoD-provided frameworks and Security Technical Implementation Guides (STIGs) to summarize a Remote Access Domain hardening strategy.
4. On your local computer, **open** a new **Internet browser window**.
5. In the address box of your Internet browser, **type** the URL **http://www.sans.org/** and **press Enter** to open the SANS Institute's Web site.
6. **Identify** the risks, threats, and vulnerabilities commonly found in the Remote Access Domain's security solution.
7. In your Lab Report file, **describe** these risks, threats, and vulnerabilities found in the Remote Access Domain's security solution.
8. In the address box of your Internet browser, **type** the URL **http://iase.disa.mil/stigs/net_perimeter/index.html#** and **press Enter** to open the Web site.
9. **Review** the DoD network hardening guidelines and other National Institute of Standards and Technology (NIST) standards.

> **▶ Note:**
> Particularly search under the **Network Other link** found toward the top of the page for relevant Remote Access Domain guidance documents.

10. In your Lab Report file, **describe** these DoD network hardening guidelines and other NIST standards.

11. In the address box of your Internet browser, **type** the URL **http://iase.disa.mil/stigs/net_perimeter/other/other.html** and **press Enter** to open the Web site.

12. **Scroll down** to the Remote Access STIGs banner, and **click** on **+Guidance Documents** to expand the options.

13. **Click** on the **Remote Access VPN STIG link** to download the ZIP file to your desktop.

14. **Double-click** the ZIP file to extract the Remote Access VPN STIG folder.

15. **Double-click** the folder to open it.

16. **Double-click** the Overview PDF file to open it. This document reviews the potential vulnerabilities and configuration recommendations for secure remote access as per DoD guidelines.

17. **Review** the following concepts from this overarching DoD standards document for secure remote access, and **discuss** these guidelines in your Lab Report file:

    - SECURITY CONSIDERATIONS FOR REMOTE ACCESS AND TELEWORK
    - ASSESSMENT, ENFORCEMENT, AND REMEDIATION SERVICES
    - ENDPOINT SECURITY
    - SECURITY READINESS REVIEW REQUIREMENTS

18. In the address box of your Internet browser, **type** the URL **http://iase.disa.mil/stigs/net_perimeter/other/other.html** and **press Enter** to **return** to the Defense Information Systems Agency (DISA) Web page.

19. If necessary, **scroll down** again to the Remote Access STIGs banner, and **click** on **+Guidance Documents** to expand the options.

20. **Review** some more remote access security checklists and guideline documents, by **clicking** through ZIPs and folders as you did in step 12 until you reach the Overview PDF for each of the following:

    - RAS Remote Access Server STIG
    - Remote Access Policy STIG
    - Remote Endpoint STIG

21. **Review** how the security controls listed in each of the Secure Remote Access checklists can help mitigate the risks, threats, and vulnerabilities within the Remote Access Domain.

22. **Review** how these security checklists and DoD guideline documents can help organizations baseline their security and achieve the compliance requirements in both government and commercial organizations.

23. **Discuss** these guidelines in your Lab Report file.

24. In your Lab Report file, **write an executive summary** that summarizes the top Remote Access Domain risks, threats, and vulnerabilities and include a description of the risk mitigation tactics you would perform to audit the Remote Access Domain for compliance. Use the U.S. DoD remote access hardening guidelines as your example for a baseline definition for compliance.

▶ Note:
This completes the lab. **Close** the **Web browser**, if you have not already done so.

Evaluation Criteria and Rubrics

The following are the evaluation criteria for this lab that students must perform:

1. Identify common risks, threats, and vulnerabilities found in the Remote Access Domain that require proper security controls for mitigation. – **[20%]**
2. Apply proper security controls and configuration standards for configuration of a secure Remote Access Domain as per Department of Defense (DoD) remote access standards. – **[20%]**
3. Identify network and security policies needed to properly secure the Remote Access Domain portion of the network infrastructure. – **[20%]**
4. Audit and assess implementation of security controls in the Remote Access Domain. – **[20%]**
5. Draft an executive summary recommending Remote Access Domain hardening solutions by implementing proper security controls at the Internet ingress/egress point within an IT infrastructure. – **[20%]**

Lab #8 - Assessment Worksheet

Auditing the Remote Access Domain for Compliance

Course Name and Number: ______________________________

Student Name: ______________________________

Instructor Name: ______________________________

Lab Due Date: ______________________________

Overview

In this lab, you learned how to audit the Remote Access Domain. You identified common risks, threats, and vulnerabilities found in the Remote Access Domain, you assessed common risks, threats, and vulnerabilities found in the Remote Access Domain, you identified network and security policies needed to properly secure the Remote Access Domain portion of the network infrastructure, and you audited and assessed the implementation of security controls in the Remote Access Domain.

Lab Assessment Questions & Answers

1. What are some common risks, threats, and vulnerabilities found in the Remote Access Domain that must be mitigated through a layered security strategy?

2. What default configuration should be placed on host-based firewalls when accessing the network remotely?

3. What risks, threats, and vulnerabilities are introduced by implementing a remote access server?

4. What is a recommended best practice when implementing a remote access policy server user authentication service?

5. What is a Remediation LAN?

6. Explain the concept of a Remediation Server and traffic separation as it relates to remote access.

7. What is a VPN? Distinguish between VPN server, VPN client, VPN router, and Secure Sockets Layer (SSL) VPNs.

8. What is the difference between a tunnel-mode VPN and a split-tunneling VPN?

9. According to the Remote Access Policy STIG, what personally owned devices are considered acceptable to perform privileged (administrative) tasks on a DoD network?

10. When connected to a public network or shared public Internet access point, what are some precautions that remote users should take to ensure confidentiality of communications?

11. What are the three types of remote access users as defined by the DoD in the Secure Remote Computing STIG?

12. What are the additional elements required of a network architecture if the enclave is to support remote access through the public Internet?

13. Name three security best practices for mobile workers as defined in the Secure Remote Computing STIG.

14. True or false: A thin client is a PC or laptop without a hard drive or storage space.

15. What are the five elements of a Remote Access Security Readiness Review?

Lab 9: Auditing the System/Application Domain for Compliance

Introduction

The System/Application Domain is arguably the most powerful of domains to secure. Compared with strictly physical domains, the System/Application Domain encompasses not only the several systems but the myriad of applications. The fact that a company's applications are likely distributed only complicates the task further. Although the systems must process data as efficiently as possible, standards and legislative requirements such as the Payment Card Industry Data Security Standard (PCI DSS) and Health Insurance Portability and Accountability Act (HIPAA) force companies to balance efficiency with compliance.

In this lab, you will learn how to audit the System/Application Domain. You will identify common risks, threats, and vulnerabilities found in the System/Application Domain, you will align the Payment Card Industry Data Security Standard (PCI DSS) standard to the System/Application Domain of security responsibility given that servers perform e-commerce credit card transactions online, you will review the PCI DSS standard for the System/Application Domain, and you will create a PCI DSS audit for a compliance checklist to identify all elements needed for assessment and compliance with the PCI DSS standard within the System/Application Domain.

Learning Objectives

Upon completing this lab, you will be able to:

- Identify common risks, threats, and vulnerabilities found in the System/Application Domain that require proper security controls for mitigation.
- Align the PCI DSS standard to the System/Application Domain of security responsibility given that servers perform e-commerce credit card transactions online.
- Review the elements of the PCI DSS standard that pertain to servers, applications, and stored personal privacy data and credit card information in the System/Application Domain.
- Create a PCI DSS audit for compliance checklist to identify all elements needed for assessment and compliance with the PCI DSS standard within the System/Application Domain.
- Draft an executive summary recommending System/Application Domain hardening solutions by implementing proper security controls at the Internet ingress/egress point within an IT infrastructure.

Deliverables

Upon completion of this lab, you are required to provide the following deliverables to your instructor:

1. Lab Report file;
2. Lab Assessments file.

Hands-On Steps

▶ Note:
This is a paper-based lab. To successfully complete the deliverables for this lab, you will need access to Microsoft® Word or another compatible word processor. For some labs, you may also need access to a graphics line drawing application, such as Visio or PowerPoint. Refer to the Preface of this manual for information on creating the lab deliverable files.

1. On your local computer, **create** the **lab deliverable files**.
2. **Review** the **Lab Assessment Worksheet**. You will find answers to these questions as you proceed through the lab steps.
3. **Consider** the following scenario:

   You are a security consultant for an information systems security firm and you have a new e-commerce client. Your client wants to know the requirements and business drivers for securing the System/Application Domain as per the PCI DSS standard. Your new client must be in compliance with the PCI DSS standard because it processes credit card transactions and obtains its customers' privacy data. The client wants you to focus on the System/Application Domain only, and you are to use the PCI DSS standard as a framework to summarize a System/Application Domain hardening strategy.

What Makes PCI DSS Special
PCI DSS is special in that an ordinary auditor cannot attest to compliance. Compliance is verified by a Qualified Security Assessor and is done annually. In the case where a company experiences only a small number of transactions, compliance is attested by answering a Self-Assessment Questionnaire. Keep this in mind as you plan to document a company's compliance.

4. On your local computer, **open** a new **Internet browser window**.
5. In the address box of your Internet browser, **type** the URL **www.sans.org** and **press Enter** to open the SANS Institute's Web site.
6. **Identify** the risks, threats, and vulnerabilities commonly found in the System/Application Domain that are a threat to credit card transaction-processing organizations.
7. In your Lab Report file, **describe** these risks, threats, and vulnerabilities commonly found in the System/Application Domain.
8. In the address box of your Internet browser, **type** the URL **https://www.pcisecuritystandards.org/security_standards/pci_dss.shtml** and **press Enter** to open the Web site.
9. **Read** the information on the **PCI SSC Data Security Standards Overview** page.

10. **Download** the **PCI DSS v3.0 standard** in PDF format at **https://www.pcisecuritystandards.org/documents/PCI_DSS_v3.pdf** or get it from your instructor. This standard applies to the System/Application Domain of an e-commerce organization that performs credit card transaction processing.

11. **Review** the PCI DSS security controls and business drivers that define requirements for the System/Application Domain's security solution.

12. **Conduct** a thorough overview of **PCI/DSS Requirement #7.1** (listed below), which says that software vendors must establish a process to identify and assign a risk ranking to newly discovered security vulnerabilities and test their payment applications for vulnerabilities. Any underlying software or systems that are provided with or required by the payment application (for example, Web servers, third-party libraries, and programs) must be included. Following are the requirements:

    - **7.1** Obtain and examine processes to identify new vulnerabilities and to test payment applications for new vulnerabilities. Verify the processes include the following:
        - **7.1.a** Verify that processes include assigning a risk ranking to identified vulnerabilities. (At minimum, the most critical, highest risk vulnerabilities should be ranked as "High.")
        - **7.1.b** Verify the processes to identify new security vulnerabilities include using outside sources for security vulnerability information.
        - **7.1.c** Verify that processes include testing of payment applications for new vulnerabilities.
        - **7.1.d** Verify that processes to identify new vulnerabilities and implement corrections into payment application apply to all software provided with or required by the payment application (for example, Web servers, third-party libraries, and programs).

13. **Conduct** a thorough overview of **PCI/DSS Requirement #7.2** (listed below), which says that software vendors must establish a process for timely development and deployment of security patches and upgrades, which includes delivery of updates and patches in a secure manner with a known chain-of-trust, and maintenance of the integrity of patch and update code during delivery and deployment. The requirements are:

    - **7.2.a** Obtain and examine processes to develop and deploy security patches and upgrades for software. Verify that processes include the timely development and deployment of patches to customers.
    - **7.2.b** Review processes to verify that patches and updates are delivered in a secure manner with a known chain-of-trust.
    - **7.2.c** Review processes to verify that patches and updates are delivered in a manner that maintains the integrity of the deliverable.
    - **7.2.d** Review processes to verify that patches and updates are integrity tested on the target system prior to installation.
    - **7.2.e** To verify that the integrity of patch and update code is maintained, run the update process with arbitrary code, and determine that the system will not allow the update to occur.

14. In the address box of your Internet browser, **type** the URL **http://iase.disa.mil/stigs/index.html** and **press Enter** to open the Web site.

15. **Review** the Security Technical Information Guides (STIGs) available at the Defense Information Systems Agency (DISA) Web site, and **review** how to properly implement security based on Department of Defense- (DoD-) recommended system application hardening guidelines.

16. **Discuss** these guidelines in your Lab Report file.

17. In the address box of your Internet browser, **type** the URL **http://iase.disa.mil/stigs/app_security/index.html** and **press Enter** to open the Web site.

> **▶ Note:**
> Do *not* click and download the presented "Application Server SRG" link in the box in the middle of the page. As you will read in the next step, you will click on the Application Security & Development link in the green banner.

18. **Click** on **Application Security & Development** in the green banner toward the top of the page.

19. **Click** on **+ Guidance Documents** under Application Security & Development.

20. **Double-click Application Security and Development STIG** to open the ZIP file.

21. **Double-click** the ZIP file to extract the folder.

22. **Double-click** the folder to open it.

23. **Double-click** the Application Security and Development STIG PDF file to open it. This STIG reviews the potential vulnerabilities and configuration recommendations for secure Web systems and applications per the DoD guidelines.

24. **Review** the following concepts from the overarching DoD standards document for systems and Web application security:

    - PROGRAM MANAGEMENT
    - DESIGN & DEVELOPMENT
    - SOFTWARE CONFIGURATION MANAGEMENT (SCM)
    - TESTING
    - DEPLOYMENT

25. In the same document, **review** the 3.10 Input Validation section:

    - 3.10.1: SQL Injection Vulnerabilities
    - 3.10.2: Integer Arithmetic Vulnerabilities
    - 3.10.3: Format String Vulnerabilities
    - 3.10.4: Command Injection Vulnerabilities
    - 3.10.5: Cross Site Scripting (XSS) Vulnerabilities
    - 3.10.6: Cross Site Request Forgery (CSRF) Vulnerabilities
    - 3.10.7: Buffer Overflow Vulnerabilities

26. **Identify** which of the security controls are listed in both the PCI DSS v3.0 standard document and the Application Security and Development STIG PDF document.

27. In your Lab Report file, **describe** some of the checklist items, provided in step 25, which might be required for the enterprise described in the scenario in step 3.

28. In your Lab Report file, **discuss** how these security checklists in PCI DSS and DoD guideline documents can help organizations baseline their security and achieve the compliance requirements in both government and commercial organizations.

29. In your Lab Report file, **write an executive summary** that summarizes the top System/Application Domain risks, threats, and vulnerabilities and include a description of the risk mitigation tactics you would perform to audit the System/Application Domain for compliance. Use the PCI DSS standard and U.S. DoD system/application hardening guidelines as your examples for a baseline definition for compliance.

▶ Note:
This completes the lab. **Close** the **Web browser**, if you have not already done so.

Evaluation Criteria and Rubrics

The following are the evaluation criteria for this lab that students must perform:

1. Identify common risks, threats, and vulnerabilities found in the System/Application Domain that require proper security controls for mitigation. – **[20%]**
2. Align the PCI DSS standard to the System/Application Domain of security responsibility given that servers perform e-commerce credit card transactions online. – **[20%]**
3. Review the elements of the PCI DSS standard that pertain to servers, applications, and stored personal privacy data and credit card information in the System/Application Domain. – **[20%]**
4. Create a PCI DSS audit for compliance checklist to identify all elements needed for assessment and compliance with the PCI DSS standard within the System/Application Domain. – **[20%]**
5. Draft an executive summary recommending System/Application Domain hardening solutions by implementing proper security controls at the Internet ingress/egress point within an IT infrastructure. – **[20%]**

Lab #9 - Assessment Worksheet

Auditing the System/Application Domain for Compliance

Course Name and Number: ______________________________

Student Name: ______________________________

Instructor Name: ______________________________

Lab Due Date: ______________________________

Overview

In this lab, you learned how to audit the System/Application Domain. You identified common risks, threats, and vulnerabilities found in the System/Application Domain, you aligned the Payment Card Industry Data Security Standard (PCI DSS) standard to the System/Application Domain of security responsibility given that servers perform e-commerce credit card transactions online, you reviewed the PCI DSS standard for the System/Application Domain, and you created a PCI DSS audit for a compliance checklist to identify all elements needed for assessment and compliance with the PCI DSS standard within the System/Application Domain.

Lab Assessment Questions & Answers

1. What are some common risks, threats, and vulnerabilities found in the System/Application Domain that must be mitigated with proper security countermeasures?

2. If your company makes software to accept credit card payments, what standard would you use to measure and audit your software security?

3. Which three PCI requirements are most relevant to the System/Application Domain?

4. Your production system is regularly backed up and some of the data is used for testing and developing a new application interface. Is this in compliance with PCI DSS?

5. Why is it a risk to use production data for development?

6. What are some options, according to PCI DSS, to protect external-facing Web applications from known attacks?

7. To perform a PCI DSS compliance audit on your e-commerce Web site, what should you incorporate into Requirement #6, "Develop and Maintain Secure Systems & Applications"?

8. What do you recommend this organization implement for privacy data storage in long-term data storage devices?

9. To perform a PCI DSS compliance audit, what elements must be in your audit checklist that pertain to the System/Application Domain?

10. Performing a vulnerability assessment on PCI DSS production systems, servers, and applications requires what applications and tools?

11. Refer to the PCI DSS Self-Assessment Questionnaire (SAQ) and Attestation of Compliance for All Merchants and all SAQ-Eligible Service Providers v1.2. There are five different SAQ validation types. Which type encompasses merchants who use imprint, standalone terminals, Point of Sale (POS) systems, and store PCI DSS privacy data in databases and storage?

12. As per the SAQ-D and Attestation of Compliance, what are the four major elements a merchant must achieve as part of PCI DSS compliance?

13. Which requirements in PCI DSS SAQ-D apply to vulnerability assessment and vulnerability management for production credit card transaction-processing servers?

14. Which requirements in PCI DSS SAQ-D apply to performing internal and external vulnerability assessment scans and penetration testing on production IT infrastructure and credit card transaction-processing servers?

15. Which requirements in PCI DSS SAQ-D apply to performing file integrity monitoring on critical cardholder servers?

Lab 10: Charting Your Career Path—Professional Certifications

Introduction

While experience certainly helps people perform to the best of their abilities, certifications can provide a benchmark and professional standard. Certifications can also help you better understand what responsibilities would accompany a position. Going further, the Department of Defense (DoD) uses industry and vendor certifications to baseline position levels. If you have a career track in mind, and guided by your experiences, you may optimize your training to achieve the DoD position you would like.

In this lab, you will create a certification and continuing education strategy in information security based on accepted certification bodies, you will identify the Department of Defense's (DoD's) 8570.01 information assurance workgroup certification definition, and you will align professional certifications to the 8570.01 information assurance and professional certification road map. You will also identify professional certifications from various certification and accreditation organizations, and you will map out a career path in information security.

Learning Objectives

Upon completing this lab, you will be able to:

- Create a certification and continuing education strategy in information security based on industry-accepted certification bodies.
- Identify the U.S. DoD's 8570.01 information assurance workgroup certification definition for various DoD-centric information assurance job positions.
- Align professional certifications to the DoD 8570.01 information assurance and professional certification road map.
- Identify professional certifications from various certification and accreditation organizations, focusing on information systems security, auditing, and ethical hacking.
- Identify and map out a career path that includes entry-level practitioner positions and graduate-level positions, so you can present this to senior management in information systems security.

Deliverables

Upon completion of this lab, you are required to provide the following deliverables to your instructor:

1. Lab Report file;
2. Lab Assessments file.

Hands-On Steps

> **▶ Note:**
> This is a paper-based lab. To successfully complete the deliverables for this lab, you will need access to Microsoft® Word or another compatible word processor. For some labs, you may also need access to a graphics line drawing application, such as Visio or PowerPoint. Refer to the Preface of this manual for information on creating the lab deliverable files.

1. On your local computer, **create** the **lab deliverable files**.
2. **Review** the **Lab Assessment Worksheet**. You will find answers to these questions as you proceed through the lab steps.
3. **Consider** the following scenario:

   While at your desk finishing up some work, your manager pops in to have a chat with you regarding your current professional certifications. He encourages you to research and explore various professional certifications in information systems security. An instructor discusses and shares various professional certifications available in information systems security, auditing, and the management sector. Finally, the instructor discusses how to map your information systems security career path by following and obtaining various professional certifications recognized by the industry.
4. On your local computer, **open** a new **Internet browser window**.
5. In the address box of your Internet browser, **type** the URL **https://www.sans.org/media/dod8570/dod8570.pdf** and **press Enter** to open a SANS Institute PDF about DoD's 8570 certification.
6. **Browse** the document.

> **Picking Your Career Goal**
> While browsing the DoD 8570 document, it's perhaps most useful to first envision where you want your career heading. Your choice of certification(s) can be strongly influenced by whether you intend to be a technical leader or a manager.
>
> It's also important to remember the document's source as you browse. The document in step 5 comes from SANS, a nongovernmental educational institute in the business of providing and maintaining information security certifications. As the document outlines DoD 8570, it associates job levels with SANS certifications.

7. In your Lab Report file, **define DoD's 8570.01 information assurance workgroup certification**.
8. Next, you will research some information systems security careers. In the address box of your Internet browser, **type** the URL **http://www.giac.org/** and **press Enter** to open the Web site.

9. **Move your cursor** to the upper right of your screen over the word **About** to reveal a menu.
10. **Download** the **Full GIAC Brochure** that explains the available certifications with training provided by the SANS Institute.
11. In your Lab Report file, **discuss** two of these.
12. In the address box of your Internet browser, **type** the URL **http://www.giac.org/certifications/steps.php** and **press Enter** to open the Web site.
13. **Review** the general certification steps toward Global Information Assurance Certification (GIAC) certification offered by the SANS Institute.
14. In your Lab Report file, **outline** these steps.
15. In the address box of your Internet browser, **type** the URL **http://www.giac.org/certifications/audit/** and **press Enter** to open the Web site.
16. **Review** the GIAC Systems and Network Auditor (GSNA) certification and track offered by the SANS Institute for auditing.
17. In your Lab Report file, **describe** what the certification and tracking are.
18. In the address box of your Internet browser, **type** the URL **www.SANS.edu**, **press Enter** to open the Web site, and then:
    - **Click** on the **Read More link** in the Engineering box at the center of the page, or **visit** the Master of Science Degree in Information Security Engineering page at **http://www.sans.edu/academics/masters-programs/msise**. In your Lab Report file, **discuss** the program goals.
    - **Click** on the **Read More** link in the Management box toward the center of the page, or **visit** the Master of Science Degree in Information Security Management page at **http://www.sans.edu/academics/masters-programs/msism**. In your Lab Report file, **discuss** the program goals.
19. In the address box of your Internet browser, **type** the URL **https://www.isaca.org/Pages/default.aspx** and **press Enter** to open ISACA's Web site.
20. **Review** the available certifications by **moving your cursor** over the **Certification tab** toward the top of the page to reveal the menu that shows the following:
    - CISA: Certified Information Systems Auditor
    - CISM: Certified Information Security Manager
    - CGEIT: Certified in the Governance of Enterprise IT
    - CRISC: Certified in Risk and Information Systems Control
21. In your Lab Report file, **discuss** each of these.

22. In the address box of your Internet browser, **type** the URL **https://www.isc2.org/** and **press Enter** to open the Web site for the International Information Systems Security Certification Consortium $(ISC)^2$.

23. **Click** on the **Credentials tab** toward the top of the $(ISC)^2$ Web site to **study** the certifications available.

24. In your Lab Report file, **discuss** each of these topics, which you'll find in a column on the left-hand side of the resulting Web page:

    - Our Credentialing Process
    - Associate of $(ISC)^2$
    - SSCP: Systems Security Certified Practitioner
    - CAP: Certified Authorization Professional
    - CSSLP: Certified Secure Software Lifecycle Professional
    - CISSP: Certified Information Systems Security Professional

Job Tips

One approach to comparing and contrasting credentials is to evaluate their popularity (how many members) and the frequency with which the credential appears as a job position requirement. Also consider that some certifying bodies require continued maintenance, often in the way of "CEUs" or continuing education units. For example, $(ISC)^2$ requires CISSP holders to submit and log 120 CEUs over a three-year span. This maintenance requirement can be considered helpful toward keeping certification holders current in their field.

25. In the address box of your Internet browser, **type** the URL **http://www.eccouncil.org/** and **press Enter** to open the Web site.

26. **Click** the **Certification tab** at the top of the EC-Council Web site.

27. Once on the EC-Council Certification page, **scroll down** the page to browse the many available certification options.

28. In your Lab Report file, **discuss** two of the certifications.

29. In your Lab Report file, **write an executive summary** outlining a career path that covers entry-level practitioner positions to graduate-level positions. **Include** a description of what career path you would like to pursue with the core information systems security foundation. In addition, **align** the professional certifications you could pursue to the DoD 8570.01 certification.

▶ Note:

This completes the lab. **Close** the **Web browser**, if you have not already done so.

Evaluation Criteria and Rubrics

The following are the evaluation criteria for this lab that students must perform:

1. Create a certification and continuing education strategy in information security based on industry-accepted certification bodies. – **[20%]**
2. Identify the U.S. DoD's 8570.01 information assurance workgroup certification definition for various DoD-centric information assurance job positions. – **[20%]**
3. Align professional certifications to the DoD 8570.01 information assurance and professional certification road map. – **[20%]**
4. Identify professional certifications from various certification and accreditation organizations, focusing on information systems security, auditing, and ethical hacking. – **[20%]**
5. Identify and map out a career path that includes entry-level practitioner positions and graduate-level positions, so you can present this to senior management in information systems security. – **[20%]**

Lab #10 - Assessment Worksheet

Charting Your Career Path—Professional Certifications

Course Name and Number: ____________________

Student Name: ____________________

Instructor Name: ____________________

Lab Due Date: ____________________

Overview

In this lab, you created a certification and continuing education strategy in information security based on accepted certification bodies, you identified the Department of Defense's (DoD's) 8570.01 information assurance workgroup certification definition, and you aligned professional certifications to the 8570.01 information assurance and professional certification road map. You also identified professional certifications from various certification and accreditation organizations, and you mapped out a career path in information security.

Lab Assessment Questions & Answers

1. Identify three vendor-centric professional certifications in security.

2. In the DoD 8570.01-M directive, which professional certifications map to the 8570.01-M directive?

3. From a career perspective, which professional certifications make sense for someone wishing to perform intrusive, penetration tests?

4. What is the primary difference between the $(ISC)^2$ SSCP® and CISSP® professional certifications from an information systems security career path perspective?

5. Why do you think it is important to take both vendor and vendor neutral professional certification exams for your career progression? Explain.

6. Pick two professional certifications that you want to pursue, and explain what the prerequisites are and in what time frame in your career path you plan on achieving them.

7. Why would an organization that is not in the DoD but does business with the DoD choose to get its employees certified using the measurement of the DoD 8570.01-M directive?

8. Explain in your own words what the significance of the $(ISC)^2$ Code of Ethics implies to information systems security professionals.

9. What Information Assurance Technical (IAT) levels in the DoD 8570.01-M map to the hands-on, entry-level professional certifications: Security+, SSCP®, Security Certified Network Professional (SCNP), Network+, and GIAC?

10. At the Information Assurance System Architect and Engineer (IASAE) level in the DoD 8570.01-M directive, what professional certification acts as the core foundation for Levels I, II, and III?

11. What are two professional certifications that can be obtained for systems and network auditing and information systems auditing?

12. If you just obtained a B.S. Degree in Information Systems Security and have one year of work experience but less than five years of work experience in information systems security, which professional certification from $(ISC)^2$ would you be eligible for?

13. If you were pursuing a management position in information systems security or information assurance, which professional certification would you obtain from $(ISC)^2$?

14. When is it a good idea to have vendor professional certifications as opposed to vendor neutral?

15. If you were responsible for designing and configuring Demilitarized Zones (DMZs), firewalls, and intrusion detection system/intrusion prevention system (IDS/IPS) security solutions, which vendor certifications would you consider?